P9-DOE-845

CLINICAL COMPANION TO

Lewis's

Medical-Surgical Nursing

Assessment and Management
of Clinical Problems

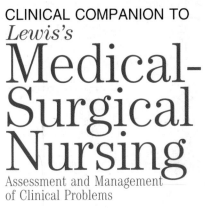

CLINICAL COMPANION TO
Lewis's
Medical-Surgical Nursing

Assessment and Management
of Clinical Problems   Eleventh Edition

Prepared By
Debra Hagler, RN, PhD, ACNS-BC, CNE, CHSE, ANEF, FAAN
Clinical Professor
Edson College of Nursing and Health Innovation
Arizona State University
Phoenix, Arizona

Mariann M. Harding, RN, PhD, CNE

Jeffrey Kwong, DNP, MPH, ANP-BC, FAANP

Dottie Roberts, RN, EdD, MACI, CMSRN, OCNS-C, CNE

Courtney Reinisch, DNP, RN, FNP-BC

ELSEVIER

Elsevier
3251 Riverport Lane
St. Louis, Missouri 63043

CLINICAL COMPANION TO LEWIS'S MEDICAL-SURGICAL   ISBN: 978-0-323551557
NURSING: ASSESSMENT AND MANAGEMENT OF
CLINICAL PROBLEMS, ELEVENTH EDITION

Copyright © 2020 by Elsevier, Inc. All rights reserved.

No part of this publication may be reproduced or transmitted in any form or by any means, electronic or mechanical, including photocopying, recording, or any information storage and retrieval system, without permission in writing from the publisher. Details on how to seek permission, further information about the Publisher's permissions policies and our arrangements with organizations such as the Copyright Clearance Center and the Copyright Licensing Agency, can be found at our website: www.elsevier.com/permissions.

This book and the individual contributions contained in it are protected under copyright by the Publisher (other than as may be noted herein).

Notice

Practitioners and researchers must always rely on their own experience and knowledge in evaluating and using any information, methods, compounds or experiments described herein. Because of rapid advances in the medical sciences, in particular, independent verification of diagnoses and drug dosages should be made. To the fullest extent of the law, no responsibility is assumed by Elsevier, authors, editors or contributors for any injury and/or damage to persons or property as a matter of products liability, negligence or otherwise, or from any use or operation of any methods, products, instructions, or ideas contained in the material herein.

Previous editions copyrighted 2017, 2014, 2011, 2007, 2004, 2000, 1996 by Mosby, Inc., an affiliate of Elsevier Inc.

Library of Congress Control Number: 2019945312

Names: Hagler, Debra, Author. | Complemented by (expression): Harding, Mariann M. Medical-Surgical Nursing. Eleventh edition.

Title: Lewis's Clinical Companion to Medical-Surgical Nursing: Assessment and Management of Clinical Problems / Prepared by Debra Hagler, Mariann M. Harding, Jeffrey Kwong, Dottie Roberts, Courtney Reinisch

Description: Eleventh edition. | St. Louis, Missouri: Elsevier, [2020] | Complemented by Lewis's Medical-Surgical Nursing / Mariann M. Harding [and four others]. Eleventh edition. [2020]. | Includes bibliographical references and index.

Senior Content Strategist: Jamie Blum
Content Development Specialist: Denise Roslonski
Publishing Services Manager: Shereen Jameel
Project Manager: Rukmani Krishnan
Design Direction: Amy Buxton

Printed in India

Last digit is the print number: 9 8 7 6 5 4 3 2

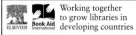

Working together
to grow libraries in
developing countries

www.elsevier.com • www.bookaid.org

The *Clinical Companion* to *Lewis's Medical-Surgical Nursing: Assessment and Management of Clinical Problems*, 11th edition, has been revised and updated as a condensed reference of essential information on almost 200 medical-surgical patient problems and clinically related topics. The 11th edition of this pocket-sized book provides nurses and nursing students with quick access to current, concise, and important information when caring for patients.

The *Clinical Companion* can be used separately as a reference or in conjunction with *Lewis's Medical-Surgical Nursing: Assessment and Management of Clinical Problems*, 11th edition.

The book is divided into three sections. Part One contains commonly encountered medical-surgical patient problems that are arranged alphabetically and organized in an easy-to-use format. The disorders are extensively cross-referenced to *Lewis's Medical-Surgical Nursing*, 11th edition, for the reader who desires additional information. Part Two contains brief explanations of common medical-surgical treatments and procedures (e.g., pacemakers, oxygen therapy) in which the role of the nurse is emphasized. Part Three contains reference material that is frequently used in clinical nursing practice (e.g., heart and breath sounds, medication administration, blood and urine laboratory values). An extensive index is provided for easy location of information.

We strongly believe the *Clinical Companion* is an invaluable source of information that will serve as an important resource in helping nurses meet the challenges and opportunities in caring for patients and their caregivers during states of altered health and well-being.

Debra Hagler
Mariann M. Harding

"Our greatest weakness lies in giving up. The most certain way to succeed is to try just one more time."
Thomas Edison

CONTENTS

Disorders

Disasters

ABDOMINAL PAIN, ACUTE

A

Description

Acute abdominal pain is pain of recent onset. It may signal a life-threatening problem requiring immediate attention. Causes include damage to organs in the abdomen and pelvis, which may lead to inflammation, infection, obstruction, bleeding, or perforation. Common causes of acute abdominal pain are listed in Table 1.

Clinical Manifestations

Pain is the most common symptom of an acute abdominal problem. Patients may have nausea, vomiting, diarrhea, constipation, flatulence, fatigue, fever, rebound tenderness, and bloating.

Diagnostic Studies

Diagnosis begins with a complete history and physical examination. Description of the pain (frequency, timing, duration, location), accompanying symptoms, and sequence of symptoms (e.g., pain before or after vomiting) provide vital clues about the problem. Physical examination should include both rectal and pelvic examinations in addition to an abdominal examination.

- Complete blood count (CBC), urinalysis, abdominal x-ray, and an electrocardiogram (ECG) are done initially, along with an ultrasound or CT scan.
- A pregnancy test is performed in women of childbearing age to rule out ectopic pregnancy.

Interprofessional Management

The goal of management is to identify and treat the cause and monitor and treat complications, especially shock. Table 42.10 in Harding et al., *Lewis' Medical-Surgical Nursing*, ed 11, outlines emergency management of the patient with acute abdominal pain.

TABLE 1 Causes of Acute Abdominal Pain	
• Abdominal compartment syndrome	• Pelvic inflammatory disease
• Acute pancreatitis	• Perforated gastric or duodenal ulcer
• Appendicitis	• Peritonitis
• Bowel obstruction	• Ruptured abdominal aneurysm
• Cholecystitis	• Ruptured ectopic pregnancy
• Diverticulitis	
• Gastroenteritis	

- A diagnostic laparoscopy may be performed to inspect the surface of abdominal organs, obtain biopsy specimens, perform laparoscopic ultrasounds, and remove organs.
- A laparotomy is used when laparoscopic techniques are inadequate. If the cause of the acute abdomen can be surgically removed (e.g., inflamed appendix) or surgically repaired (e.g., ruptured abdominal aneurysm), surgery is considered definitive therapy.

Nursing Management
Goals
The patient will have resolution of inflammation, relief of abdominal pain, freedom from complications (especially hypovolemic shock), and normal nutritional status.
Nursing Interventions
Conduct ongoing assessments of vital signs, intake and output, and level of consciousness, which are key indicators of hypovolemic shock. General care involves management of fluid and electrolyte imbalances, pain, and anxiety. Assess the quality and intensity of pain at regular intervals, and provide medication and other comfort measures. Maintain a calm environment and provide information to help allay anxiety.

General care of the preoperative patient is described in Chapter 17 of Harding et al., *Lewis' Medical-Surgical Nursing,* ed 11.

Postoperative care depends on the type of surgical procedure performed. Laparoscopic procedures result in lower rates of postoperative complications (e.g., poor wound healing, paralytic ileus), earlier diet advancement, and shorter hospital stays compared with open surgical procedures. A general nursing care plan (eNursing Care Plan 19.1) for the postoperative patient is available on the website for Chapter 19.

A nasogastric (NG) tube with low suction may be used to empty the stomach and prevent gastric distention. If the upper gastrointestinal (GI) tract was entered, drainage from the NG tube may be dark brown to dark red for the first 12 hours. Later it should be light yellowish brown or greenish. If a dark red color continues or if bright red blood is observed, notify the surgeon of the possibility of hemorrhage. "Coffee ground" granules in the drainage indicate blood that has been changed by acidic gastric secretions.

- Nausea and vomiting are common after a laparotomy and may result from the surgery, decreased peristalsis, or pain medication. Antiemetics, such as ondansetron (Zofran), promethazine, and aprepitant (Emend) may be ordered (see Nausea and Vomiting, p. 415).
- Monitor fluid and electrolyte status along with vital signs.

- Swallowed air and decreased peristalsis from decreased mobility, manipulation of abdominal organs during surgery, and anesthesia can lead to abdominal distention and gas pains. Early ambulation helps restore peristalsis, expel flatus, and reduce gas pain.

▼ **Patient and Caregiver Teaching**
Preparation for discharge begins soon after surgery. Teach the patient and caregiver about modifications in activity, care of the incision, diet, and drug therapy.

- Clear liquids are given initially after surgery, and if tolerated, the patient progresses to a regular diet.
- Normal activities should be resumed gradually, with planned rest periods. There may be restrictions on lifting.
- Both patient and caregiver should be aware of possible complications. Teach them to notify the surgeon immediately if fever is higher than 101°F (38.3°C) or if pain, weight loss, incisional drainage, or changes in bowel function occur.

ACUTE CORONARY SYNDROME

Description
Acute coronary syndrome (ACS) develops when myocardial ischemia is prolonged and not immediately reversible. ACS includes the spectrum of non-ST elevation acute coronary syndrome (unstable angina [UA] and non–ST-segment-elevation myocardial infarction [NSTEMI]), and ST-segment-elevation myocardial infarction (STEMI) (Fig. 1).

Pathophysiology
ACS is caused by the decline of a once-stable atherosclerotic plaque. The previously stable plaque ruptures, releasing substances from the lipid core into the vessel. This causes platelet aggregation and thrombus formation. The vessel may be partially blocked by a thrombus (manifesting as UA or NSTEMI) or totally blocked by a thrombus (manifesting as STEMI). What causes the plaque to suddenly become unstable is not well understood, but systemic inflammation is thought to play a role. Patients with suspected ACS need immediate hospitalization.

Unstable Angina
UA is chest pain that is new in onset, occurs at rest, or occurs with increasing frequency, duration, or less effort than the patient's chronic stable angina pattern. The pain usually lasts 10 minutes or more. The patient with chronic stable angina may develop UA, or UA may be the first clinical sign of coronary artery disease

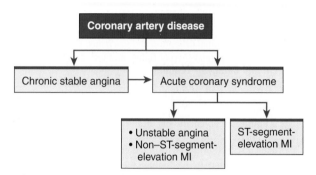

Fig. 1 Relationships among coronary artery disease, chronic stable angina, and acute coronary syndrome. *MI*, Myocardial infarction.

(CAD). Unlike chronic stable angina, UA is unpredictable and must be treated immediately.

- The patient with previously diagnosed chronic stable angina describes a significant change in the pattern of angina. It occurs with increasing frequency and is easily provoked by minimal exertion, during sleep, or even at rest.
- The patient without previously diagnosed angina describes chest pain that has progressed rapidly in the past few hours, days, or weeks, often ending in pain at rest. Ischemic electrocardiogram (ECG) changes that may be seen with UA include ST depression and/or T wave inversion.

Myocardial Infarction: ST-Elevation (STEMI) and Non–ST-Elevation (NSTEMI)

- A *myocardial infarction* (MI) occurs because of an abrupt stoppage of blood flow through a coronary artery with a thrombus caused by platelet aggregation. This causes irreversible myocardial cell death (necrosis). Serum cardiac biomarkers are released into the blood. Most MIs occur in the setting of preexisting CAD.
- A STEMI, caused by an occlusive thrombus, creates ST elevation in the ECG leads facing the area of infarction. A STEMI is an emergency. To limit the infarct size, the artery must be opened within 90 minutes of presentation to restore blood and O_2 to the heart muscle and limit the infarct size. This can be done either by percutaneous coronary intervention (PCI) or with thrombolytic (fibrinolytic) therapy. PCI is the first-line treatment, if available. The catheterization confirms which artery has the occlusive thrombus so it can be opened with a balloon

and stent. Thrombolytic therapy is done in hospitals that do not have a catheterization laboratory for PCI. If the patient does not seek treatment quickly, the STEMI will evolve.

- NSTEMI, caused by a nonocclusive thrombus, does not cause ST segment elevation on the 12-lead ECG. The ECG may or may not show ST depression and/or T wave inversion in the leads facing the area of infarction. NSTEMI patients do not go to the catheterization laboratory emergently but usually undergo the procedure within 12 to 72 hours. Thrombolytic therapy is not indicated for NSTEMI.
- Cardiac cells can withstand ischemic conditions for approximately 10 minutes before cellular death (necrosis) begins. The acute MI process evolves over time, from hours to a few days. The earliest tissue to become ischemic is the subendocardium (the innermost layer of tissue in the heart muscle). If ischemia persists, it takes around 4 to 6 hours for the entire thickness of the heart muscle to necrose. If the thrombus is not completely blocking the artery, the time to complete necrosis may be as long as 12 hours.
- The location of an MI correlates with the involved coronary circulation. For example, inferior wall infarctions result from occlusions in the right coronary artery. The majority of MIs affect the left ventricle. Damage can occur in more than 1 location (e.g., anterolateral MI, anteroseptal MI).
- The degree of collateral circulation influences the severity of the MI. A person with a long history of CAD may have developed good collateral circulation to the area surrounding the infarction site.

The body's response to cell death is the inflammatory process. Within 24 hours, leukocytes infiltrate the area. Enzymes are released from the dead cardiac cells and are important diagnostic indicators (markers) of MI. Proteolytic enzymes from neutrophils and macrophages remove necrotic tissue by the fourth day.

- The necrotic zone is identifiable by ECG changes (e.g., ST-segment elevation, pathologic Q wave) and by nuclear scanning after the onset of symptoms. The necrotic zone of a STEMI is identified by ECG changes (e.g., lowering of the initially elevated ST segments, T wave inversion and/or a pathologic Q wave) within a day or 2.
- At 10 to 14 days after MI, the new scar tissue is still weak. The heart muscle is vulnerable to increased stress during this time. At the same time, the patient's activity level may be increasing, so special caution and assessment are necessary.
- By 6 weeks after MI, scar tissue has replaced necrotic tissue and the injured area is considered healed.

Changes in the infarcted heart muscle also cause changes in the unaffected areas. To try to compensate for the damaged muscle, the normal myocardium hypertrophies and dilates. This process is called *ventricular remodeling*. Remodeling of normal myocardium can lead to the development of late heart failure (HF), especially in the person with atherosclerosis of other coronary arteries and/or an anterior MI. Angiotensin-converting enzyme (ACE) inhibitor drugs are given to limit ventricular remodeling.

Clinical Manifestations
Unstable Angina
The chest pain associated with UA is new in onset, occurs at rest, or has a worsening pattern. Women seek medical attention for symptoms of UA more often than men. Despite national efforts to increase awareness, women's symptoms related to heart problems (fatigue, shortness of breath, indigestion, anxiety) often go unrecognized.

Myocardial Infarction
Severe and persistent chest pain not relieved by rest or nitrate administration may mean the patient is having an MI.

- Pain is usually described as a heaviness, pressure, burning, crushing, tightness, or constriction. The persistent pain is unlike any other pain.
- Common locations are epigastric, substernal, or retrosternal. The pain may radiate to the neck, jaw, and arms or to the back. It may occur while the patient is active or at rest, asleep or awake, and often occurs in the early morning hours.
- The pain usually lasts for 20 minutes or more and is more severe than usual anginal pain. When epigastric pain is present, the patient may take antacids without relief.
- Some patients may not have pain but may report having "discomfort," weakness, fatigue, nausea, indigestion, or shortness of breath. Women may have atypical discomfort, shortness of breath, or fatigue.
- Patients with diabetes may have silent (asymptomatic) MIs because of cardiac neuropathy or have atypical symptoms (e.g., shortness of breath).
- An older patient may have a change in mental status (e.g., confusion), shortness of breath, pulmonary edema, dizziness, or a dysrhythmia.

The patient's skin may be ashen, clammy, and cool (cold sweat). The patient may have nausea and vomiting. Fever occurs within the first 24 hours (up to 100.4° F [38° C]) and may continue for 1 week. BP and pulse rate are elevated initially. The BP may then drop, with decreased urine output, lung crackles, hepatic engorgement, and

peripheral edema. Jugular veins may be distended, with obvious
pulsations.

Complications

- *Dysrhythmias* are the most common complication after an MI
  and are the most common cause of death in patients in the prehospital period. Dysrhythmias are caused by conditions that
  affect the myocardial cell's sensitivity to nerve impulses, such
  as ischemia, electrolyte imbalances, and sympathetic nervous
  system stimulation. Life-threatening dysrhythmias occur most
  often with anterior wall infarction, heart failure, and shock. Complete heart block is seen in a massive infarction (see Dysrhythmias, p. 195).

- *Ventricular tachycardia and ventricular fibrillation* are
  lethal dysrhythmias that most often occur within the first
  4 hours after the onset of pain. Premature ventricular contractions may precede ventricular tachycardia and fibrillation.
  Life-threatening ventricular dysrhythmias must be treated
  immediately.

- *HF* occurs when the heart's pumping action is reduced. Left-
  sided HF occurs initially with subtle signs, such as mild
  dyspnea, restlessness, agitation, or slight tachycardia. Other
  signs indicating the onset of left-sided HF include pulmonary
  congestion on chest x-ray, S3 or S4 heart sounds on auscultation
  of the heart, crackles on auscultation of the lungs, paroxysmal
  nocturnal dyspnea (PND), and orthopnea. Signs of right-sided
  HF include jugular venous distention, hepatic congestion, and
  lower extremity edema. (See Heart Failure, p. 266.)

- *Cardiogenic shock* occurs when inadequate oxygen and nutrients are supplied to the tissues because of severe left ventricular
  (LV) failure, papillary muscle rupture, ventricular septal rupture,
  LV free wall rupture, or right ventricular infarction. Cardiogenic
  shock requires aggressive management including control of
  dysrhythmias, intraaortic balloon pump therapy, and support
  of contractility with vasoactive drugs.

Other complications include papillary muscle rupture, ventricular
rupture, ventricular aneurysm, and pericarditis. (See Pericarditis,
Acute, p. 474).

Diagnostic Studies

In addition to the patient's history of pain, risk factors, and health
history, the primary diagnostic studies used to determine whether
a person has UA or an MI include an ECG and serum cardiac
markers. Other diagnostic measures can include coronary angiography, exercise stress testing, and echocardiogram.

Electrocardiogram
- When patients first present with chest pain, ST-elevations on the 12-lead ECG most likely indicate a STEMI. The ECG should be compared to a previous ECG whenever possible. ST elevation represents myocardial injury that is potentially reversible but, if not treated, will likely evolve to permanent necrosis (tissue death) of the myocardium.
- A patient with STEMI tends to have a more extensive MI that is associated with prolonged and complete coronary occlusion. A pathologic Q wave develops on the ECG.
- Patients with UA or NSTEMI may or may not have ST segment depression and/or T wave inversion on the ECG. For patients with chest pain who do not have ST segment elevation or ST-T wave changes on the ECG, it is difficult to distinguish between UA and NSTEMI until we evaluate serum cardiac biomarkers.
- A patient with UA or NSTEMI usually has transient thrombosis or incomplete coronary occlusion, and the ECG typically does not develop pathologic Q waves.
- Serial ECGs often reveal the evolution and time sequence of ischemia, injury, infarction, and resolution of the infarction.

Cardiac Biomarkers
Certain proteins, called *serum cardiac biomarkers,* are released into the blood from necrotic heart muscle after an MI.
- Cardiac-specific troponin has 2 subtypes: cardiac-specific troponin T (cTnT) and cardiac-specific troponin I (cTnI). These markers are highly specific indicators of MI and have greater sensitivity and specificity for myocardial injury than creatine kinase (CK)-MB or myoglobin.

Interprofessional Management
A patient with ACS needs rapid diagnosis and treatment to preserve cardiac muscle. Initial management of the patient with chest pain most often occurs in the emergency department (ED).
- Obtain a 12-lead ECG and start continuous ECG monitoring.
- Position the patient in an upright position unless contraindicated and start O_2 by nasal cannula to keep O_2 saturation above 93%.
- Obtain intravenous (IV) access for drug administration.
- Give sublingual nitroglycerin (NTG) and 162 to 325 mg of chewable aspirin if not given before arrival at the ED. Morphine is given for pain unrelieved by NTG.
- A high-dose statin (e.g., atorvastatin [Lipitor]) is given.
- The patient usually receives ongoing care in a critical care or telemetry unit where continuous ECG monitoring is available and dysrhythmias can be treated.

- Monitor vital signs, including pulse oximetry, frequently during the first few hours after admission and closely thereafter. Maintain bed rest and limit activity for 12 to 24 hours, with a gradual increase in activity unless contraindicated.
- If the ECG shows ST elevation, the patient with STEMI is taken directly to the cardiac catheterization laboratory in PCI-capable hospitals. Glycoprotein IIb/IIIa inhibitors may be used during PCI for STEMI patients. Thrombolytic therapy is started if the patient is unable to be quickly transported to a PCI capable hospital. Contraindications and complications with thrombolytic therapy are described in Chapter 33 of Harding et al., *Lewis' Medical-Surgical Nursing*, ed 11.
- If the ECG shows ST depression and/or T wave inversion, the patient is usually transferred to a critical care unit or telemetry unit for ongoing care. Dysrhythmias are treated according to agency protocols. Serial cardiac biomarkers are drawn until the peak level drops off.
- UA and NSTEMI patients are started on heparin. Some patients with UA or NSTEMI start on glycoprotein IIb/IIIa inhibitors (e.g., eptifibatide [Integrilin]) either before catheterization or at the time of PCI.
- For a patient with UA or NSTEMI, aspirin and heparin (unfractionated heparin [UH] or low-molecular-weight heparin [LMWH]) are recommended. Dual antiplatelet therapy (e.g., with aspirin and clopidogrel) and heparin are recommended for NSTEMI. Cardiac catheterization with possible PCI is considered as treatment for both UA and NSTEMI once the patient is stabilized and angina is controlled, or if angina returns or increases in severity.

Coronary artery bypass graft (CABG) surgery consists of the placement of conduits to transport blood between the aorta, or other major arteries, and the myocardium distal to the obstructed coronary artery (or arteries). It requires a sternotomy (opening of the chest cavity) and the use of cardiopulmonary bypass (CPB). It is a palliative treatment for CAD and not a cure. Newer techniques include minimally invasive direct coronary artery bypass, off-pump coronary artery bypass, totally endoscopic coronary artery bypass (TECAB), and transmyocardial laser revascularization. These surgical procedures and related nursing care are further discussed in Chapter 33 of Harding et al., *Lewis' Medical-Surgical Nursing*, ed 11.

Drug therapy includes IV nitroglycerin, aspirin, β-adrenergic blockers, and anticoagulation. Systemic anticoagulation may be achieved with LMWH given subcutaneously or IV UH. If PCI is anticipated, glycoprotein IIb/IIIa inhibitors may be used. ACE inhibitors are added for some patients after an MI. Calcium-channel blockers may be used if the patient is already taking adequate doses of β-blockers or does not tolerate these blockers.

Nursing Management
Goals
The patient with an MI will experience relief of pain, preservation of myocardium, effective coping with illness-associated anxiety, participation in a rehabilitation plan, and reduction of risk factors. See eNursing Care Plan 33-1 for the patient with ACS on the website.
Nursing Interventions
Priorities for nursing interventions in the initial phase include pain assessment and relief, physiologic monitoring, promotion of rest and comfort, alleviation of stress and anxiety, and understanding of the patient's emotional and behavioral reactions. Proper management of these priorities decreases the O_2 needs of a compromised myocardium. In addition, you should institute measures to avoid the hazards of immobility while encouraging rest.

- Provide nitroglycerin, morphine, and supplemental O_2 as needed to eliminate or reduce chest pain.
- Maintain continuous ECG monitoring while the patient is in the ED and intensive care unit (ICU) and after transfer to a step-down or general care unit. Dysrhythmias need to be identified and treated quickly.
- In addition to taking frequent vital signs, evaluate intake and output and perform physical assessment to detect deviations from the patient's baseline parameters. Assess lung and heart sounds and inspect for evidence of early heart failure (e.g., dyspnea, tachycardia, pulmonary congestion, distended neck veins).
- Assess oxygenation status frequently. If the patient is receiving O_2, check the nares for irritation or dryness (see Oxygen Therapy, p. 697).
- Plan nursing and therapeutic actions to ensure adequate rest periods free from interruption.
- Promote rest and comfort. Bed rest may be ordered for a few days after an MI involving a large portion of the ventricle.
- Anxiety may be present in various degrees in patients with ACS. Identify the source of anxiety and assist the patient in reducing it. If the patient is afraid of being alone, allow a caregiver to sit quietly by the bedside or check in frequently with the patient.

A

▼ **Patient and Caregiver Teaching**

The patient will need teaching at every stage of hospitalization and recovery (e.g., ED, telemetry unit, home care). The purpose of teaching is to give the patient and caregiver the tools to make informed health decisions (Table 2).

- Anticipatory guidance involves preparing both patient and caregiver for the usual course of recovery and rehabilitation. By learning what to expect, the patient gains a sense of control.
- Teach patients to check their HR. Some patients may use technology (e.g., cell phone applications, fitness trackers) to check their HR. The patient should know the limits within which to exercise. Tell the patient that the HR should return to the resting HR within a few minutes of stopping the exercise. Tell the patient to stop exercising and rest if chest pain or shortness of breath occurs. Basic physical activity guidelines for after ACS are presented in Table 33.3, Harding et al., *Lewis' Medical-Surgical Nursing*, ed 11.

TABLE 2 **Patient and Caregiver Teaching**
Acute Coronary Syndrome
Include the following information in the teaching plan for the patient with acute coronary syndrome and the caregiver.
• Signs and symptoms of angina and MI and what to do should they occur (e.g., take nitroglycerin)
• When and how to seek help (e.g., contact ERS)
• Anatomy and physiology of the heart and coronary arteries
• Cause and effect of CAD
• Definition of terms (e.g., CAD, angina, MI, sudden cardiac death, heart failure)
• Identification of and plan to decrease risk factors (see Tables 33.2–33.5, Harding et al., *Lewis' Medical-Surgical Nursing*, ed 11)
• Reasons for tests and treatments (e.g., ECG monitoring, blood tests, angiography), activity limitations and rest, diet, and drugs
• Appropriate expectations about recovery (anticipatory guidance)
• Resumption of work, physical activity, sexual activity (Table 33.21, Harding et al., *Lewis' Medical-Surgical Nursing*, ed 11)
• Measures to promote recovery and health (e.g., cardiac rehabilitation)
• Importance of the gradual, progressive resumption of activity

CAD, Coronary artery disease; *ECG,* electrocardiogram; *ERS,* emergency response system; *MI,* myocardial infarction.

- Encourage participation in an outpatient or home-based cardiac rehabilitation program.
- Include sexual counseling for cardiac patients and their partners. Tell the patient that resumption of sex depends on the emotional readiness of both the patient and partner and on the health care provider (HCP)'s assessment of recovery. It is generally safe to resume sexual activity 7 to 10 days after an uncomplicated MI. Sexual activity for most middle-aged men and women with their usual partners is considered a moderate-energy activity equivalent to climbing 2 flights of steps or walking briskly.

ACUTE RESPIRATORY DISTRESS SYNDROME

Description
Acute respiratory distress syndrome (ARDS) is a sudden and progressive form of respiratory failure in which the alveolar-capillary membrane becomes damaged and more permeable to intravascular fluid. ARDS accounts for about 10% of all adult ICU admissions. Despite supportive therapy, the mortality rate from ARDS is around 50%.

Etiology and Pathophysiology
The exact cause for the damage to the alveolar-capillary membrane is not known. Some think it is caused by stimulation of the inflammatory and immune systems. This stimulation attracts neutrophils to the pulmonary interstitium. The neutrophils release biochemical, humoral, and cellular mediators that produce changes in the lung. These changes include increased pulmonary capillary membrane permeability, collagen destruction, formation of pulmonary microemboli, and pulmonary artery vasoconstriction.

- Table 3 lists conditions that predispose patients to developing ARDS. The most common cause is sepsis. Patients with multiple risk factors are 3 or 4 times more likely to develop ARDS.
- Direct lung injury may cause ARDS, or ARDS may develop as a result of multiple organ dysfunction syndrome (MODS) (see Systemic Inflammatory Response Syndrome and Multiple Organ Dysfunction Syndrome, p. 600).
- The pathophysiologic changes in ARDS are divided into 3 phases: (1) injury (exudative) phase; (2) reparative (proliferative) phase; and (3) fibrotic (chronic or late) phase.
- The *injury (exudative) phase* usually occurs 24 to 72 hours after the initial injury and lasts up to 7 days.
- Engorgement of the peribronchial and perivascular interstitial space causes interstitial edema. Fluid in the parenchyma of the

TABLE 3	**Conditions Predisposing to Acute Respiratory Distress Syndrome**
Direct Lung Injury	**Indirect Lung Injury**
Common Causes	
• Aspiration of gastric contents or other substances • Bacterial or viral pneumonia • Sepsis	• Sepsis (especially gram-negative infection) • Severe massive trauma • Severe traumatic brain injury • Shock states (hypovolemic, cardiogenic, septic)
Less Common Causes	
• Chest trauma (blunt or penetrating) • Embolism: fat, air, amniotic fluid, thrombus • Inhalation of toxic substances • Near-drowning • O_2 toxicity • Radiation pneumonitis	• Acute pancreatitis • Cardiopulmonary bypass • Disseminated intravascular coagulation • Opioid drug overdose (e.g., heroin) • Transfusion-related acute lung injury (e.g., multiple blood transfusions) • Urosepsis

lung surrounding the alveoli crosses the alveolar membrane and enters the alveolar space. V/Q mismatch and intrapulmonary shunt develop because the alveoli fill with fluid. Blood in the capillary network cannot be oxygenated.

- Alveolar cells that produce surfactant are damaged by the changes caused by ARDS. This damage, in addition to further fluid and protein accumulation, results in surfactant dysfunction. When surfactant synthesis is decreased or surfactant is inactivated, alveoli become unstable and collapse. This causes atelectasis, further decreases lung compliance, compromises gas exchange, and worsens hypoxemia.
- Necrotic cells, protein, and fibrin form hyaline membranes that line the inside of each alveolus. These thick hyaline membranes contribute to the development of fibrosis and atelectasis, leading to a further decrease in gas exchange capability and lung compliance.
- Severe V/Q mismatch and shunting result in hypoxemia that is not responsive to increasing fraction of inspired oxygen (FiO_2). This is the classic signs of ARDS, called *refractory*

hypoxemia. Despite receiving higher concentrations of O_2, the patient's condition continues to get worse.

- The *reparative (proliferative) phase* of ARDS begins 1 to 2 weeks after the initial lung injury. During this phase, there is a continued influx of granulocytes, monocytes, and lymphocytes and fibroblasts as part of the inflammatory response.
- Increased pulmonary vascular resistance and pulmonary hypertension may occur because fibroblasts and inflammatory cells destroy the pulmonary vasculature.
- Lung compliance continues to decrease because of interstitial fibrosis. Hypoxemia worsens because of the thickened alveolar membrane.
- If this phase persists, widespread fibrosis results. If this phase is stopped, the lesions resolve.

The *fibrotic* (chronic or late) *phase* occurs 2 to 3 weeks after the initial lung injury. Not all patients who develop ARDS enter the fibrotic stage. For those that never fully recover from ARDS, the lung is completely remodeled by collagenous and fibrous tissues. Diffuse scarring of the lungs, interstitial fibrosis, and alveolar duct fibrosis result in decreased lung compliance. This reduces the surface area for gas exchange because the interstitium is fibrotic, and hypoxemia continues. Pulmonary vascular destruction and fibrosis cause varying degrees of pulmonary hypertension.

The progression of ARDS varies. Some survive the acute phase of lung injury. Pulmonary edema resolves, and complete recovery occurs within a week or so. The chance for survival is lower for those who enter the fibrotic stage. Patients may need several weeks of long-term mechanical ventilation.

Clinical Manifestations and Diagnostic Studies

At the time of the initial injury, and for 24 to 72 hours, the patient may not have respiratory symptoms. Later, the patient may exhibit mild dyspnea, tachypnea, dyspnea, cough, and restlessness. Lung auscultation may be normal or reveal fine, scattered crackles. Arterial blood gases (ABGs) may show mild hypoxemia and respiratory alkalosis caused by hyperventilation. The chest x-ray may be normal or show diffusely scattered but minimal interstitial infiltrates.

As ARDS progresses, symptoms worsen. Respiratory distress becomes evident as word of breathing (WOB) increases. Tachypnea and intercostal and suprasternal retractions may be present. Tachycardia, diaphoresis, changes in mental status, cyanosis, and pallor may be seen. Lung auscultation usually reveals scattered to diffuse crackles and coarse crackles on expiration.

- After 72 hours, the chest x-ray often shows diffuse and extensive bilateral interstitial and alveolar infiltrates.

- Refractory hypoxemia is the hallmark characteristic of ARDS. The partial pressure of oxygen in arterial blood (PaO_2) remains lower than expected despite increasing FiO_2. Hypercapnia often signifies that respiratory muscle fatigue and hypoventilation have severely affected gas exchange. Respiratory failure is imminent.
- Severe hypoxemia, hypercapnia, metabolic acidosis, and manifestations of organ dysfunction often accompany ARDS and provide additional challenges.
- Complications may develop as a result of ARDS itself or its treatment. Besides the lungs, the vital organs most often involved are the kidneys, liver, and heart. The main cause of death in ARDS is MODS, often accompanied by sepsis.

Nursing and Interprofessional Management
Goals
The overall goals for the patient with ARDS include PaO_2 within normal limits for age or at baseline on room air, O_2 saturation in arterial blood (SaO_2) > 90%, resolution of the precipitating factor(s), and clear lungs on auscultation.

The care for acute respiratory failure is applicable to ARDS (see Respiratory Failure, Acute, p. 516). Patients with ARDS are commonly cared for in critical care units. Best practices for care of the patient with ARDS include: (1) O_2 administration; (2) mechanical ventilation; (3) low tidal volume ventilation; (4) permissive hypercapnia; (5) positive end-expiratory pressure (PEEP); (6) prone positioning; and (7) extracorporeal membrane oxygenation (ECMO).

O_2 Administration. The primary goal of O_2 therapy is to correct hypoxemia (see Oxygen Therapy, p. 697). At first, the use of a high-flow system that delivers higher O_2 concentrations to maximize O_2 delivery may be all that is needed. Continuously monitor O_2 saturation (SpO_2) to assess the effectiveness of O_2 therapy.

For most patients diagnosed with ARDS, high-flow O_2 delivery, including bi-level positive airway pressure (Bi-PAP), is only a temporary measure. Patients with moderate to severe ARDS and refractory hypoxemia need mechanical ventilation (see Artificial Airways: Endotracheal Tubes, p. 663) to keep the PaO_2 at or close to near normal levels. Even with mechanical ventilation, the patient may need a FiO_2 of 70%, 80% or higher, to keep the PaO_2 at least 60 mm Hg. Most health care professionals (HCPs) agree that in the injury and reparative phases, they may have to accept a lower than normal PaO_2 (e.g., PaO_2 55–80 mm Hg) and SpO_2 (88%–95%).

Mechanical Ventilation. Mechanical ventilation is often delivered via a pressure-control type of ventilation. Pressure control ventilation helps keep the inspiratory and plateau pressures from becoming too high. This prevents alveolar overdistention and rupture. By reducing the amount of pressure going into the stiff, noncompliant lungs, we can help prevent further lung injury.

During mechanical ventilation, it is common to apply PEEP at 5 cm H_2O to compensate for loss of glottic function caused by the endotracheal tube. PEEP increases functional residual capacity, or the volume of air left in the lungs at the end of a normal expiration. PEEP also helps open up ("recruit") collapsed alveoli. PEEP can improve ventilation in respiratory units that collapse at low airway pressures. This may allow the FiO_2 to be lowered.

ECMO is used most often in specialized ICUs in major cities. Like hemodialysis, a large blood vessel is cannulated (most often the internal jugular, femoral artery, or femoral vein) and a catheter is inserted. ECMO and extracorporeal CO_2 removal pass blood across a gas-exchanging membrane outside the body and return oxygenated blood back to the body.

Positioning. Prone positioning is an option for patients with refractory hypoxemia who do not respond to other strategies to increase PaO_2. By turning the patient prone, perfusion may be better matched to ventilation. Air-filled alveoli in the anterior part of the lung become dependent. Alveoli in the posterior part of the lungs are "recruited" (given the opportunity to re-expand), improving oxygenation. Another positioning strategy to consider for management of ARDS is continuous lateral rotation therapy, which provides continuous, slow, side-to-side turning of the patient by rotating the actual bed frame < 40 degrees.

Promoting Tissue Perfusion. Maintaining fluid balance and hemodynamic stability is challenging in the patient with ARDS. Increasing pulmonary capillary permeability results in fluid in the lungs and causes pulmonary edema. At the same time, the patient may be intravascularly volume depleted and at risk for hypotension and decreased CO from mechanical ventilation and PEEP.

Hemodynamic monitoring is essential. This allows you to see trends, detect changes, and adjust therapy as needed. BP and mean arterial pressure (MAP) are important indicators of the adequacy of CO. Closely monitor BP and indicators of CO and tissue perfusion (SaO_2, mixed venous oxygen saturation) with the start of or changes in mechanical ventilation. A decrease in CO is treated by giving IV fluids, drugs, or both.

Analgesia and Sedation. The patient with ARDS may fear suffocation or death. Provide reassurance, spend time at the bedside, and ensure that the patient can obtain assistance immediately (e.g., call light and tools for alternate communication strategy while intubated). Anxiety also may be reduced through instruction in and use of progressive relaxation, guided imagery, and music therapy.

- Explain to the patient any expected sensations that may be encountered with each new experience (e.g., suctioning, drawing ABGs) so that coping strategies can be purposefully selected.

Analgesia and sedation decrease the discomfort associated with the presence of an endotracheal tube, help reduce WOB, and prevent ventilator dyssynchrony. Patients with dyssynchrony may need an adjustment of inspiratory flow rates or other settings. Patients who stay dyssynchronous despite aggressive analgesia and sedation may need a neuromuscular blocking agent (NMBA), such as vecuronium, pancuronium (Pavulon) or cisatracurium (Nimbex) to relax skeletal muscles and promote breathing with the ventilator. Remember that a patient receiving neuromuscular blockade can appear to be asleep, but still be awake and in pain. For this reason, simultaneous administration of analgesia and sedation with NMBAs is essential.

ADDISON'S DISEASE

Description
Addison's disease is a primary adrenocortical insufficiency in which all 3 classes of adrenal steroids—glucocorticoids, mineralocorticoids, and androgens—are reduced because of adrenal cortex hypofunction.

In secondary adrenocortical insufficiency, which is caused by a lack of pituitary adrenocorticotropic hormone (ACTH) secretion, corticosteroids and androgens are deficient, but mineralocorticoids rarely are.

Up to 80% of Addison's disease cases in the United States are caused by an autoimmune response which causes the adrenal cortex to be destroyed by antibodies. This results in loss of glucocorticoid, mineralocorticoid, and adrenal androgen hormones. Addison's disease can be present along with other endocrine disorders. This condition is known as *autoimmune polyglandular syndrome*.

Other causes of Addison's disease include amyloidosis, fungal infections (e.g., histoplasmosis), acquired immunodeficiency syndrome (AIDS), and metastatic cancer. Iatrogenic Addison's disease may be caused by adrenal hemorrhage, often related to anticoagulant therapy, chemotherapy, ketoconazole therapy for AIDS, or bilateral adrenalectomy.

Clinical Manifestations
Manifestations have a slow onset and include anorexia, nausea, progressive weakness, fatigue, and weight loss. Skin hyperpigmentation

is seen primarily in sun-exposed areas of the body; at pressure points; over joints; and in the creases, especially palmar creases. Other manifestations include abdominal pain, diarrhea, headache, orthostatic hypotension, salt craving, and joint pain.

Patients with adrenocortical insufficiency are at risk for *addisonian crisis* (acute adrenal insufficiency), a life-threatening emergency caused by critically low levels of adrenocortical hormones.

- The most dangerous problem is hypotension, which may cause shock, especially during stress. Circulatory collapse is often unresponsive to the usual treatment (vasopressors and fluid replacement).
- Addisonian crisis may be triggered by stress (e.g., from infection, surgery, trauma, or psychologic distress), sudden withdrawal of corticosteroid hormone therapy, adrenal surgery, or sudden pituitary gland destruction.

Diagnostic Studies

- Plasma cortisol levels are low or fail to rise over basal levels with an ACTH stimulation test. A positive response to ACTH stimulation indicates a functioning adrenal gland and points to pituitary disease rather than adrenal disease.
- Urine levels of free cortisol and aldosterone are low.
- Serum electrolytes show hyperkalemia, hypochloremia, and hyponatremia.
- CT and MRI are used to localize other causes including tumors, fungal infections, and tuberculosis, or adrenal calcification.

Nursing and Interprofessional Management

Treatment of adrenocortical insufficiency focuses on managing the underlying cause when possible. The mainstay is often lifelong hormone therapy with glucocorticoids and mineralocorticoids.

- Hydrocortisone, the most commonly used form of hormone therapy, has both glucocorticoid and mineralocorticoid properties. Glucocorticoids are usually given in divided doses, two-thirds in the morning and one-third in the afternoon. This schedule reflects normal circadian rhythm in endogenous hormone secretion and decreases the side effects associated with corticosteroid therapy. The dosage is increased in stressful situations to prevent addisonian crisis.
- Mineralocorticoids are replaced with fludrocortisone and increased dietary salt intake. Mineralocorticoids are given once daily, preferably in the morning.

- Women need androgen replacement with dehydroepiandrosterone (DHEA) as their only source of androgen production is the adrenal glands.
- Teach patients using mineralocorticoid therapy (fludrocortisone) how to take their BP, increase salt intake, and report any significant changes to their health care provider (HCP).

The patient in addisonian crisis requires immediate aggressive shock management and high-dose hydrocortisone replacement. Large volumes of 0.9% saline solution and 5% dextrose are administered to reverse hypotension and electrolyte imbalances until BP returns to normal.

- Assess vital signs and signs of fluid volume deficit and electrolyte imbalance. Monitor trends in serum glucose, sodium, and potassium.
- The patient cannot cope with stress because corticosteroids cannot be produced. Protect the patient from noise, bright light, and environmental temperature extremes.
- If hospitalization was caused by an adrenal crisis, patients usually respond to IV high-dose hydrocortisone replacement by the second day and can start oral corticosteroid replacement.

▼ **Patient and Caregiver Teaching**

The serious nature of Addison disease and the need for lifelong hormone therapy require a comprehensive teaching plan.

- Teach patients the signs and symptoms of corticosteroid deficiency and excess and to contact their HCP so that the dosage can be adjusted.
- Teach about conditions requiring increased medication. Examples of situations requiring corticosteroid adjustment are fever, influenza, tooth extraction, and rigorous physical activity, such as playing sports on a hot day or distance running.
- Teach prevention of infection and need for prompt and vigorous treatment of existing infections.
- It is critical that the patient wear a medical identification (Medic Alert) bracelet and carry a wallet card stating the patient has Addison disease, so that appropriate therapy can be initiated in an emergency.
- Patients should carry an emergency kit with 100 mg of IM methylprednisolone (Solu-Medrol), syringes, and instructions for use when hormone therapy cannot be taken orally. Have the patient verbalize instructions, practice IM injections with normal saline, and carry written instructions on when the dosage should be changed.
- Provide management instructions for patients who have diabetes and those who have elevated blood glucose levels when taking corticosteroids.

ALZHEIMER'S DISEASE

Description

Alzheimer's disease (AD) is a chronic, progressive, neurodegenerative disease of the brain. AD is the most common form of dementia and the sixth leading cause of death in the United States. Death typically occurs 4 to 8 years after diagnosis, although some patients have lived for 20 years. AD is the only cause of death among the top 10 in United States that cannot be prevented or cured, nor its progression slowed.

Pathophysiology

The exact cause of AD is unknown. Although age is the greatest risk factor, AD is not a normal part of aging, and age alone is not sufficient to cause the disease. It is believed that 11% of people age 65 years and older, and nearly one-third of those over age 85 years, have AD. When AD develops in someone younger than 60 years, it is referred to as *early-onset AD*. AD that becomes evident after the age of 60 years is called *late-onset AD*.

Characteristic findings in AD relate to changes in the brain's structure and function, including amyloid plaques, neurofibrillary tangles, loss of connections between neurons, and neuron death.

- *Amyloid plaques* consist of insoluble deposits of a protein called *β-amyloid*, other proteins, remnants of neurons, non-nerve cells, such as microglia, and other cells. In AD, the plaques develop first in brain areas used for memory and cognitive function. Eventually the cerebral cortex, especially the areas responsible for language and reasoning, is affected.
- *Neurofibrillary tangles* are abnormal collections of twisted protein threads inside nerve cells. The main component of these structures is a protein called *tau*. Normally, tau proteins maintain cellular structure by holding intracellular microtubules together. In AD, the tau protein is altered, and as a result, the microtubules twist together in a helical fashion, forming neurofibrillary tangles.

Plaques and neurofibrillary tangles are not unique to people with AD or dementia. They are also found in the brains of people without cognitive impairment. However, they are more abundant in the brains of those with AD.

The other features of AD are the loss of connections between neurons and neuron death. These processes result in structural damage. Affected parts of the brain begin to shrink in a process called *brain atrophy*. By the final stage of AD, brain tissue has shrunk significantly.

A

Genetic factors may play a critical role in the way that the brain processes the β-amyloid protein, an important risk factor for AD. Abnormally high levels of β-amyloid cause cell damage directly or through an inflammatory response and neuron death.

Diabetes, hypertension, current smoking, hypercholesterolemia, obesity, and trauma are associated with an increased risk for dementia including AD.

Clinical Manifestations

Pathologic changes often precede manifestations of dementia by at least 15 years. Early warning signs of AD are listed in Table 4. The rate of progression from mild to severe is highly variable, ranging from 3 to 20 years.

Initial manifestations are usually related to changes in cognitive functioning. Patients may have memory loss, mild disorientation,

TABLE 4   **Patient and Caregiver Teaching**
Early Warning Signs of Alzheimer's Disease (AD)
Include the following information in the teaching plan for the patient with AD and the caregiver.
1. Memory loss that affects job skills • Frequent forgetfulness or unexplainable confusion at home or in the workplace may signal that something is wrong. • This type of memory loss goes beyond forgetting an assignment, colleague's name, deadline, or phone number.
2. Problems with abstract thinking • For the patient with AD, this goes beyond challenges, such as balancing a checkbook. • The patient with AD may not be able to recognize numbers or do basic calculations.
3. Difficulty doing familiar tasks • It is normal for most people to become distracted and to forget something (e.g., leave something on the stove too long). • People with AD may cook a meal, then forget not only to serve it but also that they made it.
4. Poor or decreased judgment • Many people from time to time may choose not to dress appropriately for the weather (e.g., not bringing a coat or sweater on a cold evening). • The patient with AD may dress inappropriately in more noticeable ways, such as wearing a bathrobe to the store or a sweater on a hot day.

Continued

TABLE 4 Patient and Caregiver Teaching

Early Warning Signs of Alzheimer's Disease (AD)—cont'd

5. Problems with language
   - Most people have trouble finding the "right" word from time to time.
   - People with AD may forget simple words or substitute inappropriate words, making their speech difficult to understand.
6. Misplacing things
   - For many people, temporarily misplacing keys, purses, or wallets is a normal, albeit frustrating, event.
   - The patient with AD may put items in inappropriate places (e.g., eating utensils in clothing drawers), but have no memory of how they got there.
7. Changes in mood
   - Most people have mood changes.
   - The patient with AD tends to have more rapid mood swings for no apparent reason.
8. Changes in personality
   - As most people age, they may have some change in personality (e.g., become less tolerant).
   - The patient with AD can change dramatically, either suddenly or over time. For example, someone who is easygoing may become angry, suspicious, or fearful.
9. Loss of initiative
   - The patient with AD may become and remain uninterested and uninvolved in many or all their usual pursuits.

Adapted from Alzheimer's Association: *Early warning signs,* Chicago, The Association. *www.alz.org/alzheimers_disease_know_the_10_signs.asp.*

and/or trouble with words and numbers. Often a family member reports the patient's declining memory to the health care provider (HCP).

- Memory loss initially relates to recent events, with remote memories still intact. With time and progression of AD, memory loss includes both recent and remote memory and ultimately affects the ability to perform self-care.
- Behavioral manifestations (e.g., agitation, aggression) are from changes within the brain. The behaviors are not intentional or controllable by the person with AD. Some people develop delusions and hallucinations.
- As AD progresses, the person may develop more cognitive impairments, such as *dysphasia* (difficulty comprehending

language and oral communication), *apraxia* (inability to manipulate objects or perform purposeful acts), *visual agnosia* (inability to recognize objects by sight), and *dysgraphia* (difficulty communicating by writing).

- Later in the disease, long-term memories cannot be recalled. The person does not recognize family members and may lose the abilities to communicate and perform activities of daily living (ADLs). Some tend to wander.
- In the late or final stages, the patient is unresponsive and incontinent and needs total care.

Diagnostic Studies

The diagnosis of AD is primarily a diagnosis of exclusion. When all other possible conditions that can cause mental impairment have been excluded, the diagnosis of AD can be made.

- Comprehensive health history, physical examination, neurologic and mental status assessments, and laboratory tests are done.
- Brain imaging tests include CT or MRI scan, which may show brain atrophy in the later stages. However, this finding occurs in other diseases and in people without cognitive impairment.
- Positron emission tomography (PET) scanning can be used to differentiate AD from other forms of dementia.
- Definitive diagnosis of AD usually requires finding neurofibrillary tangles and neuritic plaques at autopsy.

Interprofessional Management

At this time, there is no cure for AD. Treatment does not stop the deterioration of brain cells. Management of AD is aimed at controlling undesirable behaviors that the patient may exhibit and providing support for the family caregivers. Table 59.11, Harding et al., *Lewis' Medical-Surgical Nursing,* ed 11, details drug therapy for AD. These drugs have no effect on overall disease progression.

- Cholinesterase inhibitors block cholinesterase, the enzyme responsible for the breakdown of acetylcholine in the synaptic cleft. Cholinesterase inhibitors include donepezil (Aricept), rivastigmine (Exelon), and galantamine (Razadyne). Rivastigmine is available as a patch.
- Memantine (Namenda) protects brain nerve cells by blocking the damaging effects of glutamate, which is released in large amounts by cells damaged by AD.
- Although antipsychotic drugs are approved for treating psychotic conditions (e.g., schizophrenia), they also have been used for the management of behavioral problems (e.g., agitation, aggressive behavior) that occur in patients with AD. However,

these drugs have been shown to increase the risk of death and cognitive decline in older patients with AD.

- Treating depression associated with AD may improve the patient's cognitive ability. Drugs include selective serotonin reuptake inhibitors (SSRIs), such as fluoxetine (Prozac), sertraline (Zoloft), fluvoxamine (Luvox CR), and citalopram (Celexa).

Nursing Management
Goals
The patient with AD will maintain functional ability for as long as possible, be in a safe environment with a minimum of injuries, have personal care needs met, and have dignity maintained. Additional information on nursing diagnoses for the patient with AD is presented in eNursing Care Plan 59-1 (available on the website).
Nursing Interventions
The diagnosis of AD is traumatic for both the patient and family.

- Assess family caregivers and their ability to accept and cope with the diagnosis. You are in an important position to assess for depression.
- Collaborate with caregivers and patients to manage manifestations, which change over time.
- Teach the caregiver to perform the tasks required to manage the patient's care.
- Adult day care is 1 option available to provide respite for the family and a safe environment for the patient.
- As the disease progresses, the demands on the caregivers eventually exceed their resources. The person with AD may need to be placed in a special dementia unit of a long-term care facility.
- Support groups for caregivers and family members can provide an atmosphere of understanding and give current information about the disease itself and related topics, such as safety, legal, ethical, and financial issues. The Alzheimer's Association has educational and support systems available (*www.alz.org*).

Hospitalization of the patient with AD can be traumatic and precipitate a worsening of the disease. Patients with AD who are hospitalized in the acute care setting need to be observed more closely, frequently oriented to place and time, and given reassurance. Anxiety or disruptive behavior may be reduced by consistent nursing staff.

A family and caregiver teaching guide based on the disease stages is provided in Table 5.

TABLE 5 Family and Caregiver Teaching

Alzheimer's Disease

Include the following instructions when teaching families and caregivers the management of the patient with Alzheimer's disease.

Mild Stage
- Many treatable (and potentially reversible) conditions can mimic dementia (see Table 59.2, Harding et al., *Lewis' Medical-Surgical Nursing,* ed 11). Try to establish a diagnosis.
- Get the patient to stop driving. Confusion and poor judgment can impair driving skills and potentially put others at risk.
- Encourage activities like visiting with friends and family, listening to music, enjoying hobbies, and exercising.
- Provide cues in the home, establish a routine, and determine a specific location where essential items (e.g., eyeglasses) need to be kept.
- Do not correct misstatements or faulty memory.
- Register with MedicAlert + Alzheimer's Association Safe Return, a program established by the MedicAlert Foundation and the Alzheimer's Association to locate those who wander from their homes.
- Make plans in terms of advance directives, care options, financial concerns, and personal preferences for care.

Moderate Stage
- Install door locks for patient safety.
- Provide protective wear for urinary and fecal incontinence.
- Ensure that the home has good lighting, install handrails in stairways and bathroom, and remove area rugs.
- Label drawers and faucets (hot and cold) to ensure safety.
- Develop ways, such as distraction and diversion, to cope with behavioral problems. Identify and reduce potential triggers (e.g., reduce stress, extremes in temperature) for disruptive behavior.
- Provide memory triggers, such as pictures of family and friends.

Severe Stage
- Provide a regular schedule for toileting to reduce incontinence.
- Provide care to meet needs, including oral care and skin care.
- Monitor diet and fluid intake to ensure their adequacy.
- Continue communication through talking and touching.
- Consider placement in a long-term care facility when providing total care becomes too difficult.

A

AMYOTROPHIC LATERAL SCLEROSIS

Amyotrophic lateral sclerosis (ALS) is a rare, progressive neuro-muscular disease marked by loss of motor neurons. ALS usually leads to death 2 to 5 years after diagnosis, but a few patients may survive for more than 10 years. This disease became known as *Lou Gehrig disease* after the famous baseball player was stricken with it in 1939. Perhaps the best-known patient with ALS is British theoretical physicist Stephen Hawking. He was diagnosed at age 21 years and lived with ALS for over 50 years, dying at age 76 years. The typical onset is between age 55 and 75 years. In ALS, motor neurons in the brainstem and spinal cord gradually degenerate for unknown reasons. Consequently, chemical and electrical messages originating in the brain never activate the muscles.

Progressive muscle weakness and atrophy are the classic sign of ALS. Early symptoms of weakness vary.

- For some, symptoms initially affect the arms or legs ("limb-onset" ALS). The person may have trouble with tasks requiring fine motor skills (e.g., writing, typing) or notice they are tripping, dropping things, or stumbling more often.
- Those who first have problems with slurred speech or swallowing have "bulbar onset" ALS.
- Muscle wasting and involuntary contractions result from the denervation of the muscles and lack of stimulation and use.
- Other symptoms include pain, sleep disorders, spasticity and hyperreflexia, drooling, emotional lability, constipation, and esophageal reflux.
- ALS does not affect a patient's intelligence, but affected people may have depression and problems with decision making and memory.
- Death often results from compromised respiratory function caused by muscle weakness and paralysis.

No cure exists for ALS and treatment options are limited. Riluzole (Rilutek) slows the progression of ALS. This drug reduces damage to motor neurons by decreasing the release of glutamate (an excitatory neurotransmitter) in the brain. Edaravone (Radicava) is a free radical scavenger that is believed to relieve effects of oxidative stress, a likely factor in progression of ALS.

Nursing interventions include: (1) facilitating communication; (2) reducing risk of aspiration; (3) facilitating early identification of respiratory insufficiency; (4) decreasing pain from muscle weakness; (5) decreasing risk of injury related to falls; and (6) providing diversional activities, such as reading and companionship.

- Help the patient and family manage the disease process, including grieving related to the loss of motor function and impending death. Discuss artificial methods of ventilation and advance directives with the patient and caregivers.

ANAL CANCER

Anal cancer is uncommon in the general population, but the incidence is increasing. In the United States around 8200 people are diagnosed with anal cancer each year. It mainly occurs in older adults, with the average age being in the early 60s. Human papillomavirus (HPV) is associated with about 80% of the cases of anal cancer. Those at high risk for anal cancer include smokers, HIV-positive homosexual men, people who are immunocompromised (e.g., posttransplant immunosuppression), and women with cervical, vaginal, or vulvar cancer.

- Frequently the initial manifestation is rectal bleeding. Other symptoms include rectal pain and sensation of a rectal mass. Some patients have no symptoms, which leads to delayed diagnosis and treatment.

It is especially important to screen high-risk persons using digital rectal examination (DRE) and anal Pap tests. In an anal Pap test, the anal lining is swabbed, and the cells examined to identify any cell changes (e.g., dysplasia, neoplasia). High-resolution anoscopy allows for visualization of the mucosa and biopsy. An endoanal (endorectal) ultrasound may be done.

Treatment of anal cancer depends on the size and depth of the lesions. Cancer therapy involves surgery or a combination of low-dose radiation and chemotherapy. Chemotherapy regimens include combinations of mitomycin, cisplatin, and fluorouracil. Options for precancerous lesions are surgical removal or treatment with topical imiquimod (Aldara) and fluorouracil. If the tumor involves the rectum and is large enough to require removing the anal sphincters, the anus will be sutured shut and a permanent ostomy created.

ANEMIA

Description

Anemia is a deficiency in the number of red blood cells (RBCs), or erythrocytes, quantity of hemoglobin (Hgb), and/or volume of packed RBCs (hematocrit). It is a prevalent condition with diverse causes, such as blood loss, impaired production of erythrocytes, or increased destruction of erythrocytes.

- Because RBCs transport O_2, erythrocyte disorders can lead to tissue hypoxia. Hypoxia accounts for many of the signs and symptoms of anemia.
- Anemia is not a specific disease; it is a manifestation of a pathologic process.
- Anemia can result from primary hematologic problems or can develop secondary to disorders in other body systems.

The various types of anemias are classified according to morphology (cell characteristics) or etiology.

- *Morphologic classification* is based on erythrocyte size and color (Table 6).
- *Etiologic classification* is related to clinical conditions causing the anemia (Table 7).

Diagnostic Studies

- Anemia is diagnosed using a complete blood count (CBC), reticulocyte count, and peripheral blood smear. Once anemia is identified, further investigation may determine its specific cause.
- Although the Hgb level is decreased in all types of anemias, other laboratory results are characteristic of specific types of anemias (Table 8).

TABLE 6 Morphologic Classification and Etiology of Anemia

RBC Morphology	Etiology
Normocytic, normochromic (normal size and color) MCV 80–95 fL, MCH 27–31 pg	Acute blood loss, hemolysis, chronic kidney disease, chronic disease, cancers, endocrine disorders, starvation, aplastic anemia, sickle cell anemia, pregnancy
Microcytic, hypochromic (small size, pale color) MCV <80 fL, MCH <27 pg	Iron-deficiency anemia, vitamin B_6 deficiency, copper deficiency, thalassemia, lead poisoning
Macrocytic (megaloblastic), normochromic (large size, normal color) MCV >95 fL, MCH >31 pg	Cobalamin (vitamin B_{12}) deficiency, folic acid deficiency, liver disease (including effects of alcohol abuse)

MCH, Mean corpuscular hemoglobin; *MCV*, mean corpuscular volume.

TABLE 7   Etiologic Classification of Anemia

Decreased RBC Production

Decreased Hemoglobin Synthesis
- Iron deficiency
- Sideroblastic anemia (decreased porphyrin)
- Thalassemias (decreased globin synthesis)

Decreased Number of RBC Precursors
- Aplastic anemia and inherited disorders (e.g., Fanconi syndrome)
- Anemia of myeloproliferative diseases (e.g., leukemia) and myelodysplasia
- Chronic diseases or disorders
- Medications and chemicals (e.g., chemotherapy, lead)
- Radiation

Defective DNA Synthesis
- Cobalamin (vitamin B_{12}) deficiency
- Folic acid deficiency

Blood Loss

Acute
- Blood vessel rupture
- Splenic sequestration crisis
- Trauma

Chronic
- Gastritis
- Hemorrhoids
- Menstrual flow

Increased RBC Destruction (Hemolytic Anemias)

Acquired (Extrinsic)
- Antibodies against RBCs
- Infectious agents (e.g., malaria) and toxins
- Physical destruction
- Disseminated intravascular coagulopathy (DIC)
- Extracorporeal circulation
- Prosthetic heart valves
- Thrombotic thrombocytopenic purpura (TTP)

Continued

TABLE 7   Etiologic Classification of Anemia—cont'd
Hereditary (Intrinsic)
• Abnormal hemoglobin (sickle cell disease)
• Enzyme deficiency (G6PD)
• Membrane abnormalities (paroxysmal nocturnal hemoglobinuria, hereditary spherocytosis)

G6PD, Glucose-6-phosphate dehydrogenase; *RBC,* red blood cell.

Clinical Manifestations

Signs and symptoms of anemia are caused by the body's response to tissue hypoxia (Table 9). Specific manifestations vary depending on how fast the anemia has evolved, its severity, and any coexisting disease. Hgb levels may determine the severity of anemia.

- *Mild anemia* (Hgb 10 to 12 g/dL [100 to 120 g/L]) may not cause symptoms. Signs and symptoms are usually caused by an underlying disease or a compensatory response to heavy exercise. Symptoms may include palpitations, dyspnea, and mild fatigue.
- In *moderate anemia* (Hgb 6 to 10 g/dL [60 to 100 g/L]), cardiopulmonary signs and symptoms (e.g., increased heart rate) may be present with rest as well as activity.
- In *severe anemia* (Hgb <6 g/dL [60 g/L]), patients display many clinical manifestations involving multiple body systems.

Nursing and Interprofessional Management

The goals of care for the patient with anemia include assuming normal activities of daily living (ADLs), maintaining adequate nutrition, and developing no complications related to anemia. See eNursing Care Plan 30.1 for the patient with anemia (available on the website).

The numerous causes of anemia require nursing interventions specific to the type of anemia and the patient's needs. General components of care for all patients with anemia may include:

- dietary and lifestyle changes that may reverse some causes of anemia;
- acute interventions, such as blood or blood product transfusions, drug therapy (e.g., erythropoietin, vitamin supplements), volume replacement, and O_2 therapy;
- assisting the patient in prioritizing activities and planning rest to accommodate energy levels and manage fatigue;
- assessing the patient's knowledge regarding adequate nutritional intake and adherence to safety precautions to prevent falls and injury;
- specific types of anemias are listed under separate headings.

TABLE 8 Laboratory Results in Anemias

Etiology of Anemia	Hgb/Hct	MCV	Reticulocytes	Serum Iron	TIBC	Transferrin	Ferritin	Bilirubin	Serum B$_{12}$	Folate
Acute blood loss	↓	N or ↓	N or ↑	N	N	N	N	N	N	N
Aplastic anemia	↓	N or slight ↑	↓	N or ↑	N or ↑	N	N	N	N	N
Chronic blood loss	↓	↓	N or ↑	↓	↑	N	N	N or ↓	N	N
Chronic disease	↓	N or ↓	N or ↓	N or ↓	↓	N or ↓	N or ↑	N	N	N
Cobalamin deficiency	↓	↑	N or ↓	N or ↑	N	Slight ↑	↑	N or slight ↑	↓	N
Folic acid deficiency	↓	↑	N or ↓	N or ↑	N	Slight ↑	↑	N or slight ↑	N	↓
Hemolytic anemia	↓	N or ↑	↑	N or ↑	N or ↓	N	N or ↑	↑	N	N
Iron deficiency	↓	↓	N or slight ↓ or ↑	↓	↑	N or ↓	↓	N or ↓	N	N
Sickle cell anemia	↓	N	↑	N or ↑	N or ↓	N	N	↑	N	↓
Thalassemia major	↓	N or ↓	↑	↑	↓	↓	N or ↑	↑	N	↓

Hgb/Hct, Hemoglobin/hematocrit; *MCV,* mean corpuscular volume; *N,* normal; *TIBC,* total iron-binding capacity.

A

TABLE 9 Manifestations of Anemia*

Body System	Mild (Hgb 10–12 g/dL [100–120 g/L])	Moderate (Hgb 6–10 g/dL [60–100 g/L])	Severe (Hgb <6 g/dL [<60 g/L])
Cardiovascular	Palpitations	Increased palpitations, "bounding pulse"	Tachycardia, increased pulse pressure, systolic murmurs, intermittent claudication, angina, heart failure, myocardial infarction
Eyes	None	None	Icteric conjunctiva and sclera*, retinal hemorrhage, blurred vision
Gastrointestinal	None	None	Anorexia, hepatomegaly, splenomegaly, difficulty swallowing, sore mouth
General	None or mild fatigue	Fatigue	Sensitivity to cold, weight loss, lethargy
Integument	None	None	Pallor, jaundice*, pruritus*
Mouth	None	None	Glossitis, smooth tongue
Musculoskeletal	None	None	Bone pain
Pulmonary	Exertional dyspnea	Dyspnea	Tachypnea, orthopnea, dyspnea at rest
Neurologic	None	"Roaring in the ears"	Headache, vertigo, irritability, depression, impaired thought processes

SEVERITY OF ANEMIA

*Caused by hemolysis.
Hgb, Hemoglobin.

ANEMIA, APLASTIC

Description

Aplastic anemia is a disease in which the patient has peripheral blood *pancytopenia* (decrease in number of all blood cell types—red blood cells [RBCs], white blood cells [WBCs], and platelets) and hypocellular bone marrow. The spectrum of the anemia can range from a moderate condition managed with erythropoietin or blood transfusions to very severe with potentially fatal hemorrhage and sepsis.

Pathophysiology

About 70% of aplastic anemias are caused by autoimmune activity by autoreactive T-lymphocytes. The cytotoxic T-cells target and destroy the patient's own hematopoietic stem cells. Other anemias may be acquired from toxic injury to bone marrow stem cells or a result of an inherited stem cell defect. Causes of aplastic anemia include chemical agents and toxins (e.g., benzene, insecticides, arsenic, alcohol); drugs (e.g., alkylating agents, antiseizure drugs, antimetabolites, antimicrobials, gold, nonsteroidal antiinflammatory drugs, thyroid medications, allopurinol); radiation; and viral or bacterial infections.

Clinical Manifestations

Aplastic anemia can manifest abruptly over days or develop insidiously over weeks and months. It can range from mild to severe. The patient may have symptoms caused by suppression of any or all bone marrow elements.

- General manifestations of anemia, such as fatigue and dyspnea, as well as cardiovascular and cerebral signs, may be seen (see Table 9).
- The patient with neutropenia (low neutrophil count) is susceptible to infection and at risk for development of septic shock and death.
- Thrombocytopenia may be manifested by bleeding (e.g., petechiae, ecchymoses, epistaxis).

Diagnostic Studies

Diagnosis is confirmed by laboratory studies.

- All marrow elements are affected (RBC, WBC, and platelet), with values often decreased (see Table 8). Reticulocyte count is low.
- Serum iron and total iron-binding capacity (TIBC) may be high as initial signs of erythroid suppression.

- Bone marrow examination is especially important in aplastic anemia. Findings include a hypocellular marrow with increased yellow marrow (fat content).

Nursing and Interprofessional Management

Management of aplastic anemia is based on identifying and removing the causative agent (when possible) and providing supportive care until pancytopenia reverses.

Nursing interventions for the patient with pancytopenia from aplastic anemia are presented in the nursing care plans (on the website) for patients with anemia (see eNursing Care Plan 30.1), thrombocytopenia (eNursing Care Plan 30.2), and neutropenia (eNursing Care Plan 30.3). Nursing actions are directed at preventing complications from infection and hemorrhage.

- The prognosis for severe untreated aplastic anemia is poor. However, advances in medical management, including hematopoietic stem cell transplantation (HSCT), steroids, and immunosuppressive therapy with antithymocyte globulin (ATG) and cyclosporine or cyclophosphamide, have significantly improved outcomes. Eltrombopag (Promacta), an oral thrombopoietin receptor agonist, can increase platelet counts. High dose cyclophosphamide, alemtuzumab, or androgens are options for select patients who do not respond other therapies.
- Treatment of choice for adults younger than 55 years of age who do not respond to immunosuppressive therapy and who have a human leukocyte antigen (HLA)–matched donor, half-matched, or unrelated donor, is HSCT. Best results are seen in younger patients who have not had previous blood transfusions. Prior transfusions increase the risk of graft rejection.
- For older adults without a HSCT donor, the treatment of choice is immunosuppression with ATG and cyclosporine, steroids, and eltrombopag. Patients who need supportive blood transfusions should be on an iron-binding agent to prevent iron overload.

ANEMIA, COBALAMIN (VITAMIN B$_{12}$) DEFICIENCY

Description

Anemia resulting from a cobalamin (vitamin B$_{12}$) deficiency is a type of megaloblastic anemia. Defective red blood cell (RBC) maturation results in large, abnormal RBCs.

Pathophysiology

Normally a protein known as *intrinsic factor* (IF) is secreted by parietal cells of the gastric mucosa. IF is required for cobalamin (extrinsic factor) absorption in the distal ileum. In *pernicious anemia,* the most common cause of cobalamin deficiency, the gastric mucosa does not secrete IF.

Cobalamin deficiency can occur in patients who have had gastrointestinal (GI) surgery, such as gastrectomy, gastric bypass, or small bowel resection involving the ileum, and in patients with Crohn's disease, ileitis, diverticula of the small intestine, and/or chronic atrophic gastritis. In these cases, cobalamin deficiency results from the loss of IF-secreting gastric mucosal surface or impaired absorption of cobalamin in the distal ileum. Cobalamin deficiency is also found in people who ingest excessive alcohol or hot tea, smokers, long-term users of histamine (H$_2$)-receptor blockers and proton pump inhibitors, and those who are strict vegetarians.

Clinical Manifestations

Manifestations of anemia related to cobalamin deficiency develop as a result of tissue hypoxia (see Table 9).

- GI manifestations include a sore red tongue, anorexia, nausea, vomiting, and abdominal pain.
- Neuromuscular manifestations include weakness, paresthesias of feet and hands, reduced vibratory and position senses, ataxia, muscle weakness, and impaired thought processes ranging from confusion to dementia.

Diagnostic Studies

Laboratory data reflective of cobalamin deficiency anemia are presented in Table 8.

- Erythrocytes appear large (macrocytic) with abnormal shapes. This structure contributes to erythrocyte destruction because the cell membrane is fragile.
- Serum cobalamin levels are reduced.
- Normal serum folate levels with low cobalamin levels suggest that megaloblastic anemia is caused by a cobalamin deficiency.
- A serum test for anti-IF antibodies may be done that is specific for pernicious anemia.
- An upper GI endoscopy and biopsy of the gastric mucosa may also be done.

Nursing and Interprofessional Management

Dietary management is not used for cobalamin replacement. Regardless of how much cobalamin is ingested, the patient is not able to absorb it when IF is lacking or if absorption in the ileum is impaired.

- Lifelong administration of cobalamin is needed. It can be given parenterally (cyanocobalamin or hydroxocobalamin) or intranasally (Nascobal). A typical treatment schedule consists of cobalamin IM daily for 2 weeks, then weekly until hematocrit is normal, and then monthly for life.
- High-dose oral cobalamin and sublingual cobalamin are also available for patients in whom GI absorption is intact.
- Long-standing neuromuscular complications may not be reversible. Physical therapy may be useful.
- Nursing interventions for the patient with anemia are also appropriate for the patient with cobalamin deficiency (see Anemia, p. 29).
- Ensure that the patient is protected from burns and trauma, because of a diminished sensation to heat and pain as a result of neurologic impairment. Follow-up evaluation is essential to assess for neurologic deficits that were not corrected by cobalamin replacement therapy.
- Because the potential for gastric cancer is increased in patients with atrophic gastritis–related pernicious anemia, the patient should have frequent screening for gastric cancer.

ANEMIA, FOLIC ACID DEFICIENCY

Folic acid (folate) deficiency can cause megaloblastic anemia. Folic acid is required for deoxyribonucleic acid (DNA) synthesis leading to the formation and maturation of red blood cells (RBCs). Common causes of folic acid deficiency are: (1) dietary deficiency, especially a lack of leafy green vegetables and citrus fruits, (2) malabsorption syndromes, (3) drugs that interfere with absorption/or use of folic acid (e.g., methotrexate); antiseizure medications (e.g., phenobarbital, phenytoin [Dilantin]), (4) chronic alcohol use and anorexia, and (5) chronic hemodialysis.

Clinical Manifestations
Clinical manifestations of folic acid deficiency are similar to those of cobalamin deficiency. The disease develops insidiously, and the patient's symptoms may be attributed to other coexisting problems, such as cirrhosis or esophageal varices.

- Gastrointestinal (GI) problems include dyspepsia and a smooth, beefy-red tongue.

- Absence of neurologic problems is an important diagnostic finding and differentiates folic acid deficiency from cobalamin deficiency.
- Laboratory findings in folic acid deficiency are presented in Table 8. The serum folate level is low (normal is 5–25 ng/mL [11–57 nmol/L]) and the serum cobalamin level is normal.

Nursing and Interprofessional Management

Folic acid deficiency is treated by replacement therapy, with a usual dosage of 1 mg/day by mouth. In malabsorption states, up to 5 mg/day may be needed. Teach the patient to eat foods high in folic acid (e.g., leafy green vegetables, breakfast cereals, breads, pasta).

Nursing interventions for the patient with anemia are also appropriate for the patient with folic acid deficiency (see Anemia, p. 29).

ANEMIA, IRON-DEFICIENCY

Description

Iron-deficiency anemia is the most common nutritional disorder in the world. Those most susceptible to iron-deficiency anemia are the very young, those on poor diets, and women in their reproductive years.

Pathophysiology

Iron deficiency may develop from inadequate dietary intake, malabsorption, blood loss, or hemolysis. Dietary iron is enough to meet the needs of men and older women. It may be inadequate for those with higher iron needs (e.g., menstruating or pregnant women).

Iron absorption occurs in the duodenum. Absorption can be altered after surgical procedures that involve removal of or bypass of the duodenum. Malabsorption syndromes may also involve disease of the duodenum, which alters or destroys the absorption surface.

Blood loss is a major cause of iron deficiency in adults. Major sources of chronic blood loss are from the gastrointestinal (GI) and genitourinary (GU) systems.

- GI bleeding is often not apparent for a prolonged period before the problem is identified. A loss of 50 to 75 mL of blood from the upper GI tract is enough for stools to appear black *(melena)*. This color results from iron in the red blood cells (RBCs).
- Common causes of GI blood loss are peptic ulcer, esophagitis, diverticula, hemorrhoids, and cancer. GU blood loss occurs

primarily from menstrual bleeding. The average monthly menstrual blood loss is about 45 mL, which causes a loss of about 22 mg of iron.
- Dialysis treatment for chronic kidney disease may induce iron-deficiency anemia because of the blood lost in the dialysis equipment and blood sampling.

Clinical Manifestations

In the early course of iron-deficiency anemia, the patient may be free of symptoms. As the disease becomes chronic, general manifestations of anemia may develop (see Table 9). In addition, specific clinical signs and symptoms related to iron-deficiency anemia may occur.
- Pallor is the most common finding, and glossitis (inflammation of the tongue) is the second most common; another finding is cheilitis (inflammation of the lips).
- The patient may report headache, paresthesia, and a burning sensation of the tongue caused by lack of iron in the tissues.

Diagnostic Studies

Laboratory abnormalities characteristic of iron-deficiency anemia are presented in Table 8. Other diagnostic studies are done to determine the cause of iron deficiency. Endoscopy and colonoscopy may be used to detect GI bleeding.

Nursing and Interprofessional Management

Consider groups who are at increased risk for development of iron-deficiency anemia, including premenopausal and pregnant women, people from lower socioeconomic backgrounds, older adults, and those who have had blood loss. Diet teaching, with an emphasis on foods high in iron and ways to maximize absorption, is important for these groups.

The main goal is to treat the underlying problem causing iron loss, reduced iron intake (e.g., malnutrition, alcohol use), or poor absorption of iron. Efforts are directed toward replacing iron. Appropriate nursing measures are presented in eNursing Care Plan 30.1, on the website.
- Teach the patient which foods are good sources of iron. If nutrition is adequate, increasing iron intake by dietary means may not be enough. Oral or occasionally parenteral iron supplements are used.
- Parenteral iron supplements require special considerations related to administration and side effects (see Drug Therapy, Iron-Deficiency Anemia in Chapter 30, Harding et al, *Lewis' Medical-Surgical Nursing*, ed 11).

- If iron deficiency is from acute blood loss, transfusion of packed RBCs may be required.

▼ **Patient and Caregiver Teaching**

- Discuss the need for diagnostic studies to identify the cause of anemia and to evaluate response to therapy.
- Stress adherence with dietary and drug therapy. To replenish the body's iron stores, the patient needs to take iron therapy for 2 to 3 months after the hemoglobin (Hgb) level returns to normal.
- Monitor patients who require lifelong iron supplementation for potential liver problems related to iron storage.

ANEURYSM, AORTIC

Description

One of the most common problems affecting the aorta is an *aneurysm*, which is a permanent, localized outpouching or dilation of the vessel wall. Aneurysms occur in men more often than in women and in whites more often than blacks. The incidence increases with age.

An *aneurysm* is a localized outpouching or dilation of the blood vessel wall. About 1.1 million adults between 55 and 84 years of age have an aneurysm. Aneurysms occur in men more often than in women.

Aneurysms may occur in more than 1 location. Aortic aneurysms may involve the aortic arch, thoracic aorta, and/or abdominal aorta. Three-fourths of aortic aneurysms occur in the abdominal aorta and one-fourth in the thoracic aorta. Most *abdominal aortic aneurysms* (AAAs) occur below the renal arteries.

Pathophysiology

A variety of disorders are associated with aortic aneurysms. The main causes are classified as degenerative, congenital, mechanical (e.g., penetrating or blunt trauma), inflammatory (e.g., aortitis [Takayasu's arteritis]), or infectious (e.g., aortitis [*Chlamydia pneumoniae,* human immunodeficiency virus]). The larger the aneurysm, the greater the risk of rupture.

- Risk factors for aortic aneurysms include age, male gender, hypertension, coronary artery disease, family history, tobacco use, high cholesterol, lower extremity peripheral artery disease (PAD), carotid artery disease, previous stroke, and excess weight or obesity. Tobacco use is the most important modifiable risk factor.

- The development of aortic aneurysm and dissection has a strong genetic component. (Aortic dissection is discussed as a separate topic.) The familial tendency is related to congenital anomalies, such as bicuspid aortic valve, coarctation of the aorta, Turner syndrome, and autosomal dominant polycystic kidney disease. Aneurysms are classified as true and false aneurysms.
- A *true aneurysm* is one in which the wall of the artery forms the aneurysm, with at least 1 vessel layer still intact. True aneurysms are further subdivided into fusiform and saccular dilations. A *fusiform aneurysm* is circumferential and relatively uniform in shape. A *saccular aneurysm* is pouchlike, with a narrow neck connecting the bulge to one side of the arterial wall.
- A *false aneurysm,* or *pseudoaneurysm,* is not an aneurysm, but a disruption of all layers of all wall layers with bleeding that is contained by surrounding anatomic structures. False aneurysms may result from trauma, infection, after peripheral artery bypass graft surgery at the site of the graft-to-artery anastomosis, or arterial leakage after removal of cannulae (e.g., femoral artery catheters, intraaortic balloon pump devices).

Clinical Manifestations

Thoracic aortic aneurysms are usually asymptomatic. When symptoms present, the most common is deep, diffuse chest pain that may extend to the interscapular area.

Aneurysms in the ascending aorta and aortic arch can cause: (1) angina from decreased blood flow to the coronary arteries; (2) transient ischemic attacks from decreased blood flow to the carotid arteries; and (3) coughing, shortness of breath, hoarseness, and/or dysphagia (difficulty swallowing) from pressure on the laryngeal nerve. Compression of the superior vena cava by the aneurysm can cause distended neck veins and face and arm edema.

AAAs are often asymptomatic, found during routine physical examination or on evaluation for an unrelated problem (e.g., abdominal x-ray). A pulsatile mass in the periumbilical area slightly to the left of midline may be present. Bruits may be auscultated over the aneurysm. Physical findings may be harder to detect in obese persons.

- AAA symptoms may mimic pain associated with abdominal or back disorders. Compression of nearby anatomic structures and nerves may cause symptoms, such as back pain, epigastric discomfort, altered bowel elimination, and intermittent claudication.
- Sometimes, aneurysms spontaneously embolize plaque, causing "*blue toe syndrome,*" (patchy mottling of the feet and toes in the presence of peripheral pulses).

Complications

Smokers with an aortic aneurysm are most likely to experience the serious complication of aortic rupture.

- If rupture occurs into the retroperitoneal space, bleeding may be controlled by surrounding structures, preventing exsanguination and death. The patient has severe back pain and may have back and/or flank ecchymosis *(Grey Turner's sign)*.
- If rupture occurs into the thoracic or abdominal cavity, the patient can die from massive hemorrhage. For patients admitted with a ruptured AAA, in-hospital mortality is high at 53%.
- The patient who reaches the hospital will be in hypovolemic shock with tachycardia; hypotension; pale, clammy skin; decreased urine output; altered sensorium; and abdominal tenderness. Simultaneous resuscitation and immediate surgical repair are needed.

Diagnostic Studies

- Chest x-rays reveal abnormal widening of the thoracic aorta. Abdominal x-rays may show calcification within the aortic wall.
- Echocardiography assesses the function of the aortic valve.
- Ultrasound is useful for aneurysm screening and to monitor aneurysm size.
- CT or MRI may help assess the location and severity of aneurysms.

Interprofessional Management

The goal of management is to prevent aneurysm rupture. Conservative therapy of small, asymptomatic AAAs (< 5.5 cm) is the best practice.

- Risk factor modification is recommended (ceasing tobacco use, decreasing BP, optimizing lipid profile, gradually increasing physical activity).
- Aneurysm size is monitored using ultrasound or CT every 6 to 12 months. Monitoring by ultrasound every 2 to 3 years is recommended for patients with AAAs smaller than 4.0 cm in diameter.
- Patients should receive medical management for hypertension, hyperlipidemia, diabetes, and other cardiovascular risk factors.

Aneurysms 5.5 cm in diameter or larger are surgically repaired. Surgical intervention may occur sooner if the patient has a genetic disorder (e.g., Marfan), if the aneurysm expands rapidly or becomes symptomatic, or if the risk of rupture is high.

- Open aneurysm repair (OAR) involves a large abdominal incision through which the surgeon: (1) cuts into the diseased aortic segment, (2) removes any thrombus or plaque, (3) sutures a synthetic graft to the aorta proximal and distal to the aneurysm, and (4) sutures the native aortic wall around the graft to act as a protective cover.

Surgical repair of an AAA is presented in Fig. 37.6 in Harding et al, *Lewis' Medical-Surgical Nursing,* ed 11.

- An alternative to OAR is the minimally invasive endovascular grafting technique. This procedure involves placement of a sutureless aortic graft into the abdominal aorta inside the aneurysm via a femoral artery cutdown.
- Endovascular aneurysm repair (EVAR) is less invasive than OAR.

The most common complication of aneurysm repair is *endoleak,* the seepage of blood back into the old aneurysm. This may result from an inadequate seal at either graft end, a tear through the graft fabric, or leakage between overlapping graft segments. Repair may require coil embolization (insertion of beads) for hemostasis.

Nursing Management

Goals

The patient undergoing aortic surgery will have normal tissue perfusion, intact motor and sensory function, and no complications related to surgical repair, such as infection, rupture, or thrombosis.

Nursing Interventions

Encourage the patient to reduce cardiovascular risk factors, including controlling BP, smoking cessation, and maintaining normal body weight and serum lipid levels. Counsel the patient about taking part in moderate physical activity.

- Before surgery, provide emotional support and teaching to the patient and caregivers. Briefly explain the disease process, the planned surgical procedure(s), preoperative routines, what to expect immediately after surgery (e.g., recovery room, tubes/drains), and usual postoperative timelines.
- After surgery, in addition to the usual goals of care for a postoperative patient (e.g., maintaining adequate respiratory function, fluid and electrolyte balance, pain control), check for graft patency and renal perfusion. Watch for and intervene to limit or treat dysrhythmias, ischemia, venous thromboembolism, infections, and neurologic complications.
- A potentially lethal complication in an emergency repair of a ruptured AAA is the development of intraabdominal hypertension (IAH) with associated abdominal compartment syndrome. Persistent IAH reduces blood flow to the viscera. IAH is confirmed by measuring the patient's intraabdominal pressure indirectly through a catheter and transducer system.

▼ **Patient and Caregiver Teaching**

Teach the patient and caregiver to gradually increase activities at home. Fatigue, poor appetite, and irregular bowel habits are common.

- Teach the patient to avoid heavy lifting for 6 weeks after surgery. Any redness, swelling, increased pain, drainage from incisions, or fever > 100°F (37.8°C) should be reported to a health care provider (HCP).
- Teach patient and caregiver to observe for changes in color or warmth of the extremities and changes in peripheral pulses.
- Sexual problems in male patients are common after aortic surgery. Referral to a urologist and counseling may be useful if erectile dysfunction occurs.

ANGINA, CHRONIC STABLE

Description

Chronic stable angina refers to chest pain that occurs intermittently over a long period with a similar pattern of onset, duration, and intensity of symptoms. Chronic stable angina is a clinical manifestation of coronary artery disease (CAD).

Angina, or chest pain, is a result of reversible myocardial ischemia that occurs when the demand for myocardial oxygen exceeds the ability of the coronary arteries to supply the heart muscle with oxygen. The primary cause of myocardial ischemia is insufficient blood flow to the myocardium through coronary arteries narrowed by atherosclerosis (see Coronary Artery Disease, p. 151).

Variants of chronic stable angina include:

- *Silent ischemia,* in which ischemia occurs in the absence of any subjective symptoms.
- *Prinzmetal's angina* (variant angina), which often occurs at rest, usually in response to spasm of a major coronary artery. This rare form of angina is seen in patients with a history of migraine headaches, Raynaud phenomenon, or heavy smoking. It is usually caused by spasm of a major coronary artery, with or without CAD.

Microvascular angina occurs in the absence of significant coronary atherosclerosis or coronary spasm, especially in women. In these patients, chest pain is related to myocardial ischemia associated with the coronary microcirculation. This is known as *coronary microvascular disease* (*MVD*), or "*syndrome X.*" Prevention and treatment of MVD follow the same recommendations as for CAD.

Pathophysiology

Myocardial cells become hypoxic within the first 10 seconds of coronary occlusion. Anaerobic metabolism begins, and lactic acid accumulates. Lactic acid irritates myocardial nerve fibers and transmits a pain message to the cardiac nerves and upper thoracic posterior nerve roots. This accounts for referred cardiac pain to the shoulders, neck, lower jaw, and arms.

- Ischemic cardiac cells are viable for about 20 minutes. With restoration of blood flow, aerobic metabolism resumes and cellular repair begins.

Clinical Manifestations

Patients may describe a pain, pressure, or ache in the chest. It is an unpleasant feeling, often described as a constrictive, squeezing, heavy, tight, or suffocating sensation (Table 10). Many people report severe indigestion or epigastric burning. Although most angina pain is substernal in location, the sensation may occur in

TABLE 10   PQRST Assessment of Angina

Use the following memory aid to obtain information from the patient who has chest pain.

	Factor	Questions to Ask Patient
P	Precipitating events	What events or activities precipitated the pain or discomfort (e.g., argument, exercise, resting)?
Q	Quality of pain	What does the pain or discomfort feel like (e.g., pressure, dull, aching, tight, squeezing, heaviness)?
R	Region (location) and radiation of pain	Can you point to where the pain or discomfort is located? Does the pain or discomfort radiate to other areas (e.g., back, neck, arms, jaw, shoulder, elbow)?
S	Severity of pain	On a scale of 0 to 10, with 0 indicating no pain and 10 being the most severe pain you could imagine, what number would you give the pain or discomfort?
T	Timing	When did the pain or discomfort begin? Has it changed since this time? Have you had pain/discomfort like this before?

the neck or radiate to locations including the jaw, neck, shoulders, and arms. Chronic angina pain usually does not change with position or breathing and is rarely described as sharp or stabbing.

- Some patients, especially women and older adults, report atypical symptoms of angina including dyspnea, nausea, and/or fatigue. This presentation is referred to as "angina equivalent."
- Often people will report pain between the shoulder blades and dismiss it as not being related to the heart.
- The pain or discomfort of chronic angina is often provoked by physical exertion, stress, or emotional upset.
- The pain usually lasts for only a few minutes (5–15 minutes) and often subsides with rest, calming down, and/or using sublingual nitroglycerin (NTG) (e.g., Nitrostat).
- An electrocardiogram (ECG) usually reveals ST-segment depression and/or T wave inversion, indicating ischemia. The ECG pattern returns to baseline when the pain is relieved.

Diagnostic Studies

Diagnostic studies used to evaluate angina are the same as those used to diagnose CAD (see Coronary Artery Disease, p. 151). For patients with known CAD and chronic stable angina, common diagnostic studies include 12-lead ECG, echocardiography, exercise stress testing, and pharmacologic nuclear imaging.

Interprofessional Management

The treatment of chronic stable angina is aimed at decreasing oxygen demand and/or increasing oxygen supply. The reduction of CAD risk factors is a priority. In addition to antiplatelet and cholesterol-lowering drug therapy, the most common interventions for chronic stable angina are nitrates, angiotensin-converting enzyme (ACE) inhibitors, β-blockers, and calcium-channel blockers.

Drug Therapy

- Aspirin is given in the absence of contraindications.
- Short-acting nitrates are first-line therapy for the treatment of angina. Nitrates produce their principal effects by dilating peripheral blood vessels, coronary arteries, and collateral vessels. Sublingual NTG tablets or spray will usually relieve pain in approximately 3 minutes and lasts approximately 30 to 60 minutes. If symptoms are unchanged or worse after 5 minutes, the patient should activate the emergency response system. Sublingual NTG can be used before undertaking an activity that the patient knows may precipitate angina.
- Long-acting nitrates, such as isosorbide dinitrate (see Table 33.12) and isosorbide mononitrate, can reduce the frequency of anginal attacks. Longer-acting nitrates are available

in oral preparations, ointments, and transdermal controlled-release patches.

- ACE inhibitors (e.g., captopril) are prescribed for patients with chronic stable angina who are at high risk for a cardiac event (e.g., ejection fraction [EF] 40% or less, diabetes, hypertension, or chronic kidney disease). These drugs result in vasodilation and reduced blood volume. Most important, they can prevent or reverse ventricular remodeling.

- Patients with left ventricular dysfunction or elevated BP or those who have had a myocardial infarction (MI) take β-blockers, such as carvedilol (Coreg), metoprolol (Lopressor), and bisoprolol (Zebeta). These medications reduce myocardial oxygen demand by decreasing myocardial contractility, heart rate (HR), systemic vascular resistance (SVR), and BP.

- Calcium-channel blockers, such as nifedipine (Procardia), verapamil (Calan), diltiazem (Cardizem), and nicardipine (Cardene), are used if β-adrenergic blocking agents are contraindicated, are poorly tolerated, or do not control symptoms. The dihydropyridines (e.g., amlodipine [Norvasc]) have more vasodilatory effects and the nondihydropyridines (e.g., verapamil [Calan], diltiazem [Cardizem]) have more rate and contractility effects.

- Ranolazine (Ranexa), a sodium current inhibitor, is used to treat chronic angina in patients who have not had an adequate response with other medications.

- Other medications, such as lipid-lowering drugs, are used to manage the underlying CAD.

Cardiac Catheterization

If a coronary blockage is amenable to treatment, coronary revascularization with percutaneous coronary intervention (PCI) may be recommended. PCI may be done at the same time as the cardiac catheterization.

- During PCI, a catheter with a deflated balloon tip is inserted into the blocked coronary artery. The deflated balloon is positioned inside the blockage and inflated. This compresses the plaque against the artery wall, resulting in vessel dilation and a larger vessel diameter. This procedure is called *balloon angioplasty*.

- *Intracoronary stents* are usually inserted to prevent abrupt closure and restenosis after balloon angioplasty. A stent is an expandable, meshlike structure designed to keep the vessel open by supporting the arterial walls. Because stents are thrombogenic, drugs are used to prevent platelet aggregation within the stent and acute stent thrombosis. Many stents are coated with a drug (e.g., paclitaxel, sirolimus) that prevents the overgrowth of new intima, which is the primary cause of stent restenosis.

- Drugs commonly used during PCI are unfractionated heparin (UH) or low-molecular-weight heparin (LMWH), a direct thrombin inhibitor (e.g., bivalirudin [Angiomax]), and/or a glycoprotein IIb/IIIa inhibitor (e.g., eptifibatide [Integrilin]) (Table 33.12). After PCI, the patient receives dual antiplatelet therapy (DAPT) (e.g., aspirin [indefinitely] and ticagrelor or clopidogrel [Plavix]) until the intimal lining grows over the stent and provides a smooth vascular surface.

The most serious complications from stent placement are abrupt closure and vascular injury. Less common complications include acute MI, stent embolization, coronary spasm, contrast medium allergy, renal compromise, bleeding (e.g., retroperitoneal), infection, stroke, and emergent coronary artery bypass graft (CABG) surgery. The possibility of dysrhythmias during and after the procedure is always present.

Nursing Management
Goals
Goals for the patient with chronic stable angina are the same as those for acute coronary syndrome (ACS) (see Acute Coronary Syndrome, p. 5).
Nursing Interventions
If your patient has angina, perform the following measures: (1) position patient upright unless contraindicated and apply supplemental O_2, (2) assess vital signs, (3) place patient on continuous ECG monitor, (4) obtain a 12-lead ECG, (5) provide prompt pain relief, first with NTG, followed by an IV opioid analgesic, if needed, (6) obtain cardiac biomarkers, (7) assess heart and breath sounds, and (8) obtain a chest x-ray.

- Ask the patient to describe the pain and to rate it on a scale of 0 to 10 before and after treatment to evaluate the effectiveness of the interventions. It is important to use the same words the patient uses to describe the symptoms (e.g., tightness, pressure).
- The patient may be anxious and may have pale, cool, clammy skin. The BP and HR may be high. Assess for other signs of pain, such as restlessness; ECG changes; high HR, respiratory rate, or BP; clutching of the bed linens; or other nonverbal cues.
- Support and reassure the patient. Use a calm approach to help reduce the patient's anxiety during an angina attack.

▼ Patient and Caregiver Teaching
Reassure the patient with a history of chronic stable angina that a long, productive life is possible.
- Heart models, video recordings, and written information are important tools for patient and caregiver teaching.

- Assist the patient to identify factors that precipitate angina and how to avoid or control these factors.
- Help the patient identify and plan to modify personal risk factors for CAD.
- Teach the patient and caregivers about diets low in sodium and saturated fats. Maintaining ideal body weight is important in controlling angina, because excess weight increases myocardial workload.
- Advise adhering to a regular, individualized exercise program that conditions rather than stresses the heart. For example, many patients can walk briskly on a flat surface at least 30 minutes a day, most days of the week.
- Teach the patient and caregivers about the proper use of NTG.
- Patients may feel a threat to their roles, identity, and self-esteem. If needed, arrange for counseling to support adjustment of the patient and caregiver to the diagnosis of CAD and resulting angina.

ANKYLOSING SPONDYLITIS

Description and Pathophysiology

Ankylosing spondylitis (AS) is a chronic inflammatory disease that primarily affects the axial skeleton, including the sacroiliac joints, intervertebral spaces, and costovertebral articulations.

The human leukocyte antigen HLA-B27 antigen is found in about 90% of whites with AS, but only 8% of those without the disease. This suggests genes play an important role in AS. Along with whites, Asians, and Hispanics are more likely to have AS than other ethnic groups.

- Inflammation in joints and adjacent tissue causes the formation of granulation tissue (pannus) and the development of dense fibrous scars that lead to joint fusion. Inflammation can affect the eyes, lungs, heart, kidneys, and peripheral nervous system.

Clinical Manifestations and Complications

Symptoms of inflammatory spine pain are the first clues to a diagnosis of AS. The patient typically reports lower back pain, stiffness, and limitation of motion that are worse during the night and in the morning but decrease with mild activity. Systemic manifestations, such as fever, fatigue, anorexia, and weight loss, are rare.

Uveitis (intraocular inflammation) is the most common nonskeletal manifestation. It can appear as an initial presentation of the disease years before joint symptoms develop. Patients may also have chest pain and sternal/costal cartilage tenderness.

Severe postural abnormalities and deformity can cause significant disability. Aortic insufficiency and pulmonary fibrosis are frequent complications. Cauda equina syndrome can also result, contributing to lower extremity weakness and bladder dysfunction. The patient is at risk for spinal fracture because of associated osteoporosis.

Diagnostic Studies

- X-rays used to diagnose AS are limited in ability to detect early sacroiliitis or subtle changes in posterior vertebrae.
- MRI can be useful in assessing early cartilage abnormalities.
- Laboratory testing is not specific, but an elevated erythrocyte sedimentation rate (ESR) and mild anemia may be seen.
- Persons with both the clinical signs of AS and the HLA-B27 antigen have an increased likelihood of being diagnosed with AS.

Interprofessional Management

Prevention of AS is not possible. However, families with other diagnosed HLA-B27–positive rheumatic diseases (e.g., acute anterior uveitis, juvenile spondyloarthritis) should be alert to signs of lower back pain and arthritis symptoms for early identification and treatment of AS.

Care of the patient is aimed at maintaining maximal mobility while decreasing pain and inflammation. Heat applications, nonsteroidal antiinflammatory drugs (NSAIDs) and salicylates, and disease-modifying antirheumatic drugs (DMARDs), such as sulfasalazine or methotrexate, can help in relieving symptoms. Etanercept, a biologic response modifier, inhibits the action of tumor necrosis factor (TNF) and has been shown to reduce active inflammation and improve spinal mobility. Additional anti-TNF agents (infliximab, adalimumab, or golimumab) may also be effective.

Good posture and stretching exercises of the back, neck, and chest are important to minimize spinal deformity. Hydrotherapy may decrease pain and facilitate spinal extension. Surgery may be needed for severe deformity and mobility impairment. Spinal osteotomy and total joint replacement are the most commonly performed procedures.

Nursing Management

A key responsibility is to teach the patient about the nature of the disease and principles of therapy. The home management program consists of local moist heat, regular exercise, and knowledgeable use of drugs.

- Discourage excessive physical exertion during periods of active inflammation.
- Evaluate chest expansion as part of baseline range-of-motion (ROM) assessment. Encourage smoking cessation to decrease the risk for lung complications in people with reduced chest expansion.
- Ongoing physical therapy should include gentle, graded stretching and strengthening exercises to preserve ROM and improve thoracolumbar flexion and extension.
- Proper positioning at rest is essential. Encourage the patient to use a firm mattress and sleep on the back with a flat pillow, avoiding positions that encourage flexion deformity.
- Stress the need to avoid spinal flexion (e.g., leaning over a desk), heavy lifting, and prolonged walking, standing, or sitting. Encourage sports that involve natural stretching, such as swimming and racquet games.
- Family counseling and vocational rehabilitation are important.

AORTIC DISSECTION

Description

Aortic dissection, often misnamed "dissecting aneurysm," is not a type of aneurysm. Rather, aortic dissection results from the creation of a false lumen between the intima (inner layer) and media (middle layer) of the arterial wall. Aortic dissection is classified according to the location of the dissection and duration of symptoms.

Type A dissection affects the ascending aorta and arch, requiring emergency surgery. Type B dissection begins in the descending aorta, allowing for potential conservative management. Dissections are also classified as acute (first 14 days), subacute (14 to 90 days), or chronic (> 90 days) based on symptom onset.

- Men are at a higher risk of developing aortic dissection than women. Women who develop aortic dissection are older and more likely than men to present with heart failure (HF), coma, or altered mental status.
- Hypertension is the most important risk factor for aortic dissection.
- Other predisposing factors include age, aortic diseases (e.g., aortitis, coarctation, arch hypoplasia), atherosclerosis, blunt trauma, tobacco use, cocaine or methamphetamine use, congenital heart disease (e.g., bicuspid aortic valve), connective tissue disorders (e.g., Marfan's syndrome), family history, history of heart surgery, and pregnancy.

Pathophysiology

Most nontraumatic aortic dissections are attributed to weakened elastic fibers in the medial layer. Chronic hypertension accelerates the degradation process. In aortic dissection, the inner wall of the aorta tears. Blood surges through this tear, causing the inner and middle layers to separate (dissect). If the blood-filled channel ruptures through the outside aortic wall, aortic dissection is often fatal.

As the heart contracts, each pulsation increases the pressure on the damaged area, which worsens the dissection. Extension of the dissection may cut off blood supply to the brain, kidneys, spinal cord, and extremities. The false lumen may remain patent, become thrombosed (clotted), rejoin the true lumen by way of a distal tear, or rupture.

Clinical Manifestations and Complications

About 80% of patients with an acute Type A aortic dissection report an abrupt onset of severe anterior chest pain or back pain. Patients with acute Type B aortic dissection are more likely to report pain in the back, abdomen, or legs. Pain location may overlap between Type A and B dissections. The pain may be described as "sharp" and "worst ever," or as "tearing," "ripping," or "stabbing." Dissection pain can be distinguished from myocardial infarction (MI) pain, which is more gradual in onset and intensity.

- Older patients are more likely to have hypotension and vague symptoms. In some cases, aortic dissection may be painless, emphasizing the importance of the physical examination.
- If the aortic arch is involved, the patient may have neurologic deficits, including altered level of consciousness and dizziness, with weakened or absent carotid and temporal pulses.
- Type A aortic dissection usually disrupts coronary artery blood flow and causes aortic valvular insufficiency.
- When either subclavian artery is involved, the pulse quality and BP readings may differ between the left and right arms.
- As dissection progresses down the aorta, the abdominal organs and lower extremities show evidence of altered tissue perfusion.

A life-threatening complication of an acute ascending aortic dissection is cardiac tamponade, which occurs when blood from the dissection leaks into the pericardial sac. Manifestations include hypotension, narrowed pulse pressure, distended neck veins, muffled heart sounds, and pulsus paradoxus.

- An aorta weakened by dissection may rupture. Hemorrhage may occur into the mediastinal, pleural, or abdominal cavity.
- Dissection can lead to occlusion of the blood supply to the spinal cord, kidneys, and abdominal structures. Spinal cord ischemia

leads to weakness and decreased sensation. Renal ischemia can lead to renal failure. Signs of abdominal (mesenteric) ischemia include abdominal pain, decreased bowel sounds, and altered bowel elimination.

Diagnostic Studies

Studies to detect aortic dissection are similar to those performed for suspected aneurysms.

- Chest x-ray indicates widening of the mediastinum and pleural effusion.
- Three-dimensional (3-D) CT scanning, transesophageal echocardiography (TEE), or MRI may be used to diagnose acute aortic dissection.

Interprofessional Management

Reducing the HR, BP, and myocardial contractility limits extension of the acute dissection.

- An IV β-blocker (e.g., esmolol [Brevibloc]) is often titrated to a target HR under 60 beats/minute, or to a systolic BP between 100 and 110 mm Hg.
- Other antihypertensive agents, such as calcium-channel blockers (e.g., diltiazem) and angiotensin-converting enzyme (ACE) inhibitors (e.g., enalapril), may be used.
- Morphine decreases sympathetic nervous system stimulation and relieves pain.
- Supportive treatment for an acute aortic dissection serves as a bridge to surgery.

Patients with acute aortic dissection are managed in the intensive care unit (ICU). An acute ascending aortic dissection is considered a surgical emergency. Otherwise, surgery is indicated when conservative therapy is ineffective or when complications (e.g., HF) occur. Because the aorta is fragile after dissection, surgical intervention is delayed when possible, to allow time for edema to decrease and to permit clotting of the blood in the false lumen.

- Surgery involves resection of the aortic segment containing the intimal tear and replacement with a synthetic graft.

Even with prompt surgical intervention, the in-hospital mortality rate for acute aortic dissection is high. Causes of death include aortic rupture, mesenteric ischemia, MI, sepsis, and multiorgan failure.

The patient with an acute or chronic type B descending aortic dissection without complications can be managed nonsurgically. Such conservative treatment includes pain relief, heart rate (HR) and BP control, and cardiovascular disease (CVD) risk factor modification along with close surveillance imaging with CT or MRI.

- Endovascular repair is a treatment option for an acute descending aortic dissection with complications (e.g., hemodynamic instability) or a chronic descending aortic dissection with complications (e.g., peripheral ischemia).

Nursing Management

Before surgery, nursing care includes keeping the patient in bed in a semi-Fowler's position and maintaining a quiet environment. These measures help keep the HR and systolic BP at the lowest possible level that maintains vital organ perfusion (typically HR <60 beats/minute and systolic BP of 100 to 120 mm Hg). Give opioids and sedatives as prescribed. Manage pain and anxiety, which can cause elevations in the HR and systolic BP.

- Titrating IV administration of antihypertensive agents requires continuous electroencephalogram (ECG) and intraarterial BP monitoring. Monitor vital signs frequently, sometimes as often as every 2 to 3 minutes, until target HR and BP are reached. Look for changes in peripheral pulses and signs of increasing pain, restlessness, and anxiety.

Postoperative care is similar to that after open aneurysm repair (see Aneurysm, Aortic, p. 41).

▼ Patient and Caregiver Teaching

- Teach patients and caregivers about taking antihypertensive drugs daily for lifelong control of HR and BP.
- Tell the patient to discuss any side effects (e.g., dizziness, depression, fatigue, erectile dysfunction) with the heath care provider (HCP) before discontinuing prescribed drugs.
- Follow-up with regularly scheduled MRI or CT scans is essential.
- Tell patients that if the pain or other symptoms return, they should contact the emergency response system (ERS) for immediate care.

APPENDICITIS

Description

Appendicitis is an inflammation of the appendix, a narrow blind tube that extends from the inferior part of the cecum. It is most common in those 10 to 30 years of age. It is the most common reason for emergency abdominal surgery.

Pathophysiology

A common cause of appendicitis is obstruction of the lumen by a fecalith (accumulated feces). Obstruction results in distention, venous engorgement, and the accumulation of mucus and bacteria, which can lead to gangrene, perforation, and peritonitis.

Clinical Manifestations and Complications

Appendicitis typically begins with dull periumbilical pain, followed by anorexia, nausea, and vomiting. The pain is persistent and continuous, eventually shifting to the right lower quadrant and localizing at McBurney's point (halfway between the umbilicus and right iliac crest).

- Further assessment reveals localized and rebound tenderness with muscle guarding. Coughing, sneezing, and deep inhalation magnify the pain.
- The patient usually prefers to lie still, often with the right leg flexed.
- A low-grade fever may develop.

If diagnosis and treatment are delayed, the appendix can rupture, and the resulting peritonitis can be fatal.

Diagnostic Studies

- White blood cell (WBC) count is usually high.
- Urinalysis is done to rule out genitourinary conditions that mimic appendicitis.
- CT scan and ultrasound may be used.

Interprofessional Management

Treatment is immediate surgical removal of the appendix (appendectomy) if the inflammation is localized. If the appendix has ruptured and there is evidence of peritonitis or an abscess, antibiotic therapy and parenteral fluids are given for 6 to 8 hours before the appendectomy to prevent sepsis and dehydration.

Nursing Management

Encourage the patient with abdominal pain to see a health care provider (HCP). Self-treatment with laxatives and enemas may cause perforation.

- Nothing should be taken by mouth to ensure that the stomach will be empty if surgery is needed.
- Postoperative nursing management is similar to postoperative care of a patient after laparotomy (see Abdominal Pain, Acute, pp. 3).
- Patients are usually discharged within 24 hours after an uncomplicated laparoscopic appendectomy. Those who had a perforation usually have a longer length of stay and need IV antibiotic therapy. Ambulation begins a few hours after surgery, and the diet is advanced as tolerated. Most patients resume normal activities 2 to 3 weeks after surgery.

ASTHMA

Description

Asthma is a lung disease characterized by bronchial hyperresponsiveness with reversible expiratory airflow limitation. Signs and symptoms vary but often include episodes of wheezing, breathlessness, chest tightness, and cough, especially at night and in the early morning. The clinical course of asthma is unpredictable, ranging from periods of adequate control to attacks with poor control of symptoms.

- Asthma affects an estimated 20.4 million adult Americans. More than 3600 people die each year from asthma. Among adults, women are more likely to have asthma than men.
- Risk factors for asthma and triggers of asthma attacks are listed in Table 11.

Pathophysiology

Asthma involves persistent but variable airway inflammation. Airflow is limited because inflammation results in bronchoconstriction, airway hyperresponsiveness (hyperactivity), and airway edema. Exposure to allergens or irritants initiates the inflammatory cascade.

- As the inflammatory process begins, mast cells in the bronchial wall release multiple inflammatory mediators, including leukotrienes, histamine, cytokines, prostaglandins, and nitric oxide.
- Inflammatory mediators have effects on the: (1) blood vessels, causing vasodilation and increasing capillary permeability (runny nose); (2) nerve cells, causing itching; (3) smooth muscle cells, causing bronchial spasms and airway narrowing; and (4) goblet cells, causing mucus production.
- The *early-phase response* in asthma occurs within 30 to 60 minutes after exposure to a trigger or irritant.
- Symptoms can recur 4 to 6 hours after the early response because of the influx of inflammatory cells and the further release of inflammatory mediators. This *late-phase response* occurs in about 50% of people with asthma.
- Bronchoconstriction with symptoms lasts for 24 hours or more. Corticosteroids are effective in treating inflammation in this phase.

Chronic inflammation may cause structural changes in the bronchial wall known as "remodeling." A progressive loss of lung function is not fully reversed by therapy.

During an asthma attack, decreased alveolar perfusion and ventilation and increased alveolar gas pressure lead to ventilation-perfusion abnormalities in the lungs.

TABLE 11   Triggers of Asthma Attacks

Air Pollutants	Occupational Exposure
• Aerosol sprays	• Agriculture, farming
• Cigarette smoke	• Paints, solvents
• Exhaust fumes	• Laundry detergents
• Oxidants	• Metal salts
• Perfumes	• Wood and vegetable dusts
• Sulfur dioxides	• Industrial chemicals and plastics
	• Pharmaceutical agents
Allergen Inhalation	**Other Factors**
• Animal dander (e.g., cats, mice, guinea pigs)	• Exercise and cold, dry air
• Cockroaches	• Stress
• House dust mites	• Hormones, menses
• Molds	• Gastroesophageal reflux disease (GERD)
• Pollens	
Drugs	**Viral or Bacterial Infection**
• Aspirin	• Sinusitis, allergic rhinitis
• Nonsteroidal antiinflammatory drugs	• Viral upper respiratory tract infection
• β-Adrenergic blockers	
Food Additives	
• Sulfites (bisulfites and metabisulfites)	
• Beer, wine, dried fruit, shrimp, processed potatoes	
• Monosodium glutamate	
• Tartrazine	

- The patient is hypoxemic early on, with decreased partial pressure of CO_2 in arterial blood ($PaCO_2$) and increased pH (respiratory alkalosis) caused by hyperventilation
- As the airflow limitation worsens with air trapping, the patient works much harder to breathe. The $PaCO_2$ normalizes as the patient tires, then increases to produce respiratory acidosis, which is an ominous sign of respiratory failure.

Clinical Manifestations

Asthma signs and symptoms can differ for each patient. The most common manifestations include cough, shortness of breath (dyspnea), wheezing, chest tightness, and variable airflow obstruction. The presence of any of these (usually in combination) can indicate that an asthma episode or attack is occurring. Attacks may last for a few minutes to several hours.

- Characteristic manifestations are wheezing, cough, dyspnea, and chest tightness. Expiration may be prolonged, with an inspiratory/expiratory (I/E) ratio of 1:3 or 1:4.
- Wheezing is an unreliable sign to gauge the severity of an attack because many patients with minor attacks wheeze loudly, whereas others with severe attacks do not wheeze.
- In some patients with asthma, cough is the only symptom. The cough may be nonproductive with secretions so thick, tenacious, and gelatinous that their removal is difficult.
- During an acute attack, the patient usually sits upright or slightly bent forward, using accessory muscles of respiration. The more difficult the breathing becomes, the more anxious the patient feels.
- Signs of hypoxemia include restlessness, increased anxiety, confusion, increased pulse and BP.
- Percussion reveals hyperresonance of the lungs. Auscultation indicates inspiratory or expiratory wheezing.
- Diminished breath sounds may indicate a significant decrease in air movement. Severely diminished breath sounds or a "silent chest" when the patient is struggling after a period of wheezing is an ominous sign, indicating severe obstruction and impending respiratory failure.

Classification of Asthma

Asthma can be classified as intermittent, mild persistent, moderate persistent, or severe persistent (Table 12). Asthma severity is used to guide treatment decisions. Patients may have different asthma classifications over the course of the disease.

Complications

In severe asthma exacerbations, the patient is dyspneic at rest and speaks in single words because of the difficulty breathing.

- The patient is often agitated, sitting forward to maximize the diaphragmatic movement and using accessory muscles in the neck to lift the chest wall. Respiratory rate may be > 30 breaths/minute and pulse > 120 beats/minute. The peak flow (PEFR [peak expiratory flow rate]) is 40% of the patient's personal best, or > 150 mL.
- A life-threatening medical emergency, *status asthmaticus* is the most extreme form of an acute asthma attack. It is characterized by hypoxia, hypercarbia, and acute respiratory failure unresponsive to treatment with bronchodilators and corticosteroids.

TABLE 12 Classification of Asthma Severity

Components of Severity	Intermittent	Persistent Mild	Persistent Moderate	Persistent Severe
ASTHMA SEVERITY				
Impairment				
Symptoms	≤2 days/wk	>2 days/wk, not daily	Daily	Continuous
Nighttime awakenings	≤2/mo	3-4/mo	>1/wk, not nightly	Often 7/wk
SABA use for symptoms	≤2 days/wk	>2 days/wk, not daily	Daily	Several times per day
Interference with normal activity	None	Minor limitation	Some limitation	Extremely limited
Lung function[a]	Normal FEV₁ between attacks FEV₁ >80% FEV₁/FVC normal	FEV₁ >80% predicted FEV₁/FVC normal	FEV₁ 60%–80% predicted FEV₁/FVC reduced by 5%	FEV₁ <60% predicted FEV₁/FVC reduced by 5%
Risk				
Attacks requiring oral corticosteroids	0-1/yr	≥2/yr even in the absence of impairment Consider severity and interval since last attack Frequency and severity may fluctuate over time Relative annual risk of exacerbation may be related to FEV₁		

Recommended Step for Initiating Treatment	Step 1	Step 2	Step 3[b]	Step 4 or 5[b]
		Reevaluate asthma control in 2–6 wk and adjust therapy accordingly		

Guidelines for Using Table

- Patients should be assigned to the most severe step in which any feature occurs. Clinical features for may overlap across steps. Determine level of severity by assessment of both impairment and risk. Assess impairment by previous 2–4 week spirometry results.
- A person's classification should change over time with treatment. After treatment, the focus switches to the level of control, not the classification of severity.
- Patients at any level of severity of chronic asthma can have mild, moderate, or severe asthma attacks. Some patients with intermittent asthma have severe and life-threatening attacks separated by long periods of normal lung function and no symptoms.

[a]Percent predicted values for FEV_1 or ratio of FEV_1/FVC. Normal FEV_1/FVC: 8–19 yr, 85%; 20–39 yr, 80%; 40–59 yr, 75%; 60–80 yr, 70%.

[b]Consider short-term corticosteroid therapy.

FEV_1, Forced expiratory volume in 1 sec; *FVC,* forced vital capacity; *SABA,* short-acting β_2-adrenergic agonist.

Source: Adapted from National Asthma Education and Prevention Program, National Heart, Lung, and Blood Institute: *Expert Panel Report 3: guidelines for the diagnosis and management of asthma,* NIH pub no 08-4051, Bethesda, Md, 2007, National Institutes of Health.

The patient may have chest tightness, a severely marked increase in shortness of breath, or suddenly be unable to speak. Hypotension, bradycardia, respiratory and/or cardiac arrest may occur. The patient must be immediately intubated, and mechanical ventilation started.

Diagnostic Studies

Underdiagnosis of asthma is common. A detailed history is important to determine if a person has had similar attacks, which are often precipitated by a known trigger.

- Spirometry determines the reversibility of bronchoconstriction. Spirometry, oximetry, and arterial blood gases (ABGs) provide information about the severity of the attack and response to treatment.
- Chest x-ray during an attack shows hyperinflation.
- Sputum specimen can be used to rule out bacterial infection.
- High serum immunoglobulin E (IgE) levels and eosinophil counts suggest atopy (allergy).
- Allergy skin testing can be used to determine sensitivity to specific allergens.

Interprofessional Management

The goal of asthma treatment is to achieve and maintain control of the disease. The health care provider (HCP) steps down the medication as the patient achieves control of the symptoms or steps it up as the symptoms worsen. The level of control is determined by the patient's spirometry results and any exacerbations or adverse treatment effects.

The classification of asthma severity (see Table 12) at initial diagnosis helps determine which types of medications are best suited to control the symptoms.

- Patients in all classifications of asthma require a rescue medication for *short-term,* immediate control of symptoms. Short-acting β_2-adrenergic agonists (SABAs) (e.g., albuterol [ProAir HFA, Proventil HFA, Ventolin HFA]) are the most effective class of drugs used as rescue medications. Patients with persistent asthma must also be on a long-term or controller medication. Inhaled corticosteroids (ICSs) (e.g., fluticasone [Flovent Diskus or HFA]) are the most effective class of drugs to treat the inflammation.
- For *long-term* control of moderate to severe persistent asthma, long-acting β_2-adrenergic agonists (LABAs) are added to daily ICSs (e.g., fluticasone [Flovent]).

Acute Asthma Exacerbations

Asthma exacerbations may be mild to life-threatening. Patients with mild or moderate asthma attacks are often seen in the community at an outpatient clinic. These attacks occur no more than twice per week, with minimal interference in day-to-day activity. The patient is alert, orientated, and speaks in sentences. The patient may describe chest tightness, varying degrees of difficulty breathing, and may report a slight increase in the use of asthma drugs. Oxygen saturation is usually > 90% on room air, and PEFR more than 50% predicted or best.

Inhaled bronchodilators and oral corticosteroids are the mainstays of treatment for mild to moderate asthma attacks. The patient's vital signs are monitored. Most improve within 60 minutes of initiation of therapy. The patient should be taught the importance of a follow-up appointment with the HCP. Oral corticosteroids will be part of the discharge plan for a moderate attack, and based on the patient's history and HCP preference, sometimes for a mild attack.

- If the patient's condition is slow to respond, does not respond, or the HCP suspects that some other condition may be occurring or contributing to the acute asthma attack, the patient should be transferred to an acute care facility.

In a severe asthmatic attack, the patient is still alert, but may be tachycardic, tachypneic, and focused on breathing with a respiratory rate > 30 breaths/minute. Accessory muscle use may be seen. The patient may be agitated from hypoxemia. If not immediately audible, auscultation of the lungs may reveal inspiratory or expiratory wheezing. The patient often sits forward to maximize diaphragmatic movement. Percussion of the lungs shows hyperresonance. PEFR is equal to or < 50% predicted or best. Symptoms may re-occur, sometimes daily, and there is interference with activities of daily living (ADLs).

A severe acute asthma attack is usually frightening enough for patients to go to the emergency department (ED). In many cases, a severe asthma attack will warrant hospital admission. Management of the patient with a severe asthma attack focuses on correcting hypoxemia and continually observing and/or improving ventilation. Supplemental O_2 is given by nasal cannula or mask to achieve a PaO_2 of at least 60 mm Hg or O_2 saturation > 93%. O_2 monitoring should be continuous with pulse oximetry.

Bedside PEFR may be used to monitor airflow obstruction. Serial PEFR results, oximetry, and measurement of ABGs give information about the severity of the attack and the response to therapy. Obtaining a PEFR during a severe asthma attack is usually not possible. However, if it can be done and is < 200 L/min, it indicates severe obstruction in all but very small adults.

- Careful monitoring of the patient's heart rate, respiratory rate and rhythm, and BP are essential. Bronchodilators and oral corticosteroids will be part of the treatment plan. The "silent chest" is an ominous clinical finding, and often signals impending respiratory failure. Immediately notify the HCP.

Drug Therapy

Drug therapy for asthma can be complex and overwhelming. Asthma drugs are divided into 2 general types: (1) quick relief, or rescue medications, to treat attacks, and (2) long-term control medications. The patient's medical history, medication plan, and severity of attack helps the HCP determine which types of drugs are best suited to control asthma symptoms. Current guidelines all suggest a stepwise approach to drug therapy.

- The mainstay of asthmatic treatment is inhalation of SABA bronchodilators. All patients need a quick relief or "rescue" medication. Short-acting SABAs, such as albuterol (ProAir HFA, Proventil HFA, Ventolin HFA), are the most effective rescue drugs for asthma.
- In patients with a moderate to severe attack, inhaled ipratropium (Atrovent) is used in conjunction with SABA. Combivent is a combination of both ipratropium and albuterol.
- Oral, and in some situations, IV corticosteroids, may given to patients who do not initially respond to SABA alone.

Patients with asthma who have frequent attacks must also be on a long-term ("controller") medication. ICSs (e.g., fluticasone [Flovent Diskus or HFA]) are the most effective long-term controllers to treat inflammation. Some ICSs are used in combination with LABA to gain better asthma control.

Nursing Management

Goals

The patient with asthma will achieve asthma control as demonstrated by minimal symptoms, acceptable activity levels (including exercise), maintaining > 80% of personal best PEFR, few or no adverse effects of therapy, no acute attacks, and adequate knowledge to carry out the plan of care.

Nursing Interventions

A goal in asthma care is to maximize the patient's ability to safely manage acute asthma attacks via an action plan developed with the HCP (see Fig. 28.9, Harding et al, *Lewis' Medical-Surgical Nursing,* ed 11).

- The patient can take 2 to 4 puffs of a SABA every 20 minutes up to 3 times as a rescue plan. Depending on the response with alleviation of symptoms or improved peak flow, continued SABA use and/or oral corticosteroids may be a part of the home management. If symptoms persist or if the patient's PEFR is > 50% of the personal best, the HCP or emergency medical services must be immediately contacted.

- When the patient is in the health care agency with an acute attack, it is important to monitor the respiratory and cardiovascular systems. This includes auscultating lung sounds and monitoring heart rate (HR) and respiratory rate, BP, pulse oximetry, and peak flow.

- An important nursing goal during an acute attack is to decrease the patient's sense of panic. Stay with the patient. A calm, quiet, reassuring attitude may help the patient relax. Position the patient comfortably (usually sitting) to maximize chest expansion.

- Maintain eye contact and use a firm, calm voice to coach the patient in pursed-lip breathing, which keeps the airways open by maintaining positive pressure.

- See eNursing Care Plan 28-1 on the website.

▼ **Patient and Caregiver Teaching**

A patient and caregiver teaching guide for the patient with asthma is presented in Table 13.

TABLE 13 Patient and Caregiver Teaching

Asthma

Include the following information in a teaching plan for the patient with asthma and the caregiver. It will help improve the patient's quality of life and promote lifestyle changes that support successful living with asthma.

What Is Asthma?
- Basic anatomy and physiology of lung
- Pathophysiology of asthma
- Relationship of pathophysiology to signs and symptoms
- Measurement and correlation of spirometry and peak expiratory flow rate

What Is Good Asthma Control?
- Personal ideas of good control
- Use Asthma Control Test available at *www.asthmacontroltest. com.*

Hindrances to Asthma Treatment and Control
- Discuss possible hindrances (e.g., denial, poor perception of asthma severity) with patient and caregiver.

Continued

TABLE 13   Patient and Caregiver Teaching
Asthma—cont'd

Environmental and Trigger Control
- Identify possible triggers and possible preventive measures (use trigger diary)
- Avoid allergens and other triggers
- Maintain good hydration

Medications
- Types (include mechanism of action)
- Use of preventive and maintenance (e.g., antiinflammatory) agents
- Write out medication list and schedule.

Asthma Action Plan (Fig. 28.9 in Harding et al., *Lewis' Medical-Surgical Nursing*, ed 11)

Correct Use of Inhaler, Spacer, Nebulizer, and Peak Flow Meter
- See Chapter 28 in Harding et al., *Lewis' Medical-Surgical Nursing*, ed 11)

Pursed-lip Breathing
For more information, visit the American Lung Association website at *http://www.lung.org/lung-disease/asthma.*

BELL'S PALSY

Description
Bell's palsy is an acute, usually temporary, facial paresis (or palsy) resulting from damage or trauma of the facial nerve (CN VII). CN VII is a mixed cranial nerve with motor, sensory, and autonomic function.

   Bell's palsy can affect 1 or both sides of the face. It is the most common facial nerve disorder.

- Most patients recover spontaneously within 2 weeks to 6 months.
- One-third of patients may have residual effects of facial weakness, involuntary movements, and persistent tearing of the eye on the affected side.

Pathophysiology

It is believed that reactivation of a dormant viral infection, such as viral meningitis, herpes simplex virus 1 (HSV-1), herpes zoster virus (HZV), or others, may trigger Bell's palsy. The viral infection causes inflammation, leading to nerve compression and the subsequent clinical features such as facial paralysis.

B

Clinical Manifestations

The onset of Bell's palsy is sudden, with a rapid onset of unilateral facial weakness over a few hours. Maximum facial weakness is seen within 2 days. Many patients have a history of a recent viral illness. Patients may report pain around and behind the ear. Other manifestations may include drooping of the eyelid and corner of the mouth, drooling, facial twitching, dryness of the eye or mouth, facial numbness, altered taste, hearing loss, and excessive tearing in 1 eye.

- A widened palpebral fissure (opening between the eyelids); flattening of the nasolabial fold; unilateral loss of taste; and inability to smile, frown, or whistle are common.
- Decreased muscle movement may alter chewing ability, and some patients may have a loss of tearing or excessive tearing.

Complications can include psychologic withdrawal because of changes in appearance, malnutrition, dehydration, mucous membrane trauma, corneal abrasions, and facial spasms and contractures.

The diagnosis and prognosis are indicated by clinical examination and observing the typical pattern of onset. Current guidelines do not support routine laboratory, imaging, or neurophysiologic testing at first presentation of Bell's palsy.

Interprofessional and Nursing Management

Care is primarily focused on relief of symptoms, protection of the eye on the affected side, and prevention of complications.

- Oral corticosteroid therapy to reduce inflammation and swelling should be started within 72 hours of onset. Some patients should receive an antiviral agent, such as acyclovir (Zovirax), in addition to the steroid therapy.
- Surgical decompression of the facial nerve remains controversial and is considered in refractory cases.

Methods of treatment include moist heat, gentle massage, electrical stimulation of the nerve, and prescribed exercises. Stimulation may maintain muscle tone and prevent atrophy.

Mild analgesics can relieve pain. Tell the patient to protect the face from cold and drafts because extreme sensitivity to pain or touch may occur.

- Maintenance of good nutrition is important. Teach the patient to chew on the unaffected side of the mouth to avoid trapping food and improve taste. Thorough oral hygiene is needed after each meal to prevent development of parotitis, caries, and periodontal disease from residual food.
- Dark glasses may be worn for protective and cosmetic reasons. Artificial tears (methylcellulose) can be instilled frequently during the day to prevent corneal drying. Ointment and an impermeable eye shield can be used at night to retain moisture. Taping the eyelids closed at night may be necessary to provide protection.
- A facial sling may be fitted by an occupational or physical therapist to support affected muscles, improve lip alignment, and facilitate eating. When function begins to return, active facial exercises are performed several times per day.

The change in physical appearance as a result of Bell's palsy can be devastating. Reassure the patient that chances for a full recovery are good.

BENIGN PAROXYSMAL POSITIONAL VERTIGO

Benign paroxysmal positional vertigo (BPPV) is a condition in which free-floating debris in the semicircular canal causes vertigo with specific head movements, such as getting out of bed, rolling over in bed, and sitting up from lying down. BPPV causes about 50% of cases of vertigo. The debris ("ear rocks") is composed of small calcium carbonate crystals that may develop in the inner ear due to head trauma, infection, or the aging process, or from an unknown cause.

Symptoms are intermittent and include dizziness, vertigo, lightheadedness, loss of balance, and nausea. There is no hearing loss. The symptoms of BPPV may be confused with those of Ménière's disease. Diagnosis is based on auditory and vestibular testing results.

A person experiencing BPPV is at risk for falls. Repositioning maneuvers may provide symptom relief. A trained health care provider (HCP) can teach the patient how to perform the maneuver. (See Chapter 21 in Harding et al, *Lewis's Medical-Surgical Nursing*, ed 11 for a description of the procedure.)

BENIGN PROSTATIC HYPERPLASIA

Description

Benign prostatic hyperplasia (BPH) is a condition in which the prostate gland increases in size, disrupting the flow of urine from the bladder through the urethra. Half of men will develop some signs of BPH by the age of 50 years. That number increases to more than 70% for men 60 to 69 years old. Symptoms of BPH can include bothersome lower urinary tract symptoms (LUTS), such as difficulty starting a urine stream, a decreased/weaker flow of urine, or urinary frequency.

B

Pathophysiology

As men age, the amount of active testosterone in the blood decreases, leaving a higher proportion of estrogen. A higher amount of estrogen within the prostate gland increases the activity of substances, including dihydroxytestosterone (DHT), that promote prostate cell growth. BPH usually develops in the inner part of the prostate. As the prostate enlarges, it gradually compresses the urethra, leading to partial or complete obstruction.

- The location of the enlargement is most significant in the development of obstructive symptoms, so even mild prostate enlargement can cause severe symptoms.
- Risk factors for BPH include aging, obesity (especially increased waist circumference), lack of physical activity, a high amount of dietary animal protein, alcohol use, erectile dysfunction (ED), smoking, and diabetes. A family history of BPH in a first-degree relative may also be a risk factor.

Clinical Manifestations

As the severity of urethral obstruction increases, the symptoms gradually worsen. Symptoms can be divided into 2 groups: obstructive and irritative.

- *Obstructive symptoms* of BPH caused by urinary retention include a decrease in the caliber and force of the urinary stream, difficulty in initiating voiding, intermittency (stopping and starting stream several times while voiding), and dribbling at the end of urination.
- *Irritative symptoms,* including urinary frequency, urgency, dysuria, bladder pain, nocturia, and incontinence, are related to inflammation and infection.

Complications

- Acute urinary retention is a sudden and painful inability to urinate. Treatment involves the insertion of a bladder catheter. Surgery may also be indicated.
- Urinary tract infections can result from incomplete bladder emptying, which provides an environment for bacterial growth.
- Calculi may develop in the bladder because of alkalinization of the residual urine.

- Hydronephrosis and pyelonephritis from back pressure of urine in an obstructed system may lead to renal failure.

Diagnostic Studies

- Physical examination including a digital rectal examination (DRE) to determine prostate size, symmetry, and consistency
- Urinalysis with culture to determine the presence of infection
- Postvoid residual urine volume to assess the degree of urine flow obstruction
- Prostate-specific antigen (PSA) blood test to rule out prostate cancer
- Uroflowmetry studies and transrectal ultrasound scan of prostate or renal ultrasound
- Cystoscopy to visualize the urethra and bladder

Interprofessional Management

The goals of collaborative care are to restore bladder drainage, relieve the patient's symptoms, and prevent or treat the complications of BPH. Treatment is generally based on the degree to which the symptoms bother the patient or the presence of complications, rather than on the size of the prostate.

- Dietary changes (decreasing intake of bladder irritants like caffeine, alcohol, carbonated drinks, artificial sweeteners, and spicy or acidic foods), avoiding medications such as decongestants and anticholinergics, and restricting evening fluid intake may reduce symptoms.
- A timed voiding schedule (also referred to as "bladder retraining") may reduce or eliminate symptoms.

If the patient has signs or symptoms that indicate an increase in obstruction, further treatment is indicated. Minimally invasive therapies are becoming more common as an alternative to watchful waiting or more invasive treatment. See Table 14 for descriptions of minimally invasive procedures and surgical treatment options.

Drug Therapy

Drugs are used to treat BPH with variable results.

- 5α-Reductase inhibitors reduce the size of the prostate gland. Finasteride (Proscar) blocks the enzyme needed to convert testosterone to DHT, the principal intraprostatic androgen. This results in a regression of hyperplastic tissue. Serum PSA levels may decrease by almost 50% in patients taking finasteride.
- Dutasteride (Avodart) is a dual inhibitor of 5α-reductase type 1 and 2 isoenzymes.
- α-Adrenergic receptor blockers are used, including, alfuzosin (Uroxatral), doxazosin (Cardura), prazosin (Minipress), silodosin (Rapaflo), and tamsulosin (Flomax). These drugs offer

TABLE 14 Treatment for Benign Prostatic Hyperplasia

Description	Advantages	Disadvantages
Minimally Invasive		
Laser Enucleation of the Prostate		
Laser beams used to rapidly vaporize and coagulate prostate tissue. Laser does not penetrate deep tissue. Two types of lasers in this class: holmium laser enucleation of the prostate (HoLEP), thulium laser enucleation of the prostate (ThuLEP).	• Outpatient procedure • Better coagulative properties in tissue compared with TURP • Comparable results to TURP and PVP • Minimal bleeding • Fast recovery time	• Catheter needed after for 24–48 hr • Irritative voiding symptoms, urinary incontinence • Hematuria • Retrograde ejaculation • May be more difficult to perform compared with PVP
Photoselective Vaporization of the Prostate (PVP)		
Procedure uses a laser beam to cut or destroy part of the prostate. May be more effective for small to moderate-sized prostates.	• Short procedure • Comparable results to TURP • Minimal bleeding • Fast recovery time • Rapid symptom improvement • Very effective	• Catheter needed up to 7 days after because of edema and urinary retention • Delayed sloughing of tissue • Takes several weeks to reach optimal effect • Retrograde ejaculation

Continued

B

TABLE 14 Treatment for Benign Prostatic Hyperplasia—cont'd

Description	Advantages	Disadvantages
Prostatic Urethral Lift (PUL)		
Permanent transprostatic implants/tension sutures placed transurethrally via cystoscope. Mechanically open the prostatic urethra by compressing the prostate tissue/parenchyma.	• Outpatient procedure • Erectile dysfunction, urinary incontinence, and retrograde ejaculation are minimal • No change in PSA since no prostate tissue ablated	• Lack of long-term durability/results • Treatment response rates slightly lower when compared with TURP • If unsuccessful, may need repeat PUL or TURP in the future
Transurethral Microwave Thermotherapy (TUMT)		
Use of microwave radiating heat to produce coagulative necrosis of the prostate.	• Outpatient procedure • Erectile dysfunction, urinary incontinence, and retrograde ejaculation are rare • Mild effects: bladder spasm, hematuria, dysuria	• Potential for damage to surrounding tissue • Urinary catheter needed after for 2–7 days • Not appropriate for men with rectal problems

Transurethral Needle Ablation (TUNA)

Low-wave radiofrequency used to heat the prostate, causing necrosis.

- Outpatient procedure
- Erectile dysfunction, urinary incontinence, and retrograde ejaculation are rare
- Precise delivery of heat to desired area
- Very little pain
- Early return to activities

- Urinary retention common
- Irritative voiding symptoms
- Hematuria for up to a week
- May need a catheter for a short time after

Transurethral Vaporization of Prostate (TUVP)

Electrosurgical modification of the standard TURP, where vaporization and desiccation are used together to destroy prostatic tissue. Can use a variety of energy delivery mediums (e.g., button, rollerball, or vaportrode).

- Minimal risks
- Minimal bleeding and sloughing

- Retrograde ejaculation
- Intermittent hematuria

Continued

B

TABLE 14   Treatment for Benign Prostatic Hyperplasia—cont'd

Description	Advantages	Disadvantages
Water Vapor Thermal Therapy Heated water vapor/steam used to destroy obstructive prostate tissue. Delivered transurethrally via handheld device with a retractable needle that releases the water vapor in 9-second doses.	• Outpatient procedure • Can be done in an outpatient office setting • Erectile dysfunction, urinary incontinence, and retrograde ejaculation are rare • Precise delivery of steam to desired area • Very little pain	• Relatively new, so lack of long-term durability/results • Irritative voiding symptoms and UTI • Hematuria
Invasive (Surgery) **_Transurethral Incision of Prostate (TUIP)_** Involves transurethral incisions into prostatic tissue to relieve obstruction. Effective for men with small to moderate prostates.	• Outpatient procedure • Minimal complications • Low occurrence of erectile dysfunction or retrograde ejaculation • Outcomes similar to TURP	• Urinary catheter needed after procedure

Transurethral Resection of Prostate (TURP)

Use of excision and cauterization to remove prostate tissue via cystoscope. Standard for treatment of BPH.

- Erectile dysfunction unlikely

- Bleeding, clot retention
- Retrograde ejaculation
- Catheter needed after

Simple Prostatectomy (open, laparoscopic, or robotic-assisted)

Surgery of choice for men with large prostates (often >100 grams), bladder damage, or other complicating factors. If open, involves an external incision with 2 possible approaches (either retropubic or perineal - see Fig. 54.6).

If laparoscopic and/or robotic-assisted, involves several small abdominal incisions and 1 slightly larger incision near the umbilicus.

- Complete visualization of the prostate and surrounding tissue

- Erectile dysfunction
- Bleeding
- Pain
- Risk of infection

BPH, Benign prostatic hyperplasia; *PSA*, prostate-specific antigen; *UTI*, urinary tract infection.

BPH symptom relief by relaxing the smooth muscle of the prostate that surrounds the urethra, but do not decrease the overall size of the prostate.

- Tadalafil (Cialis) has been shown to be effective in reducing symptoms for both BPH and ED. Saw palmetto has been shown to have no benefit over a placebo in reducing BPH symptoms. Advise patients to discuss all herbal therapies being used with their healthcare provider (HCP).

Nursing Management

The focus of nursing management is on health promotion for early detection and treatment, preoperative care, and postoperative care.

Goals

Overall preoperative goals for the patient having prostatic surgery are to have restoration of urinary drainage, resolution of any urinary tract infection, and understanding of the upcoming surgery. Overall postoperative goals are that the patient will have no complications, restoration of urinary control, complete bladder emptying, and satisfying sexual expression.

Nursing Interventions

When symptoms of prostatic hyperplasia become evident, further diagnostic screening may be necessary.

- Consuming alcohol and caffeine may increase prostatic symptoms because of the diuretic effect that increases bladder distention.
- Advise patients with obstructive symptoms to urinate every 2 to 3 hours or when they first feel the urge, to minimize urinary stasis and acute urinary retention.

Preoperative Care. Urinary drainage must be restored before surgery. A urethral catheter, such as a coudé (curved-tip) catheter, may be needed.

- Any infection of the urinary tract must be treated before surgery. Restoring drainage and encouraging a high fluid intake (2 to 3 L/day) are helpful.
- Patients are often concerned about the impact of surgery on sexual function. Provide an opportunity for the patient and his partner to express concerns.

Postoperative Care. Adjust the plan of care to the type of surgery, reasons for surgery, and patient response to surgery.

- After surgery, bladder irrigation is often done to remove clotted blood from the bladder and ensure drainage of urine. The bladder is irrigated either manually, on an intermittent basis, or as continuous bladder irrigation (CBI) with sterile normal saline solution or another prescribed solution. Monitor the inflow and outflow of the irrigant. The infusion of the continuous bladder irrigation fluid should be at a rate to keep the urine drainage light pink without clots.

- The catheter should be connected to a closed drainage system and not disconnected unless it is being removed, changed, or irrigated. Blood clots are expected for the first 24 to 36 hours. However, large amounts of bright red blood in the urine can indicate hemorrhage.

- Painful bladder spasms occur as a result of irritation of the bladder mucosa. Tell the patient not to urinate around the catheter because this increases the chance of spasm. If bladder spasms develop, check the catheter for clots. If present, remove the clots by irrigation so urine flows freely. Belladonna and opium suppositories, along with relaxation techniques, are used to relieve pain and spasms.

- Sphincter tone may be poor after catheter removal, resulting in urinary incontinence or dribbling. Sphincter tone can be strengthened by having the patient practice Kegel exercises (pelvic floor muscle technique). Continence can improve for up to 12 months.

- Observe the patient for signs of postoperative infection. If an external wound is present, the area should be observed for redness, heat, swelling, and purulent drainage. Rectal procedures, such as rectal temperatures and enemas (except insertion of well-lubricated belladonna and opium suppositories), should be avoided.

- Dietary intervention and stool softeners are important to prevent straining with bowel movements. A diet high in fiber promotes the passage of stool.

- Activities that increase abdominal pressure, such as sitting or walking for prolonged periods and straining to have a bowel movement (Valsalva maneuver), should be avoided.

▼ **Patient and Caregiver Teaching**

Discharge planning and home care issues are important aspects of care after prostate surgery.

- Instructions include: (1) caring for an indwelling catheter, if one is in place, (2) managing urinary incontinence, (3) maintaining oral fluids between 2 and 3 L/day, (4) observing for signs and symptoms of urinary tract and wound infection, (5) preventing constipation, (6) avoiding heavy lifting (more than 10 lb [more than 4.5 kg]), and (7) refraining from driving or sexual intercourse as directed by the HCP.

- Many men have retrograde ejaculation because of trauma to the internal sphincter. Semen is discharged into the bladder at orgasm and may produce cloudy urine when the patient urinates after orgasm. Discuss these changes with the patient and his partner and allow them to ask questions and express their concerns.

- Sexual counseling and treatment options may be needed if ED becomes a chronic issue.
- The bladder may take up to 2 months to return to its normal capacity. Teach the patient to drink at least 2 to 3 L of fluid per day and to urinate every 2 to 3 hours to flush the urinary tract. Teach the patient to avoid or limit bladder irritants such as caffeine products, citrus juices, and alcohol.
- Advise the patient to discuss the need for a yearly DRE with his HCP if he has not had complete removal of the prostate. Hyperplasia or cancer can occur in the remaining prostatic tissue.

BLADDER CANCER

Description

Bladder cancer is the most common cancer of the urinary system. Ninety percent of cases occur in those over the age of 55 years. Bladder cancer is far more common in men than in women and in whites than in blacks or Hispanics.

The most frequent cancerous tumor of the urinary tract is transitional cell cancer of the bladder. Most bladder tumors are papillomatous growths within the bladder.

About one-half of bladder cancers are related to cigarette smoking. Other risk factors include exposure to dyes used in the rubber and other industries. Others at risk include women treated with radiation for cervical cancer; patients who received cyclophosphamide, docetaxel, or gemcitabine; and those who have indwelling catheters for long periods. People with chronic, recurrent urinary tract stones, often bladder, and chronic lower urinary tract infections (UTIs) have an increased risk of squamous cell cancer of the bladder.

Clinical Manifestations

Microscopic or gross, painless hematuria (chronic or intermittent) is the most common clinical finding. Dysuria, frequency, and urgency may occur because of bladder irritability.

Diagnostic Studies

- When cancer is suspected, obtain urine specimens to identify cancer or atypical cells.
- Ultrasound, CT, or MRI may be used to detect bladder cancer.
- Cystoscopy and biopsy are used to confirm a diagnosis of bladder cancer.

Pathologic grading systems are used to classify the cancer potential of tumor cells, on a scale ranging from well-differentiated to undifferentiated.

Nursing and Interprofessional Management

The majority of bladder cancers are diagnosed at an early stage when the cancer is treatable. Low-stage, low-grade, superficial bladder cancers are most common and most responsive to treatment.

Surgical therapies include a variety of procedures:

- *Transurethral resection of the bladder tumor* (TURBT) is used for superficial lesions of the bladder's inner lining. This procedure is also used to control bleeding in the patient who is a poor operative risks or who has advanced tumors. The primary disadvantages of this approach are reoccurrence of the bladder cancer at another site and potential for scarring and/or limited ability to hold urine with repeated TURBT procedures.
- A *partial or radical cystectomy with urinary diversion* is the treatment of choice when the tumor is invasive or involves the trigone (area where ureters insert into the bladder) and the patient is free from metastases beyond the pelvic area.
- A *partial cystectomy* includes resection of the part of the bladder wall containing the tumor, along with a margin of normal tissue.
- A *radical cystectomy* involves removal of the bladder, prostate, and seminal vesicles in men and the bladder, uterus, cervix, urethra, anterior vagina, and ovaries in women.

Postoperative management for any of these procedures includes instructions to drink large amounts of fluid for the first week after the procedure, avoid alcoholic beverages, use opioid analgesics and stool softeners if necessary, and take sitz baths to promote muscle relaxation and reduce urinary retention. Administer opioid analgesics for a brief period after the procedure, along with stool softeners.

Radiation therapy is used with cystectomy or as the primary therapy when the cancer is inoperable or when the patient refuses surgery. Chemotherapeutic or immune-stimulating agents can be delivered into the patient's bladder through a urethral catheter, usually at weekly intervals for 6 to 12 weeks. Intravesical agents are instilled directly into the bladder and retained for about 2 hours. The position of the patient may be changed every 15 minutes during the instillation for maximum contact in all areas of the bladder.

- Bacille Calmette-Guérin (BCG), a weakened strain of *Mycobacterium bovis,* is the treatment of choice for carcinoma in situ. A weakened strain of BCG stimulates the immune system rather than acting directly on cancer cells in the bladder.

- When BCG fails, α-interferon, in addition to BCG, may be used. Other treatments that can be used when BCG fails include mitomycin, epirubicin, gemcitabine, valrubicin, and thiopeta (an alkylating agent).

After intravesical therapy, most patients have irritative voiding symptoms and hemorrhagic cystitis. Encourage patients to increase daily fluid intake and to quit smoking. Assess the patient for a secondary UTI and stress the need for routine urologic follow-up care. The patient may have fears or concerns about sexual activity or bladder function.

BONE TUMORS

Description
Primary *bone tumors*, both benign and malignant, are rare in adults. They account for only about 3% of all tumors. Metastatic bone cancer, in which the cancer has spread from another site, is more common.

- Benign bone tumors, such as osteochondroma, osteoclastoma, and enchondroma, are often removed by surgery.
- Primary bone cancer is called *sarcoma*. The more common types of primary bone cancer are osteosarcoma, chondrosarcoma, and Ewing's sarcoma. Primary malignant tumors occur most often during childhood and young adulthood. They cause bone destruction and have rapid metastasis.

Osteochondroma
Osteochondroma is the most common primary benign bone tumor. It is characterized by an overgrowth of cartilage and bone near the end of the bone at the growth plate. It is more often found in the pelvis, scapula, or long bones of the leg.

- Clinical manifestations of osteochondroma include a painless, hard, and immobile mass; lower-than-normal-height for age; sore muscles near the tumor; 1 leg or arm longer than the other; and pressure or irritation with exercise. Patients may be asymptomatic.
- Diagnosis is confirmed using x-ray, CT scan, and MRI.
- No treatment is necessary. If the tumor is causing pain or neurologic manifestations because of compression, surgical removal is usually done. Patients should have regular screening examinations to detect progression to cancer.

Osteosarcoma
- Osteosarcoma is an extremely aggressive bone cancer that rapidly metastasizes. It usually occurs in the pelvis or metaphyseal

region of long bones of the extremities, especially in the distal femur, proximal tibia, and proximal humerus. It is the most common malignant bone tumor affecting children and young adults, and is often associated with Paget's disease and prior radiation.

- The gradual onset of pain and swelling in the affected bone are the most common manifestations. The pain may be worse at night and increase with activity. A minor injury does not cause the cancer but may bring the condition to medical attention.
- Diagnosis is confirmed from tissue biopsy, increased serum alkaline phosphatase and calcium levels, and x-ray, CT or positron emission tomography (PET) scans, and MRI findings.
- Metastasis is present in 10% to 20% of people when they are diagnosed with osteosarcoma.

Preoperative chemotherapy may decrease tumor size before surgery. Limb-salvage surgical procedures are usually considered if there is a clear (no cancer present) 6- to 7-cm margin surrounding the lesion. Adjunct chemotherapy after surgery has increased the 5-year survival rate to 70% in patients without metastasis. Chemotherapy includes combinations of methotrexate, doxorubicin, cisplatin, ifosfamide, cyclophosphamide, and etoposide.

Metastatic Bone Cancer

Metastatic bone cancer is the most common type of malignant bone tumor. It occurs as a result of metastasis from a primary tumor. Common sites for the primary tumor include the breast, colon, prostate, lungs, kidney, and thyroid. Metastatic bone lesions are often found in the spine, ribs, or pelvis.

- Pathologic fractures at the site of metastasis are common because the bone is weak. Serum calcium levels rise as calcium is released from damaged bones.
- Radionuclide bone scans may detect metastatic lesions before they are visible on x-ray. The lesions may occur at any time (even years later) after treatment of the primary tumor.
- Bone metastasis should be suspected in any patient who has local bone pain and a history of cancer.
- Palliative treatment consists of radiation and pain management. Surgical stabilization may be indicated if there is a fracture or impending fracture. Prognosis depends on the primary type of cancer and if other sites of metastasis are present.

Nursing Management: Bone Cancer

Nursing care of the patient with bone cancer is similar to care provided to the patient with cancer of any other body system Anemia and decreased mobility may cause weakness. Use careful handling and support of the affected extremity to prevent pathologic fractures.

- Monitor the tumor site for swelling, changes in circulation, and decreased movement, sensation, or joint function.
- Pain caused by the tumor pressing against nerves and other organs near the bone can be very severe. Carefully monitor the patient's pain and ensure adequate pain medication. Sometimes radiation therapy is used to shrink the tumor and decrease the pain.
- The patient may be reluctant to take part in activities because of weakness and fear of pain. Provide rest periods between activities.
- Assist the patient and family in adjusting to the prognosis associated with bone cancer.
- Special attention is needed for problems of pain and disability, side effects of chemotherapy, and postoperative care (e.g., after spinal cord decompression or amputation).

BRAIN TUMORS

Description

Brain tumors may be primary, arising from tissues within the brain, or secondary, as a metastasis from cancer elsewhere in the body. Secondary tumors are more common. The cancers that most often metastasize to the brain are lung and breast.

Brain tumors are generally classified according to the tissue from which they arise. *Meningiomas* are the most common primary brain tumor. Other common brain tumors are gliomas (e.g., astrocytoma, glioblastoma [most common form of glioma]).

- More than half of brain tumors are malignant. They infiltrate the brain tissue and are not amenable to complete surgical removal. Other tumors may be histologically benign but are located such that complete removal is not possible.
- Brain tumors rarely metastasize outside the central nervous system (CNS) because they are contained by structural (meninges) and physiologic (blood-brain) barriers. (For a comparison of the most common brain tumors, see Table 56.12, Harding et al., *Lewis' Medical-Surgical Nursing,* ed 11.)

Clinical Manifestations

A wide range of manifestations are possible with brain tumors, depending on the location and size.

- Headache is common. Tumor-related headaches tend to be worse at night and may awaken the patient. The headaches are usually dull and constant but may be throbbing.

- Seizures are common with gliomas and brain metastases. Brain tumors can cause nausea and vomiting from increased intracranial pressure (ICP). See Increased Intracranial Pressure, p. 331.
- Cognitive problems, including memory problems and mood or personality changes, is common with brain metastases. Expanding tumors may produce signs of increased ICP, cerebral edema, or obstruction of cerebrospinal fluid (CSF) pathways.

Diagnostic Studies

- Extensive history and a comprehensive neurologic examination are essential.
- MRI and positron emission tomography (PET) scans allow for detection of very small tumors.
- CT (with contrast) and brain scanning assist in tumor location.
- Other tests include angiography, magnetic resonance spectroscopy, functional MRI, PET scans, and single-photon emission computed tomography (SPECT).

Correct diagnosis of a brain tumor is made by obtaining tissue for histologic study. In most patients, tissue is obtained at time of surgery.

Interprofessional Management

Surgical removal is the preferred treatment for brain tumors. Outcome depends on the type, size, and location of the tumor. Meningiomas and oligodendrogliomas can usually be completely removed. The more invasive gliomas and medulloblastomas can be only partially removed. Even if complete tumor removal is not possible, surgery can reduce the tumor mass to decrease ICP, provide symptom relief, and extend survival time.

Radiation therapy is used as a follow-up measure after surgery. Radiation seeds can also be implanted into the brain. Cerebral edema and rapidly increasing ICP may be complications of radiation therapy, but they can be managed with high doses of corticosteroids (dexamethasone or methylprednisolone [Solu-Medrol]).

- Stereotactic radiosurgery delivers a highly concentrated dose of radiation precisely to a location within the brain. It may be used when conventional surgery has failed or is not an option because of the tumor location.

Normally the blood-brain barrier prohibits the entry of most drugs into brain tissue. Cancerous tumors can cause a breakdown of the blood-brain barrier in the area, thus allowing chemotherapy drugs to reach the tumor. Temozolomide (Temodar) is an oral chemotherapy agent that can cross the blood-brain barrier. Chemotherapy drug–laden biodegradable wafers implanted during surgery can deliver chemotherapy directly to the tumor site. Intrathecal administration also allows direct delivery of chemotherapeutic drugs to the CNS.

Bevacizumab (Avastin) is used to treat patients with glioblastoma when this type of brain cancer continues to progress after standard therapy. Bevacizumab is a targeted therapy agent that inhibits the action of vascular endothelial growth factor (substance that helps form new blood vessels).

Nursing Management

Goals
The patient with a brain tumor will maintain normal ICP, maximize neurologic functioning, achieve control of pain and discomfort, and be aware of the long-term implications with respect to prognosis and cognitive and physical functioning.

Nursing Interventions
Behavioral changes associated with a frontal lobe lesion, such as loss of emotional control, confusion, memory loss, and depression, are often not perceived by the patient but can be disturbing and frightening to the family. Assist the caregiver and family in understanding what is happening.

- Care of the confused patient with behavioral instability can be a challenge. Use a calm and reassuring approach, closely supervise activity, and provide padded side rails.
- Minimize environmental stimuli. Create a routine and use reality orientation for the confused patient.
- Seizures often occur with brain tumors. Institute seizure precautions for the protection of the patient (see Seizure Disorders, p. 538).
- Motor and sensory dysfunctions interfere with the activities of daily living. Encourage the patient to provide as much self-care as physically possible. Self-image often depends on the patient's ability to take part in care within the limitations of the physical deficits.
- Motor (expressive) or sensory (receptive) dysphasia may occur. Disturbances in communication can be frustrating for the patient and may interfere with your ability to meet patient needs. Establish a communication system that can be used by both the patient and staff.
- Tumors in the temporal lobe can cause hallucinations, which may be confused with dementia or delirium.
- Nutritional intake may be decreased because of the patient's inability to eat, loss of appetite, or loss of desire to eat. Assess the nutritional status of the patient and ensure adequate nutritional intake. The patient may need encouragement to eat or may need enteral or parenteral nutrition (see Enteral Nutrition, p. 685, and Parenteral Nutrition, p. 710).

Social workers and home health nurses may be needed to aid the caregiver with discharge planning and to help the family adjust to role changes and psychosocial and socioeconomic factors. Issues related to palliative and end-of-life care must be discussed with both the patient and family.

B

BREAST CANCER

Description

Breast cancer is the most common cancer in women in the United States except for skin cancer and is second only to lung cancer as the leading cause of death from cancer in women. In the United States, over 255,180 new cases of invasive breast cancer and over 60,000 cases of in situ breast cancer are diagnosed annually. About 2470 new cases of breast cancer are diagnosed in men annually.

Etiology and Risk Factors

Risk factors for breast cancer appear to be cumulative and interactive (Table 15). A breast cancer risk assessment tool for health care providers (HCPs) is available through the National Cancer Institute (*www.cancer.gov/bcrisktool*).

- The use of combined hormone therapy (estrogen plus progesterone) increases the risk of breast cancer after as little as 2 years use and increased the risk of having a larger, more advanced breast cancer at diagnosis. The use of estrogen therapy alone for longer than 15 years (for women with a prior hysterectomy) increases a woman's long-term risk for breast cancer.
- A link also exists between oral contraceptive use and increased risk of breast cancer. However, the risk decreases as soon as use is stopped and is gone after 10 years.
- About 5% to 10% of all breast cancers are hereditary and are associated with mutations in 2 genes: *BRCA1* and *BRCA2*.
- Modifiable risk factors include excess weight gain during adulthood, sedentary lifestyle, smoking, dietary fat intake, obesity, and alcohol intake. Environmental factors, such as radiation exposure, may play a role.

In general, breast cancer arises from the epithelial lining of the ducts (*ductal carcinoma*) or from the epithelium of the lobules (*lobular carcinoma*). Breast cancers may be in situ (within the duct) or invasive (arising from the duct and invading through the wall of the duct).

Breast cancer can be classified as noninvasive or invasive, and as ductal or lobular (Table 16).

TABLE 15   Risk Factors for Breast Cancer

Risk Factor	Comments
Age ≥50 yr	Majority found in postmenopausal women After age 60 yr, increase in incidence
Alcohol consumption	Women who drink ≥1 alcoholic beverage per day may have an increased risk
Benign breast disease with atypical epithelial hyperplasia, lobular carcinoma in situ	Atypical changes in breast biopsy increase risk
Early menarche (before age 12 yr), late menopause (after age 55 yr)	A long menstrual history increases risk
Exposure to ionizing radiation	Radiation damages DNA (e.g., prior treatment for Hodgkin's lymphoma)
Family history	Breast cancer in a first-degree relative, particularly when premenopausal or bilateral
Female	Women account for 99% of breast cancer cases
First full-term pregnancy after age 30 yr, nulliparity, no breast feeding	Prolonged exposure to unopposed estrogen increases risk
Genetic factors (BRCA1, BRCA2, P53, PTEN, PALB2, ATM, CHEK2, NBM)	Gene mutations play a role in up to10% of breast cancer cases
Hormone use	Use of estrogen and/or progesterone as hormone therapy, especially in postmenopausal women
Long-term heavy smoking	May increase risk particularly in women who begin smoking before first pregnancy
Personal history of breast, colon, endometrial, or ovarian cancer	Personal history significantly increases risk of breast cancer, risk of cancer in other breast, and recurrence
Physical inactivity	Risk increases most after menopause
Weight gain and obesity after menopause	Fat cells store estrogen, which increases the risk of developing breast cancer

TABLE 16   Classification of Breast Cancer

Based on Tissue Type
- Ductal carcinoma (affects milk ducts)
  - Medullary
  - Tubular
  - Colloid (mucinous)
- Lobular carcinoma (affects milk-producing glands)
- Other
  - Inflammatory
  - Paget's disease
  - Phyllodes tumor

Based on Invasiveness
Noninvasive (In Situ)
- Ductal carcinoma in situ (DCIS)
- Pure Paget's disease

Invasive (Spreading to Other Locations)
- Invasive ductal carcinoma
- Invasive lobular carcinoma

Based on Hormone Receptor and Genetic Status
Estrogen and Progesterone Receptor Status
- Estrogen receptor–positive
- Estrogen receptor–negative
- Progesterone receptor–positive
- Progesterone receptor–negative

HER-2 Genetic Status
- HER-2–positive
- HER-2–negative

HER-2, Human epidermal growth factor receptor 2.

- Factors that affect cancer prognosis are tumor size, axillary node involvement (the more nodes involved, the worse the prognosis), tumor differentiation (morphology of malignant cells), estrogen and progesterone receptor status, and human epidermal growth factor receptor 2 (HER-2) status, which is a genetic marker.

Clinical Manifestations

Breast cancer is usually detected as a lump in the breast or mammographic abnormality. It occurs most often in the upper outer quadrant of the breast because that is the location of most of the glandular tissue.

- If palpable, breast cancer is characteristically hard and may be irregularly shaped, poorly delineated, nonmobile, and nontender.
- A small number of breast cancers cause clear or bloody nipple discharge, usually unilateral. Nipple retraction may occur.
- Plugging of the dermal lymphatics can cause skin thickening and exaggeration of the usual skin markings, giving skin the appearance of an orange peel (peau d'orange).
- In large cancers, infiltration, induration, and dimpling of the overlying skin may occur.

Recurrence may be local or regional (skin or soft tissue near mastectomy site, axillary lymph nodes) or distant (most commonly bone, brain, lung, and liver).

Diagnostic Studies

Screening

- Physical examination of breast and lymphatics
- Mammography and ultrasound
- Breast MRI
- Biopsy including fine-needle aspiration and stereotactic core biopsy

Postdiagnosis

Axillary lymph node dissection is often performed. An examination of the nodes can help determine if cancer has spread to the axilla. The more nodes involved, the greater the risk of recurrence.

Lymphatic mapping and *sentinel lymph node (SLN) biopsy* help the surgeon identify the lymph node(s) that drain from the tumor site (sentinel node). Assessment of this node can be used to determine the extent of tumor spread. If the SLNs are positive, a complete *axillary lymph node dissection* (ALND) may be done.

- The larger the tumor, the poorer the prognosis. In general, poorly differentiated tumors appear morphologically disorganized and are more aggressive.
- Estrogen and progesterone receptor status helps determine treatment decisions and prognosis. Receptor-positive tumors: (1) often show histologic evidence of being well differentiated, (2) have a lower chance for recurrence, (3) often have a diploid (more normal) DNA content and low proliferative indices, and (4) are frequently hormone dependent and responsive to hormone therapy. Receptor-negative tumors: (1) are often poorly differentiated histologically, (2) frequently recur, (3) have a high incidence of aneuploidy (abnormally high or low DNA content) and higher proliferative indices, and (4) are usually unresponsive to hormone therapy.

- DNA content (ploidy status) correlates with tumor aggressiveness. Diploid tumors have been shown to have a significantly lower risk of recurrence than aneuploid tumors.
- Overexpression of the HER-2 receptor has been associated with a greater risk for recurrence and a poorer prognosis in patients with breast cancer. About 10% to 20% of metastatic breast cancers produce excessive HER-2.
- Genomic assays (MammaPrint, Oncotype DX, PAM50 [Prosigna], EndoPredict, and the Breast Cancer Index) are used to analyze the activity of a group of genes.

A person whose breast cancer tests negative for all 3 receptors (estrogen, progesterone, and HER-2) has *triple-negative breast cancer,* an aggressive tumor with a poorer prognosis. The incidence of triple-negative breast cancer is higher in Hispanics, blacks, younger women, and women with a *BRCA1* mutation.

Interprofessional Management

Prognostic factors are considered in treatment decisions. Tumor size (T), nodal involvement (N), and presence of metastasis (M) are used to stage breast cancer with the TNM system (see TNM Classification System, p. 761). The stages range from 0 to IV, with stage 0 being in situ cancer with no lymph node involvement and no metastasis. Stage IV indicates metastatic spread, regardless of tumor size or lymph node involvement.

Surgical Therapy

The most common surgical options for resectable breast cancer are: (1) breast-conserving surgery (lumpectomy, segmental mastectomy), and (2) mastectomy with or without reconstruction. Most women diagnosed with early-stage breast cancer (tumors smaller than 4 to 5 cm) are candidates for either treatment choice.

Breast-conserving surgery (lumpectomy) usually involves removal of the entire tumor along with a margin of normal tissue. After surgery, radiation therapy is delivered to the entire breast, ending with a boost to the tumor bed. If the risk for recurrence is high, chemotherapy may be given before radiation therapy.

A *total* or *simple mastectomy* removes the entire breast. *Modified radical mastectomy* includes removing the breast and axillary lymph nodes while preserving the pectoralis major muscle. See Table 51.7, Harding et al., *Lewis' Medical-Surgical Nursing,* ed 11, for treatment options, side effects, complications, and patient issues related to surgical procedures for breast cancer.

Radiation Therapy

Radiation therapy may be used for breast cancer as treatment to prevent local tumor recurrences after breast-conserving surgery, prevent local and nodal recurrences after mastectomy, or palliate pain caused by local, regional, and distant recurrence.

- A minimally invasive method of delivering internal radiation therapy uses a balloon catheter to insert radioactive seeds into the breast after the tumor is removed.

Chemotherapy

Many breast cancers are responsive to cytotoxic drugs. A combination of drugs is most often superior to a single drug. The incidence and severity of the side effects that accompany chemotherapy are influenced by the drug combinations, schedule, and doses (see Chemotherapy, p. 674). Chemotherapy may be given preoperatively.

Hormone Therapy

Estrogen can promote growth of breast cancer cells if cells are estrogen-receptor (ER) positive. Hormonal therapy can block the source of estrogen, promoting tumor regression. It may be used as an adjuvant to primary treatment or in patients with recurrent or metastatic cancer.

Hormone receptor assays can identify women who are likely to respond to hormone therapy. Hormonal therapy can block ERs or suppress estrogen synthesis through inhibiting aromatase, an enzyme needed for estrogen synthesis (Table 17).

- Antiestrogens include tamoxifen, toremifene (Fareston), and fulvestrant (Faslodex).
- Aromatase inhibitor drugs include anastrozole (Arimidex), letrozole (Femara), and exemestane (Aromasin) and are used in the treatment of breast cancer in postmenopausal women.
- Raloxifene (Evista) is a selective ER modulator that has both estrogen-agonistic effects on bone and estrogen-antagonistic effects on breast tissue.

Immunotherapy and Targeted Therapy

Trastuzumab (Herceptin) is a monoclonal antibody to HER-2. After the antibody attaches to the antigen, it is taken into the cells and eventually kills them. It can be used alone or in combination with chemotherapy to treat patients with breast cancer whose tumors overexpress the HER-2 gene.

Other drugs that target HER-2 include pertuzumab (Perjeta) and ado-trastuzumab emtansine (Kadcyla), which is trastuzumab connected to a chemotherapy drug called *DM1*. Lapatinib (Tykerb) works inside the cell by blocking the function of the HER-2 protein. Using 2 of these agents together for neoadjuvant therapy has been proven to increase the number of tumors that become undetectable.

Drugs in other classes used to treat breast cancer include everolimus (Afinitor) and palbociclib (Ibrance). Everolimus works by blocking mammalian target of rapamycin (mTOR), a protein that normally promotes cell growth and division. Palbociclib is a kinase

TABLE 17 Drug Therapy

Breast Cancer

Drug Class	Mechanism of Action	Indications
Hormone Therapy		
Aromatase Inhibitors		
anastrozole (Arimidex) exemestane (Aromasin) letrozole (Femara)	Prevents production of estrogen by inhibiting aromatase	Estrogen receptor (ER)-positive breast cancer in postmenopausal women only
Estrogen Receptor Blockers		
fulvestrant (Faslodex)	Blocks ERs	ER-positive breast cancer in postmenopausal women only
tamoxifen	Blocks ERs	ER-positive breast cancer in premenopausal and postmenopausal women Used as a preventive measure in high-risk premenopausal and postmenopausal women
toremifene (Fareston)	Blocks ERs	ER-positive breast cancer in postmenopausal women only
Estrogen Receptor Modulator		
raloxifene (Evista)	In breast blocks the effect of estrogen. In bone promotes effect of estrogen and prevents bone loss	Postmenopausal women

B

Continued

TABLE 17 **Drug Therapy**

Breast Cancer—cont'd

Drug Class	Mechanism of Action	Indications
Immunotherapy and Targeted Therapy		
ado-trastuzumab emtansine (Kadcyla)	Trastuzumab connected to a chemotherapy drug called DM1	HER-2-positive breast cancer
everolimus (Afinitor)	Binds to mammalian target of rapamycin (mTOR), thereby suppressing T cell activation and proliferation	ER-positive, HER-2-negative breast cancer in postmenopausal women
lapatinib (Tykerb)	Inhibits HER-2 tyrosine kinase and EGFR tyrosine kinase	HER-2-positive breast cancer
abemaciclib (Verzenio) palbociclib (Ibrance) ribociclib (Kisqali)	Kinase inhibitors	ER-positive, HER-2-negative breast cancer in postmenopausal women
neratinib (Nerlynx) pertuzumab (Perjeta) trastuzumab (Herceptin)	Blocks HER-2 receptor	HER-2-positive breast cancer

EGFR, Epidermal growth factor receptor; *HER-2,* human epidermal growth factor receptor 2.

inhibitor that prevents cells from dividing, thus slowing cancer growth.

Follow-up and Survivorship Care

After treatment for breast cancer, the patient will have ongoing survivorship care.

- A history and physical examination is recommended 1 to 4 times per year as clinically appropriate for 5 years, then annually thereafter.
- Teach breast cancer survivors to perform monthly breast self-examination (BSE) and chest wall self-examination and report any changes to their HCP. Local recurrence of breast cancer is usually at the surgical site.

- Breast cancer survivors should have an annual mammogram. Other breast imaging studies, such as a breast ultrasound or breast MRI, should only be done as an adjunct to mammography and not for annual routine surveillance.

Nursing Management

Goals

The patient with breast cancer will actively take part in the decision-making process related to treatment, adhere to the therapeutic plan, communicate about and manage the side effects of adjuvant therapy, access and benefit from the support provided by significant others and the HCPs, and adhere to recommended follow-up and surveillance after treatment.

Nursing Interventions

The times of waiting for the initial biopsy results and waiting for the HCP to make treatment recommendations are difficult for patients and their families. Even after the HCP has discussed treatment options, the patient often relies on you to clarify and expand on these options.

- Explore the woman's usual decision-making processes, help her evaluate the advantages and disadvantages of the options, provide information relevant to the decision(s), and support the patient and family once decisions are made.
- Regardless of the surgery planned, provide the patient with enough information to ensure informed consent. Preoperative teaching includes turning and deep breathing, a review of post-operative exercises, and an explanation of the recovery period from the time of surgery until the first postoperative visit.

The woman who has breast-conserving surgery usually has an uncomplicated postoperative course with variable pain intensity. After ALND or a mastectomy, patients are generally discharged home with drains in place. Teach the patient and family (including a return demonstration) how to manage the drains at home.

- Restoring arm function on the affected side after mastectomy and axillary lymph node dissection is a key nursing goal.
- Place the woman in a semi-Fowler's position with the arm on the affected side elevated on a pillow. Flexing and extending the fingers should begin in the recovery room, with progressive increases in activity.
- Postoperative arm and shoulder exercises are instituted gradually.
- Postoperative discomfort can be minimized by administering analgesics about 30 minutes before initiating exercises. When able to shower, the warm water on the affected shoulder often has a muscle-relaxing effect and reduces joint stiffness.

Lymphedema (accumulation of lymph in soft tissue) can occur as a result of excision or radiation of the lymph nodes. The patient may have heaviness, pain, impaired motor function in the arm, and numbness and paresthesia of the fingers. Help the patient understand that lymphedema can occur at any point after treatment. Teach measures to prevent or reduce lymphedema including:

- No BP readings, venipunctures, or injections on the affected arm.
- The affected arm should not be dependent for long periods of time, and caution should be used to prevent infection, burns, or compromised circulation on the affected side.
- If trauma to the arm occurs, the area should be washed thoroughly with soap and water and observed. A topical antibiotic ointment and a bandage or other sterile dressing may be applied.

Frequent and sustained elevation of the arm, regular use of a custom-fitted pressure sleeve, and treatment with an inflatable sleeve (pneumomassage) may also be helpful.

It is important to remain sensitive to the complex psychologic impact that a diagnosis of cancer and subsequent breast surgery can have on a woman and her family. Help meet the woman's psychologic needs by the following:

- Help her identify sources of support and strength, such as her partner, family, and spiritual practices.
- Provide a safe environment for the expression of the full range of feelings.
- Encourage the patient to identify and learn individual coping strengths.
- Promote communication between the patient and her family and/ or friends.
- Provide accurate and complete answers to questions about the disease, treatment options, and reproductive or lactation issues (if appropriate).
- Make resources available for mental health counseling.
- Offer information about community resources, such as local or national breast cancer organizations.

Breast reconstruction is discussed in Chapter 51, Harding et al., *Lewis' Medical-Surgical Nursing,* ed. 11.

▼ **Patient and Caregiver Teaching**
- Explain the specific follow-up plan to the patient, emphasizing the importance of ongoing monitoring and self-care.
- Immediately after surgery, advise the patient of symptoms to report to the HCP, including fever, inflammation at the surgical site, erythema, postoperative constipation, and unusual swelling.
- For women who have had a mastectomy without breast reconstruction, a variety of garment choice products are available,

including camisoles with soft breast prosthetic inserts as well as a fitted prosthesis with bra.

- A preoperative sexual assessment provides baseline data that can be used to plan postoperative interventions.
- The spouse, sexual partner, or family members may need assistance in dealing with their emotional reactions to the diagnosis and surgery so that they can support the patient.
- Depression and anxiety may occur with the continued stress and uncertainty of a cancer diagnosis. The support of family and friends and participation in a cancer support group are important aspects of care that are often helpful in improving quality of life and have a significant impact on survival.
- Additional information on expected outcomes for the patient after breast cancer surgery is presented in eNursing Care Plan 51-1 (available on the website).

BRONCHIECTASIS

Description

Bronchiectasis is characterized by permanent, abnormal dilation of medium-sized bronchi. It is a result of inflammatory changes that destroy elastic and muscular structures supporting the bronchial wall. There is a continuing cycle of inflammation, airway damage, and remodeling, enhanced by the accumulation of neutrophils in the airways.

Airways become colonized with microorganisms (e.g., Pseudomonas), which causes the bronchial walls to weaken and pockets of infection to begin to form stasis of thickened mucus occurs along with impaired movement by the cilia, resulting in a reduced ability to clear mucus from the lungs.

Cystic fibrosis is the main cause of bronchiectasis in children. In adults, the main cause is bacterial infections of the lungs that are either not treated or receive delayed treatment. Other causes include obstruction of an airway with mucus plugs, impairment of pulmonary defenses, inflammatory bowel disease, rheumatoid arthritis, and immune disorders (e.g., acquired immunodeficiency syndrome [AIDS]).

Clinical Manifestations

The hallmark is persistent cough with consistent production of purulent, thick sputum. Recurrent infections injure blood vessels, causing hemoptysis.

- Other manifestations are pleuritic chest pain, dyspnea, wheezing, clubbing of digits, weight loss, and anemia.
- Lung auscultation reveals a variety of adventitious sounds (e.g., crackles, wheezes).

Diagnostic Studies

A person with a chronic productive cough and copious purulent sputum (which may be blood streaked) should be suspected of having bronchiectasis.

- A CT scan is considered the gold standard for diagnosing bronchiectasis.
- Chest x-ray shows nonspecific abnormalities.
- Spirometry usually shows an obstructive pattern, including a decrease in forced expiratory volume in 1 second (FEV_1) and in the ratio of FEV_1 to forced vital capacity (FVC).
- Bronchoscopy may be used with localized bronchiectasis to diagnose obstruction.
- Sputum may provide additional information regarding active infection. Sputum samples are frequently found to contain *Haemophilus influenzae, Staphylococcus aureus,* or *Pseudomonas aeruginosa.*

Nursing and Interprofessional Management

Bronchiectasis is hard to treat. Therapy is aimed at treating acute flare-ups and preventing a decline in lung function. Choice of antibiotic primarily depends on culture results or most likely organism. Bronchodilators or anticholinergics are given to prevent bronchospasm and stimulate mucus clearance.

- Maintaining good hydration is important to liquefy secretions. Unless there are contraindications, the patient is to drink at least 3 L of fluid daily.
- Direct hydration of the respiratory system may help in expectorating secretions. Often nebulized hypertonic saline may be ordered for a more aggressive effect. At home, a steamy shower can prove effective.
- Chest physiotherapy and other airway clearance techniques facilitate expectoration of sputum.
- Teach the patient to reduce exposure to excessive air pollutants and irritants, avoid cigarette smoking, and obtain pneumococcal and influenza vaccinations.
- Teach the patient and caregiver manifestations to report to the health care provider (HCP). These include increased sputum production, bloody sputum, increasing dyspnea, fever, chills, and chest pain.

- If hemoptysis occurs in the acute care setting, contact the HCP immediately. Elevate the head of the bed and place the patient in a side-lying position with the suspected bleeding side down.
- Good nutrition may be difficult to maintain because the patient is often anorexic. Oral hygiene to cleanse the mouth and remove dried sputum crusts may improve the patient's appetite.

BURNS

Description

Burns are tissue injuries caused by heat, chemicals, electric current, or radiation. An estimated 486,000 Americans seek medical care each year for burns. The highest fatality rates occur in children aged 4 years and younger and adults older than age 65 years.

Pathophysiology

Immediately after the burn injury occurs, there is increased blood flow to the area surrounding the wound. This is followed by the release of various vasoactive substances from burned tissue, which results in increased capillary permeability. Fluid then shifts from the intravascular compartment to the interstitial space, producing edema, hypovolemia, and (potentially) shock. After several days, diuresis from fluid mobilization occurs and healing begins.

Types of Burn Injury

Various types of burns may be seen alone or in combination with other burns.

- *Thermal burns* are caused by flame, flash, scald, or contact with hot objects. Severity depends on the temperature of the burning agent and duration of contact.
- *Chemical burns* are the result of tissue injury and destruction from acids, alkalis (e.g., cement, oven cleaner), and organic compounds, such as petroleum products.
- *Smoke and inhalation injury* results from inhalation of hot air or noxious chemicals that damage the respiratory tract. These injuries include metabolic asphyxiation (carbon monoxide poisoning), upper airway injury, and lower airway injury.
- *Electrical burns* result from the intense heat of an electric current.

Classification of Burn Injury

The treatment of burns is related to the severity of injury. A variety of methods exist for determining burn severity.

1. Depth of burn is described according to the depth of skin destruction (epidermis, dermis, or subcutaneous tissue). Table 18

TABLE 18 Classification of Burn Injury Depth

Classification	Appearance	Possible Cause	Structures Involved
Partial-Thickness Skin Destruction			
Superficial (first-degree) burn	Erythema, blanching on pressure, pain and mild swelling, no vesicles or blisters (although after 24 hr skin may blister and peel)	Quick heat flash Superficial sunburn	Superficial epidermal damage with hyperemia. Tactile and pain sensation intact.
Deep (second-degree) burn	Fluid-filled vesicles that are red, shiny, wet (if vesicles have ruptured). Severe pain caused by nerve injury. Mild to moderate edema	Chemicals Contact burns Electric current Flame Flash Scald Tar, cement	Epidermis and dermis involved to varying depths. Skin elements, from which epithelial regeneration occurs, remain viable.
Full-Thickness Skin Destruction			
Third- and fourth-degree burns	Dry, waxy white, leathery, or hard skin. Visible thrombosed vessels. Insensitivity to pain because of nerve destruction. Possible involvement of muscles, tendons, and bones	Chemical Electric current Flame Scald Tar, cement	All skin elements and local nerve endings destroyed. Coagulation necrosis present. Surgical intervention required for healing.

compares the various burn classifications according to the depth of injury.

2. Extent of the burn wound is calculated as percent of total body surface area (TBSA) affected. Two common methods for determining the extent of a burn include:
   - *Lund-Browder chart,* which is considered the most accurate because it takes into account patient age in proportion to relative body area size (Fig. 2A).
   - *Rule of Nines chart,* which is often used for initial assessment because it is easy to remember (see Fig. 2B).

3. Severity of the burn injury is also determined by the location of the burn wound. For example, face and neck burns may inhibit respiratory function. Hands, feet, joint, and eye burns may limit self-care and functioning.

4. Age of the patient, preburn medical history, and circumstances or complicating factors affect the patient's ability to recover from the tremendous demands of burn injury. The patient with diabetes or peripheral vascular disease is at high risk for poor healing, especially with foot and leg burns.

The American Burn Association (ABA) has established referral criteria to determine which burn injuries should be treated in burn centers with specialized facilities (Table 19).

Clinical Manifestations

Burns can be organized chronologically into 3 phases: emergent (resuscitative), acute (wound healing), and rehabilitative (restorative).

Emergent Phase

The greatest initial threat to a patient with a major burn is hypovolemic shock. Shivering (a result of heat loss or anxiety) and a paralytic ileus (if the burn area is large) may also be present. Full-thickness and deep partial-thickness burns are initially painless because nerve endings have been destroyed. Superficial to moderate partial-thickness burns are very painful. Blisters are common in partial-thickness burns. Unconsciousness or altered mental status is the result of smoke inhalation or head trauma. Complications may include respiratory distress, dysrhythmias, venous thromboembolism, and acute tubular necrosis. The emergent phase ends when fluid mobilization and diuresis begin.

Acute Phase

Partial-thickness wounds form eschar. After eschar is removed, reepithelialization begins at wound margins and appears as red or pink scar tissue. Wound closure and healing usually occur within 10 to 21 days. Separation of eschar from full-thickness wounds takes longer, and these wounds require surgical debridement and skin

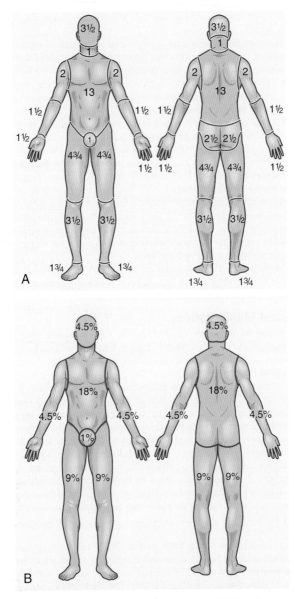

Fig. 2 (A) Lund-Browder chart. (B) Rule of Nines chart.

TABLE 19   Burn Center Referral Criteria

Burn injuries that should be referred to a burn center include the following:

1. Partial-thickness burns >10% of total body surface area (TBSA).
2. Burns that involve the face, hands, feet, genitalia, perineum, or major joints
3. Third-degree burns in any age group
4. Electrical burns, including lightning injury
5. Chemical burns
6. Inhalation injury
7. Burn injury in patients with preexisting medical disorders that could complicate management, prolong recovery, or affect mortality risk (e.g., heart or kidney disease)
8. Patients with burns and concomitant trauma (e.g., fractures) when the burn injury poses the greatest risk of morbidity or mortality. If the trauma poses the greater immediate risk, the patient may be initially stabilized in a trauma center before being transferred to a burn center. The HCP will need to use judgment, in consultation with the regional medical control plan and triage protocols.
9. Burn injury in children in hospitals without qualified personnel or equipment needed to care for them
10. Burn injury in patients who will require special social, emotional, or long-term rehabilitative intervention

Source: American Burn Association: Guidelines for the operation of burn centers. Retrieved from *http://www.ameriburn.org/Chapter14.pdf.*

grafting. Wound infection is a serious complication. Other possible complications include extreme disorientation and delirium, contractures, Curling's ulcer, hyperglycemia, and pneumonia.

Rehabilitative Phase

Mature healing of burns occurs in about 12 months when suppleness has returned, and the color has faded to a slightly lighter hue than the surrounding unburned tissue. New scar tissue shrinks, causing a contracture if not prevented with range-of-motion (ROM) exercises. The healing site, which is extremely sensitive to trauma, may itch. Complications are skin and joint contractures and hypertrophic scarring.

Diagnostic Studies

- Serum electrolytes, especially sodium (Na^+) and potassium (K^+), to monitor fluid and electrolyte shifts

- Chest x-ray, arterial blood gases (ABGs), and sputum for inhalation injury
- Urine output and serum creatinine to evaluate fluid replacement and detect acute tubular necrosis and/or renal ischemia
- Complete blood count (CBC) to detect anemia and immunologic response to injury
- White blood cell (WBC) count and wound cultures if infection is suspected

Nursing and Interprofessional Management

Burn management can be classified into 3 phases: emergent, acute, and rehabilitative (Table 20).

Emergent Phase

Patient survival depends on rapid and thorough assessment and intervention.

- Assess adequacy of airway management and fluid therapy, provide pain medication and wound care, and offer support to patient and family. Begin feeding patient by most appropriate route as soon as possible.
- Standard pulse oximetry (SpO_2) does not distinguish oxyhemoglobin from carboxyhemoglobin. For patients with suspected or confirmed carbon monoxide exposure, use a carbon monoxide pulse oximetry (SpCO) device.

Acute Phase

Major interventions are wound care, excision and grafting, pain management, physical and occupational therapy, nutritional therapy, and psychosocial care.

- Wound care consists of ongoing observation, assessment, cleansing, debridement, and dressing reapplication.
- Pain assessment and management are critical.

Rehabilitative Phase

Care of the person with burns can be very intense over a long period of time. Nurses should seek support from co-workers, a manager, or the employee assistance program as needed.

Encourage the patient and caregiver to actively participate in care.

- Continue to encourage patient to perform physical and occupational therapy routines.
- Apply water-based moisturizers that penetrate the dermis on healed areas to keep skin supple.
- Assist patients in adapting to a realistic, yet positive appraisal of the situation. Stress what they *can* do instead of what they *cannot* do.

▼ Patient and Caregiver Teaching

- Describe the burn injury healing process and phases of burn management.

TABLE 20 Interprofessional Care

Burn Injury

Emergent Phase	Acute Phase	Rehabilitation Phase
Fluid Therapy	**Fluid Therapy**	• Continue to teach patient and caregiver about wound care.
• Assess fluid needs.	• Continue to replace fluids, depending on patient's clinical response.	• Continue to encourage and aid patient in resuming self-care.
• Begin IV fluid replacement.		• Continue to prevent or minimize contractures.
• Insert indwelling urinary catheter.	**Wound Care**	• Assess risk for scarring (surgery, physical and occupational therapy, splinting, pressure garments).
• Monitor urine output.	• Continue daily shower and wound care.	
	• Continue debridement (if needed).	• Discuss possible reconstructive surgery.
Wound Care	• Assess wound daily and adjust dressing protocols as needed.	• Prepare for discharge home or transfer to rehabilitation hospital.
• Start daily shower and wound care.	• Observe for complications (e.g., infection).	• Discuss possible need for home care nursing.
• Debride as needed.	**Early Excision and Grafting**	
• Assess extent and depth of burns.	• Provide temporary allografts.	
• Give tetanus toxoid or tetanus antitoxin.	• Provide permanent autografts.	
	• Care for donor sites.	
Pain and Anxiety	**Pain and Anxiety**	
• Assess and manage pain and anxiety.	• Continue to assess for and treat pain and anxiety.	

B

Continued

TABLE 20 Interprofessional Care—cont'd

Burn Injury

Emergent Phase	Acute Phase	Rehabilitation Phase
Physical and Occupational Therapy • Place patient in position that prevents contracture formation and reduces edema. • Assess need for splints.	**Physical and Occupational Therapy** • Begin daily therapy program for maintenance of range of motion. • Assess need for splints and anticontracture positioning. • Encourage and aid patient with self-care as possible.	
Nutritional Therapy • Assess nutritional needs and begin feeding patient by most appropriate route as soon as possible.	**Nutritional Therapy** • Continue to assess diet to support wound healing.	
Respiratory Therapy • Assess oxygenation needs. • Provide supplemental O_2 as needed. • Intubate if needed. • Monitor respiratory status.	**Respiratory Therapy** • Continue to assess oxygenation needs. • Continue to monitor respiratory status. • Monitor for signs of complications (e.g., pneumonia).	

B

Psychosocial Care

- Provide support to patient and caregiver during initial crisis phase.

Psychosocial Care

- Provide ongoing support, counseling, and teaching to patient and caregiver about physical and emotional aspects of care and recovery.
- Begin discharge planning.

Drug Therapy

(see Table 24.11, Harding et al, Medical-Surgical Nursing, ed 11)

- Assess need for drugs (e.g., antibiotics).
- Continue to monitor effectiveness and adjust dosage as needed.

- Explain therapeutic interventions, precautionary measures, gowning and hand washing, and visiting policy to elicit cooperation and decrease anxiety.
- Teach the patient to watch for injuries or signs and symptoms of infection in new skin.
- Teach caregivers how to perform dressing changes to ensure proper technique and increase their sense of control.
- Stress exercise and appropriate physical therapy. Plan a daily program with the patient and offer appropriate resources to provide a continuing activity program.
- Anticipatory guidance decreases anxiety and inaccurate perceptions. Help the patient and caregiver know what to expect during recovery and set realistic future expectations. Assist the patient and caregivers to establish contact with family and patient support groups, such as the Phoenix Society *(www.phoenix-society.org)*.

CARDIOMYOPATHY

Description

Cardiomyopathy (CMP) is a group of diseases that directly affect myocardial structure or function. CMP is classified as primary or secondary:

- *Primary CMP* refers to conditions in which the cause of the heart disease is unknown. The heart muscle is the only portion of the heart involved, and other cardiac structures are unaffected.
- In *secondary CMP,* the myocardial disease is caused by another disease process. Common causes of secondary CMP are coronary artery disease (CAD), myocarditis, hypertension, cardiotoxic agents (alcohol, cocaine), valve disease, and metabolic and autoimmune disorders.

Three major types of CMP are *dilated, hypertrophic,* and *restrictive.* Each type has its own pathogenesis, clinical presentation, and treatment (Table 21). CMP that leads to cardiomegaly and heart failure (HF) is the main reason for heart transplants.

Dilated Cardiomyopathy

Pathophysiology

Dilated CMP is the most common type. It appears with diffuse inflammation and rapid degeneration of heart fibers. It results in ventricular dilation, impairment of systolic function, atrial enlargement, and blood stasis in the left ventricle. The ventricular walls do not hypertrophy.

TABLE 21   Types of Cardiomyopathy

Dilated	Hypertrophic	Restrictive
Cardiac Output		
Decreased	Normal or decreased	Normal or decreased
Cardiomegaly		
Moderate to severe	Mild to moderate	Mild
Contractility		
Decreased	Increased or decreased	Normal or decreased
Dysrhythmias		
Sinus tachycardia, atrial and ventricular dysrhythmias	Atrial and ventricular dysrhythmias	Atrial and ventricular dysrhythmias
Major Manifestations		
Fatigue, weakness, palpitations, dyspnea	Exertional dyspnea, fatigue, angina, syncope, palpitations	Dyspnea, fatigue
Outflow Tract Obstruction		
None	Increased	None
Valvular Incompetence		
Atrioventricular (AV) valves, especially mitral	Mitral valve	AV valves

C

- Dilated CMP often follows infectious myocarditis. Some evidence links dilated CMP with an autoimmune process or genetic causes. Other common causes include alcohol, cocaine, hypertension, and CAD.

Clinical Manifestations

Signs and symptoms of dilated CMP may develop acutely after an infection or slowly over time. Most affected people eventually develop HF. Symptoms can include fatigue, dyspnea at rest, paroxysmal nocturnal dyspnea, and orthopnea. Dry cough, abdominal bloating, and anorexia may occur as the disease progresses. Signs can include an irregular heart rate with an abnormal S_3 and/or S_4, pulmonary crackles, edema, pallor, hepatomegaly, heart murmurs, dysrhythmias, and jugular venous distention.

Diagnostic Studies

A diagnosis is made on the basis of patient history and exclusion of other causes of HF.

- Doppler echocardiography is usually the basis for the diagnosis of dilated CMP.
- Chest x-ray may show cardiomegaly with pulmonary venous hypertension and pleural effusion.
- The electrocardiogram (ECG) may reveal tachycardia, bradycardia, and dysrhythmias with conduction disturbances.
- Serum levels of b-type natriuretic peptide (BNP) are increased in the presence of HF.
- Heart catheterization confirms or excludes CAD, and multiple gated acquisition (MUGA) nuclear scan determines ejection fraction (EF).

Nursing and Interprofessional Management

The goals of therapy are to keep the patient at an optimal level of functioning and out of the hospital. Interventions focus on controlling HF by enhancing myocardial contractility and decreasing preload and afterload. Observe for signs and symptoms of worsening HF, dysrhythmias, and embolus formation.

Drug and nutritional therapy and cardiac rehabilitation may help alleviate symptoms of HF and improve cardiac output (CO) and quality of life. Monitor for drug effectiveness.

- Nitrates and loop diuretics decrease preload.
- Angiotensin-converting enzyme (ACE) inhibitors reduce afterload.
- β-Adrenergic blockers (e.g., metoprolol [Lopressor]) and aldosterone antagonists (e.g., spironolactone [Aldactone]) control the neurohormonal stimulation that occurs in HF.
- Antidysrhythmics (e.g., amiodarone) and anticoagulants are used as indicated.
- Anticoagulation therapy reduces the risk of systemic embolization from clots that form in the heart chambers.
- The use of statins (e.g., atorvastatin [Lipitor]) in ischemic and idiopathic dilated CMP improves survival and heart function while reducing inflammatory markers.
- A patient with secondary dilated CMP must be treated for the underlying disease process. For example, the patient with alcohol-induced dilated CMP must abstain from alcohol.
- All patients with CMP are at risk for infective endocarditis from any procedure that may cause bacteremia. Teach the patient about the need for prophylactic antibiotics.

Patients may also benefit from nondrug therapies. Cardiac resynchronization therapy and an implantable cardioverter-defibrillator may be used. A ventricular assist device (VAD) allows the heart to rest and recover from acute HF. It may also serve as a bridge to heart transplantation.

- The patient with terminal or end-stage CMP may consider heart transplantation. Currently, approximately 50% of heart transplantations performed are for treatment of CMP. Heart transplant recipients have a good prognosis.
- Encourage caregivers to learn cardiopulmonary resuscitation (CPR). Teach them when and how to activate emergency care.

Hypertrophic Cardiomyopathy

Pathophysiology

Hypertrophic cardiomyopathy (HCM) is asymmetric left ventricular hypertrophy without ventricular dilation. HCM is more common in men than in women. It is usually diagnosed in young adulthood and is often seen in active, athletic persons. HCM is the most common cause of sudden cardiac death (SCD) in otherwise healthy young people.

- The main characteristics of HCM result from massive ventricular hypertrophy: rapid, forceful contraction of the left ventricle; impaired relaxation (diastole); and obstruction to aortic outflow (not present in all patients). The end result is poor filling of the stiff ventricle. Decreased ventricular filling and obstruction to outflow result in decreased CO, especially during exertion.

Clinical Manifestations

Patients may be asymptomatic. The most common symptom is dyspnea, caused by an elevated left ventricular diastolic pressure. Other manifestations include fatigue, angina, syncope (especially during exertion), and dysrhythmias.

- Common dysrhythmias include atrial fibrillation, ventricular tachycardia, and ventricular fibrillation.
- Clinical findings on examination may be unremarkable. On chest palpation, the apical impulse can be exaggerated and displaced to the left. Auscultation may reveal an S_4 and a systolic murmur between the apex and sternal border at the fourth intercostal space.

Diagnostic Studies

- Echocardiogram is the primary diagnostic tool to confirm HCM, showing left ventricular hypertrophy, wall motion abnormalities, and diastolic dysfunction.
- Heart catheterization and nuclear stress testing may help in diagnosing and guiding treatment.

Nursing and Interprofessional Management

Goals of care are to improve ventricular filling by reducing ventricular contractility and relieving left ventricular outflow obstruction. This can be achieved with β-blockers (e.g., metoprolol) or calcium-channel blockers (e.g., verapamil).

- Amiodarone or sotalol (Betapace) are effective antidysrhythmic drugs. However, their use does not prevent SCD. Patients at risk for SCD need implantable cardioverter-defibrillator.
- Atrioventricular pacing can reduce the degree of outflow obstruction by causing the septum to move away from the left ventricular wall.
- Patients with severe symptoms unresponsive to therapy may be candidates for surgical treatment (ventriculomyotomy and myectomy) of the hypertrophied septum. Most patients have an improvement in symptoms and exercise tolerance after surgery.
- An alternative nonsurgical procedure to reduce symptoms is percutaneous transluminal septal myocardial ablation (PTSMA). Ablation of the septal wall decreases the obstruction to flow, and the patient's symptoms decrease.
- Vasodilators, such as nitroglycerin, may worsen the chest pain by decreasing venous return and further increasing obstruction of blood flow from the heart.

Nursing interventions focus on relieving symptoms, observing for and preventing complications, and providing emotional support.

- Teaching should focus on helping the patients plan to adjust their lifestyle to avoid strenuous activity and dehydration. Any activity that causes an increase in systemic vascular resistance (thus increasing obstruction to forward blood flow) is dangerous.
- Rest and elevation of the feet to improve venous return to the heart can help manage chest pain.

Restrictive Cardiomyopathy

Pathophysiology

Restrictive cardiomyopathy is a disease of the heart muscle that impairs diastolic filling and stretch. Several pathologic processes may be involved, including myocardial fibrosis, hypertrophy, and infiltration, which produce stiffness of the ventricular wall. The ventricles resist filling and require high diastolic filling pressures to maintain CO.

Clinical Manifestations

Classic manifestations of restrictive CMP are fatigue, exercise intolerance, and dyspnea. Other manifestations may include angina, orthopnea, syncope, palpations, and signs of HF.

Diagnostic Studies

Chest x-ray may appear normal or show cardiomegaly with pleural effusions and pulmonary congestion.

- ECG may show tachycardia at rest. The most common dysrhythmias are atrial fibrillation and atrioventricular block.
- Echocardiography may show a left ventricle of normal size with a thickened wall, a slightly dilated right ventricle, and dilated atria.
- Endomyocardial biopsy, CT scan, and nuclear imaging may help determine a diagnosis.

Nursing and Interprofessional Management

No specific treatment for restrictive CMP exists. Interventions are aimed at improving diastolic filling and the underlying disease process. Treatment includes conventional therapy for HF and dysrhythmias. Heart transplantation may be an option.

Nursing care is similar to the care of a patient with HF. As with HCM, teach patients to avoid situations, such as strenuous activity and dehydration, that impair ventricular filling and increase systemic vascular resistance.

CARPAL TUNNEL SYNDROME

Description

Carpal tunnel syndrome (CTS) is caused by compression of the median nerve, which enters the hand through the narrow confines of the carpal tunnel. The carpal tunnel is formed by ligaments and bones. This condition is often caused by pressure from trauma or edema because of inflammation of a tendon (tenosynovitis), cancer, rheumatoid arthritis, or soft tissue masses, such as ganglion cysts.

- CTS is associated with hobbies or occupations that require continuous wrist movement (e.g., musicians, carpenters, computer users).
- Women are affected more often than men, possibly because of a smaller carpal tunnel. Hormones may be involved because CTS often occurs during the premenstrual period, pregnancy, and menopause.

Clinical Manifestations

Manifestations are impaired sensation, pain, numbness, or weakness in the distribution of the median nerve and clumsiness in performing fine hand movements. Numbness and tingling may awaken the patient at night. Shaking the hands will often relieve these symptoms. Physical signs of CTS include Tinel's sign and Phalen's sign.

- *Tinel's sign* can be elicited by tapping over the median nerve as it passes through the carpal tunnel in the wrist. A positive response is a sensation of tingling in the distribution of the median nerve over the hand.
- *Phalen's sign* can be elicited by allowing the wrists to fall freely into maximum flexion and maintain the position for more than 60 seconds. A positive response is a sensation of tingling in the distribution of the median nerve over the hand.

In late stages, there is atrophy of the thenar muscles around the base of the thumb, resulting in recurrent pain and eventual dysfunction of the hand.

Nursing and Interprofessional Management

Teach employees and employers about risk factors for CTS to prevent its occurrence. Adaptive devices, such as wrist splints, may relieve pressure on the median nerve. Special keyboard pads and mice are available for computer users. Other ergonomic changes include workstation modifications, change in body position, and frequent breaks from work-related activities.

Early symptoms of CTS can usually be relieved by stopping the aggravating movement and by resting the hand and wrist by immobilizing them in a hand splint. Splints worn at night help keep the wrist in a neutral position and may reduce night pain and numbness. Injection of a corticosteroid drug directly into the carpal tunnel may give short-term relief.

If symptoms persist for more than 6 months, surgery is generally recommended, which involves severing the band of tissue around the wrist to reduce pressure on the median nerve. Surgery is done in an outpatient setting under local anesthesia. Endoscopic carpal tunnel release is performed through a small puncture incision(s) in the wrist and palm.

- After surgery, assess the neurovascular status of the hand regularly.
- Teach the patient about wound care and the appropriate assessments to perform at home.

Although symptoms may be relieved after surgery, full recovery may take months.

CATARACT

Description

A cataract is an opacity within the lens of 1 or both eyes, causing a gradual decline in vision. Cataract removal is the most common surgical procedure in the United States.

Pathophysiology

Although most cataracts are age-related (senile cataracts), they can be associated with other factors. These include blunt or penetrating trauma, smoking, alcohol use, radiation or ultraviolet light exposure, certain drugs (e.g., steroids), and ocular inflammation. Patients with diabetes tend to develop cataracts at a younger age.

- In senile cataract formation, altered metabolic processes within the lens cause water accumulation and changes in the lens fiber structure. These changes affect lens transparency and vision.

Clinical Manifestations

- Patients may have decreased vision, abnormal color perception, and glare.
- Visual decline is gradual and the rate of cataract development varies.

Diagnostic Studies

- Lens opacity is observed by ophthalmoscopic or slit lamp microscopic examination
- Visual acuity measurement
- Glare testing
- Keratometry and A-scan ultrasound if surgery is planned

Interprofessional Management

Currently no treatment "cures" cataracts other than surgical removal.

- Helpful palliative measures include a changing eyeglass prescription, using strong reading glasses or magnifiers, increasing the amount of light for reading, and avoiding nighttime driving if glare is worse at night.
- When these measures no longer provide an acceptable level of visual function, the patient is a candidate for surgery. Removal of the lens may also be medically necessary in patients with increased intraocular pressure and diabetic retinopathy.

Almost all patients have an intraocular lens (IOL) implanted at the time of cataract extraction surgery. The patient's eye may be covered with a patch or protective shield, which is removed during the first postoperative visit. IOL implants provide immediate visual improvement for most patients.

Nursing Management

Goals

- Preoperatively, the patient will make an informed decision and experience minimal anxiety.

- Postoperatively, the patient will avoid falls while the operative eye that is patched limits depth perception, understand and adhere with therapy, maintain an acceptable level of physical and emotional comfort, and remain free of infection and other complications.

Nursing Interventions

For the patient who chooses not to have surgery, suggest vision enhancement techniques and a modification of activities and lifestyle to accommodate the visual deficit.

For the patient who elects surgery, provide information, support, and reassurance about the surgical and postoperative experience to reduce or alleviate anxiety. Postoperatively, offer mild analgesics for slight scratchiness or mild eye pain.

▼ **Patient and Caregiver Teaching**
- Suggest ways of modifying activities and the environment to maintain safe functioning. Suggestions may include getting assistance with stairs, removing area rugs and other obstacles, preparing meals for freezing before surgery, and obtaining audio books for diversion until visual acuity improves.
- Written and verbal discharge teaching should include eye care, activity restrictions, medications, follow-up visit schedule, and signs of possible complications (Table 22).

TABLE 22   Patient and Caregiver Teaching

After Eye Surgery

Include the following information in the teaching plan for the patient and caregiver after eye surgery.
- If a patch is used, the patient will not have depth perception until the patch is removed. Ask for assistance to walk on uneven ground or on stairs.
- Use proper hygiene to ensure that medications, dressings, and/or surgical wounds are not contaminated during eye care.
- Report signs and symptoms of infection (such as redness, increased or purulent drainage) to allow for early treatment.
- Follow postoperative restrictions on head positioning, bending, coughing, and Valsalva maneuver to prevent increased intraocular pressure.
- Instill eye medications using aseptic techniques and adhere to prescribed eye medication routine to prevent infection.
- Monitor pain, take pain medication, and report pain not relieved by medication.
- Schedule recommended postoperative appointments to maximize visual outcomes.

- Patients may have difficulty with self-care activities, especially if vision in the unoperated eye is poor. Include the patient's caregiver in your teaching. Provide an opportunity for the patient and caregiver to do return demonstrations of any self-care activities.

CELIAC DISEASE

Description

Celiac disease is an autoimmune disease that causes damage to the small intestinal mucosa. It is triggered by ingesting gluten, a protein in wheat, barley, and rye.

Celiac disease is not the same as the disease *tropical sprue,* a chronic disorder occurring primarily in tropical areas. Tropical sprue causes disruption of jejunal and ileal tissue, resulting in malnutrition. It is treated with folic acid and tetracycline.

Celiac disease affects about 1 in 100 people worldwide. First-degree relatives of someone with celiac disease have a 4% to 15% chance of developing the disorder. It is associated with other autoimmune diseases, particularly rheumatoid arthritis, type 1 diabetes and thyroid disease. It is slightly more common in women. Symptoms often begin in childhood. Many people seek treatment for nonspecific complaints for years before celiac disease is diagnosed.

Pathophysiology

Three factors necessary for the development of celiac disease are a genetic predisposition, gluten ingestion, and an immune-mediated response.

- About 90% to 95% of patients with celiac disease have human leukocyte antigen (HLA) allele HLA-DQ2, and the other 5% to 10% have HLA-DQ8. However, not everyone with these genetic markers develops the disease.
- Tissue destruction that occurs with celiac disease is the result of chronic inflammation activated by the ingestion of gluten found in wheat, rye, and barley.
- Damage is most severe in the duodenum, probably because it is the site of the highest concentration of gluten. The inflammation lasts as long as gluten ingestion continues.

Clinical Manifestations

Classic manifestations of celiac disease include foul-smelling diarrhea, abdominal pain, flatulence, abdominal distention, and symptoms of malnutrition. Atypical signs and symptoms include joint pain, osteoporosis, dental enamel hypoplasia, fatigue, peripheral neuropathy, and reproductive problems.

- A pruritic, vesicular skin lesion called *dermatitis herpetiformis* may be present as a rash on the buttocks, scalp, face, elbows, and knees.
- Weight loss, muscle wasting, and other signs of malnutrition may be present. Patients may exhibit lactose intolerance.
- Iron-deficiency anemia is common.

Diagnostic Studies
Celiac disease is confirmed by a combination of findings from the history and physical examination, serologic testing, and histologic analysis of small intestine biopsy specimens.

Nursing and Interprofessional Management
A gluten-free diet is the only effective treatment for celiac disease. Most patients need to maintain a gluten-free diet for the rest of their lives. In patients with refractory celiac disease who do not respond to the gluten-free diet alone, corticosteroids may be used.

Periodic nutrition evaluations and laboratory monitoring are done to monitor for anemia and malnutrition. The patient should undergo bone density screening every 2 to 3 years.

- Refer all patients for a dietary consultation. Reinforce that continued gluten consumption will result in chronic inflammation, which can lead to as anemia and osteoporosis.
- Dietary gluten comes from wheat, barley, rye, and oats (oats do not contain gluten but can become contaminated with gluten during milling). Gluten is also found in some medications, food additives, preservatives, and stabilizers.
- Many restaurants now indicate gluten-free menu options.
- The National Celiac Association website *(https://nationalceliac. org/)* and the Celiac Disease Foundation *(www.celiac.org)* provide suggestions for maintaining a gluten-free diet and living with celiac disease.

CERVICAL CANCER

Description and Etiology
Cervical cancer was once a common cause of cancer death. However, with early detection (Pap test, human papilloma virus [HPV] testing), the mortality rate from cervical cancer has significantly declined. Around 13,240 women in the United States are diagnosed with cervical cancer each year and 4100 women will

die. While Hispanic women are the most likely to be diagnosed with cervical cancer, black women have the highest mortality rate from cervical cancer.

- Risk factors for cervical cancer include: (1) infection with high-risk strains of HPV 16 and 18, (2) immunosuppression, (3) using oral contraceptive pills (OCPs) for a long period of time, (4) being exposed to the drug diethylstilbestrol (DES), (5) giving birth to many children, and (6) smoking.

The progression from normal cervical cells to dysplasia and on to cervical cancer occurs over years. There is a strong relationship between sexual exposure to HPV and cervical dysplasia. A vaccine can protect against cervical cancer that is caused by HPV types 16 and 18.

Clinical Manifestations

Early cervical cancer often has no symptoms. Unusual discharge, abnormal uterine bleeding, or postcoital bleeding eventually occur.

- Vaginal discharge that is thin and watery becomes dark and foul-smelling as the disease advances.
- Vaginal bleeding is initially spotting, but it becomes heavier and more frequent.
- Pain is a late symptom and is followed by weight loss, anemia, and cachexia.

Diagnostic Studies

- Pap test, colposcopy, and biopsy
- HPV testing can identify high-risk HPV types 16 and 18, of which 80% are associated with cervical cancer

Interprofessional Management

Vaccination against HPV provides an opportunity for primary prevention of cervical cancer. Inform both parents and patients about the need to complete the HPV vaccination series before the first sexual contact. It should be given at age 11 to 12 years, when the immune system has a good response to of the vaccine.

Currently 2 vaccines are available to protect against high-risk HPV types: (1) Gardasil, which protects against types 6, 11, 16, and 18; and (2) Gardasil 9. It protects against HPV types 6, 11, 16, 18, and 5 other HPV types. These vaccines are given in 2 to 3 IM doses (depending on the patient's age) over a 6-month period. They have few side effects.

Treatment options for cervical cancer can include surgery or a combination of chemotherapy and irradiation.

- For patients with advanced disease, bevacizumab (Avastin), a targeted therapy drug, may be used in addition to cisplatin-based chemotherapy. Bevacizumab is an angiogenesis inhibitor. It works by interfering with development of the blood vessels that supply nutrients to cancer cells.

- Surgical procedures include hysterectomy, radical hysterectomy, and, rarely, pelvic exenteration (Table 23).

TABLE 23 Surgical Procedures Involving the Female Reproductive System

Type of Surgery	Description
daVinci	Minimally invasive surgery using robotics for major gynecologic procedures.
Dilation and curettage (D&C)	Dilation of cervix and scraping of endometrium.
Endometrial ablation	An outpatient procedure using hot or cold energy to destroy the endometrial lining of the uterus in cases of abnormal uterine bleeding (AUB).
Hysterectomy	
Abdominal supracervical hysterectomy	Removal of uterus only with cervix remaining intact.
Radical hysterectomy	Panhysterectomy, partial vaginectomy, and dissection of lymph nodes in pelvis.
Total abdominal hysterectomy (TAH)	Uterus and cervix removed using a pfannenstiel incision (bikini cut).
Total abdominal hysterectomy and bilateral salpingo-oophorectomy (TAH-BSO)	Uterus, cervix, fallopian tubes, and ovaries removed using a pfannenstiel or a vertical incision.
Vaginal hysterectomy	Uterus and cervix removed through a cut in the top of vagina.
Laparoscopic hysterectomy	Laparoscope (video camera and small surgical instruments).
• Laparoscopic-assisted vaginal hysterectomy (LAVH)	Incision made at top of vagina. Uterus and cervix removed through the vagina. Laparoscope inserted into abdomen to assist in the procedure.
• Laparoscopic supracervical hysterectomy	Uterus removed using only laparoscopic instruments. Cervix is left intact.

TABLE 23 Surgical Procedures Involving the Female Reproductive System—cont'd	
Type of Surgery	**Description**
Hysteroscopy	Video done with D&C to check for abnormal uterine lining, AUB, polyps.
Myomectomy	Removal of fibroid from the uterus, leaving the uterus in place.
Pelvic exenteration	Radical hysterectomy, total vaginectomy, removal of bladder with diversion of urinary system and resection of colon and rectum with colostomy.
Vaginectomy	Removal of vagina.
Vulvectomy	Removal of part or all the vulva.
• Skinning vulvectomy	Removal of top layer of vulvar skin where the cancer is found. Skin grafts from other parts of the body may be needed to cover the area.
• Simple vulvectomy	Entire vulva is removed.
• Radical vulvectomy	Entire vulva, including clitoris, labia majora and minora, and nearby tissue, is removed. Nearby lymph nodes may be removed.

C

Nursing Management: Cervical Cancer and Other Cancers of the Female Reproductive System

In addition to cervical cancer, malignant tumors of the female reproductive system can be found in the endometrium, ovaries, vagina, and vulva. Management of the patient with any cancer of the female reproductive system includes many similar interventions.

Goals

The patient with a malignant tumor of the female reproductive system will take part in treatment decisions, achieve satisfactory pain and symptom management, recognize and report problems promptly, maintain preferred lifestyle as long as possible, and continue to practice cancer detection strategies.

Nursing Management

Teach women the importance of routine screening for cancers of the reproductive system. Cancer can be prevented when screening reveals precancerous conditions of the vulva, cervix, endometrium, and rarely the ovaries. Assist women to view routine cancer screening as an important self-care activity.

- Teaching women about risk factors for cancers of the reproductive system is important. Limiting sexual activity during adolescence, HPV vaccination against cervical cancer, using condoms, having fewer sexual partners, and not smoking reduce the risk of cervical cancer.

Hysterectomy. Preoperatively, the patient is prepared for surgery with the standard perineal or abdominal preparation. A vaginal douche and enema may be given according to surgeon preference. The bladder should be emptied before the patient is sent to the operating room. An indwelling catheter is often inserted.

- After a hysterectomy, abdominal distention may develop from the sudden release of pressure on the intestines when a large tumor is removed or from paralytic ileus because of anesthesia and pressure on the bowel. Food and fluids may be restricted if the patient is nauseated. Ambulation will help relieve abdominal flatus.
- Initiate venous thromboembolism (VTE) prophylaxis. Apply intermittent pneumatic compression devices and administer anticoagulant therapy. Minimize stasis and pooling of blood with frequent position changes and avoiding the high Fowler's position or pressure under the knees. Pay special attention to patients with varicosities. Encourage leg exercises to promote circulation.
- Teach the patient what to expect after surgery (e.g., she will not menstruate). Intercourse should be avoided until the wound is healed (about 4 to 6 weeks).
- If a vaginal hysterectomy was done, tell the patient that she may have a temporary loss of vaginal sensation which should return in several months.
- Heavy lifting should be avoided for 2 months. Teach the patient to avoid activities that may increase pelvic congestion, such as dancing and walking swiftly, for several months. However, activities, such as swimming, may be both physically and mentally helpful.
- See also eNursing Care Plan 53-1: Patient Having Abdominal Hysterectomy (on the website).

Salpingectomy and Oophorectomy. Postoperative care of the woman who has undergone removal of a fallopian tube (salpingectomy) or an ovary (oophorectomy) is similar to that for any patient having abdominal surgery. When both ovaries are removed (bilateral oophorectomy), surgical menopause results. Symptoms of menopause may be more severe because of the sudden withdrawal of hormones.

Pelvic Exenteration. When other forms of therapy do not control cancer spread and no metastases have been found outside the pelvis, pelvic exenteration may be done. This radical surgery usually involves removal of the uterus, ovaries, fallopian tubes, vagina, bladder, urethra, and pelvic lymph nodes. In some situations, the descending colon, rectum, and anal canal may also be removed. Postoperative care involves that of a patient who has had a radical hysterectomy, an abdominal perineal resection, and an ileostomy or colostomy. Physical, emotional, and social adjustments to life on the part of the woman and her family are great. Changes include urinary or fecal diversions in the abdominal wall, a reconstructed vagina, possible lymphedema, and the onset of menopausal symptoms.

- Much understanding and support are needed from the nursing staff during a long recovery period. Gently encourage the patient to regain independence.

C

CHLAMYDIAL INFECTIONS

Description

Chlamydia trachomatis infection is the most common reportable sexually transmitted infection (STI) in the United States. *Chlamydia,* a gram-negative bacterium, is transmitted through exposure to sexual fluids during vaginal, anal, or oral sex. Ejaculation does not have to occur for it to be transmitted. Numerous different strains of *C. trachomatis* cause urogenital infections (e.g., nongonococcal urethritis [NGU] in men and cervicitis in women), ocular trachoma, and lymphogranuloma venereum.

High-risk groups and risk factors include women and adolescents, new or multiple sexual partners, sexual partners who have had multiple partners, history of STIs and cervical ectopy, coexisting STIs, and inconsistent or incorrect use of a condom.

The incubation period for chlamydia is 1 to 3 weeks. Infection with Chlamydia does not provide protection from reinfection, so people treated for chlamydia can be reinfected.

Clinical Manifestations

Patients with chlamydia often have no symptoms.

- Men may have pain with urination or a urethral discharge. Rarely, men can have pain or swelling of the testicles caused by infection of the epididymis.
- In women, manifestations of cervicitis include mucopurulent discharge (mucus with pus), bleeding, dysuria, and pain with intercourse.

Symptoms of rectal chlamydia include anorectal pain, discharge, bleeding, pruritus, tenesmus, mucus-coated stools, or painful bowel movements.

Complications

Complications often develop from poorly managed, inaccurately diagnosed, or undiagnosed *Chlamydia*.

- In men, rare complications may result in epididymitis with possible infertility.
- In women, infection may result in pelvic inflammatory disease, which damages fallopian tubes and increases the risk for ectopic pregnancy (pregnancy outside of uterus), infertility, and chronic pelvic pain.

Diagnostic Studies

Chlamydia can be diagnosed by collecting urine or swab specimens from the endocervix or vagina (women), urethra (men), oropharynx, or rectum. The most common test is the nucleic acid amplification test (NAAT).

Interprofessional and Nursing Management

Because of the high prevalence of asymptomatic infections, regular screening for *Chlamydia* in high-risk populations is recommended.

Doxycycline (Vibramycin) or azithromycin (Zithromax) is used to treat patients and their partners. Treatment of pregnant women usually prevents transmission to the fetus.

- All sexual contacts within 60 days should be evaluated and treated to prevent reinfection and further transmission.
- Teach patients to abstain from sexual contact for 7 days after treatment, or until all partners have been treated and have also abstained from sexual contact for 7 days.
- Review the ways to reduce risk of acquiring a repeat or new STI in the future.

See Nursing Management: Sexually Transmitted Infections, pp. 547.

CHOLELITHIASIS/CHOLECYSTITIS

Description

The most common disorder of the biliary system is *cholelithiasis* (stones in the gallbladder). The stones may lodge in the neck of the gallbladder or in the cystic duct. *Cholecystitis* (inflammation of the gallbladder) may be acute or chronic, and it is usually associated with gallstones.

Gallbladder disease is a common health problem in the United States. Up to 10% of American adults have cholelithiasis.

- Gallstones are more common in women, especially multiparous women and those older than 40 years of age. Postmenopausal women on estrogen replacement therapy and younger women on oral contraceptives are at an increased risk. Other factors that seem to increase the incidence of gallbladder disease are sedentary lifestyle, familial tendency, and obesity.
- The incidence of gallbladder disease is especially high in Native Americans.

Pathophysiology

The cause of gallstones is unknown. They develop when the balance that keeps cholesterol, bile salts, and calcium in solution changes so that these substances precipitate. Conditions that upset this balance include infection and changes in cholesterol metabolism. Mixed cholesterol stones, which are mainly cholesterol, are the most common.

The stones may stay in the gallbladder or migrate to the cystic duct or common bile duct. They cause pain as they pass through the ducts and may lodge in the ducts and cause obstruction. Stasis of bile in the gallbladder can lead to cholecystitis.

Cholecystitis is most often associated with obstruction from gallstones or biliary sludge. Cholecystitis in the absence of obstruction occurs most often in older adults and patients who are critically ill. Once a calculous cholecystitis is present, secondary infection with enteric pathogens, including *Escherichia coli, Enterococcus faecalis, Klebsiella, Pseudomonas,* and *Proteus,* is common. Perforation occurs in severe cases.

- During an acute attack of cholecystitis, the gallbladder is edematous and hyperemic and it may be distended with bile or pus. The cystic duct may become occluded.
- The wall of the gallbladder becomes scarred after an acute attack. Decreased functioning occurs if large amounts of tissue become fibrotic.

Clinical Manifestations

Severity of symptoms depends on whether the stones are stationary or mobile and whether obstruction is present.

- When a stone is lodged in the ducts or when stones are moving through the ducts, spasms may produce severe pain, termed *biliary colic.* The pain can be accompanied by tachycardia, diaphoresis, and prostration. The severe pain may last up to 1 hour, and when it subsides there is residual tenderness in the right upper quadrant.
- The attacks of pain frequently occur 3 to 6 hours after a high-fat meal or when the patient lies down.

- When total obstruction occurs, symptoms related to bile block-age occur. These include steatorrhea, pruritus, dark amber urine, bleeding tendencies, and jaundice.

Manifestations of cholecystitis vary from indigestion to moderate to severe pain, fever, and jaundice. Initial symptoms include indigestion and pain and tenderness in the right upper quadrant, which may be referred to the right shoulder and scapula. Pain may be acute and is accompanied by restlessness, diaphoresis, and nausea and vomiting.

- Symptoms of chronic cholecystitis include a history of fat intolerance, dyspepsia, heartburn, and flatulence.

Complications

Complications of cholecystitis include gangrenous cholecystitis, subphrenic abscess, pancreatitis, *cholangitis* (inflammation of biliary ducts), biliary cirrhosis, fistulas, and rupture of the gallbladder, which can cause bile peritonitis.

Diagnostic Studies

- Ultrasonography is used to diagnose gallstones.
- Endoscopic retrograde cholangiopancreatography (ERCP) allows for visualization of the gallbladder, cystic duct, common hepatic duct, and common bile duct. Bile taken during ERCP is sent for culture to identify any possible infecting organism.
- Percutaneous transhepatic cholangiography may locate stones in the bile ducts.
- Laboratory tests reveal increased serum enzymes and pancreatic enzymes, increased white blood cell (WBC) count, increased direct and indirect bilirubin levels, and urinary bilirubin.

Interprofessional Management

The treatment of gallstones in cholelithiasis depends on the stage of disease. Bile acids (cholesterol solvents), such as ursodeoxycholic (ursodiol) and chenodeoxycholic (chenodiol), are used to dissolve stones, but the stones may recur. ERCP with sphincterotomy (papillotomy) may be used for stone removal. ERCP allows for visualization of the biliary system, placement of stents, and sphincterotomy.

Extracorporeal shock-wave lithotripsy (ESWL) may be used to treat cholelithiasis. In this procedure, a lithotriptor uses high-energy shock waves to disintegrate gallstones.

Drug therapy for gallbladder disease includes analgesics, anticholinergics (antispasmodics), fat-soluble vitamins, and bile salts. Morphine may be used initially for pain management. Cholestyramine, used to provide relief from pruritus, is a resin that binds bile salts in the intestine, increasing their excretion in the feces.

During an acute episode of cholecystitis, treatment focuses on pain control, control of possible infection with antibiotics, and maintenance of fluid and electrolyte balance. Treatment is mainly supportive and symptomatic. A cholecystostomy may be used to drain purulent material from the obstructed gallbladder.

- If nausea and vomiting are severe, nasogastric (NG) tube insertion and gastric decompression may prevent further gallbladder stimulation.
- Anticholinergics may be administered to decrease secretions and counteract smooth muscle spasms.

Laparoscopic cholecystectomy is the preferred surgical procedure for symptomatic gallstones. The gallbladder is removed through 1 of 4 small punctures in the abdomen. Most patients have minimal postoperative pain and are discharged the day of surgery or the day after. In most cases, they can resume normal activities and return to work within 1 week.

Nursing Management
Goals
The overall goals are that the patient with gallbladder disease will have relief of pain and discomfort, no complications postoperatively, and no recurrent attacks of cholecystitis or gallstones.
Nursing Interventions
Nursing actions for the patient undergoing conservative therapy include relieving pain, relieving nausea and vomiting, providing comfort and emotional support, maintaining fluid and electrolyte balance and nutrition, making accurate assessments to ensure effective treatment, and observing for complications.

The patient with acute cholecystitis or gallstones often has severe pain. Give the drugs ordered to relieve the pain as needed before it becomes more severe. Observe for signs of obstruction of the ducts by stones, including jaundice; clay-colored stools; dark, foamy urine; steatorrhea; fever; and increased WBC count.

Postoperative nursing care after a laparoscopic cholecystectomy includes monitoring for complications, such as bleeding, making the patient comfortable, and preparing the patient for discharge.

- Patients may report referred pain to the shoulder because of the CO_2 that the health care provider (HCP) used to inflate the abdominal cavity during surgery. CO_2 can irritate the phrenic nerve and diaphragm, causing some difficulty breathing. Placing the patient in Sims' position (left side with right knee flexed) helps move the gas pocket away from the diaphragm. Encourage deep breathing, movement, and ambulation.
- If the patient has a T tube, maintain the system drainage and observe for bile drainage.

TABLE 24   Patient & Caregiver Teaching

Postoperative Laparoscopic Cholecystectomy

Include the following instructions in the patient's postoperative teaching plan.
- Remove the bandages on the puncture site the day after surgery, and you can shower.
- Notify your surgeon if any of the following signs and symptoms occurs:
  - Redness, swelling, bile-colored drainage or pus from any incision
  - Severe abdominal pain, nausea, vomiting, fever, chills
- You can gradually resume normal activities.
- Return to work within 1 week of surgery.
- You can resume your usual diet, but a low-fat diet is usually better tolerated for several weeks after surgery.

▼ **Patient and Caregiver Teaching**
- When the patient has conservative therapy, teach about a diet is low in fat. The patient may need to take fat-soluble vitamin supplements. If needed, review a weight-reduction diet.
- Teach the patient indications of biliary obstruction (stool and urine changes, jaundice, and pruritus).
- The patient who undergoes a laparoscopic cholecystectomy is discharged soon after the surgery, so home care and teaching are important (Table 24).

CHRONIC OBSTRUCTIVE PULMONARY DISEASE

Description

Chronic obstructive pulmonary disease (COPD) is a preventable, treatable, but often progressive disease characterized by persistent airflow limitation. COPD is associated with an enhanced inflammatory response in the airways and lungs, primarily caused by cigarette smoking and other noxious particles and gases. Previous definitions of COPD encompassed 2 types of obstructive airway disease, emphysema and chronic bronchitis, but neither term is part of the current definition of COPD.

More than 16 million people in the United States have COPD. Cardiovascular diseases often occur along with COPD, because smoking is a primary risk factor for both.

- *Emphysema* is the destruction of the alveoli without fibrosis. The term explains only 1 of several structural abnormalities in COPD.

- *Chronic bronchitis,* the presence of cough and sputum production for at least 3 months in each of 2 consecutive years, is an independent disease that may precede or follow the development of airflow limitation.
- People with COPD may have asthma. Asthma may be a risk factor for the development of COPD. There is a considerable overlap between these disorders, particularly among older adults, who may have components of both diseases. This disorder is called *asthma-COPD overlap syndrome.*

Etiology

Many factors influence the development and progression of COPD.

- Cigarette smoking is the major risk factor for developing COPD. It affects about 20% of smokers. The irritating effect of cigarette smoke causes hyperplasia of cells, which increases mucus production. Hyperplasia reduces airway diameter and makes it harder to clear secretions. Smoking reduces ciliary activity and destroys alveolar walls.
- *Passive smoking* is the exposure of nonsmokers to cigarette smoke, also known as *environmental tobacco smoke* (ETS) or secondhand smoke. In adults, ETS is associated with decreased pulmonary function, increased respiratory symptoms, and severe lower respiratory tract infections (e.g., pneumonia). ETS is associated with increased risk for nasal sinus cancer and lung cancer.
- High levels of urban air pollution are harmful to people with existing lung disease.
- If a person has intense or prolonged exposure to various dusts, vapors, irritants, or fumes in the workplace, symptoms of lung impairment consistent with COPD can develop. If a person has occupational exposure and smokes, the risk of COPD increases.
- Another risk factor is exposure to coal and other biomass fuels used for indoor heating and cooking.
- Severe recurring respiratory tract infections in childhood have been associated with reduced lung function and increased respiratory symptoms in adulthood. It is unclear whether the development of COPD is related to recurrent infections in adults.
- Asthma may be a risk factor for COPD development.
- Genetic factors influence which smokers get the disease. α_1-*Antitrypsin (AAT) deficiency* is a genetic risk factor for COPD. The main function of AAT, an α_1-protease inhibitor, is to protect normal lung tissue from attack by proteases during inflammation related to cigarette smoking and infections.

Pathophysiology

COPD is characterized by chronic inflammation of the airways, lung parenchyma (respiratory bronchioles and alveoli), and pulmonary blood vessels. The pathogenesis of COPD is complex and involves many mechanisms. The defining feature of COPD is airflow limitation not fully reversible during forced exhalation. This is caused primarily by loss of elastic recoil and airflow obstruction caused by mucus hypersecretion, mucosal edema, and bronchospasm.

The inflammatory process starts with inhalation of noxious particles (e.g., cigarette smoke) that causes the release of inflammatory mediators that damage lung tissue.

- The predominant inflammatory cells are neutrophils, macrophages, and lymphocytes. These cells attract other inflammatory mediators (e.g., leukotrienes) and proinflammatory cytokines (e.g., tumor necrosis factor).
- After the inhalation of oxidants in tobacco or air pollution, protease activity (which breaks down the connective tissue of the lungs) increases and antiproteases (which protect against the breakdown) are inhibited.
- Inability to expire air is the main characteristic of COPD. As the peripheral airways become obstructed, air is progressively trapped during expiration. The chest hyperexpands and becomes barrel shaped since the respiratory muscles are not able to function effectively.
- Gas exchange abnormalities result in hypoxemia and hypercapnia (increased CO_2). As air trapping increases and alveoli are destroyed, bullae (large air spaces in the parenchyma) and blebs (air spaces adjacent to pleurae) form. There is a significant ventilation-perfusion (V/Q) mismatch, and hypoxemia results.
- Excess mucus production, resulting in a chronic productive cough, is caused by an increased number of mucus-secreting goblet cells, enlarged submucosal glands, dysfunction of cilia, and stimulation from inflammatory mediators.
- Pulmonary vascular changes resulting in mild to moderate pulmonary hypertension may occur late in the course of COPD.

Clinical Manifestations

COPD typically develops slowly. A diagnosis of COPD should be considered in a patient with chronic cough or sputum production, dyspnea, and a history of exposure to risk factors for the disease (e.g., tobacco smoke, occupational dusts and chemicals).

- A chronic intermittent cough, often the first symptom to develop, may later be present every day.

- Dyspnea with exertion is often progressive. In the late stages, dyspnea may be present at rest. Wheezing and chest tightness vary by time of the day or from day to day, especially in patients with more severe disease.
- The patient with advanced COPD often has fatigue, anorexia, and weight loss.
- During physical examination, a prolonged expiratory phase, wheezes, or decreased breath sounds are noted in all lung fields. The anterior-posterior diameter of the chest is increased *(barrel chest)* from chronic air trapping. The patient may assume a tripod position and use pursed-lip breathing.
- Over time, hypoxemia may develop with hypercapnia. The bluish-red color of the skin results from polycythemia and cyanosis. Polycythemia develops from increased production of red blood cells as the body tries to compensate for chronic hypoxemia.

Complications

Cor pulmonale results from pulmonary hypertension. In COPD, pulmonary hypertension is caused mainly by constriction of pulmonary vessels in response to alveolar hypoxia and acidosis. Chronic hypoxia also stimulates erythropoiesis, which causes polycythemia. This results in increased viscosity of the blood. When pulmonary hypertension develops, the pressure on the right side of the heart must increase to push blood into the lungs. Eventually right-sided heart failure develops (see Cor Pulmonale, p. 150).

A *COPD exacerbation* is the acute worsening of the patient's usual patterns of dyspnea, cough, and/or sputum production. The main causes of exacerbations are bacterial or viral infections. Exacerbations are common and increase in frequency (averaging 1–2 per year) as the disease progresses.

- Teach the patient and caregiver early recognition of the cardinal symptoms of exacerbations (increase in dyspnea, sputum volume, or sputum purulence) to promote early treatment and thus prevent hospitalization and possible acute respiratory failure.
- Other complaints include malaise, insomnia, increased wheezing, fatigue, depression, confusion, fever, and decreased exercise tolerance. Exacerbations are managed with short-acting bronchodilators, oral systemic corticosteroids, and antibiotics.

Acute respiratory failure may occur in patients with severe COPD who have exacerbations. Be alert for signs of increasing severity, such as use of accessory muscles, central cyanosis, edema in the lower extremities, unstable BP, right-sided heart failure, and altered alertness. Often, patients with COPD wait too long to contact a health care provider (HCP) after first experiencing symptoms suggesting an exacerbation. Stopping bronchodilator or corticosteroid medications may also precipitate respiratory failure. (Respiratory failure is discussed in Chapter 67, Harding et al., *Lewis' Medical-Surgical Nursing,* ed 11.)

Diagnostic Studies

- A forced expiratory volume in 1 minute/forced vital capacity ratio (FEV_1/FVC) $< 70\%$ along with the appropriate symptoms can help diagnose COPD. A lower value of FEV_1 indicates more severe COPD.
- A history and physical examination are extremely important in the diagnostic workup.
- Chest x-rays may show a flat diaphragm because of hyperinflation of lungs.
- Electrocardiogram (ECG) can be used to determine right- and left-sided ventricular failure.
- Sputum culture and sensitivity are done during an acute exacerbation.
- Arterial blood gases (ABGs) in later stages usually indicate low partial pressure of oxygen in arterial blood (PaO_2), elevated partial pressure of carbon dioxide in arterial blood ($PaCO_2$), decreased or low normal pH, and increased bicarbonate (HCO_3^-) levels.

Interprofessional Management

Most patients with COPD are treated as outpatients. They are hospitalized for an acute exacerbation or a complication, such as pneumonia, heart failure, or acute respiratory failure.

Evaluate the patient's exposure to environmental or occupational irritants, and determine ways to control or avoid them. The person with COPD and anyone who smokes should receive an influenza immunization yearly. The pneumococcal vaccine is recommended for patients with COPD and smokers 19 years of age or older.

- Treat exacerbations of COPD as soon as possible, especially if the patient is in the severe stages.
- Stopping cigarette smoking can have the biggest impact on reducing the risk of developing COPD and on decreasing progression of the disease in any stage of COPD. Smoking cessation techniques are discussed in Chapter 10 of Harding et al., *Lewis' Medical-Surgical Nursing,* ed 11.

Drugs for COPD can reduce symptoms, increase exercise capacity, improve overall health, and reduce the number and severity of exacerbations. Drugs are stepped up but usually not stepped down, as in asthma, because in COPD continual symptoms are probably present.

- Bronchodilator drugs commonly used are β_2-adrenergic agonists, anticholinergic agents, and methylxanthines (see Table 28.7, Harding et al., *Lewis' Medical-Surgical Nursing,* ed 11). When the patient has mild COPD or intermittent symptoms, a short-acting bronchodilator is used as needed. In the moderate stage of COPD, a long-acting bronchodilator is also used.
- In patients with COPD associated with an $FEV_1 < 60\%$, regular treatment with inhaled corticosteroids (ICSs) is often prescribed with a long-acting β-agonist (LABA). Examples of combinations of ICSs with LABAs are fluticasone/salmeterol (Advair) and budesonide/formoterol (Symbicort).
- Roflumilast (Daliresp) is an oral medication used to decrease the frequency of exacerbations in patients with severe COPD and chronic bronchitis. This drug is a phosphodiesterase inhibitor. It is an antiinflammatory agent that suppresses the release of cytokines and other inflammatory mediators and inhibits the production of reactive oxygen radicals.

Long-term continuous (more than 15 hr/day) O_2 therapy (LTOT) increases survival and improves exercise capacity and mental status in hypoxemic patients with COPD (see Oxygen Therapy, p. 697).

The main types of breathing exercises commonly taught are pursed-lip breathing and diaphragmatic breathing. Patients with moderate to severe COPD and marked hyperinflation may be poor candidates for diaphragmatic breathing.

Airway clearance techniques loosen mucus and secretions for clearance by coughing. A variety of treatments can be used to achieve airway clearance. Respiratory therapists, physical therapists, and nurses are involved in performing these techniques. See Chapter 28 of Harding et al., *Lewis' Medical-Surgical Nursing,* ed 11, for more information on airway clearance techniques.

- Weight loss and muscle wasting are common in the patient with severe COPD. To decrease dyspnea and conserve energy, the patient should rest at least 30 minutes before eating and use a bronchodilator before meals. A diet high in calories and protein, moderate in carbohydrates, and moderate to high in fat is recommended. Food can be divided into 5 or 6 small meals a day.

Surgical Therapy

Four different surgical procedures have been used in severe COPD. One type of surgery is *lung volume reduction surgery,* which is done to reduce the size of the lungs by removing the most diseased lung tissue so that the remaining healthy lung tissue can perform better. A second procedure, *bronchoscopic lung volume reduction surgery*, involves placing one-way valves in the airways. The valves let air out of diseased parts of the lung, but not in. Another surgical procedure is a *bullectomy*, which is used for patients with emphysematous COPD who have large bullae (>1 cm). The bullae are usually resected via thoracoscope. A fourth surgical procedure is *lung transplantation,* which benefits carefully selected patients with advanced COPD.

Nursing Management

Goals

The overall goals are that the patient with COPD will have relief from symptoms, ability to perform activities of daily living (ADLs) and improved exercise tolerance, no complications related to COPD, knowledge and ability to implement a long-term treatment plan, prevention of disease progression, and overall improved quality of life.

See eNursing Care Plan 28-2 (available on the website) for specific goals related to the care of the patient with COPD.

Nursing Interventions

Counsel the patient regarding smoking cessation, because it is the only way to slow the progression of COPD. Avoiding or controlling exposure to occupational and environmental pollutants and irritants is another preventive measure to maintain healthy lungs. Early diagnosis and treatment of respiratory tract infections and COPD exacerbations help prevent progression of the disease.

- Patients with COPD should avoid people who are sick, practice good hand-washing techniques, take drugs as prescribed, exercise regularly, and maintain a healthy weight. Influenza and pneumococcal vaccines are recommended.
- The patient with COPD needs acute intervention for exacerbations of COPD, pneumonia, cor pulmonale, and acute respiratory failure.

▼ Patient and Caregiver Teaching

Teaching is the most important aspect of long-term care of the patient with COPD (Table 25). In pulmonary rehabilitation (PR), an interprofessional team works to individualize the treatment plan for the patient with COPD.

- Components of PR vary but usually include exercise training, smoking cessation, nutrition counseling, and teaching.
- Other important topics include health promotion, psychologic counseling, and vocational rehabilitation. Smoking cessation is critical.

Energy conservation is an important component in COPD rehabilitation. Exercise training of the upper extremities may improve muscle function and reduce dyspnea. Alternative energy-saving practices for ADLs and scheduled rest periods should be planned.

- Walking or other endurance exercises (e.g., cycling) combined with strength training are the best interventions to strengthen muscles and improve the patient's endurance. Teach the patient

TABLE 25   Patient and Caregiver Teaching

Chronic Obstructive Pulmonary Disease (COPD)

Include the following information in the teaching plan to assist the patient with COPD and the caregiver to improve quality of life through promoting lifestyle practices that support successful living with COPD.

What Is COPD?

- Basic anatomy and physiology of lung
- Basic pathophysiology of COPD
- Signs and symptoms of COPD, exacerbation
- How to tell COPD from the common cold, flu, pneumonia
- Tests to assess breathing

C

Breathing and Airway Clearance Exercises

- Pursed-lip breathing (see Table 28.12, Harding et al., *Lewis' Medical-Surgical Nursing*, ed 11)
- Airway clearance technique—huff cough (see Table 28.21, Harding et al., *Lewis' Medical-Surgical Nursing*, ed 11)

Energy Conservation Techniques

- Daily activities (e.g., bathing, grooming, shopping, traveling)
- Consultation with physical therapist and occupational therapist

Medications

- Types (include mechanism of action and types of devices)
- Establishing medication schedule
- Correct use of inhalers, spacer, and nebulizer
- Reason for use of O_2 equipment
- Guide for home O_2 use and equipment

Psychosocial/Emotional Issues

Open discussion (sharing with patient, caregiver, and family)

- Concerns about interpersonal relationships (e.g., intimacy)
- Problems with emotions (e.g., depression, anxiety, panic)
- Dependency

Treatment decisions

Support and rehabilitation groups

COPD Management Plan

Nurse and patient develop and write up COPD management plan that meets individual needs.

- Focus on self-management
- Need to report changes
- Cause of acute exacerbations

Continued

| TABLE 25   Patient and Caregiver Teaching |

Chronic Obstructive Pulmonary Disease (COPD)—cont'd

- Recognition of signs and symptoms of respiratory infection, heart failure
- Reduce risk factors, especially smoking cessation
- Exercise program of walking and arm strengthening
- Yearly follow-up evaluations

Healthy Nutrition (see Table 28.22 in Harding et al., Lewis' Medical-Surgical Nursing, ed 11)

- Ways to lose or gain weight, as appropriate
- Consultation with dietitian

For more information, see American Lung Association at *www.lung. org/lung-disease/copd.*

coordinated walking with slow, pursed-lip breathing. Encourage the patient to walk 15 to 20 minutes/day at least 3 times a week, with gradual increases.
- Modifying sexual activity can contribute to a healthy psychologic well-being. Using an inhaled bronchodilator before sexual activity can help ventilation.
- Adequate sleep is extremely important. The patient who is a restless sleeper, snores, stops breathing while asleep, and has a tendency to fall asleep during the day may need to be tested for sleep apnea.
- Healthy coping is a challenge for the patient and family. As the disease progresses, patients with COPD frequently have to deal with lifestyle changes that may involve decreased ability to care for themselves, decreased energy for social activities, and loss of a job. Support groups at local chapters of the American Lung Association, hospitals, and clinics may be helpful.

CIRRHOSIS

Description

Cirrhosis, the end stage of liver disease, is characterized by the extensive degeneration and destruction of liver cells. The most common causes of cirrhosis in the United States are chronic hepatitis C infection and alcohol-induced liver disease.

- Malnutrition, biliary obstruction, right-sided heart failure, and chronic liver diseases, such as nonalcoholic fatty liver disease (NAFLD), also cause cirrhosis. NAFLD can be a complication of metabolic syndrome (see Metabolic Syndrome, p. 401).
- Biliary causes of cirrhosis include primary biliary cirrhosis and primary sclerosing cholangitis. Primary sclerosing cholangitis is a chronic inflammatory condition affecting the liver and bile ducts.

Pathophysiology

Damaged liver cells try to regenerate, but a disorganized process results in abnormal blood vessel and bile duct architecture. The overgrowth of new and fibrous connective tissue distorts the liver's normal lobular structure, resulting in lobules of irregular size and shape with impeded blood flow and poor function.

Clinical Manifestations

Patients may be unaware of their liver condition because there are few symptoms in early-stage disease. Early symptoms may include fatigue or an enlarged liver. Later manifestations may be severe and result from liver failure and portal hypertension. Jaundice, peripheral edema, and ascites develop gradually. Other late signs and symptoms include skin lesions, hematologic and endocrine problems, and peripheral neuropathies. In advanced stages, the liver becomes small and nodular. (See Fig. 3 for systemic clinical manifestations of cirrhosis.)

- *Jaundice* occurs because of the decreased ability of the liver to conjugate and excrete bilirubin.
- *Skin lesions*, such as *spider angiomas*, that occur on the nose, cheeks, upper trunk, and neck and a redness of the palms of the hands, known as "palmar erythema," are from an increase in circulating estrogen because the liver cannot metabolize steroid hormones.
- *Hematologic disorders*, such as anemia, leukopenia, and thrombocytopenia, may be caused by splenomegaly that results from backup of blood from the portal vein into the spleen (portal hypertension). Coagulation problems result from the liver's inability to produce prothrombin and other essential clotting factors.
- *Endocrine problems* result because adrenocortical hormones, estrogen, and testosterone cannot be metabolized by a damaged liver. Men lose masculine sex characteristics as a result of increased estrogen levels, and amenorrhea may occur in younger women. Hyperaldosteronism causes sodium and water retention and potassium loss.

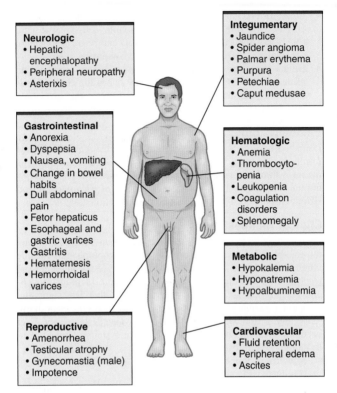

Fig. 3 Systemic clinical manifestations of liver cirrhosis.

- *Peripheral neuropathy* is probably caused by a dietary deficiency of thiamine, folic acid, and cobalamin.

Complications

Major complications of cirrhosis are portal hypertension with resultant esophageal and/or gastric varices, peripheral edema, abdominal ascites, hepatic encephalopathy (coma), and hepatorenal syndrome.

Structural changes from cirrhosis obstruct blood flow in and out of the liver, causing *portal hypertension,* an increased pressure within the liver's circulatory system, and *esophageal* and *gastric varices.*

- Collateral channels often form in the lower esophagus, anterior abdominal wall, parietal peritoneum, and rectum. Varicosities develop where collateral and systemic circulations join, resulting in esophageal and gastric varices, *caput medusae* (ring of varices around the umbilicus), and hemorrhoids.

- *Esophageal varices* are a complex of tortuous veins at the end of the esophagus. *Gastric varices* are found in the upper part of the stomach. These fragile collateral vessels tolerate high pressure poorly, and bleed easily.
- Bleeding esophageal varices are the most life-threatening complication of cirrhosis. Patients may have melena or hematemesis. There may be slow oozing or massive bleeding, which is a medical emergency.

Peripheral edema occurs in the lower extremities and presacral area. Peripheral edema results from decreased colloidal osmotic pressure from impaired liver synthesis of albumin and increased portacaval pressure from portal hypertension.

Ascites is the accumulation of serous fluid in the peritoneal or abdominal cavity by 3 mechanisms. The first mechanism is portal hypertension which causes proteins to move from the blood vessels into the lymph space and then leak into the peritoneal cavity. A second mechanism is fluid shifting because of hypoalbuminemia and decreased colloidal oncotic pressure, which results from the liver's inability to synthesize albumin. A third mechanism is hyperaldosteronism, which results when aldosterone is not metabolized by damaged hepatocytes, causing increased renal reabsorption of sodium and water.

- Ascites is manifested by abdominal distention with weight gain. In severe ascites, the umbilicus may be everted. Abdominal striae with distended abdominal wall veins may be present.
- Patients may have signs of dehydration (e.g., dry tongue and skin, sunken eyeballs, muscle weakness) and decreased urinary output.
- Hypokalemia is common and is caused by an excessive loss of potassium from hyperaldosteronism and the use of diuretic therapy to treat ascites.

Hepatic encephalopathy is a neuropsychiatric manifestation of liver disease. When blood is shunted past the liver by way of collateral vessels or the liver is unable to convert ammonia to urea, the levels of ammonia in the systemic circulation rise. Ammonia crosses the blood-brain barrier and produces toxic neurologic manifestations.

- Factors that increase ammonia in the circulation include GI hemorrhage, constipation, infection, hypokalemia, hypovolemia, dehydration, and metabolic alkalosis.
- Hepatic encephalopathy causes changes in neurologic and mental responsiveness, ranging from sleep problems to trouble concentrating to deep coma. *Asterixis* (flapping tremors), is a

rapid flexion and extension movement of the hands when the arms and hands are held stretched out.

Hepatorenal syndrome is a type of renal failure with advancing azotemia, oliguria, and intractable ascites.

- There is no structural abnormality of the kidneys. Portal hypertension along with liver decompensation results in splanchnic and systemic vasodilation and decreased arterial blood volume. As a result, renal vasoconstriction occurs and renal failure follows.
- In the patient with cirrhosis, this syndrome frequently follows diuretic therapy, GI hemorrhage, or paracentesis.

Diagnostic Studies

- Liver function studies demonstrate an elevation in alkaline phosphatase, aspartate aminotransferase (AST), alanine aminotransferase (ALT), and γ-glutamyl transferase (GGT).
- Prothrombin time is prolonged. Serum albumin and protein levels are decreased and bilirubin and globulin levels are increased.
- Ultrasound elastography and biopsy (percutaneous needle) can help determine severity of cirrhosis.

Interprofessional Management

The goal of treatment is to slow the progression of cirrhosis and prevent and treat any complications. Management of ascites focuses on sodium restriction (2 g/day), diuretic therapy (e.g., a potassium-sparing diuretic combined with a loop diuretic), and fluid removal (paracentesis) for those patients with impaired respiration or abdominal pain.

The main goal related to esophageal varices is to prevent bleeding and hemorrhage. The patient who has esophageal varices should avoid ingesting alcohol, aspirin, and nonsteroidal antiinflammatory drugs (NSAIDs). Patients with varices at risk of bleeding may take a nonselective β-adrenergic blocker (nadolol [Corgard] or propranolol [Inderal]) to decrease high portal pressure.

- When variceal bleeding occurs, the first step is to stabilize the patient and manage the airway. IV therapy may include blood products. A combination of drug therapy and endoscopic therapy is more successful than either approach alone. Drug therapy may include somatostatin analog octreotide (Sandostatin) or vasopressin.
- At the time of endoscopy, band ligation or sclerotherapy may be used to prevent varices from rebleeding. Balloon tamponade may be used to control hemorrhage that cannot be controlled on initial endoscopy.

- Supportive measures during an acute variceal bleed include giving fresh frozen plasma and packed red blood cells (RBCs), vitamin K, and proton pump inhibitors (e.g., pantoprazole [Protonix]). Lactulose and rifaximin (Xifaxan) may be administered to prevent hepatic encephalopathy from breakdown of blood and the release of ammonia in the intestine. Antibiotics are given to prevent bacterial infection.

Transjugular intrahepatic portosystemic shunt (TIPS) is a procedure where a catheter is placed in the jugular vein to create a tract (shunt) between the systemic and portal venous systems. This redirects portal blood flow, reduces portal venous pressure, and decompresses the varices, thus controlling bleeding and alleviating ascites. Shunting procedures tend to be used more after a second major bleeding episode than during an initial bleeding episode.

The goal of management of hepatic encephalopathy is to reduce ammonia formation. Lactulose, a drug that traps ammonia in the gut, reduces ammonia formation in the intestines. We can give it orally, as an enema, or through a nasogastric (NG) tube. The drug's laxative effect expels the ammonia from the colon. Antibiotics, such as rifaximin, may also be given, particularly in patients who do not respond to lactulose.

Specific nutritional therapy varies with the degree of liver damage and the danger of encephalopathy; generally, the diet is high in calories (3000 cal/day) and carbohydrates with sodium restricted. Protein restriction is rarely needed in patients with cirrhosis and persistent hepatic encephalopathy. For many patients, malnutrition is a more serious clinical problem than hepatic encephalopathy.

Nursing Management
Goals
The patient with cirrhosis will have relief of discomfort, have minimal to no complications (ascites, esophageal varices, hepatic encephalopathy), and return to as normal a lifestyle as possible.
Nursing Interventions
Prevention and early treatment of cirrhosis focus on reducing or eliminating risk factors.

- Urge patients to abstain from alcohol. Encourage those with a chronic alcohol use history to enroll in support programs that help patients maintain sobriety.
- Adequate nutrition is essential to promote liver regeneration.
- Identify and treat acute hepatitis early so that it does not progress to chronic hepatitis and cirrhosis.

Nursing care for the patient with cirrhosis focuses on conserving the patient's strength while maintaining muscle strength. Modify the activity and rest schedule according to signs of clinical improvement (e.g., decreasing jaundice, improvement in liver function studies).

- Anorexia, nausea and vomiting, pressure from ascites, and poor eating habits all interfere with adequate intake of nutrients. Make between-meal snacks available. Offer preferred foods when possible.
- Assess the patient for progression of jaundice and pruritus. Check urine and stool color.
- Record intake and output, daily weights, and measurements of extremities and abdominal girth to help monitor edema.
- A semi-Fowler's or Fowler's position allows for maximal respiratory efficiency when dyspnea is a problem. Use pillows to support arms and chest.
- When the patient is taking diuretics, monitor serum electrolyte levels.
- Meticulous skin care is needed because edematous tissues are subject to breakdown. Use an alternating air pressure mattress or other special mattress. Adhere to a turning schedule (minimum of every 2 hours). Support the abdomen with pillows.
- Have the patient void immediately before a paracentesis to prevent bladder puncture. After the procedure, monitor for hypovolemia and electrolyte changes. Check the dressing for bleeding and leakage.
- Observe for signs of bleeding from esophageal or gastric varices, such as hematemesis and melena. If hematemesis occurs, assess the patient for hemorrhage, call the health care provider (HCP), and be ready to assist with treatments to control bleeding.

▼ Patient and Caregiver Teaching

Explain that cirrhosis is a chronic illness and requires continual health care. Teach the symptoms of complications and when to seek medical attention to enable prompt treatment.

- Teach the patient to avoid potentially hepatotoxic over-the-counter drugs, because the diseased liver is unable to metabolize them.
- Encourage abstinence from alcohol because continued use increases the rate of liver disease progression and risk of liver complications.
- Instruct the patient with esophageal or gastric varices to avoid aspirin and NSAIDs to prevent hemorrhage.
- Teach the patient with portal hypertension and varices that straining at stool, coughing, sneezing, and retching and vomiting may increase the risk of variceal hemorrhage.

COLORECTAL CANCER

Description

Of cancers that affect both men and women, colorectal cancer (CRC) is the third leading cause of cancer-related deaths and the third most common cancer in men and women. CRC is more common in men. Mortality rates are highest among black men and women. The risk of CRC increases with age, with about 90% of new cases detected in people older than 50 years.

Pathophysiology

No single risk factor accounts for most cases of CRC. The risk is highest in people with first-degree relatives with CRC and people with inflammatory bowel disease (IBD). About 20% of cases occur in patients with a family history of CRC.

About 30% to 50% of people with CRC have an abnormal *KRAS* gene. The *KRAS* gene, which is primarily involved in regulating cell division, belongs to a class of genes known as *oncogenes*. When mutated, oncogenes have the potential to cause normal cells to become cancerous.

- Maintaining a healthy weight, being physically active, limiting alcohol use, not smoking, and eating a diet with large amounts of fruits, vegetables, and grains may decrease the risk of CRC.

CRC usually starts as a polyp that on the inner lining of the colon or rectum that grows over a period of 10 to 20 years. Most polyps are adenomas, which arise from the cells that make mucus. As the tumor grows, the cancer invades and penetrates the wall of colon or rectum. Eventually cancer cells gain access to the lymph nodes and vascular system and spread to distant sites. Since venous blood leaving the colon and rectum flows through the portal vein and the inferior rectal vein, the liver is a common site of metastasis. The cancer spreads from the liver to other sites, including the lungs, bones, brain, and adjacent structures.

Clinical Manifestations and Complications

CRC develops slowly, and symptoms do not appear until the disease is advanced. Common manifestations include iron-deficiency anemia, rectal bleeding, abdominal pain, and change in bowel habits. (See Fig. 4.)

- Early disease: none or nonspecific findings (fatigue, weight loss).
- More advanced disease: abdominal tenderness, palpable abdominal mass, hepatomegaly, ascites.

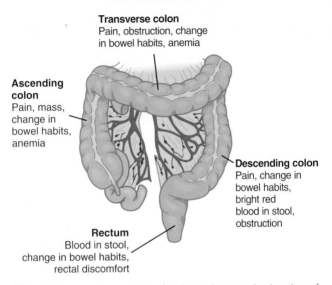

Transverse colon
Pain, obstruction, change
in bowel habits, anemia

**Ascending
colon**
Pain, mass,
change in
bowel habits,
anemia

Descending colon
Pain, change in
bowel habits,
bright red
blood in stool,
obstruction

Rectum
Blood in stool,
change in bowel habits,
rectal discomfort

Fig. 4 Signs and symptoms of colorectal cancer by location of
primary cancer.

Bleeding can occur with both right- and left-sided CRC. Bleeding
on the right side is more common than the left side. It is often unrecognized and an early manifestation is often anemia. Hematochezia
(fresh blood in the stool) is more often caused by left-sided CRC
than right-sided CRC.

Right-sided cancers are more likely to cause diarrhea. Left-sided
cancers are usually detected later and could present with bowel
obstruction Complications of CRC include obstruction, bleeding,
perforation, peritonitis, and fistula formation.

Diagnostic Studies

Because cancer symptoms do not become evident until the disease is
advanced, regular screening is advocated to detect and remove
polyps before they become cancerous. Beginning at age 45 years,
both men and women at average risk for developing CRC should
have screening tests to detect both polyps and cancer based on 1
of these testing schedules:

- flexible sigmoidoscopy (every 5 years)
- colonoscopy (every 10 years)
- double-contrast barium enema (every 5 years)
- CT colonography (virtual colonoscopy) (every 5 years)

Tests that primarily find cancer include the following:
- high sensitivity fecal occult blood test (FOBT) (every year), or
- fecal immunochemical test (FIT) (every year)
- stool deoxyribonucleic acid (DNA) test (every 3 years)

Complete blood count (CBC), coagulation studies, and liver function tests are done when the diagnosis is confirmed by colonoscopy and biopsy.
- CT scan or MRI of abdomen and pelvis is used to detect liver metastases.
- Carcinoembryonic antigen (CEA) serum test is used as a baseline to follow the progress of the patient after surgery or chemotherapy.

Interprofessional Management

Prognosis and treatment correlate with the pathologic staging of the disease. The TNM staging system is the most commonly used method to stage the tumor (see p. 761, Part Three). Prognosis worsens with greater size and depth of tumor, lymph node involvement, and metastasis.

Surgical Therapy

Surgical goals include complete resection of the tumor with adequate margins of healthy tissue, a thorough exploration of the abdomen to detect spread, removal of all lymph nodes that drain the cancer area, restoration of bowel continuity so that normal bowel function will return, and prevention of surgical complications.
- Polypectomy during colonoscopy can be used to resect CRC in situ.
- The site of the tumor determines the site of the resection (e.g., right hemicolectomy, left hemicolectomy).
- Surgery for stage I cancer includes removal of the tumor and at least 5 cm of intestine on either side of the tumor, plus removal of nearby lymph nodes. The remaining cancer-free ends are sewn back together. Laparoscopic surgery is sometimes used for stage I tumors, especially those in the left colon.
- Low-risk stage II tumors are treated with wide resection and reanastomosis, but chemotherapy is used in addition to surgery for high-risk stage II tumors.
- Stage III tumors are treated with surgery and chemotherapy.

In treating rectal cancer, there are 3 major options: (1) local excision, (2) abdominal-perineal resection (APR) with a permanent colostomy, and (3) low anterior resection (LAR) to preserve sphincter function. The surgical decision is based on the location and stage of the cancer and the likelihood of restoring normal bowel function and continence. Most patients with rectal cancer require APR or LAR.

Chemotherapy and Targeted Therapy

Chemotherapy can be used to shrink the tumor before surgery, as adjuvant therapy after colon resection, and as palliative treatment for nonresectable disease (see Chemotherapy, p. 674). Current protocols include varying doses of fluorouracil and leucovorin alone or in combination with oxaliplatin (Eloxatin) or irinotecan (Camptosar). The preferred protocol includes oxaliplatin. Oral fluoropyrimidines (e.g., capecitabine [Xeloda]) in combination with oxaliplatin are an alternative to fluorouracil/leucovorin.

Several targeted therapies have a role in treating metastatic CRC. Angiogenesis inhibitors, which inhibit the blood supply to tumors, include aflibercept (Zaltrap), bevacizumab (Avastin), and ramucirumab (Cyramza). Cetuximab (Erbitux) and panitumumab (Vectibix) block the epidermal growth factor receptor. These drugs are often given with a combination chemotherapy regimen (e.g., fluorouracil/leucovorin/oxaliplatin).

Regorafenib (Stivarga) is a multikinase inhibitor that blocks several enzymes that promote cancer growth. It, or Lonsurf, a combination of trifluridine and tipiracil, are given to patients with metastatic CRC who are no longer responding to other therapies. Trifluridine impairs DNA function and angiogenesis. Tipiracil prevents the rapid metabolism of trifluridine, thus increasing its bioavailability.

Radiation Therapy

Radiation therapy may be used as an adjuvant to surgery and chemotherapy or as a palliative measure for patients with metastatic cancer. As a palliative measure, its primary goal is to reduce tumor size and provide symptomatic relief (see Radiation Therapy, p. 712).

Nursing Management

Goals

The patient with CRC will have normal bowel elimination patterns, quality of life appropriate to disease progression, relief of pain, and feelings of comfort and well-being.

Nursing Interventions

Encourage patients older than 50 years to have regular screening for CRC. Help identify those at high risk who need screening at an earlier age.

- Endoscopic and radiographic procedures can only reveal polyps when the bowel has been adequately prepared. Provide teaching about bowel cleansing for outpatient diagnostic procedures, and give cleansing preparations to inpatients.

Preoperative Care. Nursing care for patients with a colon resection is similar to care for patients undergoing a laparotomy (see Abdominal Pain, Acute, p. 3). Patients who have had an APR will have a permanent ostomy. Provide emotional support to cope with the diagnosis of cancer and the impending changes in body appearance and function.

Postoperative Care. Many patients have immediate reanastomosis of bowel and require general postoperative care. Patients with more extensive surgery (e.g., APR) may have an open wound and drains and a permanent stoma.

Postoperative care includes sterile dressing changes, care of drains, and patient and caregiver teaching about the stoma. Consult with a wound, ostomy, and continence nurse (WOCN) before surgery to select the ostomy site on the abdomen, and then provide follow-up care and teaching.

- A patient who has open and packed wounds requires meticulous postoperative care. Reinforce dressings and change them frequently during the first several hours postoperatively. Carefully assess all drainage for amount, color, and consistency. Examine the wound regularly and record bleeding, excessive drainage, and unusual odor.
- The patient may have phantom rectal sensation because the sympathetic nerves responsible for rectal control are not severed during the surgery. Assess to distinguish phantom sensations from the pain of a developing perineal abscess.
- Sexual problems are a possible complication of APR. Although the likelihood of sexual problems depends on the surgical technique used, the surgeon should discuss the possibility with the patient.

▼ **Patient and Caregiver Teaching**
- Patients with colostomies need to know how to care for them.
- Teach about diet, incontinence products, and strategies for managing bloating, diarrhea, and bowel evacuation.
- Patients undergoing sphincter-sparing surgery may need antidiarrheal drugs or bulking agents to control diarrhea. A dietitian should help the patient choose foods that are less likely to cause diarrhea.
- Teach the patient and caregiver about community resources and services available for assistance.

CONJUNCTIVITIS

Conjunctivitis is an infection or inflammation of the conjunctiva. Conjunctivitis may be caused by bacteria or viruses. Inflammation can result from exposure to allergens or chemical irritants. The tarsal conjunctiva (lining of the lid's interior surface) may become inflamed from a long-term foreign body in the eye, such as a contact lens. See Table 26 for a comparison of clinical manifestations and management of the different types of conjunctivitis.

TABLE 26 Types of Conjunctivitis

Description	Clinical Manifestations	Management
Bacterial		
• Acute bacterial conjunctivitis (pinkeye) • More common in children • *Staphylococcus aureus* is most common cause.	• Discomfort, pruritus, redness, mucopurulent drainage • Generally spreads to unaffected eye	• Usually self-limiting, but antibiotic drops will shorten course. • Careful hand washing • Individual or disposable towels help prevent spread
Viral		
• Caused by many different viruses • Adenovirus conjunctivitis contracted by direct contact and in contaminated swimming pools	• Tearing, foreign body sensation, redness, mild photophobia • Usually mild and self-limiting but can be severe with increased discomfort and subconjunctival hemorrhaging	• Treatment is palliative, ice packs and dark glasses • Topical corticosteroids for temporary relief
Chlamydial		
• *Chlamydia trachomatis* serotypes A-C cause trachoma, a major cause of blindness worldwide.	• Mucopurulent ocular discharge, irritation, redness, lid swelling	• Antibiotic therapy • Patients with AIC have a high risk of concurrent chlamydial genital infection

- Adult inclusion conjunctivitis (AIC) caused by *C. trachomatis* serotypes D-K is increasing with rise in chlamydial infections. AIC does not lead to blindness

Allergic

- Conjunctivitis may develop after exposure to pollens, animal dander, ocular solutions, contact lenses, or other allergens.

- Itching (defining symptom), burning, redness, and tearing

and other sexually transmitted infections (STIs). Refer for STI testing and treatment.

- Artificial tears to dilute allergen and wash from eye
- Topical antihistamines and corticosteroids
- Teach to avoid known allergens.

C

CONSTIPATION

Description

Constipation is characterized by difficult or infrequent bowel movements, often accompanied by excessive exertion during defecation or a feeling of incomplete evacuation. Constipation is a symptom, not a disease. It can be acute, usually lasting < 1 week, or chronic, lasting over 3 months.

Risk factors associated with chronic constipation include a low fiber diet, decreased physical activity, or ignoring the defecation urge. Ignoring the urge to defecate for a prolonged period can cause the muscles and mucosa of the rectum to become insensitive to the presence of feces. In addition, the prolonged retention of feces results in drying of stool because of water absorption. The harder and drier the feces, the harder it is to expel. Emotions, including anxiety, depression, and stress, affect the GI tract and can contribute to constipation.

Clinical Manifestations

Constipation varies from a mild discomfort to a more severe acute event mimicking an "acute abdomen." Stools are absent or hard, dry, and difficult to pass. Abdominal distention, bloating, increased flatulence, and a sensation of increased rectal pressure may be present.

- Hemorrhoids are a common complication of chronic constipation. They result from venous engorgement resulting from repeated Valsalva maneuvers (straining) and venous compression from hard impacted stool (see Hemorrhoids, p. 283).
- In the presence of obstipation (severe constipation with no passage of gas or stool) or fecal impaction secondary to constipation, colonic perforation may occur. Perforation, which is life-threatening, causes abdominal pain, nausea, vomiting, fever, and a high white blood cell (WBC) count.

Diagnostic Studies

In most patients, the diagnosis of constipation is based on findings from a thorough history and physical examination.

- Diagnostic testing may include abdominal x-rays, barium enema, colonoscopy, sigmoidoscopy, rectal balloon expulsion test, anorectal manometry, defecography with barium or fluoroscopy, and colonic transit tests.

Interprofessional Management

Increasing dietary fiber, fluid intake, and exercise can prevent many cases of constipation. Laxatives and enemas are an option. All promote bowel movements, but each class works differently. Which one a patient receives depends on the severity and duration of the constipation and the patient's health.

- Daily bulk-forming laxatives (psyllium) can prevent constipation because they work like dietary fiber and do not cause dependence.
- In patients with chronic constipation who do not respond to diet and lifestyle modifications, osmotic laxatives are the next recommended treatment.
- Stimulant laxatives are given to patients who do not respond to osmotic laxatives.
- Methylnaltrexone (Relistor) and naloxegol (Movantik) are peripherally acting opioid receptor antagonists that reduce constipation caused by opioid use.
- Enemas are fast-acting and beneficial for immediate treatment of constipation but must be used cautiously.

Biofeedback therapy may benefit patients who are constipated as a result of anismus (uncoordinated contraction of the anal sphincter during straining). A patient with severe constipation related to a motility or mechanical disorder may require more intensive treatment, including surgery.

Nursing Management

Encourage patients to exercise the abdominal muscles and contract the abdominal muscles several times each day. Sit-ups and straight-leg raises can improve abdominal muscle tone.

- Teach the patient and caregiver the importance of diet and activity to prevent constipation. Stress a high-fiber diet, increased fluid intake, and a regular exercise program.
- Teach the patient to establish a regular time to defecate and not suppress the urge.
- Discourage the patient from using laxatives and enemas.

Defecation is easiest when the person is sitting on a commode with the knees higher than the hips. The sitting position allows gravity to aid defecation, and flexing the hips straightens the angle between the anal canal and the rectum so that stool is expelled more easily.

- Place a footstool in front of the toilet to promote flexion of the thighs.
- For a patient in bed sitting on a bedpan, elevate the head of the bed as high as the patient can tolerate. Provide as much privacy as possible and offer an odor eliminator.

COR PULMONALE

Description

Cor pulmonale is enlargement of the right ventricle (RV) caused by a primary disorder of the respiratory system. Cor pulmonale may be present with or without overt cardiac failure.

- The most common cause of cor pulmonale is chronic obstructive pulmonary disease (COPD) (see p. 126). Almost any disorder that affects the respiratory system can cause cor pulmonale.

Clinical Manifestations and Diagnostic Tests

- Manifestations are often masked by the symptoms of the pulmonary condition. Common signs and symptoms include exertional dyspnea, tachypnea, cough, and fatigue.
- Physical signs include evidence of right ventricular hypertrophy on the electrocardiogram (ECG) and increased intensity of the second heart sound. Chronic hypoxemia leads to polycythemia and increased total blood volume and viscosity of the blood.
- If heart failure accompanies cor pulmonale, manifestations include peripheral edema, weight gain, distended neck veins, full bounding pulse, and enlarged liver.

Diagnostic tests may include arterial blood gases (ABGs), arterial O_2 saturation by pulse oximetry (SpO_2), b-type natriuretic peptide (BNP) level, ECG, chest x-ray, CT scan, MRI, and cardiac catheterization.

Nursing and Interprofessional Management

Early identification is essential before irreversible changes to the heart develop. Management is directed at treating the underlying pulmonary problem. Long-term O_2 therapy to correct the hypoxemia reduces vasoconstriction and pulmonary hypertension.

- Fluid, electrolyte, and acid-base imbalances must be corrected. Diuretics and a low-sodium diet decrease plasma volume and reduce the heart's workload. Diuretics must be used with extreme caution. In some cases, decreases in fluid volume from diuresis can worsen heart function.
- Bronchodilator therapy is needed if the underlying respiratory problem is caused by an obstructive disorder.
- Other treatments include those for pulmonary hypertension, such as vasodilator therapy, calcium-channel blockers, and anticoagulants.

Nursing management of cor pulmonale resulting from COPD is similar to that described for COPD (see pp. 132).

CORONARY ARTERY DISEASE

Description

Coronary artery disease (CAD) is a type of blood vessel disorder that is included in the general category of atherosclerosis. *Atherosclerosis* is derived from 2 Greek words: *athero,* meaning "fatty mush," and *skleros,* meaning "hard." It can occur in any artery in the body. When the atheromas (fatty deposits) form in the coronary arteries, the disease is called *CAD*.

- The terms *arteriosclerotic heart disease (ASHD)*, *cardiovascular heart disease (CVHD)*, *ischemic heart disease (IHD)*, and *coronary heart disease (CHD)* are other terms used to describe CAD.
- Cardiovascular disease is the major cause of death in the United States. CAD is the most common type of cardiovascular disease and accounts for the majority of these deaths.
- Patients with CAD may be asymptomatic or develop *chronic stable angina (chest pain).*
- CAD may evolve to the more serious conditions of unstable angina (UA) and myocardial infarction (MI), which are referred to as "acute coronary syndrome" (ACS). (See Acute Coronary Syndrome, p. 5.)

Fig. 1 on p. 6 shows the relationship among the clinical manifestations of CAD.

Risk factors for CAD are grouped as nonmodifiable or modifiable (Table 27).

Pathophysiology

Atherosclerosis is characterized by lipid deposits within the intima of the artery. Inflammation and endothelial injury play a central role in the development of atherosclerosis.

- The endothelial lining can be injured by tobacco use, hyperlipidemia, hypertension, diabetes, hyperhomocystinemia, and infection causing a local inflammatory response.
- C-reactive protein (CRP), a protein produced by the liver, is a nonspecific marker of systemic inflammation. It is increased in many patients with CAD.
- CAD takes many years to develop. When the patient becomes symptomatic, the disease process is usually well advanced. Stages of development in atherosclerosis are: (1) fatty streak, (2) fibrous plaque resulting from smooth muscle cell proliferation, and (3) complicated lesion.

Normally some arterial anastomoses or connections, called *collateral circulation,* exist within the coronary circulation (Fig. 5).

C

TABLE 27 Risk Factors for Coronary Artery Disease (CAD)	
Nonmodifiable Risk Factors	**Modifiable Risk Factors**
<ul><li>Increasing age</li><li>Gender (highest incidence of CAD is among middle-aged men, but for men over age 45 yrs and women over age 55 yrs, the risk of CAD increases for both genders)</li><li>Ethnicity (more common in white than black men)</li><li>Genetic predisposition and family history of heart disease</li></ul>	**Major**<ul><li>Serum lipids:<ul><li>Total cholesterol >200 mg/dL</li><li>Triglycerides ≥150 mg/dL[a]</li><li>LDL cholesterol >130 mg/dL</li><li>HDL cholesterol <40 mg/dL in men or <50 mg/dL in women[a]</li></ul></li><li>BP > 120/80 mm Hg[a]</li><li>Diabetes</li><li>Tobacco use</li><li>Physical inactivity</li><li>Obesity: Waist circumference ≥102 cm (≥40 in) in men and ≥88 cm (≥35 in) in women[a]</li></ul>**Contributing**<ul><li>Diabetes</li><li>Psychosocial risk factors (e.g., depression, hostility</li><li>High homocysteine levels</li><li>Substance abuse</li></ul>

[a]Three or more of these risk factors meet the criteria for metabolic syndrome. Metabolic syndrome is discussed in Chapter 40 of Harding et al., *Lewis' Medical-Surgical Nursing*, ed 11.

HDL, High-density lipoprotein; *LDL*, low-density lipoprotein.

- When blockages in coronary arteries occur over a long period, there is a greater chance of collateral circulation developing, and the heart muscle may still receive adequate blood and oxygen.
- With rapid-onset CAD, there is not enough time to develop collateral circulation. Reduced blood flow results in more severe ischemia or infarction.

Clinical Manifestations

CAD is a progressive disease. Patients may be asymptomatic for many years or may develop chronic stable angina. When the demand

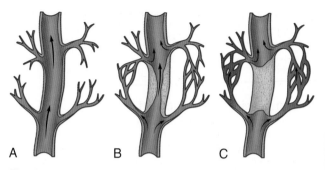

Fig. 5 Vessel occlusion with collateral circulation. (A) Open, functioning coronary artery. (B) Partial coronary artery closure, with collateral circulation being established. (C) Total coronary artery occlusion with collateral circulation bypassing the occlusion to supply blood to the myocardium.

C

for myocardial oxygen exceeds the ability of the coronary arteries to supply the heart with oxygen, myocardial ischemia occurs.

- *Angina,* or chest pain, is a symptom of reversible myocardial ischemia. The primary reason for insufficient blood flow is narrowing of coronary arteries by atherosclerosis.
- Chronic stable angina refers to chest pain that occurs intermittently over a long period with the same pattern of onset, duration, and intensity of symptoms (see Angina, Chronic Stable, p. 45).

When ischemia is prolonged and not immediately reversible, ACS develops and encompasses the spectrum of UA, non–ST-segment-elevation myocardial infarction (NSTEMI), and ST-segment-elevation myocardial infarction (STEMI) (see Fig. 1 on p. 6).

Diagnostic Studies

- Chest x-ray to detect cardiac enlargement, cardiac calcifications, and pulmonary congestion.
- The 12-lead electrocardiogram (ECG) detects heart rhythm, pacemaker activity, conduction abnormalities, heart position, atrial and ventricular size, and ischemia/injury/infarction.
- Serum lipid levels to screen for risk factors.
- Exercise or stress testing to detect ST-segment and T wave changes that indicate ischemia with exercise.
- Ambulatory 24- to 48-hour ECG monitoring to identify silent ischemia.
- Nuclear imaging studies to determine myocardial perfusion, contractility, and ejection fraction.

- Positron emission tomography (PET) to identify and quantify ischemia and infarction.
- Angiography studies to visualize coronary arteries and help determine treatment and prognosis.
- Echocardiography with exercise to diagnose coronary artery stenosis.

Interprofessional Management

People who have modifiable risk factors should be encouraged to make lifestyle changes to prevent, modify, or slow CAD progression. Lifestyle changes, including a low-saturated-fat, high-fiber diet; avoiding tobacco; and increase in physical activity, can promote regression in the course of coronary atherosclerosis and a reduction in coronary events.

- A physical activity program should be designed to improve physical fitness by following the FITT formula: *f*requency (how often), *i*ntensity (how hard), *t*ype (isotonic), and *t*ime (how long). Everyone should aim for at least 30 minutes of moderate physical activity on most days of the week. The American Heart association (AHA) encourages people to increase their daily physical activity and lower the chance of developing heart disease simply by walking.
- Dietary recommendations focus on ways to lower low-density lipoprotein (LDL) cholesterol. They emphasize a decrease in saturated fat and cholesterol and an increase in complex carbohydrates (e.g., whole grains, fruit, vegetables) and fiber.

Drug Therapy

People with serum cholesterol levels higher than 200 mg/dL are at risk for CAD. Treatment usually begins with dietary caloric restriction (if overweight), decreased dietary fat and cholesterol intake, and increased physical activity. Serum lipid levels are reassessed after 6 weeks of diet therapy. If they remain elevated, additional dietary options and drug therapy may be considered. The statin drugs are the most widely used lipid-lowering drugs. •Guidelines for the treatment of high cholesterol recommend that the following groups of people receive statin therapy: (1) patients with known cardiovascular disease (CVD), (2) patients with primary elevations of LDL cholesterol levels to 190 mg/dL or greater (e.g., familial hypercholesterolemia), (3) patients between 40 and 75 years of age with diabetes and LDL cholesterol levels between 70 and 189 mg/dL, and (4) patients between 40 and 75 years of age with LDL cholesterol levels between 70 and 189 mg/dL and a 10-year risk for CVD of at least 7.5%.

Statin drugs inhibit the synthesis of cholesterol in the liver by blocking hydroxymethylglutaryl coenzyme A (HMG-CoA) reductase. Examples include lovastatin, pravastatin (Pravachol), simvastatin (Zocor), fluvastatin (Lescol), atorvastatin (Lipitor), and rosuvastatin (Crestor). These drugs primarily lower LDL cholesterol and increase high-density lipoprotein (HDL). Niacin, a water-soluble B vitamin, also interferes with the synthesis of LDL and triglyceride levels.

Fibric acid derivatives, such as gemfibrozil (Lopid), are effective in lowering very-low-density lipoprotein (VLDL) levels and triglycerides, while increasing HDL levels. Drugs that increase lipoprotein removal by increasing conversion of cholesterol to bile acids include cholestyramine, colestipol (Colestid), and colesevelam (Welchol). Ezetimibe (Zetia) inhibits the absorption of dietary and biliary cholesterol. It may be combined with a statin to promote greater reductions in LDL.

- PCSK9 inhibitors are a newer class of cholesterol-lowering drugs. Examples are evolocumab (Repatha) and alirocumab (Praluent), given subcutaneously every 2 weeks. They are used in addition to diet and maximum statin therapy for adults with familial hypercholesterolemia and for patients intolerant of statin drugs.
- Drug therapy for hyperlipidemia often continues for a lifetime. Diet modification minimizes the need for drug therapy.

Antiplatelet therapy with low-dose aspirin (81 mg) is recommended for people who have CAD and for most people at risk for CAD unless contraindicated (e.g., history of GI bleeding). People who are aspirin-intolerant may consider taking clopidogrel (Plavix).

Nursing Management

Management of CAD risk factors in CAD may prevent, modify, or slow the disease progression. of the disease. Risk screening involves obtaining a thorough health history. Question the patient about a family history of heart disease in parents and siblings. Note any cardiovascular symptoms.

Assess environmental factors, such as eating habits, type of diet, and level of exercise, to identify lifestyle patterns. Include a psychosocial history to determine tobacco use, alcohol intake, recent life-stressing events (e.g., loss of a spouse), and the presence of any negative psychologic states (e.g., anxiety, depression, anger). The place and type of employment provide important information on the kind of activity performed, exposure to pollutants or noxious chemicals, and the degree of stress associated with work.

- Identify patient attitudes and beliefs about health and illness that may relate to misconceptions about risks and treatment of heart disease.

- Knowing the patient's educational background and health literacy is helpful for planning a teaching approach.
- Encourage the patient to make lifestyle choices that decrease cardiac risk factors.

CROHN'S DISEASE

Crohn's disease is an autoimmune disorder that, along with ulcerative colitis, is referred to as *inflammatory bowel disease* (IBD). See Inflammatory Bowel Disease, p. 337, for a discussion of the disorder.

CUSHING SYNDROME

Description
Cushing syndrome is a clinical condition that results from chronic exposure to excess corticosteroids, particularly glucocorticoids. The most common cause of Cushing syndrome is iatrogenic administration of *exogenous* corticosteroids (e.g., prednisone). About 85% of the cases of *endogenous* Cushing syndrome are caused by an adrenocorticotropic hormone (ACTH)–secreting pituitary tumor *(Cushing disease)*. Less common causes of Cushing syndrome include adrenal or other tumors.

Clinical Manifestations
Manifestations are seen in most body systems related to excess levels of corticosteroids. Although signs of glucocorticoid excess usually predominate, symptoms of mineralocorticoid and androgen excess can occur.
- Corticosteroid excess causes pronounced changes in physical appearance. Weight gain, the most common feature, results from an accumulation of adipose tissue in the trunk (centripetal obesity), face ("moon face"), and cervical areas ("buffalo hump").
- Hyperglycemia occurs because of glucose intolerance associated with cortisol-induced insulin resistance and increased gluconeogenesis by the liver.
- Muscle wasting leads to muscle weakness, especially in the extremities.
- Loss of bone protein matrix leads to osteoporosis with pathologic fractures (e.g., vertebral compression fractures) and bone and back pain.

- Loss of collagen makes the skin weaker, thinner, and easier to bruise. Purplish-red striae appear on the abdomen, breast, or buttocks.
- Mineralocorticoid excess may cause hypertension, whereas adrenal androgen excess may cause pronounced acne, with hirsutism and menstrual disorders in women.

Diagnostic Studies
- Plasma cortisol levels may be elevated without diurnal variation.
- A 24-hour urine collection for free cortisol is done. Urine cortisol levels higher than 100 mcg/24 hours in adults indicate Cushing syndrome. If these results are borderline, a low-dose dexamethasone suppression test is done.
- High or normal plasma ACTH levels indicate Cushing disease, while low or undetectable levels indicate an adrenal or medication cause.
- Other findings on diagnostic tests associated with Cushing syndrome include hyperglycemia, hypokalemia, glycosuria, hypercalciuria, and osteoporosis.
- CT scan and MRI of the pituitary and adrenal glands may be done.

Interprofessional Management
The primary goal is to normalize hormone secretion. The standard treatment for a pituitary adenoma is surgical removal of the pituitary tumor using the transsphenoidal approach. Radiation therapy may be used for patients who are not good surgical candidates. Adrenalectomy is indicated for adrenal tumors or hyperplasia. Patients with ectopic ACTH-secreting tumors (usually located in the lung or pancreas) are also treated surgically.

- When the patient is a poor candidate for surgery or prior surgery has failed, then drug therapy may be tried. The goal of drug therapy is inhibition of adrenal function (medical adrenalectomy). Drugs that inhibit corticosteroid synthesis include ketoconazole and mitotane.

If Cushing syndrome has developed because of prolonged administration of corticosteroids (e.g., prednisone), the following alternatives may be tried: (1) gradually discontinuing corticosteroid therapy, (2) reducing corticosteroid dose, and (3) converting to alternate-day dosing.

Nursing Management
Goals
The patient with Cushing syndrome will have relief of symptoms with no serious complications, maintain a positive self-image, and actively take part in the therapeutic plan.

Nursing Interventions

Therapy for Cushing syndrome has many side effects, so assessment focuses on signs and symptoms of hormone and drug toxicity and complicating conditions (e.g., cardiovascular disease, diabetes, infection).

- Monitor vital signs, glucose, and daily weights.
- Assess for pain, loss of function, and purulent drainage. Signs and symptoms of inflammation (e.g., fever, redness) may be absent.
- Monitor for signs of thromboembolic phenomena, such as sudden chest pain, dyspnea, and tachypnea.

Another important focus of nursing care is providing emotional support. Changes in appearance, such as truncal obesity, bruising, hirsutism in females, and gynecomastia in males, can be distressing. Remain sensitive to the patient's feelings and offer respect and unconditional acceptance. Reassure the patient that the physical changes and much of the emotional lability will resolve when hormone levels return to normal.

If treatment involves surgical removal of a pituitary adenoma, an adrenal tumor, or one or both adrenal glands, nursing care will include preoperative and postoperative care.

Preoperative Care. Before surgery, hypertension and hyperglycemia need to be controlled, with hypokalemia corrected by diet and potassium supplements. A high-protein meal plan helps correct protein depletion. Preoperative teaching should include information about the expected postoperative care.

Postoperative Care. Because of hormone fluctuations, the patient's BP, fluid balance, and electrolyte levels tend to be unstable after surgery. High doses of corticosteroids (hydrocortisone) are administered IV during surgery and for several days afterward to ensure adequate responses to the stress of the procedure.

- Report any rapid or significant changes in BP, respirations, or heart rate (HR).
- Carefully monitor fluid intake and output and assess for potential imbalance.
- If corticosteroid dosage is tapered too rapidly after surgery, acute adrenal insufficiency may develop. Vomiting, increased weakness, dehydration, and hypotension are signs of hypocortisolism. The patient may have painful joints, pruritus, or peeling skin and may have severe emotional problems.
- After surgery, the patient usually remains on bed rest until the BP stabilizes.
- Be alert for subtle signs of postoperative infections. Provide meticulous care when changing the dressing and during procedures that involve access to body cavities, circulation, or areas under skin.

▼ **Patient and Caregiver Teaching**

Discharge instructions are based on the patient's lack of endogenous cortisol and resulting inability to react physiologically to stressors. Lifetime replacement therapy is required for many patients. It may take several months to satisfactorily adjust the hormone dose.

- Teach patients to always wear a medical identification (Medic Alert) bracelet and carry instructions in a wallet or purse. Teach the patient to avoid exposure to extreme temperatures, infections, and emotional situations.
- Stress may precipitate acute adrenal insufficiency because the remaining adrenal tissue cannot meet an increased hormonal demand. Teach patients to adjust their corticosteroid replacement in accordance with stress levels.
- If the patient cannot adjust their own medication or if weakness, fainting, fever, or nausea and vomiting occur, the patient should contact the health care provider (HCP).

CYSTIC FIBROSIS

Description

Cystic fibrosis (CF) is an autosomal recessive, multisystem disease characterized by altered function of the exocrine glands involving primarily the lungs, pancreas, biliary tract, and reproductive tract.

Severity and progression of CF vary. With early diagnosis and improvements in therapy, the prognosis has been significantly improved. The median predicted survival in 1970 was for 16 years, but has increased to more than 37 years.

Pathophysiology

CF results from mutations in a gene found on chromosome 7 that produces a protein called CF transmembrane regulator (CFTR). CFTR regulates sodium and chloride channels in the epithelial surface of the airways, pancreatic ducts, and sweat gland ducts. Mutations in the *CFTR* gene alter the CFTR in such a way that the channel is blocked.

- Cells that line the passageways of the lungs, pancreas, and other organs make abnormally thick, sticky mucus. This mucus plugs up the ducts, ultimately resulting in organ failure.
- The hallmark of respiratory involvement is its effect on the airways. The disease progresses from being a disease of the small airways *(chronic bronchiolitis)* to involving the larger airways, and finally destroys lung tissue. CF is also characterized by persistent airway infection that cannot be eradicated. Lung disorders

include chronic bronchiolitis and bronchiectasis, blebs, large cysts, and hemoptysis from erosion of pulmonary arteries.

- Pancreatic insufficiency is caused by mucus plugging the pancreatic duct, which results in atrophy of the gland and progressive fibrotic cyst formation. Because the pancreatic digestive enzymes cannot reach the intestine, malabsorption of nutrients occurs. Fat malabsorption results in steatorrhea, and protein malabsorption results in failure to grow and gain weight.
- CF-related diabetes results from fibrotic scarring of the pancreas.

Clinical Manifestations

Manifestations vary depending on the disease severity. Carriers are not affected by the gene mutation. Median age at diagnosis of CF is 5 months.

- In the adult, a common symptom is frequent cough that becomes persistent and produces viscous, purulent sputum.
- Over time exacerbations (increased cough and sputum, weight loss) become frequent, bronchiectasis worsens, and the recovery of lost lung function is less complete, which may ultimately lead to respiratory failure.
- Affected persons have delayed puberty. Affected women may be infertile.
- Pneumothorax is an uncommon but serious complication caused by the formation of bullae and blebs. CF-related diabetes, bone disease, and liver disease are additional complications.

Diagnostic Studies

- Sweat chloride test (pilocarpine iontophoresis method) is the gold standard for diagnosing CF. Persons with CF excrete 4 times the normal amount of sodium and chloride in their sweat.
- A genetic test is often used if the results from a sweat test are uncertain.

Nursing and Interprofessional Management

A team should be involved in the care of a patient with CF, including a nurse, physician, respiratory and physical therapists, dietitian, and social worker. Goals for the patient with CF include adequate airway clearance, reduced risk factors associated with respiratory infections, adequate nutritional support, ability to perform activities of daily living (ADLs), recognition and treatment of complications, and active participation in a therapeutic regimen. Management is focused on relieving airway obstruction and controlling infection.

- Agents that degrade the DNA in CF sputum (e.g., inhaled dornase alfa [Pulmozyme]) increase airflow and reduce the number

of acute exacerbations. Inhaled hypertonic saline (7%) increases osmolality, allowing water to collect on airway surfaces. It is effective in clearing mucus and decreases the frequency of exacerbations.
■ Airway clearance techniques include chest physiotherapy (CPT), positive expiratory pressure (PEP) devices, and breathing exercises. Drainage of thick bronchial mucus is assisted by aerosol and nebulization treatments that dilate the airways, liquefy mucus, and promote clearance.
■ The use of antibiotics should be carefully guided by sputum culture results.

Management of pancreatic insufficiency includes pancreatic enzyme replacement (e.g., pancrelipase [Pancreaze, Creon, Ultresa, Viokace, Zenpep]) administered before each meal and snack. Fat-soluble vitamins need to be supplemented. Added dietary salt is needed when sweating is excessive during hot weather, in the presence of fever, or from intense physical activity. Hyperglycemia may require treatment with insulin.

■ Aerobic exercise also seems to be effective in clearing airways.
■ There is a higher incidence of depression among persons with CF. Issues such as fertility, decreased life expectancy, costs of health care, and career choices may lead to depression.

▼ Patient and Caregiver Teaching
■ Sexuality is an important issue to discuss with the young adult. Delayed development of secondary sex characteristics and menses is common.
■ Genetic counseling is appropriate for those considering having children.
■ Living with a chronic disease can be emotionally overwhelming. Community resources and the Cystic Fibrosis Foundation may be helpful.

DEMENTIA

Description
Dementia is a disorder characterized by a decline from previous level of function in 1 or more cognitive domains: complex attention, executive function, language, learning and memory, perceptual-motor, and social cognition. The cognitive decline interferes with ability to function and perform daily activities. This decline does not occur with onset of an acute state of confusion, such as delirium, or the onset of another major mental disorder, such as depression.

- There are many causes of dementia. Alzheimer's disease (AD) is the most common form.
- As the average life span increases, the number of patients diagnosed with dementia is increasing. In 2018, 5.7 million Americans over age 65 years were living with AD. It is expected this number will reach 14 million by 2050.

Pathophysiology

The 2 most common causes of dementia are neurodegenerative conditions (e.g., AD) and vascular disorders. Dementia is sometimes caused by treatable conditions that initially may be reversible, such as vitamin B_1 and B_{12} deficiencies, thyroid disorders, subarachnoid hemorrhage, prescribed drugs (e.g., anticholinergics, hypnotics), cocaine, alcohol use, and head injury. However, with prolonged exposure or disease, irreversible changes may occur.

Vascular dementia is loss of cognitive function resulting from ischemic or hemorrhagic brain lesions caused by cardiovascular disease. Vascular dementia may be caused by a single stroke (infarct) or by multiple strokes.

Clinical Manifestations

Dementia associated with neurologic degeneration is often gradual and progressive. Vascular dementia often results in a more abrupt onset and progression.

- An acute (days to weeks) or subacute (weeks to months) pattern of change may indicate an infectious or metabolic cause of dementia, including encephalitis, meningitis, hypothyroidism, or drug-related dementia.

Other clinical manifestations of dementia are discussed with AD (see Alzheimer's Disease, pp. 22).

Diagnostic Studies

- Comprehensive medical, neurologic, and psychologic histories help in determining the presence and cause of dementia.
- Physical examination and neuroimaging techniques (CT or MRI) may be performed to rule out some causes of dementia.
- Dementia is often diagnosed when 2 or more brain functions, such as memory loss or language skills, are significantly impaired.

Nursing and Interprofessional Management

Management of dementia is similar to management of the patient with AD (see Alzheimer's Disease, pp. 22). One form of dementia, vascular dementia, can often be prevented. Preventive measures include treatment of risk factors such as hypertension, diabetes, smoking, hypercholesterolemia, and dysrhythmias. Drugs that are used for patients with AD are also useful for patients with vascular dementia.

DIABETES INSIPIDUS

Description

Diabetes insipidus (DI) is caused by a deficiency of production or secretion of antidiuretic hormone (ADH) or a decreased renal response to ADH. The decrease in ADH results in fluid and electrolyte imbalances caused by increased urine output and increased plasma osmolality. Depending on the cause, DI may be transient or a lifelong condition.

There are several types of DI. *Central DI* (also known as *neurogenic DI*) results from an interference with ADH synthesis, transport, or release. Causes include brain tumor or surgery, central nervous system (CNS) infections, and head injury. It is the most common form of DI.

Nephrogenic DI occurs when there is adequate ADH, but there is a decreased response to ADH in the kidney. Causes include drug therapy (especially lithium), renal damage, and hereditary renal disease.

Psychogenic DI, a less common condition, is associated with excessive water intake. This can be caused by a structural lesion in the thirst center or a psychologic disorder.

Clinical Manifestations

The main characteristic of DI is large quantities of urine (2 to 20 L/day) with a very low specific gravity (<1.005) and urine osmolality (100 mOsm/kg). Serum osmolality is increased as a result of hypernatremia, which is caused by pure water loss in the kidney.

- Most patients compensate for fluid loss by drinking great amounts of water (polydipsia) so that serum osmolality is normal or only moderately increased. The patient may be tired from nocturia and may have generalized weakness.
- Central DI is usually acute and accompanied by excess fluid loss.
- Although the clinical manifestations of nephrogenic DI are similar, the onset and amount of fluid losses are less dramatic than with central DI.

- Severe dehydration can result if oral fluid intake cannot keep up with urinary losses. This is manifested by poor tissue turgor, hypotension, tachycardia, and hypovolemic shock.
- The patient may also show CNS manifestations ranging from irritability and mental dullness to coma, which are related to rising serum osmolality and hypernatremia. Uncorrected hypernatremia can cause brain shrinkage and intracranial bleeding.

Diagnostic Studies

- Water deprivation test distinguishes central DI from nephrogenic DI. Patients with central DI exhibit a dramatic increase in urine osmolality with this test, from 100 to 600 mOsm/kg, and a significant decrease in urine volume. The patient with nephrogenic DI is not able to increase urine osmolality to >300 mOsm/kg.
- Measuring ADH levels after an analog of ADH (e.g., desmopressin [DDAVP]) is given also distinguishes central DI from nephrogenic DI. If the cause is central DI, the kidneys will respond to the hormone by concentrating urine. If the kidneys do not respond in this way, the cause is nephrogenic.

Nursing and Interprofessional Management

Management of the patient with DI includes early detection, maintenance of adequate hydration, and patient teaching for long-term management. A therapeutic goal is maintaining fluid and electrolyte balance.

For central DI, fluid and hormone therapy are needed. Fluids are replaced orally or IV, depending on the patient's condition. Monitor serum glucose levels because hyperglycemia and glucosuria can lead to osmotic diuresis, which increases the fluid volume deficit.

- Monitor level of consciousness, BP, heart rate, and urine output and specific gravity hourly in the acutely ill patient.
- Maintain an accurate record of intake and output and daily weights to determine fluid volume status.
- Desmopressin (DDAVP), a synthetic analog of ADH, is the hormone replacement of choice for central DI. Other ADH replacement drugs include aqueous vasopressin.

Treatment for nephrogenic DI revolves around dietary measures (low-sodium diet) and thiazide diuretics. Limiting sodium intake to no more than 3 g/day often helps decrease urine output. When a low-sodium diet and thiazide drugs are not effective, indomethacin may be prescribed. Indomethacin, a nonsteroidal antiinflammatory drug (NSAID), helps increase renal responsiveness to ADH.

DIABETES MELLITUS

Description

Diabetes mellitus (DM) is a chronic multisystem disease characterized by hyperglycemia from abnormal insulin production, impaired insulin use, or both. Currently in the United States, an estimated 29.1 million people, or 9.3% of the population, have DM, and 86 million people have prediabetes. About 8.1 million people with DM are unaware that they have the disease.

- Diabetes is the leading cause of adult blindness, end-stage renal disease, and nontraumatic lower limb amputations.
- Adults with diabetes have heart disease death rates and risk for strokes that are 2 to 4 times higher than adults without diabetes.
- The 2 most common types of diabetes are type 1 DM and type 2 DM (Table 28).

Type 1 Diabetes Mellitus

Type 1 DM, formerly known as "juvenile-onset diabetes" or "insulin-dependent diabetes mellitus" (IDDM), accounts for approximately 5% to 10% of all cases of diabetes. This type generally affects people younger than 40 years of age, although it can occur at any age.

Pathophysiology. Type 1 diabetes is an autoimmune disorder in which the body develops antibodies against insulin and/or the pancreatic β-cells that produce insulin. This eventually results in insufficient insulin for survival.

- A genetic predisposition and exposure to a virus may contribute to the pathogenesis of immune-related type 1 diabetes.

Once the pancreas can no longer make enough insulin to maintain normal glucose, the onset of symptoms is usually rapid.

- The patient usually has a history of recent and sudden weight loss and the classic symptoms of *polydipsia* (excessive thirst), *polyuria* (frequent urination), and *polyphagia* (excessive hunger).
- The person with type 1 diabetes requires a supply of insulin from an outside source *(exogenous insulin)* to sustain life. Without insulin, the patient develops *diabetes-related ketoacidosis* (DKA), a life-threatening condition resulting in metabolic acidosis.

Type 2 Diabetes Mellitus

Type 2 DM was formerly known as "adult-onset diabetes mellitus" (AODM) or "non–insulin-dependent diabetes mellitus" (NIDDM). This type accounts for 90% to 95% of person with diabetes.

Pathophysiology. In type 2 diabetes, the pancreas continues to produce some endogenous (self-made) insulin. However, the body

TABLE 28	Comparison of Type 1 and Type 2 Diabetes Mellitus	
Factor	Type 1 Diabetes Mellitus	Type 2 Diabetes Mellitus
Age at onset	More common in young people but can occur at any age	More common in adults but can occur at any age. Incidence increasing in children
Type of onset	Signs and symptoms usually abrupt, but disease process may be present for several years	Insidious, may go undiagnosed for years
Prevalence	Accounts for 5%–10% of all types of diabetes	Accounts for 90%–95% of all types of diabetes
Endogenous insulin	Absent	Initially increased in response to insulin resistance. Secretion decreases over time
Environmental factors	Virus, toxins	Obesity, lack of exercise
Islet cell antibodies	Often present at onset	Absent
Primary defect	Absent or minimal insulin production	Insulin resistance, decreased insulin production over time, and changes in adipokines production
Symptoms	Polydipsia, polyuria, polyphagia, fatigue, weight loss without trying	Often none. Fatigue, recurrent infections. May also have polyuria, polydipsia, and polyphagia
Ketosis	Present at onset or during insulin deficiency	Not present except during infection or stress
Insulin therapy	Required for all	Required for some. Disease is progressive and insulin treatment may need to be added to treatment plan
Nutrition status	Thin, normal, or obese	Often overweight or obese. May be normal
Nutrition therapy	Essential	Essential
Vascular and neurologic complications	Frequent	Frequent

either does not produce enough insulin or does not use it effectively, or both. The presence of endogenous insulin is the major pathophysiologic distinction between type 1 and type 2 diabetes.

Genetic mutations that lead to insulin resistance and a higher risk for obesity have been found in many people with type 2 diabetes. Persons who have a first-degree relative with the disease are 10 times more likely to develop type 2 diabetes. Four major metabolic abnormalities play a role in the development of type 2 diabetes.

- The first factor is *insulin resistance,* which describes a condition in which body tissues do not respond to the action of insulin because insulin receptors are unresponsive, insufficient in number, or both. Entry of glucose into the cell is impeded, resulting in hyperglycemia.
- A second factor is a marked decrease in the ability of the pancreas to make insulin as the β-cells become fatigued from the compensatory overproduction of insulin or when β-cell mass is lost.
- A third factor is inappropriate glucose production by the liver. Instead of properly regulating the release of glucose in response to blood levels, the liver does so in a haphazard way that does not correspond to the body's needs at the time.
- A fourth factor is alteration in the production of hormones and cytokines by adipose tissue (adipokines). Adipokines play a role in glucose and fat metabolism and likely contribute to the pathophysiology of type 2 diabetes.

Persons with metabolic syndrome are at an increased risk for the development of type 2 diabetes. Overweight persons with metabolic syndrome can reduce their risk for diabetes through a program of weight loss and regular physical activity (see Metabolic Syndrome, p. 401).

Disease onset in type 2 diabetes is usually gradual, with signs and symptoms of hyperglycemia developing when about 50% to 80% of β-cells no longer secrete insulin. Many people are diagnosed on routine laboratory testing or when they undergo treatment for other conditions and elevated glucose or glycosylated hemoglobin (A1C) levels are found.

Prediabetes

Persons diagnosed with prediabetes are at increased risk for the development of type 2 diabetes. *Prediabetes,* an intermediate stage between normal glucose homeostasis and diabetes, is defined as impaired glucose tolerance (IGT), impaired fasting glucose (IFG), or both.

- A diagnosis of IGT is made if the 2-hour oral glucose tolerance test (OGTT) values are 140 to 199 mg/dL (7.8 to 11.0 mmol/L).

IFG is diagnosed when fasting blood glucose levels are 100 to 125 mg/dL (5.56 to 6.9 mmol/L).

People with prediabetes usually do not have symptoms. However, long-term damage to the body, especially the heart and blood vessels, may already be occurring. It is important for adults to undergo screening and understand risk factors for diabetes.

- Encourage those with prediabetes to have their blood glucose and A1C tested regularly and to self-monitor for symptoms of diabetes, such as polyuria, polyphagia, and polydipsia.
- Maintaining a healthy weight, exercising regularly, and eating a healthy diet reduce the risk of developing overt diabetes in people with prediabetes.

Clinical Manifestations

Type 1 Diabetes
Because the onset of type 1 DM is rapid, the initial manifestations are usually acute. The osmotic effect of excess glucose produces polydipsia and polyuria. Polyphagia is a consequence of cellular malnourishment when insulin deficiency prevents use of glucose for energy. Weight loss, weakness, and fatigue may also occur.

Type 2 Diabetes
Manifestations of type 2 DM are often nonspecific, including fatigue, recurrent infections, prolonged wound healing, and vision problems. Polydipsia, polyuria, and polyphagia may also occur.

Acute Complications
Acute complications arise from events associated with hyperglycemia and hypoglycemia (also referred to as *insulin reaction*). It is important for the health care provider (HCP) to distinguish between hyperglycemia and hypoglycemia because hypoglycemia worsens rapidly and constitutes a serious threat if action is not immediately taken. Table 29 compares hyperglycemia and hypoglycemia.

Diabetic Ketoacidosis
Diabetes-related ketoacidosis (DKA) is caused by a profound deficiency of insulin and is characterized by hyperglycemia, ketosis, acidosis, and dehydration. Precipitating factors include illness and infection; inadequate insulin dosage; undiagnosed type 1 diabetes; lack of education, understanding, or resources; and neglect.

- DKA is most likely to occur in type 1 diabetes. It may be seen in type 2 during severe illness or stress when the pancreas cannot meet the extra demand for insulin. If left untreated, death is inevitable.
- Manifestations of DKA include dehydration signs (e.g., poor skin turgor, dry mucous membranes), tachycardia, orthostatic

TABLE 29 Comparison of Hyperglycemia and Hypoglycemia

Hyperglycemia	Hypoglycemia
Manifestations	
• Elevated blood glucose • Increase in urination • Increase in appetite followed by lack of appetite • Weakness, fatigue • Blurred vision • Headache • Glycosuria • Nausea and vomiting • Abdominal cramps • Progression to DKA or HHS • Mood swings	• Blood glucose <70 mg/dL (3.9 mmol/L) • Cold, clammy skin • Numbness of fingers, toes, mouth • Tachycardia • Emotional changes • Headache • Nervousness, tremors • Faintness, dizziness • Unsteady gait, slurred speech • Hunger • Changes in vision • Seizures, coma
Causes	
• Illness, infection • Corticosteroids • Too much food • Too little or no diabetes medication • Inactivity • Emotional, physical stress • Poor absorption of insulin	• Alcohol intake without food • Too little food—delayed, omitted, inadequate intake • Too much diabetes medication • Too much exercise without adequate food intake • Diabetes medication or food taken at wrong time • Loss of weight without change in medication • Use of β-adrenergic blockers interfering with recognition of symptoms
Clinical Course	
• More gradual onset • Definition of elevated glucose varies by person, based on personal glucose targets	• More rapid onset • Pattern of manifestations changes over time

D

Continued

TABLE 29   Comparison of Hyperglycemia and Hypoglycemia—cont'd

Hyperglycemia	Hypoglycemia
Treatment	
• Get medical care • Continue diabetes medication as prescribed • Check blood glucose frequently and check urine for ketones; record results • Drink fluids at least on an hourly basis • Contact the health care provider (HCP) about ketonuria	• Follow the Rule of 15. Conscious person: Give 15 g of a simple (fast-acting) carbohydrate (fruit juice or regular soft drink). Recheck the blood glucose 15 minutes later. If the value is still below 70 mg/dL, have the patient ingest 15 g more of carbohydrate and recheck the blood glucose in 15 minutes. Have the patient ingest a complex carbohydrate after recovery to prevent a rebound hypoglycemic attack. If no significant improvement occurs after 2 or 3 doses of 15 g of simple carbohydrate, contact the HCP. • Worsening symptoms or unconscious patient: Subcutaneous or IM injection of 1 mg glucagon, or IV administration of 25–50 mL of 50% glucose.
Preventive Measures	
• Take prescribed dose of medication at proper time • Accurately give insulin, noninsulin injectables, OA • Make healthy food choices • Follow sick-day rules when ill • Check blood glucose routinely • Wear or carry diabetes identification	• Take prescribed dose of medication at proper time • Accurately give insulin, noninsulin injectables, OA • Coordinate eating with medications • Eat adequate food intake needed for calories for exercise

TABLE 29 Comparison of Hyperglycemia and Hypoglycemia—cont'd	
Hyperglycemia	**Hypoglycemia**
	• Be able to recognize symptoms and treat them immediately • Carry simple carbohydrates • Teach family and caregiver about symptoms and treatment • Check blood glucose routinely • Wear or carry diabetes identification

DKA, Diabetic ketoacidosis; *HHS*, hyperosmolar hyperglycemic syndrome; *OAs*, oral agents.

D

hypotension with a weak and rapid pulse, vomiting, Kussmaul respirations, and a sweet fruity odor of acetone on the breath.

■ Laboratory findings include a blood glucose level of 250 mg/dL (13.9 mmol/L) or greater, arterial blood pH < 7.30, and serum bicarbonate level < 16 mEq/L (16 mmol/L). A moderate to large amount of ketones are found in the urine or serum.

Hyperosmolar Hyperglycemia Syndrome

Hyperosmolar hyperglycemia syndrome (HHS) is a life-threatening syndrome that can occur in the patient with DM who is able to make enough insulin to prevent DKA but not enough to prevent severe hyperglycemia, osmotic diuresis, and extracellular fluid depletion.

■ The main difference between HHS and DKA is that the patient with HHS usually has enough circulating insulin to avoid ketoacidosis. Because HHS produces fewer symptoms in the earlier stages, blood glucose levels can climb quite high before the problem is noted. The higher blood glucose levels increase serum osmolality and cause severe neurologic manifestations, such as somnolence, coma, seizures, hemiparesis, and aphasia.

■ HHS is less common than DKA. It often occurs in patients > 60 years of age with type 2 diabetes. Common causes of HHS are urinary tract infections, pneumonia, sepsis, and any acute illness. HHS is more common among patients with newly diagnosed type 2 diabetes.

- Laboratory values include a blood glucose level above 600 mg/dL (33.33 mmol/L) and a marked increase in serum osmolality. Ketone bodies are absent or minimal in both blood and urine.

Hypoglycemia

Hypoglycemia, or low blood glucose, occurs when there is too much insulin in proportion to available glucose in the blood. This causes the blood glucose level to drop below 70 mg/dL. Manifestations include shakiness, palpitations, nervousness, diaphoresis, anxiety, hunger, and pallor. Manifestations of hypoglycemia can mimic alcohol intoxication. Untreated hypoglycemia can progress to loss of consciousness, seizures, coma, and death.

Chronic Complications

Chronic complications are primarily those of end-organ disease arising from damage to the blood vessels from chronic hyperglycemia. *Angiopathy,* or blood vessel disease, is one of the leading causes of diabetes-related deaths. These chronic blood vessel problems are divided into 2 categories: macrovascular complications and microvascular complications.

Macrovascular Complications

Macrovascular complications are diseases of the large and medium-sized blood vessels that occur with greater frequency and an earlier onset in people with diabetes. Risk factors associated with macrovascular complications, such as obesity, smoking, hypertension, high fat intake, and sedentary lifestyle, can be reduced. Insulin resistance appears to play a role in the development of cardiovascular disease and is implicated in the pathogenesis of essential hypertension and dyslipidemia.

Microvascular Complications

Microvascular complications result from thickening of the vessel membranes in the capillaries and arterioles (small vessels) in response to chronic hyperglycemia. The areas most noticeably affected are the eyes (retinopathy), kidneys (nephropathy), and nerves (neuropathy).

Diabetes-related retinopathy is estimated to be the most common cause of new cases of adult blindness.

- In *nonproliferative retinopathy,* the most common form, partial occlusion of the small blood vessels in the retina causes micro-aneurysms to develop in the capillary walls. Capillary fluid leaks, causing retinal edema and eventually hard exudates or intraretinal hemorrhages. Vision may be affected if the macula is involved.
- *Proliferative retinopathy* is more severe and involves the retina and vitreous. When retinal capillaries are occluded, new, fragile blood vessels form. Eventually light does not reach the retina as

vessels break and bleed. A tear or retinal detachment may occur. If the macula is involved, vision is lost. Treatment involves laser photocoagulation.

Diabetes-related nephropathy is a microvascular complication associated with damage to the small blood vessels that supply the glomeruli of the kidney. It is the leading cause of end-stage renal disease in the United States. Tight blood glucose control is critical to prevent or delay diabetes-related nephropathy. Hypertension significantly accelerates the progression of nephropathy, so aggressive BP management is indicated. See Hypertension, p. 313.

- Patients with diabetes are screened for nephropathy annually to assess for albuminuria and measure the albumin-to-creatinine ratio. Serum creatinine is also measured to give an estimate glomerular filtration rate and the degree of kidney function.

Neuropathy is nerve damage that occurs because of the metabolic alterations associated with diabetes. About 60% to 70% of patients with diabetes have some degree of neuropathy. More than 60% of nontraumatic amputations in the United States are done for people with diabetes. Screening for neuropathy should begin at the time of diagnosis in patients with type 2 diabetes and 5 years after diagnosis in patients with type 1 diabetes.

Two major categories of diabetes-related neuropathy are *sensory neuropathy,* which affects the peripheral nervous system and is the more common type of neuropathy, and *autonomic neuropathy,* which can affect nearly all body systems.

- The most common form of sensory neuropathy is distal symmetric neuropathy, which affects the hands or feet. Characteristics include loss of sensation, abnormal sensations, pain, and paresthesias. The pain, which is often described as burning, cramping, crushing, or tearing, is usually worse at night. The paresthesias may be associated with tingling, burning, and itching sensations.
- Autonomic neuropathy can lead to hypoglycemia unawareness, bowel incontinence and diarrhea, and urinary retention. Delayed gastric emptying *(gastroparesis),* a complication of autonomic neuropathy, can cause nausea, vomiting, gastroesophageal reflux, and persistent feelings of fullness. Cardiovascular abnormalities, such as postural hypotension, painless myocardial infarction, and resting tachycardia, can occur. Erectile dysfunction (ED) in men with diabetes is well recognized and common, often being the first manifestation of autonomic neuropathy.

Control of blood glucose is the only treatment for diabetic neuropathy. It is effective in many but not all cases. Drug therapy may be used to treat neuropathic symptoms, particularly pain.

Diagnostic Studies

The diagnosis of diabetes can be made through 1 of the following 4 methods. In the absence of unequivocal hyperglycemia, criteria 1 to 3 should be confirmed by repeat testing.

1. A1C level of 6.5% or greater
2. Fasting plasma glucose (FPG) level at or above 126 mg/dL (7.0 mmol/L). *Fasting* is defined as no caloric intake for at least 8 hours.
3. Two-hour plasma glucose level at or above 200 mg/dL (11.1 mmol/L) during an OGTT, using a glucose load of 75 g
4. In a patient with classic symptoms of hyperglycemia (polyuria, polydipsia, unexplained weight loss) or hyperglycemic crisis, a random plasma glucose of at least 200 mg/dL (11.1 mmol/L)

Interprofessional Management

The goals of diabetes management are to reduce symptoms, promote well-being, prevent acute complications related to hypo- or hyperglycemia, and prevent or delay the onset and progression of long-term complications. Nutritional therapy, drug therapy, exercise, and self-monitoring of blood glucose are the tools used in the management of diabetes. The major types of glucose-lowering agents (GLAs) used in the treatment of diabetes are insulin, oral agents (OA)s, and noninsulin injectable agents. For a majority of patients, drug therapy is needed.

Drug Therapy: Insulin

Exogenous (injected) insulin is needed when the patient has inadequate insulin to meet specific metabolic needs. People with type 1 diabetes require exogenous insulin to survive. People with type 2 diabetes usually controlled with diet, exercise, and/or OAs may require exogenous insulin during periods of severe stress, such as illness or surgery. When patients with type 2 diabetes cannot maintain satisfactory blood glucose levels, exogenous insulin is added.

Human insulin is made using genetic engineering. The insulin is derived from common bacteria (e.g., *Escherichia coli*) or yeast cells using recombinant DNA technology. Insulins differ in their onset, peak action, and duration of effect. They are categorized as rapid-acting, short-acting, intermediate-acting, and long-acting insulin.

Examples of insulin regimens ranging from 1 to 4 injections per day are presented in Table 48.4 in Harding et al., *Lewis' Medical-Surgical Nursing,* ed 11.

- The insulin approach that most closely mimics endogenous insulin production is the basal-bolus plan (often called *intensive* or *physiologic insulin therapy*). It consists of multiple daily insulin injections (or an insulin pump) together with frequent self-monitoring of blood glucose (or a continuous glucose monitoring system).

- To manage postprandial blood glucose levels, the timing of rapid- and short-acting insulin in relation to meals is crucial. Rapid-acting synthetic insulin analogs, which include aspart (NovoLog), glulisine (Apidra), and lispro (Humalog), have an onset of action of about 15 minutes. They should be injected within 15 minutes of mealtime. The rapid-acting analogs most closely mimic natural insulin secretion in response to a meal.
- A rapid-acting inhaled insulin (Afrezza) can be administered at the beginning of each meal or within 20 minutes after starting a meal. It is not a substitute for long-acting insulin.
- In addition to mealtime insulin, people with type 1 diabetes must also use a long- or intermediate-acting (background) insulin to control blood glucose levels between meals and overnight.
- Combination insulin therapy involves mixing short- or rapid-acting insulin with intermediate-acting insulin to provide both mealtime and basal coverage with 1 injection. Premixed formulas are available for this regimen, but optimal blood glucose control is not as likely because there is less flexibility in dosing.

The steps in administering a subcutaneous insulin injection are outlined in Table 48.5 in Harding et al., Lewis' *Medical-Surgical Nursing,* ed 11.

Continuous subcutaneous insulin infusion can be administered through an insulin pump, a small battery-operated device that resembles a standard pager in size and appearance. Every 2 or 3 days the insertion site is changed. A major advantage of the pump is the potential for tight glucose control.

Nursing Care Related to Insulin Therapy. Nursing responsibilities for the patient receiving insulin include proper administration, assessment of patient's response to insulin therapy, and teaching the patient about administration of, adjustment to, and side effects of insulin.

- Assess the patient who is new to insulin and evaluate their ability to manage insulin therapy safely. This includes the ability to understand the interaction of insulin, diet, and activity and to recognize and appropriately treat the symptoms of hypoglycemia.
- The patient or the caregiver must be able to prepare and inject the insulin. If not able, additional resources will be needed.
- Follow-up assessment of the patient who has been using insulin therapy includes inspection of insulin sites for *lipodystrophy* (atrophy of subcutaneous tissue) and other reactions, a review of the insulin preparation and injection technique, a history

pertaining to hypoglycemic episodes, and assessment of the patient's method for handling hypoglycemic episodes.

Drug Therapy: Oral and Noninsulin Injectable Agents

OAs and noninsulin injectable agents work to improve the mechanisms by which the body produces and uses insulin and glucose (Fig. 6). These drugs work on the 3 defects of type 2 diabetes: insulin resistance, decreased insulin production, and increased hepatic glucose production. These drugs may be used in combination with agents from other classes or with insulin to achieve blood glucose targets.

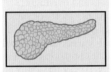

Pancreas

Sulfonylureas, meglitinides, DPP-4 inhibitors, and GLP-1 receptor agonists
↑ Insulin production

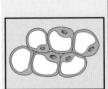

Adipose tissue

Muscle

Biguanides and thiazolidinediones
↑ Uptake and use of glucose
↓ Insulin resistance

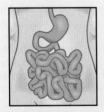

Stomach and small intestine

α-Glucosidase inhibitors
Delay absorption of starches
DPP-4 inhibitors
↑ Activity of incretins
GLP-1 receptor agonists and amylin
↓ Gastric emptying

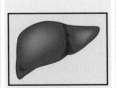

Liver

Biguanides, thiazolidinediones, and DPP-4 inhibitors
↓ Hepatic glucose production

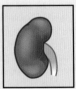

Kidney

SGLT inhibitors
↓ Glucose reabsorption

Fig. 6 Sites and methods of action of type 2 diabetes drugs. *DPP-4,* Dipeptidyl peptidase-4; *GLP-1,* glucagon-like peptide-1; *SGLT,* sodium-glucose co-transporter.

Metformin, a biguanide, reduces glucose production by the liver, but also enhances insulin sensitivity and improve glucose transport into cells. Metformin is the most effective first-line treatment for type 2 diabetes. Many other types of OAs and noninsulin injectable agents (Table 30) are used in the treatment of type 2 diabetes.

Nursing Care Related to Oral and Noninsulin Injectable Agents. Your responsibilities for the patient taking oral and noninsulin injectable agents are similar to those for the patient taking insulin. Proper administration, assessment of the patient's use of and response to these drugs, and teaching the patient and family are all essential nursing actions.

- Your assessment is valuable in determining the most appropriate drug for a patient. This includes assessing the patient's mental status, eating habits, home environment, attitude toward diabetes, and medication history.
- Teach the importance of diet and activity plans.

Nutritional Therapy

Nutritional therapy is a cornerstone of diabetes care. Guidelines from the American Diabetes Association (ADA) indicate that within the context of an overall healthy eating plan, a person with DM can eat the same foods as a person who does not have diabetes. This means that the same principles of good nutrition that apply to the general population also apply to people with diabetes. See Table 48.8, which describes nutritional therapy for patients with diabetes, Harding et al., *Lewis' Medical-Surgical Nursing,* ed 11.

- *Type 1 diabetes.* People with type 1 diabetes base their meal planning on usual food intake and preferences balanced with insulin and exercise patterns. Day-to-day consistency in timing and amount of food eaten makes it much easier to manage blood glucose levels, especially for those persons using conventional, fixed insulin regimens. Rapid-acting insulin doses can be adjusted before the meal depending on current blood glucose level and the carbohydrate content of the meal. Multiple daily injections or the use of an insulin pump allows considerable flexibility in food selection, and regimens can be adjusted for variations in eating and exercise habits.
- *Type 2 diabetes.* Nutritional therapy in type 2 diabetes should emphasize achieving glucose, lipid, and BP goals. Modest weight loss has been associated with improved insulin resistance and blood glucose control.

Most often, a dietitian initially teaches the principles of the nutritional therapy regimen as part of an interprofessional diabetes care team. When patients do not have access to a dietitian, you may need to assume responsibility for teaching basic dietary management to patients with diabetes.

TABLE 30 Drug Therapy

Oral Agents and Noninsulin Injectable Agents

Type	Mechanism of Action	Side Effects
Oral Agents		
α-Glucosidase Inhibitors		
acarbose (Precose) miglitol (Glyset)	Delays absorption of complex carbohydrates (starches) from GI tract	Gas, abdominal pain, diarrhea
Biguanides		
metformin (Fortamet Glucophage, Glucophage XR, Glumetza, Riomet)	Decreases rate of hepatic glucose production. Augments glucose uptake by tissues, especially muscles	Diarrhea, lactic acidosis. Must be held 1–2 days before IV contrast media given and for 48 hr after
Dipeptidyl Peptidase-4 (DPP-4) Inhibitors		
alogliptin (Nesina) linagliptin (Tradjenta) saxagliptin (Onglyza) sitagliptin (Januvia)	Enhances activity of incretins Stimulates release of insulin from pancreatic β-cells. Decreases hepatic glucose production	Pancreatitis, allergic reactions
Dopamine Receptor Agonists		
bromocriptine (Cycloset)	Activates dopamine receptors in central nervous system. Unknown how it improves glucose levels	Orthostatic hypotension
Meglitinides		
nateglinide (Starlix) repaglinide (Prandin)	Stimulates a rapid and short-lived release of insulin from the pancreas	Weight gain, hypoglycemia

TABLE 30   Drug Therapy

Oral Agents and Noninsulin Injectable Agents—cont'd

Type	Mechanism of Action	Side Effects
Sodium-Glucose Co-Transporter 2 (SGLT2) Inhibitors		
canagliflozin (Invokana) dapagliflozin (Farxiga) empagliflozin (Jardiance) ertugliflozin (Steglatro)	Decreases renal glucose reabsorption and increases urinary glucose excretion	Increased risk of genital and urinary tract infections. Hypoglycemia
Sulfonylureas		
glimepiride (Amaryl) glipizide (Glucotrol, Glucotrol XL) glyburide (DiaBeta, Glynase)	Stimulates release of insulin from pancreatic islets. Decreases glycogenolysis and gluconeogenesis. Enhances cellular sensitivity to insulin	Weight gain, hypoglycemia
Thiazolidinediones		
pioglitazone (Actos) rosiglitazone (Avandia)	Increases glucose uptake in muscle. Decreases endogenous glucose production	Weight gain, edema. *pioglitazone:* may increase risk for bladder cancer and worsen heart failure. *rosiglitazone:* may increase risk for cardiovascular events (e.g., myocardial infarction, stroke)

D

Continued

TABLE 30 Drug Therapy

Oral Agents and Noninsulin Injectable Agents—cont'd

Type	Mechanism of Action	Side Effects
Combination Oral Therapy		
Actoplus Met, Actoplus Met XR	Same as for metformin and pioglitazone	See side effects for individual drugs
Duetact	Same as for pioglitazone and glimepiride	Same as above
Glucovance	Same as for metformin and glyburide	Same as above
Glyxambi	Same as for empagliflozin and linagliptin	Same as above
Janumet, Janumet XR	Same as for metformin and sitagliptin	Same as above
Jentadueto	Same as for linagliptin and metformin	Same as above
Kazano	Same as for alogliptin and metformin	Same as above
Kombiglyze	Same as for saxagliptin and metformin	Same as above
Oseni	Same as for alogliptin and pioglitazone	Same as above
PrandiMet	Same as for metformin and repaglinide	Same as above
Segluromet	Same as for metformin and ertugliflozin	Same as above
Steglujan	Same as for sitagliptin and ertugliflozin	Same as above
Synjardy	Same as metformin and empagliflozin	Same as above
Xigduo	Same as for dapagliflozin and metformin	Same as above
Noninsulin Injectable Agents		
Amylin Analogs[a]		
pramlintide (Symlin)	Slows gastric emptying, decreases glucagon secretion and endogenous glucose output from liver. Increases satiety	Hypoglycemia, nausea, vomiting, decreased appetite, headache

TABLE 30 Drug Therapy

Oral Agents and Noninsulin Injectable Agents—cont'd

Type	Mechanism of Action	Side Effects
Glucagon-Like Peptide-1 (GLP-1) Receptor Agonists[b]		
albiglutide (Tanzeum) dulaglutide (Trulicity) exenatide (Byetta) exenatide extended-release (Bydureon) liraglutide (Victoza) lixisenatide (Adlyxin) semaglutide (Ozempic)	Stimulates release of insulin, decrease glucagon secretion, and slow gastric emptying. Increase satiety	Nausea, vomiting, hypoglycemia, diarrhea, headache

[a]Given subcutaneously only in abdomen or thigh.
[b]Given subcutaneously.

Exercise

Regular, consistent exercise is an essential part of diabetes and pre-diabetes management. Encourage patients to be active every day and to seek medical clearance before starting a new or more intensive exercise program. The ADA recommends that people with diabetes engage in at least 150 minutes weekly (30 minutes, 5 days/wk) of a moderate-intensity aerobic physical activity. Encourage people with type 2 diabetes to perform resistance training 3 times a week in the absence of contraindications.

Exercise decreases insulin resistance and can have a direct effect on lowering blood glucose levels. It also contributes to weight loss, which further decreases insulin resistance, and in addition it may help reduce triglyceride and low-density lipoprotein (LDL) cholesterol levels, increase high-density lipoprotein (HDL), reduce BP, and improve circulation.

- People who use drugs that can cause hypoglycemia should exercise about 1 hour after a meal or that they have a 10- to 15-g carbohydrate snack and check their blood glucose before exercising. It is preferable not to increase caloric intake for exercise.

Blood Glucose Monitoring

Self-monitoring of blood glucose is a critical part of diabetes management. By providing a current blood glucose reading, self-monitoring lets the patient make decisions about food intake, activity patterns, and medication dosages.

Because incorrect monitoring technique can cause errors in management strategies, comprehensive patient teaching is essential. Initial instruction should be followed up with regular reassessment. Table 48.11 in Harding et al., *Lewis' Medical-Surgical Nursing*, ed 11, presents instructions for teaching the patient to perform self-monitoring of blood glucose.

Management of Acute Complications

Diabetic Ketoacidosis

If fluid and electrolyte imbalances are not severe and blood glucose levels can be safely monitored at home, DKA can be managed on an outpatient basis. Emergency management of DKA is needed when fluid imbalance is potentially life-threatening. The aim of fluid and electrolyte therapy is to replace extracellular and intracellular water and to correct deficits of sodium, chloride, bicarbonate, potassium, phosphate, magnesium, and nitrogen.

- IV insulin administration is directed toward correcting hyperglycemia and hyperketonemia. Insulin is immediately started by a continuous infusion.
- Although initial serum potassium may be normal or high, levels can rapidly decrease once therapy starts as insulin drives potassium into the cells, leading to life-threatening hypokalemia.

Hyperosmolar Hyperglycemic Syndrome

HHS constitutes a medical emergency with a high mortality rate. Therapy is similar to that for DKA except that HHS requires more fluid replacement.

- Insulin is given immediately by IV infusion.
- Electrolytes are monitored and replaced as needed. Assess vital signs, intake and output, tissue turgor, laboratory values, and cardiac monitoring to monitor the efficacy of fluid and electrolyte replacement.

Hypoglycemia

At the first sign of hypoglycemia, check the blood glucose if possible. If it is below 70 mg/dL (3.9 mmol/L), immediately begin treatment for hypoglycemia. If the patient has symptoms of hypoglycemia and monitoring equipment is not available, or if the patient has a history of chronic poor glucose control, assume it is hypoglycemia and begin treatment.

- Hypoglycemia is treated by ingesting 15 g of a simple (fast-acting) carbohydrate, such as 4 to 6 ounces of fruit juice or regular soft drink. Avoid overtreatment with large quantities of quick-acting carbohydrates, such as candy bars, to avoid a rapid fluctuation to hyperglycemia.
- Recheck the blood glucose 15 minutes later. If the value is still below 70 mg/dL, have the patient ingest 15 g more of

carbohydrate and recheck the blood glucose in 15 minutes. Because of the potential for rebound hypoglycemia after an acute episode, have the patient ingest a complex carbohydrate after recovery to prevent another hypoglycemic attack.

- If no significant improvement occurs after 2 or 3 doses of 15 g of simple carbohydrate, contact the HCP.

Once acute hypoglycemia has been reversed, explore the reasons why the situation developed with the patient. This assessment may indicate a need for additional patient teaching to avoid future episodes of hypoglycemia.

Nursing Management
Goals
The patient with diabetes will engage in self-care behaviors to actively manage their diabetes, have few or no episodes of acute hyperglycemic or hypoglycemic emergencies, maintain blood glucose levels at normal or near-normal levels, reduce the risk for chronic complications of diabetes, and adjust lifestyle to accommodate the diabetes regimen with a minimum of stress. The goal is for the patient with diabetes to safely and effectively fit diabetes into life, rather than living life around diabetes.

Nursing Interventions
Your role in health promotion is to identify, monitor, and teach the patient at risk for diabetes.

Management of Acute Illness and Surgery. Emotional and physical stress can increase blood glucose levels and result in hyperglycemia. Acute illness, injury, and surgery may evoke a counterregulatory hormone response resulting in hyperglycemia. When patients with diabetes are ill, they should check blood glucose at least every 4 hours. Teach acutely ill patients who have type 1 diabetes with a blood glucose level above 240 mg/dL (13.3 mmol/L) to test the urine for ketones every 3 to 4 hours.

- Patients should contact the HCP when glucose levels are above 300 mg/dL for 2 tests in a row or urine ketone levels are moderate to high.
- If patients can eat normally, they should continue with the regular meal plan while increasing the intake of noncaloric fluids, such as broth, water, dietary gelatin, and other decaffeinated beverages, and continue taking oral agents and insulin as prescribed.
- If illness causes the patient to eat less than normal, drug therapy should be continued as prescribed while supplementing food intake with carbohydrate-containing fluids. Examples include low-sodium soups, juices, and regular, sugar-sweetened decaffeinated soft drinks. Notify the HCP if the patient is unable to keep down fluid or food.

- Adjustments in the diabetes plan during the intraoperative period can be made to ensure glycemic control. The patient is given IV fluids and insulin (if needed) immediately before, during, and after surgery when there is no oral intake.
- When caring for an unconscious surgical patient receiving insulin, be alert for hypoglycemic signs, such as sweating, tachycardia, and tremors.

Ambulatory Care. Successful diabetes management requires ongoing interaction among the patient, family, and interprofessional health care team. It is important that a certified diabetes educator (CDE) be involved in the care of the patient and family.

Persons with diabetes face lifestyle choices that affect the food they eat, their activities, and demands on their time and energy. In addition, they face the challenge of preventing or dealing with the devastating complications of diabetes. Careful assessment of what it means to have diabetes is the starting point for patient teaching.

The potential for infection requires diligent skin care and dental hygiene. Routine care includes toothbrushing and flossing and regular bathing, with an emphasis on foot care. Skin injuries should be treated promptly. If the injury does not begin to heal within 24 hours or signs of infection develop, the HCP should be notified at once.

▼ **Patient and Caregiver Teaching**

The goals of diabetes self-management education are to match the level of self-management to the patient's ability so that they can become the most active participant possible. Those who actively manage their diabetes care have better outcomes than those who do not. Guidelines for patient and caregiver teaching for management of diabetes are listed in Table 31.

- Assess the patient's knowledge base frequently so that gaps in knowledge or inaccurate ideas can be quickly corrected.
- Tell the patient to carry medical identification at all times.

TABLE 31   **Patient & Caregiver Teaching**

Management of Diabetes Mellitus

Component	What to Teach
Disease process	• Introduce the pancreas and the islets of Langerhans. • Describe how insulin is made and what affects its production. • Discuss the relationship of insulin and glucose. • Explain the difference between type 1 and type 2 diabetes.

TABLE 31   Patient & Caregiver Teaching

Management of Diabetes Mellitus—cont'd

Component	What to Teach
Physical activity	• Discuss the effect of regular exercise on managing blood glucose and improving cardiovascular function and general health.
Menu planning	• Stress the importance of a well-balanced diet as part of a diabetes management plan. • Explain the impact of carbohydrates on blood glucose levels.
Medication	• Ensure that the patient understands the proper use of prescribed medication (e.g., insulin, oral agents, noninsulin injectables [see Table 31]). • Account for a patient's physical or other limitations or inabilities for self-medication. If necessary, involve the family or caregiver in proper use of medication. • Discuss all side effects and safety issues about medication.
Monitoring blood glucose	• Teach correct blood glucose monitoring. • Include when to check blood glucose levels, how to record them, and how to adjust insulin levels, if necessary.
Risk reduction	• Ensure that the patient understands and appropriately responds to the signs and symptoms of hypoglycemia and hyperglycemia (see Table 29). • Stress the importance of proper foot care, regular eye examinations, and consistent glucose monitoring. • Teach the patient about the effect that stress can have on blood glucose.
Psychosocial	• Help the patient identify resources that are available to help with the adjustment and answer questions about living with a chronic condition, such as diabetes.

D

DIARRHEA

Description

Diarrhea is the passage of at least 3 loose or liquid stools per day. It may be acute, lasting 14 days or less, or persistent, lasting > 14 days. Chronic diarrhea lasts 30 days or longer.

Pathophysiology

The primary cause of acute diarrhea is ingesting infectious organisms. Viruses cause most cases of infectious diarrhea in the United States. Bacterial infections are also common. *Escherichia coli* O157:H7 is a common cause of bloody diarrhea in the United States. It is transmitted by undercooked beef or chicken contaminated with the bacteria or by fruits and vegetables exposed to contaminated manure. *Giardia lamblia* is the most common intestinal parasite that causes diarrhea in the United States.

Infectious organisms attack the intestines in different ways. Some organisms (e.g., *Rotavirus, Norovirus, G. lamblia*) change the secretion and/or absorption of the enterocytes of the small intestine without inflammation. Other organisms (e.g., *Clostridium difficile*) impair absorption by destroying cells, causing inflammation in the colon, and producing toxins that cause damage.

Patients receiving broad-spectrum antibiotics (e.g., carbapenems, cephalosporins, piperacillin/tazobactam are susceptible to infections with pathogenic strains of *C. difficile. C. difficile* infection (CDI) causes the most serious antibiotic-associated diarrhea and is a common cause of hospital-acquired GI illness in the United States.

Diarrhea is not always caused by infection. Drugs and specific food intolerances can also cause diarrhea. Diarrhea from celiac disease and short bowel syndrome result from malabsorption in the small intestine.

Clinical Manifestations

Infections that attack the upper GI tract (e.g., *Norovirus* organisms, *G. lamblia*) usually produce large-volume, watery stools; cramping; and periumbilical pain. Patients have either a low-grade or no fever and often have nausea and vomiting before the diarrhea begins. Infections of the colon and distal small bowel (e.g., *Shigella, Salmonella, C. difficile*) produce fever and frequent bloody diarrhea with a small volume.

Leukocytes, blood, and mucus may be present in the stool, depending on the causative agent. Severe diarrhea produces life-threatening dehydration, electrolyte problems (e.g., hypokalemia), and acid-base imbalances (metabolic acidosis). CDI can progress to severe colitis and intestinal perforation.

Diagnostic Studies

Most cases of diarrhea resolve quickly. Stool cultures are only indicated for patients who are very ill, have a significant fever, have diarrhea longer than 3 days or were exposed during an outbreak. Those with travelers' diarrhea lasting 14 days or longer should be evaluated for parasitic infections.

- Stools are examined for blood, mucus, white blood cells (WBCs), and parasites, and cultures are done to identify infectious organisms.
- CDI is detected by enzyme immunoassay (EIA).
- In a patient with chronic diarrhea, measurement of stool electrolytes, pH, and osmolality may help determine whether diarrhea is related to decreased fluid absorption or increased fluid secretion.
- Measurement of stool fat and undigested muscle fibers may indicate fat and protein malabsorption conditions, including pancreatic insufficiency.
- Blood cultures should be done in those with signs of sepsis or systemic infection (e.g., high fever) or who are immunocompromised.

Interprofessional Management

Treatment depends on the cause. Foods and drugs that cause diarrhea should be avoided. Acute infectious diarrhea is usually self-limiting. The major concerns are preventing transmission, replacing fluid and electrolytes, and protecting the skin.

Oral solutions containing glucose and electrolytes (e.g., Gatorade, Pedialyte) may be sufficient to replace losses from mild diarrhea. In severe diarrhea, parenteral administration of fluids, electrolytes, vitamins, and nutrition may be necessary.

Antidiarrheal agents may be given to coat and protect mucous membranes, absorb irritating substances, inhibit GI motility, decrease intestinal secretions, or decrease central nervous system (CNS) stimulation to the GI tract.

- Antidiarrheal agents have limited short-term use. They coat and protect mucous membranes, absorb irritating substances, inhibit intestinal transit, decrease intestinal secretions, or decrease CNS stimulation of the GI tract. They are used cautiously in inflammatory bowel disease because of the danger of *toxic megacolon* (colonic dilation to > 5 cm).
- Regardless of the cause, antidiarrheal medications should be given only for a short period. Antibiotics are rarely used to treat infectious diarrhea.

CDI is a particularly hazardous health care–associated infection (HAI). The risk for contracting CDI is highest in patients receiving antimicrobial, chemotherapy, gastric acid-suppressing, or immuno-suppressive agents. Its spores can survive for up to 70 days on objects including commodes, telephones, thermometers, bedside tables, and floors. CDI can be transmitted from patient to patient by health care workers who do not adhere to infection control precautions.

- CDI is treated with either oral vancomycin (125 mg, 4 times a day) or fidaxomicin (200 mg twice daily) are recommended for 10 days. All nonessential antibiotics, stool softeners, laxatives, and antidiarrheal agents should be stopped.
- Metronidazole is an option when patients are unable to be treated with vancomycin or fidaxomicin.

Nursing Management: Acute Infectious Diarrhea
Goals
The patient with infectious diarrhea will have no transmission of the microorganism causing the diarrhea, cessation of diarrhea and resumption of normal bowel patterns, normal fluid and electrolyte and acid-base balance, normal nutritional status, and no perianal skin breakdown.
Nursing Interventions
Consider all cases of acute diarrhea to be infectious until the cause is known.

- Use strict infection control precautions to prevent the illness from spreading to others. Wash your hands before and after contact with each patient and when handling any body fluids.
- Provide private rooms for patients with CDI and ensure that visitors and health care providers (HCPs) wear gloves and gowns.
- Ensure surfaces and equipment are disinfected with a 10% bleach solution or a disinfectant labeled as *C. difficile* sporicidal.

▼ Patient and Caregiver Teaching
- Teach the patient and caregiver the principles of hygiene, infection control precautions, and potential dangers of an illness that is infectious to themselves and others.
- Discuss proper food handling, cooking, and storage.

DISSEMINATED INTRAVASCULAR COAGULATION

Description
Disseminated intravascular coagulation (DIC) is a serious bleeding and thrombotic disorder that results from abnormally initiated and accelerated clotting. Subsequent decreases in clotting factors and platelets may lead to uncontrollable hemorrhage. The term

DIC can be misleading because it only suggests that blood is clotting. However, there is also profuse bleeding from depletion of platelets and clotting factors.

Pathophysiology

DIC is an abnormal response of the normal clotting cascade stimulated by a disease process or disorder. Major physiologic assaults known to predispose patients to acute DIC include shock, septicemia, abruptio placentae, cancers, severe head injury, heatstroke, and pulmonary emboli. The underlying disease must be treated for DIC to resolve.

- DIC can occur as an acute, catastrophic condition, or it may exist at a subacute or chronic level. Each condition may have multiple triggering mechanisms to start the clotting cascade.

Tissue factor released at the site of tissue injury or some cancers enhances normal coagulation mechanisms. Abundant intravascular thrombin, the most powerful coagulant, is made. It catalyzes the conversion of fibrinogen to fibrin and enhances platelet aggregation. There is widespread fibrin and platelet deposition in capillaries and arterioles, causing thrombosis. Excess clotting activates the fibrinolytic system, which in turn breaks down newly formed clots, creating fibrin-split (fibrin-degradation) products (FSPs), which inhibit normal blood clotting. Ultimately the blood loses its ability to form a stable clot at injury sites, which predisposes the patient to hemorrhage.

- Chronic and subacute DIC is most often seen in patients with long-standing illnesses, such as cancer or autoimmune diseases. Occasionally these patients have subclinical disease manifested only by laboratory abnormalities.

Clinical Manifestations

Bleeding in a person with no previous history or obvious cause should be investigated further because it may be one of the first manifestations of acute DIC. Other nonspecific manifestations include weakness, malaise, and fever. There are both bleeding and thrombotic manifestations in DIC (Fig. 7).

- *Bleeding manifestations* include petechiae, oozing blood, tachypnea, hemoptysis, tachycardia, hypotension, bloody stools, hematuria, dizziness, headache, changes in mental status, and bone and joint pain.
- *Thrombotic manifestations* are a result of fibrin or platelet deposition in the microvasculature. Manifestations include ischemic tissue necrosis (e.g., gangrene), acute respiratory distress syndrome (ARDS), cardiovascular and electrocardiogram (ECG) changes, kidney damage, and paralytic ileus.

D

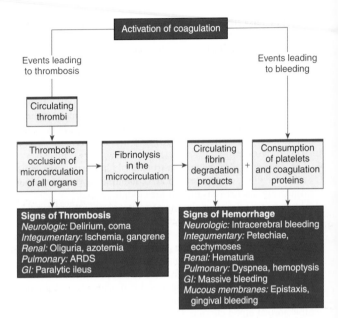

Fig. 7 The sequence of events that occur during disseminated intra-vascular coagulation (DIC). *ARDS,* Acute respiratory distress syndrome; *GI,* gastrointestinal.

Diagnostic Studies

Diagnostic findings include:

- prolonged prothrombin time and partial thromboplastin time;
- prolonged activated partial thromboplastin time and thrombin time;
- reduced fibrinogen, antithrombin III (AT III), and platelets;
- elevated FSPs and elevated D-dimers (cross-linked fibrin fragments);
- reduced levels of factors V, VII, VIII, X, and XIII.

For comparison of laboratory results in DIC with other types of thrombocytopenia, see Table 30.12, Harding et al., *Lewis' Medical-Surgical Nursing,* ed 11.

Interprofessional Management

It is important to diagnose DIC quickly, stabilize the patient if needed (e.g., with oxygenation or volume replacement), treat the underlying causative disease or problem, and control the ongoing thrombosis and bleeding. Depending on its severity, a variety of methods are used to manage DIC.

- If chronic DIC is diagnosed in a patient who is not bleeding, treatment of the underlying disease may be sufficient to reverse DIC (e.g., chemotherapy when DIC is caused by cancer).
- When the patient with DIC is bleeding, therapy is directed toward providing support with needed blood products while treating the primary disorder. Blood product support is usually reserved to stabilize the patient with life-threatening hemorrhage. Platelets are given to correct thrombocytopenia, and cryoprecipitate replaces factor VIII and fibrinogen. Fresh frozen plasma (FFP) replaces all clotting factors except platelets and provides a source of antithrombin.
- A patient with thrombosis is often treated by anticoagulation with unfractionated heparin or low-molecular-weight heparin. Heparin is used in the treatment of DIC only when the benefit (reducing clotting) outweighs the risk of bleeding. Antithrombin III (AT III) (ATnativ) may be useful in fulminant DIC, although it increases the risk of bleeding.
- Chronic DIC does not respond to oral anticoagulants, but can be controlled with long-term use of heparin.

Nursing Management

Be alert to the possible development of DIC. The cause of DIC needs to be managed while you provide supportive care.

- Assess for signs of external bleeding (e.g., petechiae, oozing at IV or injection sites) and internal bleeding (e.g., changes in mental status, increasing abdominal girth, pain) and any indications that microthrombi may be causing clinically significant organ damage (e.g., decreased renal output).
- Handle the patient gently to minimize tissue damage and protect the patient from additional bleeding.
- Administer blood products and medications correctly.

DIVERTICULOSIS/DIVERTICULITIS

Description

Diverticula are saccular dilations or outpouchings of the mucosa that develop in the colon. *Diverticulosis* is the presence of multiple noninflamed diverticula. *Diverticulitis* is inflammation of 1 or more diverticula, resulting in perforation into the peritoneum. Clinically, diverticular disease covers a spectrum from asymptomatic, uncomplicated diverticulosis to diverticulitis with complications, such as perforation, abscess, fistula, and bleeding.

- Diverticula are common, especially in older adults, but most people never develop diverticulitis.
- The disease is more prevalent in populations with diets low in fiber and high in refined carbohydrates. Diverticula are uncommon in vegetarians.
- Other risk factors for development of diverticula are obesity, inactivity, smoking, excessive alcohol use, and immunosuppression.

Pathophysiology

Diverticula may occur anywhere in the GI tract but are most common in the left (descending, sigmoid) colon. They seem to occur at weak points in the intestinal wall, such as where the blood vessels pass through the muscle layer.

The cause is thought to include both genetic and environmental factors. The disease is more prevalent in Western, industrialized populations, where people tend to consume diets low in fiber and high in refined carbohydrates. The cause of diverticulosis of the sigmoid colon is thought to be associated with high intraluminal pressures from a deficiency in dietary fiber intake.

Clinical Manifestations and Complications

Most patients with diverticulosis have no symptoms. Those with symptoms typically have abdominal pain, bloating, flatulence, and changes in bowel habits. In more serious situations, the diverticula bleed or diverticulitis develops.

The most common signs and symptoms of diverticulitis are acute pain in the left lower quadrant, distension, decreased or absent bowel sounds, nausea, vomiting, and systemic symptoms of infection (fever, leukocytosis with a shift to the left). Older adults with diverticulitis may be afebrile, with a normal white blood cell (WBC) count and little, if any, abdominal tenderness.

Diverticulitis can cause erosion of the bowel wall and perforation into the peritoneum. A localized abscess develops when the body walls off the perforated area. Peritonitis develops if it cannot be contained. Bleeding can be extensive but usually stops spontaneously.

Diagnostic Studies

- History and physical examination
- Abdominal and chest x-rays to rule out other causes of acute abdominal pain

- Sigmoidoscopy or colonoscopy
- CT scan with contrast to confirm the diagnosis

Nursing and Interprofessional Management: Diverticulosis and Diverticulitis

A high-fiber diet, mainly from fruits and vegetables with a decreased intake of fat and red meat, is the best way to prevent diverticular disease. High levels of physical activity seem to decrease the risk. Currently, there is no evidence to support the theory that diverticulitis can be prevented by avoiding nuts and seeds.

In acute diverticulitis, the goal of treatment is to let the colon rest and the inflammation subside. Some patients can be managed at home with a clear liquid diet, bedrest, and analgesics. Hospitalization is needed if symptoms are severe, the patient is unable to tolerate oral fluids, there are systemic manifestations of infection (fever, significant leukocytosis), or the patient has co-morbid conditions (e.g., immunosuppression).

If hospitalized, the patient is kept on NPO status, placed on bedrest, and given IV fluids and antibiotics. Observe for signs of abscess, bleeding, and peritonitis, and monitor the WBC count. Give analgesics as needed. Maintain strict intake and output records. If needed, a nasogastric (NG) tube with low suction will provide decompression. When the acute attack subsides, give oral fluids first and then progress the diet to semisolids.

Patients with reoccurring diverticulitis or complications, such as an abscess or obstruction, may have a resection of the involved colon with a primary anastomosis. If the health care provider (HCP) is not able to anastomose the colon, then the patient will have a temporary diverting colostomy. After the colon heals, the temporary colostomy can be "taken down" and the ends of the colon reconnected.

Patient Teaching

Teach patients with diverticular disease to avoid increased intraabdominal pressure because it may precipitate an attack.

- Factors that increase intraabdominal pressure are straining at stool, vomiting, bending, lifting, and wearing tight, restrictive clothing.
- Provide the patient with a full explanation of the condition.
- Teach about the importance of following a high-fiber diet. Encourage a fluid intake of at least 2 L/day. Explain that the patient does not have to avoid nuts, seeds, and corn.
- Weight reduction is important for the obese person with diverticular disease.

DYSMENORRHEA

Description

Dysmenorrhea is painful menses with abdominal cramping. The degree of pain and discomfort varies. The 2 types of dysmenorrhea are primary (no pathologic condition exists) and secondary (pelvic disease is the underlying cause). Dysmenorrhea is one of the most common gynecologic problems.

Pathophysiology

Primary dysmenorrhea begins in the first few years after menarche, typically with the onset of regular menstrual cycles. It is usually related to increased levels of prostaglandin, a hormone that is found in the endometrium.

- Endometrial stimulation by estrogen and progesterone increases prostaglandin production. Prostaglandin stimulates the uterus to contract. Uterine contractions and constriction of small endometrial blood vessels cause tissue ischemia and sensitize pain receptors, resulting in painful menstrual cramps. As menstruation continues, prostaglandin levels decrease each day and cramping lessens.

Secondary dysmenorrhea usually occurs after adolescence, most commonly at 30 to 40 years of age, and worsens as the woman ages. Common pelvic conditions that cause secondary dysmenorrhea include endometriosis, chronic pelvic inflammatory disease, and uterine leiomyomas (fibroids).

Clinical Manifestations

In *primary dysmenorrhea,* symptoms start 12 to 24 hours before the onset of menses. The pain is most severe the first day of menses and rarely lasts more than 2 days.

- Manifestations include lower abdominal colicky, cramping pain that often radiates to the lower back and upper thighs. The abdominal pain is often accompanied by nausea, diarrhea, loose stools, fatigue, and headache.

In *secondary dysmenorrhea,* usually the woman previously had little to no pain during the menstrual cycle. The pain, which may be unilateral, is often more constant in nature and continues for a longer time than with primary dysmenorrhea.

- Signs and symptoms such as *dyspareunia* (painful intercourse), painful defecation, or irregular bleeding may occur at times other than menstruation.

Diagnostic Studies

Evaluation begins with a complete health history and a pelvic examination.

- If the pelvic examination is normal and the history reveals an onset shortly after menarche with symptoms only associated with menses, the probable diagnosis is primary dysmenorrhea.
- If a specific cause is evident, the diagnosis is secondary dysmenorrhea.

Interprofessional and Nursing Management

Nonsteroidal antiinflammatory drugs (NSAIDs) (e.g., naproxen [Naprosyn]) inhibit prostaglandins. Oral contraceptives may be used to decrease estrogen and progesterone, lower prostaglandin levels, decrease monthly endometrial lining proliferation, and decrease menstrual flow.

- Teach the patient that applying heat to the abdomen or back and taking NSAIDs may relieve acute pain.
- Suggest pain-relieving practices, such as relaxation breathing, guided imagery, and yoga.
- Encourage regular exercise, which may reduce endometrial hyperplasia and subsequent prostaglandin production.

DYSRHYTHMIAS

Description

Dysrhythmias are abnormal cardiac rhythms that result from disorders of impulse formation, impulse conduction, or both. Promptly assess abnormal cardiac rhythms and the patient's response to the rhythm.

Normally, the sinoatrial (SA) node is the natural pacemaker of the heart. A pacemaker from a site other than the SA node may be fired in 2 ways.

- If the SA node fires more slowly than a secondary pacemaker, the electrical signals from the secondary pacemaker may "escape." The secondary pacemaker will then fire automatically at its intrinsic rate. These secondary pacemakers may start from the atrioventricular (AV) node at a rate of 40 to 60 times per minute or the His-Purkinje system at a rate of 20 to 40 times per minute.
- Another way that secondary pacemakers can start is when they fire more rapidly than the normal pacemaker of the SA node. *Triggered beats* (early or late) may come from an *ectopic focus* (area outside the normal conduction pathway) in the atria, AV node, or ventricles. This results in a dysrhythmia, which replaces the normal sinus rhythm.

Dysrhythmias occur as the result of various abnormalities and disease states. The cause of a dysrhythmia influences the patient's treatment. Common causes of dysrhythmias are presented in Table 32.

TABLE 32   Common Causes of Dysrhythmias[a]

Heart Conditions
- Accessory pathways
- Cardiomyopathy
- Conduction defects
- Heart failure
- Myocardial ischemia, infarction
- Valve disease

Other Conditions
- Acid-base imbalances
- Alcohol
- Caffeine, tobacco
- Connective tissue disorders
- Drowning
- Drug effects (e.g., antidysrhythmia drugs, stimulants, β-adrenergic blockers) or toxicity
- Electric shock
- Electrolyte imbalances (e.g., hyperkalemia, hypocalcemia)
- Emotional crisis
- Herbal supplements (e.g., areca nut, wahoo root bark, yerba maté)
- Hypoxia
- Metabolic conditions (e.g., thyroid dysfunction)
- Sepsis, shock
- Toxins

[a]List is not all-inclusive.

A systematic approach to assessing a cardiac rhythm is described in Table 33.

Types of Dysrhythmias

The characteristics of common dysrhythmias are described in Part Three (Reference Appendix) on pp. 740. Examples of electrocardiogram (ECG) tracings of common dysrhythmias are presented in Chapter 35 of Harding et al., *Lewis' Medical-Surgical Nursing*, ed 11.

Sinus Bradycardia

Sinus bradycardia occurs when the SA node discharges at a rate < 60 beats/minute. It may be a normal rhythm in aerobically trained athletes or in some people during sleep. It also occurs in response to carotid sinus massage, Valsalva maneuver, hypothermia, increased intraocular pressure, vagal stimulation, and the administration of certain drugs (e.g., β-adrenergic blockers, calcium channel

TABLE 33   Approach to Assessing Heart Rhythm

When assessing a heart rhythm, use a consistent and systematic approach. One such approach includes the following:

1. Look for the P wave. Is it upright or inverted? Is there 1 for every QRS complex or more than 1? Are atrial fibrillatory or flutter waves present?
2. Evaluate the atrial rhythm. Is it regular or irregular?
3. Calculate the atrial rate.
4. Measure the duration of the PR interval. Is it normal duration or prolonged? Is it consistent in its duration before each QRS?
5. Evaluate the ventricular rhythm. Is it regular or irregular?
6. Calculate the ventricular rate.
7. Measure the duration of the QRS complex. Is it of normal duration or prolonged?
8. Assess the ST segment. Is it isoelectric (flat), elevated, or depressed?
9. Measure the duration of the QT interval. Correct for heart rate (cQT) to determine if it is normal or prolonged.[a]
10. Note the T wave. Is it upright or inverted?

Additional questions to consider include the following:

1. What is the dominant or underlying rhythm and/or dysrhythmia?
2. What is the clinical significance of your findings?
3. What is the treatment for the particular rhythm?

[a]A website for calculating the cQT interval for heart rate is available *(www.mdcalc. com/corrected-qt-interval-qtc)*.

blockers). Disease states associated with sinus bradycardia are hypothyroidism, increased intracranial pressure, hypoglycemia, and inferior wall myocardial infarction (MI).

- Symptomatic bradycardia refers to a heart rate (HR) that is < 60 beats/minute and causes the patient to have symptoms of inadequate perfusion (e.g., fatigue, dizziness, chest pain, syncope).
- If bradycardia is caused by drugs, these may have to be held, discontinued, or reduced. For the patient with symptoms, treatment consists of giving IV atropine (anticholinergic drug). If atropine is ineffective, transcutaneous pacing or a dopamine or epinephrine infusion are options. The patient may need a permanent pacemaker.

Sinus Tachycardia

Sinus tachycardia involves an HR of 101 to 180 beats/minute from the SA node, occurring as a result of vagal inhibition or sympathetic stimulation. This dysrhythmia is associated with stressors, such as

exercise, fever, pain, hypotension, hypovolemia, anemia, hypoglycemia, myocardial ischemia, heart failure (HF), hyperthyroidism,
and anxiety. It can be an effect of drugs, such as epinephrine, norepinephrine, caffeine, theophylline, nifedipine, or hydralazine.
Pseudoephedrine, which is found in many over-the-counter cold
remedies, can also cause tachycardia.

- The clinical significance of sinus tachycardia depends on the
  patient's tolerance of the increased HR. The patient may have
  dizziness, dyspnea, and hypotension because of decreased cardiac output (CO). An increased HR increases myocardial O_2
  consumption. Angina or an increase in infarction size may occur
  with sinus tachycardia in those with coronary artery disease
  (CAD) or an acute MI.
- The underlying cause of tachycardia guides the treatment. For
  example, if the patient is experiencing tachycardia from pain,
  effective pain management is important to treat the tachycardia.
  In clinically stable patients, vagal maneuvers can be tried. IV β-
  blockers (e.g., metoprolol), adenosine (Adenocard), or calcium-
  channel blockers (e.g., diltiazem) can reduce HR and decrease
  myocardial O_2 consumption. Clinically unstable patients may
  need synchronized cardioversion.

Premature Atrial Contraction

Premature atrial contraction (PAC) is a contraction starting from
an ectopic focus in the atrium (in a location other than the SA
node) sooner than the next expected sinus beat. The ectopic focus
starts in the left or right atrium and travels across the atria by an
abnormal pathway, creating a distorted P wave. At the AV node,
it may be stopped (nonconducted PAC), delayed (lengthened PR
interval), or conducted normally. If the impulse moves through
the AV node, in most cases it is conducted normally through the
ventricles.

In a normal heart, a PAC can result from emotional stress or physical fatigue, or from caffeine, tobacco, or alcohol use. A PAC can
also result from hypoxia, electrolyte imbalances, hyperthyroidism,
chronic obstructive pulmonary disease (COPD), and heart disease,
including CAD and valvular disease.

- HR varies with the underlying rate and frequency of PACs, and
  the rhythm is irregular.
- In persons with healthy hearts, isolated PACs are not significant.
  Patients may report palpitations or a sense that the heart "skipped
  a beat."
- In persons with heart disease, frequent PACs may indicate
  enhanced automaticity of the atria or a reentry mechanism. Such
  PACs may warn of or start more serious dysrhythmias (e.g., supraventricular tachycardia).

- Treatment depends on the patient's symptoms. Withdrawal of sources of stimulation, such as caffeine or sympathomimetic drugs (e.g., epinephrine, dopamine), may be needed. β-Blockers may be used to decrease PACs.

Paroxysmal Supraventricular Tachycardia

Paroxysmal supraventricular tachycardia (PSVT), also known as *supraventricular tachycardia* (SVT) or *atrial tachycardia*, is a dysrhythmia starting in an ectopic focus anywhere above the bifurcation of the bundle of His (see Fig. 35.13). Identifying the ectopic focus is often hard even with a 12-lead ECG, since it requires recording the dysrhythmia as it starts.

PSVT occurs because of a reentrant phenomenon (reexcitation of the atria when there is a one-way block). Usually a PAC triggers a run of repeated premature beats. Paroxysmal refers to an abrupt onset and ending. A brief period of asystole (absence of all cardiac electrical activity) may follow the termination. AV block may prevent some of the impulses from being conducted to the ventricles. PSVT can occur with Wolff-Parkinson-White (WPW) syndrome or "preexcitation" with extra conduction or accessory pathways. HR is 151 to 220 beats/minute and rhythm is regular. Some degree of AV block may be present.

- Clinical significance depends on the associated symptoms. A prolonged episode and HR above 180 beats/minute decreases CO, resulting in hypotension, dyspnea, and angina.
- Treatment for PSVT includes vagal stimulation and drug therapy. Common vagal maneuvers include Valsalva, carotid massage, and coughing. IV adenosine is the drug of choice to convert PSVT to a normal sinus rhythm. This drug has a short half-life (10 seconds) and is well tolerated. IV β-blockers and calcium-channel blockers (e.g., diltiazem, verapamil) are also options. If vagal stimulation and drug therapy are ineffective and the patient becomes hemodynamically unstable, synchronized cardioversion is used.

Atrial Flutter

Atrial flutter is an atrial tachydysrhythmia identified on the ECG by recurring, regular, sawtooth-shaped flutter waves that originate from a single ectopic focus in the right atrium. Atrial flutter is associated with CAD, hypertension, mitral valve disorders, pulmonary embolus, chronic lung disease, cor pulmonale, cardiomyopathy, hyperthyroidism, and the use of drugs, such as digoxin, quinidine, and epinephrine.

- The atrial rate is 250 to 350 beats/minute. The ventricular rate varies depending on the conduction ratio. In 2:1 conduction, the ventricular rate is typically about 150 beats/minute. Atrial and ventricular rhythms are usually regular.

- High ventricular rates (>100 beats/minute) can decrease CO and cause serious consequences, such as HF. The primary treatment goal is to slow ventricular response by increasing AV block. Drugs used to control the ventricular rate include calcium-channel blockers and β-blockers.
- Electrical cardioversion may be done to convert the atrial flutter to sinus rhythm in an emergency (i.e., when the patient is clinically unstable) and electively.
- Antidysrhythmic drugs can convert atrial flutter to sinus rhythm (e.g., ibutilide [Corvert]) or to maintain sinus rhythm (e.g., amiodarone, flecainide, dronedarone [Multaq]).
- Radiofrequency catheter ablation in an electrophysiologic (EPS) laboratory is the treatment of choice for atrial flutter.

Atrial Fibrillation

Atrial fibrillation is a consequence of total disorganization of atrial electrical activity associated with multiple ectopic foci. It results in loss of effective atrial contraction. The dysrhythmia may be paroxysmal (i.e., beginning and ending spontaneously) or persistent (lasting longer than 7 days).

Atrial fibrillation is the most common, clinically significant dysrhythmia with respect to morbidity, mortality, and economic impact. Its prevalence increases with age. Atrial fibrillation usually occurs with underlying heart disease. It often develops acutely with thyrotoxicosis, alcohol intoxication, caffeine use, electrolyte problems, stress, or heart surgery.

- The atrial rate may be as high as 350 to 600 beats/minute. Chaotic, fibrillatory waves replace the P waves. The ventricular rate varies, and the rhythm is usually irregular.
- Atrial fibrillation results in a decrease in CO secondary to ineffective atrial contractions and/or rapid ventricular response. Thrombi may form in the atria because of blood stasis. An embolized clot may pass to the brain, causing a stroke.

The goals of treatment include a decrease in ventricular response to <100 beats/minute, prevention of cerebral embolic events, and conversion to sinus rhythm, if possible. Drugs used for rate control include calcium-channel blockers (e.g., diltiazem), β-blockers (e.g., metoprolol), amiodarone, and digoxin (Lanoxin). Amiodarone is often used for maintenance of sinus rhythm after cardioversion.

Electrical cardioversion may convert atrial fibrillation to normal sinus rhythm.

- If a patient is in atrial fibrillation for longer than 48 hours, anticoagulation therapy is needed for 3 to 4 weeks before the cardioversion and for several weeks after successful cardioversion.

- For patients with drug-refractory atrial fibrillation or those who do not respond to electrical conversion, radiofrequency catheter ablation (similar to the procedure for atrial flutter) and the Maze procedure (surgical intervention that interrupts ectopic electrical signals) may be used.
- Left atrial appendage occlusion is a surgical strategy to prevent blood clot formation in patients who have atrial fibrillation but cannot use oral anticoagulants.

First-Degree Atrioventricular Block

In first-degree AV block, every impulse from the atria is conducted to the ventricles, but the time of AV conduction is prolonged. After the impulse moves through the AV node, the ventricles usually respond normally. First-degree AV block is associated with increasing age, MI, CAD, rheumatic fever, hyperthyroidism, vagal stimulation, and drugs such as digoxin, β-blockers, calcium-channel blockers, and flecainide.

- HR is normal and rhythm is regular.
- Patients with first-degree AV block are asymptomatic.
- There is no treatment for first-degree AV block. Treatment of associated conditions may be considered.

Second-Degree Atrioventricular Block, Type I (Mobitz I, Wenckebach)

A type I second-degree AV block is characterized by gradual lengthening of the PR interval. It occurs because of an AV conduction time that is increasingly prolonged until an atrial impulse is nonconducted and a QRS complex is blocked (missing). Type I AV block may result from use of digoxin or β-blockers. It may be associated with CAD. It is usually the result of myocardial ischemia or inferior MI. It is generally transient and well tolerated. However, it may be a warning signal of a more serious AV conduction disturbance (e.g., complete heart block).

- The rhythm appears on the ECG in a pattern of grouped beats.
- If the patient is symptomatic, atropine is used to increase HR, or a temporary pacemaker may be needed, especially if the patient has had an MI.

Second-Degree Atrioventricular Block, Type II (Mobitz II)

In type II second-degree AV block, the P wave is nonconducted without progressive PR lengthening. This usually occurs when a bundle branch block is present. On conducted beats, the PR interval is constant. In a second-degree heart block, a certain number of impulses from the SA node are not conducted to the ventricles. This occurs in ratios of 2:1, 3:1, and so on when there are 2 P waves to 1 QRS complex, 3 P waves to 1 QRS complex, and so on. It may occur with varying ratios. Type II AV block is associated with rheumatic heart disease, CAD, anterior MI, and drug toxicity.

D

- The atrial rate is usually normal. The ventricular rate depends on the intrinsic rate and degree of AV block. The atrial rhythm is regular, but the ventricular rhythm may be irregular.
- Type II AV block often progresses to third-degree AV block and is associated with a poor prognosis.
- Reduced HR frequently results in decreased CO with subsequent hypotension and myocardial ischemia.
- Transcutaneous pacing or the insertion of a temporary pacemaker may be necessary before the insertion of a permanent pacemaker if the patient becomes symptomatic (e.g., hypotension, angina) (see Pacemakers, p. 707). Atropine is not an effective drug for this dysrhythmia.

Third-Degree Atrioventricular Block (Complete Heart Block)

Third-degree AV block is a form of AV dissociation in which no impulses from the atria are conducted to the ventricles. The atria are stimulated and contract independently of the ventricles. Ventricular rhythm is an escape rhythm from above or below the bifurcation of the bundle of His. This rhythm is associated with severe heart disease, including CAD, MI, myocarditis, cardiomyopathy, and some systemic diseases, such as amyloidosis and scleroderma. Drugs such as digoxin, β-blockers, and calcium-channel blockers can cause third-degree AV block.

- Atrial rate is usually a sinus rate of 60 to 100 beats/minute. Ventricular rate depends on the site of the block. If it is in the AV node, the rate is 40 to 60 beats/minute, and if it is in the Purkinje system, it is 20 to 40 beats/minute. Atrial and ventricular rhythms are regular but unrelated to each other.
- Third-degree AV block usually results in reduced CO with subsequent ischemia and heart failure.
- Symptomatic patients need a temporary transcutaneous pacemaker until a permanent pacemaker can be inserted. Atropine is not effective for this dysrhythmia. Epinephrine and dopamine are temporary measures to increase HR and support BP before pacemaker insertion (see Pacemakers, p. 707).

Premature Ventricular Contractions

Premature ventricular contractions (PVCs) originate in an ectopic focus in the ventricles. PVCs are a premature occurrence of the QRS complex, which is wide and distorted in shape. PVCs that start from different foci appear different in shape from each other and are termed *multifocal PVCs.* When every other beat is a PVC, the condition is called *ventricular bigeminy.* When every third beat is a PVC, the condition is called *ventricular trigeminy.* Two consecutive PVCs are called *couplets. Ventricular tachycardia* (VT) appears as 3 or more consecutive PVCs. A PVC falling on the T wave of a preceding beat is termed the *R-on-T phenomenon* and is considered to be dangerous because it may precipitate VT or ventricular fibrillation (VF).

PVCs are associated with stimulants such as caffeine, alcohol, nicotine, epinephrine, and digoxin. They are also associated with electrolyte imbalances, hypoxia, fever, exercise, and emotional stress. Disease states associated with PVCs include MI, cardiomyopathy, mitral valve prolapse, HF, and CAD.

- HR varies depending on the intrinsic rate and number of PVCs. Rhythm is irregular because of premature beats.
- PVCs are usually not harmful in the patient with a normal heart. In heart disease, PVCs may reduce CO and precipitate angina and HF. PVCs in CAD or acute MI represent ventricular irritability.
- Treatment relates to the cause of the PVCs (e.g., oxygen therapy for hypoxia, electrolyte replacement). Assessing the patient's hemodynamic status is important to determine if drug therapy is indicated. Drug therapy includes β-blockers, lidocaine, or amiodarone.

Ventricular Tachycardia

VT is seen on the ECG as a run of 3 or more PVCs that occurs when an ectopic focus or foci fire repetitively. VT is a life-threatening dysrhythmia because of the associated decrease in CO and the possibility of the development of VF. VT is associated with MI, CAD, significant electrolyte imbalances, hypoxemia, cardiomyopathy, mitral valve prolapse, long QT syndrome, digitalis toxicity, and central nervous system disorders. The dysrhythmia can be seen in patients who have no evidence of cardiac disease.

- The ventricular rate is 150 to 250 beats/minute.
- VT can be stable (patient has a pulse) or unstable (patient is pulseless). Sustained VT causes a severe decrease in CO because of decreased ventricular diastolic filling times and loss of atrial contraction. This results in hypotension, pulmonary edema, decreased cerebral blood flow, and cardiopulmonary arrest.
- VT must be treated quickly, even if it occurs only briefly and stops abruptly. Episodes may recur if prophylactic treatment is not started.
  Different forms of VT exist:
- If the patient is hemodynamically stable and has *monomorphic VT* (QRS complexes have same shape, size, and direction) with preserved left ventricular function, then IV procainamide, amiodarone, or lidocaine is used. These drugs can also be used if the VT is polymorphic with a normal baseline QT interval.
- *Polymorphic VT* with a prolonged baseline QT interval is treated with IV magnesium, isoproterenol, phenytoin, or antitachycardia pacing. Drugs that prolong the QT interval (e.g., dofetilide

[Tikosyn]) should be stopped. Cardioversion is used when drug therapy is ineffective.

- VT without a pulse is lethal and is treated in the same way as VF.

Ventricular Fibrillation

VF is a severe derangement of the heart rhythm characterized on the ECG by irregular waveforms of various shapes and amplitudes. This pattern represents the firing of multiple ectopic foci in the ventricle. Mechanically, the ventricle is simply "quivering," and no effective contraction or CO occurs. This dysrhythmia is lethal. VF occurs in acute MI and myocardial ischemia and in chronic diseases, such as CAD and cardiomyopathy. It may occur during cardiac pacing or cardiac catheterization procedures because of catheter stimulation of the ventricle. It may also occur with coronary reperfusion after thrombolytic therapy. Other clinical associations are electrical shock, hyperkalemia, hypoxemia, acidosis, and drug toxicity.

- HR is not measurable. Rhythm is irregular and chaotic.
- VF results in an unresponsive, pulseless, and apneic state. If VF is not treated quickly, the patient will not recover.
- Treatment consists of immediate initiation of cardiopulmonary resuscitation (CPR) and advanced cardiac life support (ACLS) with the use of defibrillation and definitive drug therapy (e.g., epinephrine, amiodarone). There should be no delay in starting chest compressions and using a defibrillator once available.

EATING DISORDERS

Description

Eating disorders are psychiatric conditions associated with physiologic alterations. Patients with eating disorders may be hospitalized for fluid and electrolyte problems; dysrhythmias; and nutritional, endocrine, and metabolic disorders. Menstrual problems may occur in women of childbearing age.

The 3 most common types of eating disorders are *anorexia nervosa* (AN), *bulimia nervosa,* and *binge-eating disorder.* Binge-eating disorder is less severe than bulimia nervosa and AN. Persons with binge-eating disorder do not have a distorted body image and are often overweight or obese.

Anorexia Nervosa

AN is characterized by restricting energy intake, difficulties in maintaining an appropriate weight, an intense fear of gaining weight or being fat, and distorted body image. People with AN generally restrict the number of calories and the types of food they eat. Some people exercise compulsively, purge via vomiting and laxatives, and/or binge eat. AN manifests as unwillingness to maintain a healthy weight, refusal to eat, continuous dieting, detailed food rituals, and avoiding social situations. Common assessment findings include signs of malnutrition, extreme thinness, hypothermia, and muscle weakness.

Diagnostic studies often show osteopenia or osteoporosis, iron-deficiency anemia, and a high blood urea nitrogen level from marked intravascular volume depletion and abnormal renal function.

- Lack of potassium in the diet and loss of potassium in the urine lead to potassium deficiency. Manifestations of potassium deficiency include muscle weakness, dysrhythmias, and renal failure.
- Leukopenia, hypoglycemia, and decreased sodium, magnesium, and phosphorus may be present.

Treatment involves a combination of nutritional support and psychiatric care. Nutritional care focuses on reaching and maintaining a healthy weight, normal eating patterns, and perception of hunger and satiety.

Hospitalization may be needed if the patient has complications that cannot be managed in an outpatient therapy program. Nutritional repletion must be closely supervised to ensure consistent and ongoing weight gain. Refeeding syndrome is a rare but serious complication of behavioral refeeding programs. The use of enteral or parenteral nutrition may be needed (see Enteral Nutrition, p. 685, and Parenteral Nutrition, p. 710).

Improved nutrition is not a cure for AN. The underlying psychiatric issues must be addressed by identifying problematic personal and family interactions, followed by personal and family counseling.

Bulimia Nervosa

Bulimia nervosa is a disorder characterized by episodes of binge eating with compensatory behaviors to avoid weight gain (vomiting, laxative misuse, overexercise). The person with bulimia is concerned with body image and often goes to great lengths to conceal abnormal eating habits. They may have normal weight for height or the weight may fluctuate with bingeing and purging.

- Signs of frequent vomiting include macerated knuckles, swollen salivary glands, broken blood vessels in the eyes, and dental problems.
- Abnormal laboratory values, including hypokalemia, metabolic alkalosis, and increased serum amylase, may occur from frequent vomiting.

The cause of bulimia is unclear but is thought to be similar to that of AN. Substance use, anxiety, affective disorders, and personality changes have been reported among people with bulimia.

- Combination treatment with psychologic counseling and nutritional therapy is essential.
- Fluoxetine (Prozac) is the only U.S. Food and Drugs Administration (FDA)-approved antidepressant for treating bulimia nervosa. Antidepressants are not helpful for all patients with bulimia.
- Education and emotional support for the patient and the family are vital. Support groups, such as the National Association of Anorexia Nervosa and Associated Disorders (ANAD) (*www.anad.org*), may be helpful.

ENCEPHALITIS

Description
Encephalitis is a serious, sometimes fatal, acute inflammation of the brain. It is usually caused by a virus. Many different viruses have been implicated in encephalitis; some are associated with seasons of the year or geographic areas. Ticks and mosquitoes transmit epidemic encephalitis, whereas nonepidemic encephalitis may occur as a complication of measles, chickenpox, or mumps.

- Herpes simplex virus (HSV) encephalitis is the most common form of nonepidemic viral encephalitis.
- Cytomegalovirus encephalitis occurs in patients with acquired immunodeficiency syndrome (AIDS).

Clinical Manifestations and Diagnostic Studies
Infection can be acute or subacute. The onset is typically nonspecific, with fever, headache, nausea, and vomiting. Signs of encephalitis appear on day 2 or 3 and may range from minimal changes in mental status to coma.

- Almost any central nervous system (CNS) abnormality can occur, including hemiparesis, tremors, seizures, dysphasia, cranial nerve palsies, personality changes, memory impairment, and amnesia.
- Diagnostic findings related to viral encephalitis are shown in Table 34.
- Brain imaging techniques include CT, MRI, and positron emission tomography (PET).
- Polymerase chain reaction (PCR) tests can be used to detect HSV and West Nile encephalitis.

TABLE 34 Comparison of Cerebral Inflammatory Conditions

Feature	Meningitis	Encephalitis	Brain Abscess
Cause	Bacteria[a] (*Streptococcus pneumoniae, Neisseria meningitidis*, group B streptococci, viruses, fungi	Bacteria, fungi, parasites, herpes simplex virus (HSV), other viruses (e.g., West Nile virus)	Streptococci, staphylococci (acquired through bloodstream)
CSF (reference interval)			
• Pressure (70–150 mm H_2O)	Increased *Bacterial:* 200–500 mm H_2O *Viral:* ≤250 mm H_2O	Normal to slight increase	Increased
• WBC count (0–5 cells/μL)	*Bacterial:* >1000/μL (mainly neutrophils) *Viral:* 25–500/μL (mainly lymphocytes)	500/μL, neutrophils (early), lymphocytes (later)	25–300/μL (neutrophils)
• Protein (15–45 mg/dL [0.15–0.45 g/L])	*Bacterial:* >500 mg/dL *Viral:* 50–500 mg/dL	Slight increase	Normal
• Glucose (40–70 mg/dL [2.2–3.9 mmol/L])	*Bacterial:* decreased at 5–40 mg/dL *Viral:* normal or low at >40 mg/dL	Normal	Low or absent
• Appearance	*Bacterial:* turbid, cloudy *Viral:* clear or cloudy	Clear	Clear
Diagnostic studies	CT scan, Gram stain, smear, culture, PCR assay[b]	CT scan, EEG, MRI, PET, PCR, IgM antibodies to virus in serum or CSF	CT scan
Treatment	Antibiotics, dexamethasone, supportive care, prevention of ↑ ICP	Supportive care, prevention of ↑ ICP, acyclovir (Zovirax) for HSV infection	Antibiotics, incision and drainage Supportive care

[a]See also Meningitis, Bacterial on p. 397.
[b]PCR testing is used to detect viral RNA or DNA.
CSF, Cerebrospinal fluid; *DNA,* deoxyribonucleic acid; *EEG,* electroencephalography; *ICP,* intracranial pressure; *IgM,* immunoglobulin M; *PCR,* polymerase chain reaction; *PET,* positron emission tomography; *RNA,* ribonucleic acid; *WBC,* white blood cell.

E

West Nile virus infection should be strongly considered in adults older than 50 years who develop encephalitis or meningitis in summer or early fall. The best diagnostic test to identify West Nile virus is a blood test that detects viral ribonucleic acid (RNA).

Nursing and Interprofessional Management

Mosquito control to prevent encephalitis includes cleaning rain gutters, removing old tires, draining bird baths, and removing water where mosquitoes can breed. Insect repellant should be used outdoors during mosquito season.

Management of encephalitis, including West Nile virus infection, is symptomatic and supportive. Initially many patients require intensive care. Acyclovir is used to treat HSV encephalitis. For maximal benefit, treatment should be started before the onset of coma. Prophylactic treatment with antiseizure drugs may be used in severe cases of encephalitis.

ENDOCARDITIS, INFECTIVE

Description

Infective endocarditis (IE) is an infection of the endocardial (innermost) surface of the heart and the heart valves. In the United States, there are around 40,000 to 50,000 new cases of IE per year.

IE is most often classified by cause (e.g., IV drug abuse, fungal endocarditis) or site of involvement (e.g., prosthetic valve endocarditis).

- In the past, IE was classified as "subacute" or "acute." The subacute form affects those with preexisting valve disease over a period of months. In contrast, the acute form affects those with healthy valves and appears as a rapidly progressive illness.

Pathophysiology

IE occurs when blood flow allows organisms to contact and infect previously damaged heart valves or other endothelial surfaces. About 30% of cases of IE are caused by *Staphylococcus aureus.* Other bacterial causes include *Streptococcus viridans* and *Coagulase Negative Staphylococci.*

Principal risk factors include valve placement, hemodialysis, and IV drug use. IE typically develops in 3 stages: (1) bacteremia, (2) adhesion, and (3) vegetation.

Vegetations, the primary lesions of IE, consist of fibrin, leukocytes, platelets, and microbes, which adhere to the valve surface or endocardium. The loss of portions of this vegetation into the circulation results in embolization. Up to 30% of persons with IE will develop embolization. This occurs when left-sided heart vegetations move to various organs (e.g., kidney, spleen, brain) and extremities. Right-sided heart lesions embolize to the lungs, resulting in pulmonary emboli.

The infection may spread locally to cause damage to valves or their supporting structures. This results in dysrhythmias, valve dysfunction, and eventual invasion of the myocardium, leading to heart failure (HF), sepsis, and heart block.

At 1 time, rheumatic heart disease was the most common cause of IE. Now, it accounts for < 20% of cases. The main contributing factors to IE are: (1) aging (more than 50% of older people have calcified aortic stenosis), (2) IV drug abuse, (3) use of prosthetic valves, (4) use of intravascular devices resulting in health care–associated infections (e.g., methicillin-resistant *S. aureus* [MRSA]), and (5) renal dialysis.

Clinical Manifestations

The clinical manifestations are nonspecific and can involve multiple organ systems. Ninety percent of patients have fever. Fever may be low grade or may be absent in older adults or those who are immunocompromised. Other symptoms include chills, weakness, malaise, fatigue, and anorexia. Patients may have arthralgias, myalgias, back pain, abdominal discomfort, weight loss, headache, and clubbing of fingers in subacute forms of IE.

Vascular signs may include splinter hemorrhages (black longitudinal streaks) in the nail beds. Petechiae, from fragmentation and microembolization of vegetative lesions are common on the conjunctivae, lips, buccal mucosa, and palate and over the ankles, feet, and antecubital and popliteal areas. *Osler's nodes* (painful, tender, red or purple, pea-size lesions) may be on the fingertips or toes. *Janeway's lesions* (flat, painless, small, red spots) may be found on the palms and soles. Eye examination may show hemorrhagic retinal lesions called *Roth's spots*.

Most patients with IE have a new or worsening systolic murmur. HF is common, occurring in up to 80% of patients with aortic valve IE and 50% of those with mitral valve IE.

Septic embolism is a potential complication of IE. Embolic events occur in more than 50% of patients. The central nervous system is the most often affected organ system, followed by extremities, spleen, and kidney.

Diagnostic Studies

A health history should be obtained with inquiry made regarding any recent dental, urologic, surgical, or gynecologic procedures including normal or abnormal obstetric delivery. Note any previous history of intravenous drug abuse (IVDA), heart disease, recent heart catheterization, heart surgery, intravascular device placement, renal dialysis, or infections (e.g., skin, respiratory, urinary tract).

- Blood culture of 3 samples drawn 1 hour apart from 3 different sites will be positive in more than 90% of patients.
- A mild leukocytosis occurs in acute IE.
- Erythrocyte sedimentation rate (ESR) and C-reactive protein (CRP) levels may be elevated.
- Chest x-ray can detect an enlarged heart.
- Echocardiography can visualize vegetations.
- Electrocardiogram (ECG) may show first- or second-degree heart block because the valves lie in close proximity to the atrioventricular (AV) node.
- Cardiac catheterization may be used to evaluate valve functioning.

Interprofessional Management
Prophylactic Treatment
Antibiotic prophylaxis is recommended for high cardiac risk conditions including prosthetic heart valves, history of endocarditis, surgically constructed systemic-pulmonary shunts, congenital heart disease, and heart valve disease after heart transplantation. Specific antibiotic regimens are recommended for dental, respiratory, gastrointestinal (GI) and genitourinary (GU) procedures (see Table 36.2, Harding et al., *Lewis' Medical-Surgical Nursing,* ed 11).
Drug Therapy
Accurate identification of the causative organism is the key to successful treatment. Complete removal of the organisms generally takes weeks, and relapses are common. IV antibiotic therapy is based on blood cultures.

- Blood cultures that stay positive indicate inadequate or inappropriate antibiotics, aortic root or myocardial abscess, or the wrong diagnosis (e.g., an infection elsewhere).
- Fever that persists is treated with aspirin, acetaminophen, fluids, and rest.
- Complete bed rest is usually not needed unless the temperature remains elevated or there are signs of HF.
- Endocarditis coupled with HF responds poorly to antibiotic therapy and valve replacement, so it can be life-threatening.

Nursing Management
Goals
The patient with IE will have normal or baseline cardiac function, perform activities of daily living without fatigue, and understand the therapeutic regimen to prevent recurrence of endocarditis.

Nursing Interventions

The incidence of IE can be decreased by identifying people who are at risk for the disease. Tell the patient to avoid people with infections, especially upper respiratory tract infections, and to report cold, flu, and cough symptoms. Stress the importance of avoiding excessive fatigue, planning rest periods, using good oral hygiene, and scheduling regular dental visits.

IE generally requires treatment with antibiotics for 4 to 6 weeks. After initial treatment in the hospital, the patient may continue treatment in the home setting.

- Patients who receive outpatient IV antibiotics require vigilant home nursing care. Teach the patient or caregiver about monitoring body temperature because persistent, prolonged temperature elevations may indicate ineffective drug therapy.
- The patient needs adequate periods of physical and emotional rest. Bed rest may be needed when fever is present or there are complications (e.g., heart damage). Otherwise the patient may perform moderate activity.
- Monitor laboratory data, including blood cultures, to determine antibiotic effectiveness. Assess IV lines for patency and any signs of complications (e.g., phlebitis). Give antibiotics as scheduled and monitor for adverse drug reactions.
- To prevent problems related to decreased mobility, teach the patient to wear elastic compression gradient stockings, perform range-of-motion (ROM) exercises, and cough and deep breathe every 2 hours.
- The patient may have anxiety and fear associated with the illness. Implement strategies to help the patient cope.

▼ **Patient and Caregiver Teaching**
- Instruct the patient about symptoms that may indicate another infection, such as fever, fatigue, malaise, and chills.
- Teach the patient about the importance of prophylactic antibiotic therapy before invasive procedures.
- Explain the relationship of follow-up care, good nutrition, and early treatment of common infections (e.g., colds) to maintaining good health.

ENDOMETRIAL CANCER

Description

Endometrial cancer is the most common gynecologic cancer. If endometrial cancer is diagnosed in the early stage, it has a low mortality rate.

- The major risk factor for endometrial cancer is exposure to unopposed estrogen. Obesity is a risk factor because adipose cells store estrogen, thus increasing the amount of circulating estrogen. Other risk factors include increasing age, never being pregnant, early menarche, late menopause, smoking, diabetes, and a patient or family history of hereditary nonpolyposis colorectal cancer
- Pregnancy, use of oral contraceptives and intrauterine devices (IUDs), and physical exercise are associated with reduced risk.

Pathophysiology

Endometrial cancer arises from the endometrial lining. Most tumors are adenocarcinomas. If endometrial cancer is not diagnosed in early stages, it can invade the myometrium (muscle of the uterus) and the regional lymph nodes.

If metastasis occurs, common sites include the lung, liver, bone, and brain. Prognosis depends on the tumor size, cell type, degree of invasion into the myometrium, and metastasis.

Clinical Manifestations and Diagnostic Studies

- Early manifestations include abnormal uterine bleeding, especially in postmenopausal women.
- Later symptoms include dysuria, dyspareunia, unintentional weight loss and pelvic pain.

Endometrial biopsy is the primary diagnostic procedure for endometrial cancer.

Interprofessional Management

Treatment of endometrial cancer in the early stage is a total hysterectomy and bilateral salpingo-oophorectomy with lymph node biopsies. These may be done by less invasive types of surgery, including robotics and laparoscopy. Surgery may be followed by external irradiation either to the pelvis or abdomen or internal radiation (brachytherapy) intravaginally for local or distant metastasis. Chemotherapy and hormonal therapy may be needed for advanced or recurrent disease.

Nursing Management: Cancers of the Female Reproductive Tract

See Cervical Cancer, p. 116.

ENDOMETRIOSIS

Description

Endometriosis is a common gynecologic condition in which endometrial tissue accumulates outside the uterus. The most frequent sites are in or near the ovaries, uterosacral ligaments, and uterovesical peritoneum (Fig. 8). The endometrial tissue responds to the hormones of the ovarian cycle and undergoes a "mini-menstrual cycle" similar to that of the uterine endometrium. Endometriosis can cause considerable pain.

- Endometriosis is a common cause of infertility and increases the risk of ovarian cancer. The cause of endometriosis is unknown.

Clinical Manifestations

Patients with endometriosis have a wide range of manifestations. The severity of symptoms does not always correlate with the degree of disease found.

- The most common signs and symptoms are secondary dysmenorrhea, infertility, pelvic pain, dyspareunia, and irregular bleeding.
- Less common symptoms include backache, painful bowel movements, and dysuria.
- With menopause, the ovaries no longer make estrogen, and the symptoms may disappear.

E

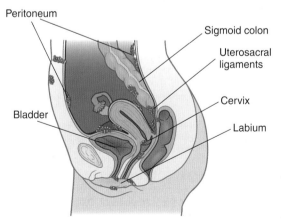

Fig. 8 Common sites of endometriosis.

Diagnostic Studies

Diagnosis is frequently confirmed by patient history and the palpation of firm nodular lumps in the adnexa on bimanual examination. Laparoscopic examination is necessary for a definitive diagnosis. MRI is now being used more often before surgery to determine if the gynecologic symptoms the woman is having are from endometriosis.

Interprofessional and Nursing Management

Treatment is influenced by the patient's age, desire for pregnancy, symptom severity, and the extent and location of the disease. When symptoms are not disruptive, a "watch and wait" approach is used.

Drugs can reduce symptoms. Pain may be relieved with nonsteroidal antiinflammatory drugs such as ibuprofen, naproxen (Naprosyn), and diclofenac (Voltaren). Endometriosis can be controlled but not cured by drug therapy. Persistent lesions give rise to subsequent recurrences once the menstrual cycle is reestablished.

- Continuous use (for 9 months) of combined oral contraceptives causes regression of endometrial tissue.
- Gonadotropin-releasing hormone (GnRH) agonists, such as leuprolide acetate (Lupron) and nafarelin (Synarel), result in amenorrhea. Side effects are the same as those of menopause (hot flashes, vaginal dryness, emotional lability). Loss of bone density can occur in women who stay on the therapy longer than 6 months.

The only cure for endometriosis is surgical removal of all endometrial tissue by means of laparoscopic laser surgery or laparotomy. Definitive surgery involves removal of the uterus, fallopian tubes, ovaries, and as many endometrial implants as possible. GnRH agonist therapy can be given for 4 to 6 months to reduce the size of the lesions before surgery.

- Explore the patient's feelings about maintaining her ovarian function. Each woman should be actively involved in making the decision about preserving part or all of her ovaries if surgically possible.
- For women wishing to get pregnant, conservative surgical therapy is used to remove implants that may block the fallopian tube. Adhesions are removed from the tubes, ovaries, and pelvic structures.

If conservative surgery is the treatment selected, nursing care is similar to general preoperative and postoperative care of a patient undergoing laparotomy (see Abdominal Pain, Acute, p. 3). If definitive surgery is planned, nursing care is similar to care of the patient undergoing an abdominal hysterectomy (see Hysterectomy, p. 120).

ESOPHAGEAL CANCER

Description

Esophageal cancer is not common. However, the rates are increasing. In the United States, around 17,280 new cases are diagnosed and 15,850 deaths occur from esophageal cancer each year. The overall 5-year survival rate is 19%. Risk factors include Barrett's esophagus, smoking, excessive alcohol intake, obesity, and occupational exposure to asbestos or cement dust.

Pathophysiology

Most esophageal cancers are adenocarcinomas. The others are squamous cell tumors. Adenocarcinomas arise from the glands lining the esophagus and resemble cancers of the stomach and small intestine.

- Most tumors occur in the middle and lower portions of the esophagus. The tumor may penetrate the muscular layer and extend outside the esophageal wall.
- The tumor usually appears as an ulcerated lesion. Many patients have advanced disease at the time of diagnosis.
- Obstruction of the esophagus occurs in the later stages.
- Achalasia, a condition of slow esophageal emptying, is associated with squamous cell cancer.

Clinical Manifestations

The onset of symptoms is usually late relative to tumor growth.

- Progressive dysphagia is the most common symptom. It may be a substernal feeling that food is not passing. Initially dysphagia occurs with meat, then with soft foods, and eventually with liquids.
- Pain develops later in the substernal, epigastric, or back and usually increases with swallowing. The pain may radiate to the neck, jaw, ears, and shoulders.
- If the tumor is in the upper third of the esophagus, symptoms such as sore throat, choking, and hoarseness may occur. Weight loss is common.
- When esophageal stenosis (narrowing) is severe, regurgitation of blood-flecked esophageal contents is common.

Complications may include hemorrhage from cancer eroding through the esophagus and into the aorta. Esophageal perforation into the lung or trachea may develop. The liver and lung are common metastatic sites.

Diagnostic Studies

- Esophagram (barium swallow) may detect narrowing at the tumor site.

E

- Endoscopic biopsy is required for diagnosis.
- Endoscopic ultrasonography (EUS) is important in staging esophageal cancer.

Interprofessional Management

Treatment depends on the tumor location and whether metastasis has occurred. The best results may be obtained with a combination of surgery, endoscopic ablation, chemotherapy, and radiation therapy.

- Surgical approaches may be open (thoracic or abdominal incision) or minimally invasive (e.g., laparoscopic vagal nerve–sparing surgery).
- Endoscopic approaches use photodynamic therapy, endoscopic mucosal resection (EMR), or radiofrequency ablation.

Palliative therapy consists of restoring swallowing function and maintaining nutrition and hydration. Dilation and stent placement can relieve obstruction.

Nutritional Therapy

After esophageal surgery, parenteral fluids are given. A swallowing study is often done before the patient takes oral fluids. When fluids are permitted, water (30 to 60 mL) is given hourly, with gradual progression to small, frequent, bland meals. The patient should be in an upright position during and 2 hours after meals to prevent regurgitation. Observe the patient for intolerance to the feeding or leakage into the mediastinum. Pain, increased temperature, and dyspnea may indicate leakage.

- A jejunostomy, gastrostomy, or esophagostomy tube may be placed to feed the patient.

Nursing Management

Goals

The overall goals are that the patient with esophageal cancer will have relief of symptoms, including pain and dysphagia, achieve optimal nutritional intake, and experience a quality of life appropriate to stage of disease and prognosis.

Nursing Interventions

In addition to general preoperative teaching and preparation, pay attention to the patient's nutritional needs. Many patients are poorly nourished because of the inability to ingest adequate food and fluids. Teaching should include information about chest tubes (if a thoracic approach is used), IV lines, nasogastric (NG) and feeding tubes, turning, coughing, and deep breathing. Meticulous oral care is essential.

Postoperative care should include assessment of drainage; maintenance of the NG tube; oral and nasal care; and prevention of respiratory complications by turning, coughing, and deep breathing, with incentive spirometry every 2 hours, and placing the patient in a semi-Fowler's position to prevent gastric reflux and aspiration.

▼ **Patient and Caregiver Teaching**

- Provide emotional and physical support, provide information, clarify test results, and maintain a positive attitude with respect to the patient's immediate recovery and long-term survival.
- Refer the patient to a home health nurse as needed for continued care (e.g., gastrostomy teaching and follow-up wound care).

FIBROCYSTIC BREAST CHANGES

Description

Fibrocystic breast changes include the development of excess fibrous tissue, hyperplasia of the epithelial lining of the mammary ducts, proliferation of mammary ducts, and cyst formation. These benign changes are the most frequently occurring breast disorder. Fibrocystic changes occur most frequently in women between 30 and 50 years old but often begin as early as the age of 20 years. They are not associated alone with increased breast cancer risk.

Fibrocystic changes are the most common breast disorder, occurring in more than 50% of women in North America. Fibrocystic changes most often occur in women with premenstrual abnormalities, nulliparous women, women with a history of spontaneous abortion, nonusers of oral contraceptives, and women with early menarche and late menopause.

Pathophysiology

Fibrocystic changes are thought to be heightened responsiveness of breast tissue to circulating estrogen and progesterone. These changes produce pain from chronic inflammation, edema, nerve irritation, and fibrosis.

- Masses or nodules are often found in the upper, outer quadrants. They usually occur bilaterally.
- Symptoms of fibrocystic changes often worsen in the premenstrual phase and subside after menstruation.

Clinical Manifestations and Diagnostic Studies

Manifestations of fibrocystic breast changes include 1 or more palpable lumps that are round, well delineated, and freely movable within the breast. Discomfort ranges from tenderness to pain.

- The lump usually increases in size and tenderness before menstruation. Cysts may enlarge or shrink rapidly.

- Nipple discharge is often green or dark brown, not bloody.
- Pain and nodularity tend to subside after menopause unless estrogen replacement is used.

Mammography may help distinguishing fibrocystic changes from breast cancer. However, in some women the breast tissue is so dense that it is difficult to obtain a mammogram. Ultrasound may be more useful in differentiating a cystic mass from a solid mass.

Nursing and Interprofessional Management

With discovery of a discrete breast mass, aspiration or surgical biopsy may be indicated. If the nodularity is recurrent, a wait of 7 to 10 days may be planned to note any changes related to the menstrual cycle.

- An excisional biopsy should be done if no fluid is found on aspiration, the fluid is hemorrhagic, or a residual mass remains.

Many types of treatment have been suggested for a fibrocystic condition. Some relief for cyclic pain may occur by reducing intake of caffeine and dietary fat; taking vitamin E or gamma-linolenic acid (evening primrose oil); and continually wearing a supportive bra. Compresses, ice, analgesics, and antiinflammatory drugs may also help. Prescription medication such as oral contraceptives and danazol may also be used. However, the androgenic side effects of danazol (acne, edema, hirsutism) may make this therapy unacceptable.

▼ **Patient and Caregiver Teaching**

Your role in the care of the patient with fibrocystic breast changes is primarily one of teaching.

- Teach the patient to expect recurrences of the cysts in 1 or both breasts until menopause, and that cysts may enlarge or become painful just before menstruation. In addition, offer reassurance that cysts do not "turn into" cancer.
- Encourage the woman with cystic changes to get regular follow-up care. Teach her breast self-examination (BSE) to self-monitor changes. Severe fibrocystic changes may make palpation of the breast more difficult. Teach her to report any changes in symptoms or changes found during the BSE so they can be evaluated.

FIBROMYALGIA

Description

Fibromyalgia is a chronic central pain syndrome marked by widespread, nonarticular musculoskeletal pain and fatigue with multiple tender points. People with fibromyalgia may have nonrestorative sleep, morning stiffness, irritable bowel syndrome, and anxiety.

Fibromyalgia affects more than 3.7 million Americans, most of whom are women ages 40 to 75 years.

Fibromyalgia and systemic exertion intolerance disease (SEID), formerly called *chronic fatigue syndrome*, share many common features (see Table 82, p. 599).

Pathophysiology

Fibromyalgia is a disorder involving abnormal central processing of nociceptive pain input. The increased pain experienced by the patient is caused by abnormal sensory processing in the central nervous system (CNS).

Multiple physiologic abnormalities have been found, including increased levels of substance P in the spinal fluid, low blood flow to the thalamus, dysfunction of the hypothalamic-pituitary-adrenal (HPA) axis, low levels of serotonin and tryptophan, and abnormalities in cytokine function.

- Serotonin and substance P play a role in mood regulation, sleep, and pain perception. Changes in the HPA axis can lead to depression and a decreased response to stress.
- Genetic factors contribute to the development of fibromyalgia, as a familial tendency exists. Recent illness or trauma may be a trigger.

Clinical Manifestations

Widespread burning pain fluctuates through the course of a day. The patient often cannot determine whether pain occurs in the muscles, joints, or soft tissues.

- Head or facial pain often results from stiff or painful neck and shoulder muscles. This pain can accompany temporomandibular joint dysfunction.
- Physical examination characteristically reveals point tenderness at 11 or more of 18 identified sites (Fig. 9).
- Cognitive effects range from difficulty concentrating to memory lapses and a feeling of being overwhelmed when dealing with multiple tasks. Many persons report migraine headaches. Depression and anxiety often occur.
- Numbness or tingling in the hands or feet (paresthesia) often accompanies fibromyalgia. Restless legs syndrome is common.
- Women with fibromyalgia may have more difficult menstruation, with worse disease symptoms during this time.
- Irritable bowel syndrome with diarrhea or constipation, abdominal pain, and bloating can occur. In addition, increased urinary frequency and urgency may occur.

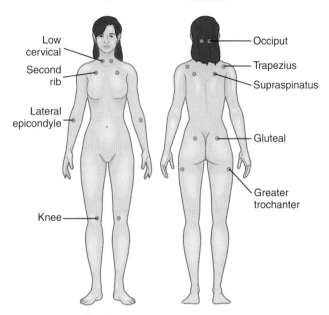

Fig. 9 Tender points in fibromyalgia.

Diagnostic Studies

A definitive diagnosis is often difficult to establish. Laboratory results may serve to rule out other suspected disorders.

- Muscle biopsy may reveal a nonspecific moth-eaten appearance or fiber atrophy.

The American College of Rheumatology classifies a person as having fibromyalgia if 2 criteria are met: (1) pain in 11 of the 18 tender points on palpation, and (2) a history of widespread pain for at least 3 months.

Interprofessional Management

Treatment is symptomatic and requires a high level of patient motivation. Teach the patient to be an active participant in treatment. Rest can help the pain, aching, and tenderness.

Drug therapy for the chronic widespread pain associated with fibromyalgia includes pregabalin (Lyrica), duloxetine (Cymbalta), and milnacipran (Savella). Low-dose tricyclic antidepressants (TCAs), selective serotonin reuptake inhibitors (SSRIs), or benzodiazepines (e.g., diazepam ([Valium]) may be prescribed. If the TCA is not well tolerated, similar drugs can be substituted, such as doxepin, imipramine (Tofranil), or trazodone.

- SSRI antidepressants (e.g., sertraline [Zoloft] or paroxetine [Paxil]) tend to be reserved for patients who also have depression. Antidepressants and muscle relaxants (e.g., baclofen) have sedative effects that can help with nighttime rest for the patient with fibromyalgia.
- Long-acting opioids generally are not recommended unless fibromyalgia is refractory to other therapies.
- In some patients, pain may be managed with over-the-counter (OTC) analgesics, such as acetaminophen (Tylenol), ibuprofen, or naproxen (Aleve), used in combination with a TCA. Nonopioids, such as tramadol (Ultram), may also be used. In addition, zolpidem (Ambien) or trazodone is sometimes prescribed for short-term intervention in the patient with severe sleep problems.

Because of the chronic nature of fibromyalgia and the need to maintain an ongoing rehabilitation program, the patient needs information and consistent support from the interprofessional team. Massage combined with ultrasound or the application of alternating heat and cold packs soothes tense, sore muscles and increases blood circulation.

- Gentle stretching can be done by a physical therapist and practiced by the patient at home to relieve muscle tension and spasm.
- Limit intake of muscle irritants, such as sugar, caffeine, and alcohol.
- Pain and the related symptoms of fibromyalgia can cause significant stress. Effective relaxation strategies include biofeedback, guided imagery, and autogenic training. Counseling and a support group may be helpful.

F

FLAIL CHEST

Description

Flail chest results from the fracture of 3 or more consecutive ribs in 2 or more separate locations that cause an unstable segment. It can also be caused by fracture of the sternum and several consecutive ribs.

Pathophysiology

The affected (flail) area moves in the opposite direction with respect to the intact part of the chest. During inspiration, the affected part is sucked in, and during expiration it bulges out. This paradoxical chest movement prevents adequate ventilation of the lung in the injured area and increases the work of breathing.

Clinical Manifestations and Diagnostic Studies

A flail chest is usually apparent on physical examination.

- The patient has rapid, shallow respirations and tachycardia.
- Movement of the thorax is asymmetrical and uncoordinated. The patient may ventilate poorly, and try to splint the chest to assist with breathing. Observation of abnormal chest cavity movement, palpation for crepitus near the rib fractures, and chest x-ray all assist in the diagnosis.

Interprofessional Management

Initial therapy consists of ensuring adequate ventilation and supplemental O_2 therapy. The goal is to promote lung expansion and ensure adequate oxygenation. Analgesia can help promote adequate respiration. Although many patients can be managed without mechanical ventilation, intubation and ventilation may be needed. In cases of extreme chest trauma, surgical fixation of the flail segment may be done.

FRACTURE

Description

A *fracture* is a disruption or break in the continuity of the structure of bone. Traumatic injuries cause most fractures, although some fractures are caused by a disease process (pathologic fractures from cancer or osteoporosis).

Fractures are described as *open* or *closed* depending on communication with the external environment. In an open fracture, the skin is broken, exposing the bone and causing soft tissue injury. In a closed fracture, the skin is intact over the site.

- Fractures can also be classified as complete or incomplete. Fractures are *complete* if the break goes completely through the bone and *incomplete* if the break occurs partly across a bone shaft but the bone is still intact. An incomplete fracture is often the result of bending or crushing forces applied to a bone.
- Fractures are also described according to the direction of the fracture line. Types include linear, oblique, transverse, longitudinal, and spiral fractures.
- Fractures can also be classified as *displaced* or *nondisplaced.* In a displaced fracture, the 2 ends of the broken bone are separated and out of their normal positions.

- Displaced fractures are often comminuted (more than 2 fragments) or oblique. In a nondisplaced fracture, the periosteum is intact and the bone is still in alignment. Nondisplaced fractures are usually transverse, spiral, or greenstick.

Illustrations of the various classifications of fractures can be found in Figs. 62.6 and 62.7 in Harding et al., *Lewis' Medical-Surgical Nursing,* ed 11.

Clinical Manifestations

Manifestations include immediate localized pain, decreased function, and inability to bear weight on or use the affected part.

- The patient guards the extremity (protects it against movement). Obvious bone deformity may be visible.

Complications

The majority of fractures heal without complications.

- Direct complications include problems with bone infection, bone union, and avascular necrosis.
- Indirect complications include compartment syndrome, venous thromboembolism (VTE), fat embolism syndrome (FES), breakdown of skeletal muscle (rhabdomyolysis), and hypovolemic shock.
- Most musculoskeletal injuries are not life threatening. Death after a fracture is usually caused by damage to underlying organs and vascular structures or complications of the fracture or immobility.
- Open fractures, fractures with severe blood loss, and fractures that damage vital organs (e.g., lung, heart) are medical emergencies requiring immediate attention.

Diagnostic Studies

- History and physical examination
- X-ray examination
- CT scan and MRI

Interprofessional Management

The goals of treatment are anatomic realignment of bone fragments through reduction of the fracture, immobilization to maintain realignment, and restoration of function of the injured part.

- If a fracture is suspected, the extremity is immobilized in the position in which it is found. Unnecessary movement increases soft tissue damage and may convert a closed fracture to an open fracture or create further injury to adjacent nerves and blood vessels.

F

Fracture Reduction

Closed reduction is the nonsurgical, manual realignment of bones to their anatomic position. Traction and countertraction are manually applied to bone fragments to restore position, length, and alignment.

- Closed reduction is usually done with the patient under local or general anesthesia. After reduction, the injured part is immobilized by casting, traction, external fixation, splints, or orthoses (braces) to maintain alignment until healing occurs.

Open reduction is correction of bone alignment through a surgical incision. It usually includes internal fixation of the fracture with the use of wires, screws, pins, plates, intramedullary rods, or nails.

- The main risks of open reduction are infection, complications associated with anesthesia, and effects of preexisting medical conditions (e.g., diabetes). However, open reduction with internal fixation (ORIF) facilitates early ambulation, which decreases the risk of complications related to prolonged immobility.

Traction devices apply a pulling force on the fractured extremity while countertraction pulls in the opposite direction. The 2 most common types of traction are skin traction and skeletal traction.

- *Skin traction* is generally used for short-term treatment (48 to 72 hours) until skeletal traction or surgery is possible. Tape, boots, or slings are applied directly to the skin to help decrease muscle spasms in the injured extremity. *Buck's traction* is a type of skin traction device that is used sometimes for the patient with a hip, knee, or femur fracture.
- *Skeletal traction* is used to align injured bones and joints or treat joint contractures and congenital hip dysplasia. It provides a long-term pull that keeps injured bones and joints aligned. Skeletal traction requires the insertion of a pin or wire into the bone to align and immobilize the injured body part. Fracture alignment depends on correct positioning and alignment of the patient while the traction forces remain constant. For extremity traction to be effective, forces must be pulling in the opposite direction *(countertraction)*.
- Countertraction is supplied by the patient's body weight or may be augmented by elevating the end of the bed.

Fracture Immobilization

A cast is a temporary immobilization device which allows the patient to perform many normal activities of daily living (ADLs) while providing enough immobilization to ensure stability. A cast generally incorporates the joints above and below a fracture. Synthetic casting materials are often used because they are light in weight and dry more quickly than plaster of Paris.

Immobilization of an acute fracture or soft tissue injury of the upper extremity is often accomplished by use of the: (1) sugar-tong splint, (2) posterior splint, (3) short-arm cast, or (4) long-arm cast. See Fig. 62.11 in Harding et al., *Lewis' Medical-Surgical Nursing,* ed 11.

An *external fixator* is composed of metal pins and wires that are inserted into the bone and attached to external rods to stabilize the fracture while it heals. It can be used to apply traction or to immobilize reduced fragments when the use of a cast or traction is not appropriate. Ongoing assessment for pin loosening and infection is critical. Infection signaled by exudate, redness, tenderness, and pain may require removal of the device.

Internal fixation devices (pins, plates, intramedullary rods, and metal and bioabsorbable screws) are surgically inserted to realign and maintain bony fragments. These metal devices are biologically inert and made from stainless steel, vitallium, or titanium. Proper alignment is evaluated by x-ray studies at regular intervals.

Other Therapy

Electrical bone growth stimulation can promote healing, especially with fracture nonunion or delayed union.

Central and peripheral muscle relaxants, such as carisoprodol (Soma), cyclobenzaprine, or methocarbamol (Robaxin), may be used to manage pain associated with muscle spasms. Give tetanus and diphtheria toxoid or tetanus immunoglobulin to the patient with an open fracture who has not been previously immunized or whose immunization is expired. Bone-penetrating antibiotics, such as a cephalosporin (e.g., cefazolin), are used prophylactically before surgery.

Proper nutrition is essential to ensure optimal soft tissue and bone. The patient's diet must include ample protein (e.g., 1 g/kg body weight daily), vitamins (especially B, C, and D), and calcium, phosphorus, and magnesium.

Nursing Management

Goals

The patient with a fracture will have healing with no associated complications, have acceptable pain relief, and achieve maximal rehabilitation potential.

Nursing Interventions

Patients with fractures may be treated in an emergency department or a physician's office and released to home care, or they may require hospitalization. Specific nursing measures depend on the type of treatment used and setting in which patients are placed.

Preoperative Care. If surgical intervention is needed, patients must be prepared. In addition to the usual preoperative nursing care, teach patients about immobilization and assistive devices. Discuss expected activity limitations after surgery. Assure patients that

F

nursing staff will help meet personal needs until they can resume self-care.

- Review pain management strategies

Postoperative Care. Frequent neurovascular assessments of the affected extremity are needed to detect early and subtle changes. Closely monitor limitations of movement or activity related to turning, positioning, and extremity support.

- Minimize pain and discomfort through proper alignment and positioning.
- Frequently observe dressings, casts, and wound drainage systems for bleeding or drainage. Report increased or purulent drainage to the health care provider (HCP). Whenever the contents of a drainage system are measured or emptied, use sterile technique to avoid contamination.

Plan care to prevent possible complications of immobility. Prevent constipation by increasing activity, maintaining a high fluid intake, and providing a diet high in bulk and roughage. Maintain a regular time for elimination. If these measures are not effective in maintaining the patient's normal bowel pattern, give stool softeners, laxatives, or suppositories as necessary.

- Renal stones can develop because of bone demineralization related to reduced mobility. Unless contraindicated, maintain a fluid intake of 2500 mL/day.
- Rapid deconditioning of the cardiovascular system can occur from prolonged bed rest, resulting in orthostatic hypotension and decreased lung capacity. Unless activity is contraindicated, these effects can be decreased by having the patient sit on the side of the bed, allowing the lower limbs to dangle over the bedside, and having the patient perform standing transfers.
- When the patient is allowed to increase activity, assess for orthostatic hypotension. Also assess patients for signs of VTE.

When slings are used with traction, inspect exposed skin areas regularly. Observe skeletal traction pin sites for signs of infection. Pin site care often includes regularly cleansing with chlorhexidine, rinsing with sterile saline, and drying the area with sterile gauze.

▼ **Patient and Caregiver Teaching**

Teaching is important to prevent complications. In addition to specific instructions for cast care and recognition of complications, encourage the patient to contact the HCP if questions arise. Validate patient and caregiver understanding of instructions before discharge.

For further information on rehabilitation management of fractures, including the use of assistive devices such as walkers and crutches, see Chapter 62 in Harding et al., *Lewis' Medical-Surgical Nursing,* ed 11, and see the specific types of fractures discussed in this *Companion.*

FRACTURE, HIP

Description

Hip fractures are common in older adults, with 95% of these caused by a fall. More than 320,000 patients are admitted to hospitals each year because of a hip fracture. Up to 37% of those patients die within 1 year of injury. Many older adults develop disabilities that require long-term care. By age 90 years, about 33% of all women and 17% of all men will have had a hip fracture. In adults over 65 years old, hip fracture occurs more often in women than in men because of osteoporosis.

A fracture of the hip refers to a fracture of the proximal (upper) third of the femur, which extends up to 5 cm below the lesser trochanter.

- Fractures within the hip joint capsule are called *intracapsular fractures.* Intracapsular fractures (femoral neck) are further identified by their specific locations: capital, subcapital, and transcervical. These fractures are associated with osteoporosis and minor trauma.

- *Extracapsular fractures* occur outside the joint capsule. They are *intertrochanteric* if they occur in a region between the greater and lesser trochanter or *subtrochanteric* if they occur below the lesser trochanter. Most are caused by severe direct trauma or a fall.

Clinical Manifestations

Manifestations of a hip fracture are external rotation, muscle spasm, shortening of the affected extremity, and severe pain and tenderness in the region of the fracture site. Displaced femoral neck fractures may disrupt the blood supply to the femoral head, which can result in avascular necrosis.

Interprofessional Management

Initially the affected extremity may be immobilized by Buck's traction until the patient's physical condition is stable and surgery can be done. Buck's traction can be used for 24 to 48 hours to relieve painful muscle spasms.

Surgical treatment allows early mobilization and decreases the risk of major complications. The type of surgery depends on the location of the fracture, severity of the fracture, and person's age. Better outcomes are associated with surgery performed within 24 hours of injury.

- Surgical options include: (1) repair with internal fixation devices (e.g., hip compression screw, intramedullary devices),

(2) replacement of part of the femoral head with a prosthesis (partial hip replacement), and (3) total hip replacement (involves both the femur and acetabulum).

These types of surgical repair are shown in Figs. 62.19 and 62.20 in Harding et al., *Lewis' Medical-Surgical Nursing,* ed 11.

Nursing Management

Preoperative Management

Before surgery, severe muscle spasms can increase pain. Analgesics or muscle relaxants, comfortable positioning unless contraindicated, and properly adjusted traction can help manage spasms.

- Plans for discharge begin as the patient enters the hospital because the length of postoperative stay is only a few days.

Postoperative Management

Similar principles of patient care apply to any of the surgical procedures for hip fractures. In the initial postoperative period, assess vital signs and intake and output and monitor respiratory activities such as deep breathing and coughing. Assess pain and give pain medication. Observe the dressing and incision for signs of bleeding and infection.

Neurovascular impairment is possible. Assess the patient's extremity for motor function, temperature and color, sensation, distal pulses, capillary refill, edema, and pain.

- Decrease edema by elevating the leg whenever the patient is in bed or a chair.
- Pain in the affected extremity can be reduced by maintaining limb alignment with pillows between the knees when turning the patient to the nonoperative side. Avoid turning patient to the affected side unless approved by the surgeon.
- The patient can exercise the unaffected leg and both arms. Encourage patient to use overhead trapeze bar and the opposite side rail to help in position changes. A physical therapist can teach the patient how to perform out-of-bed and chair transfers.
- If hemiarthroplasty or total joint replacement was done by a *posterior approach* (accessing the hip joint from the back), measures to prevent dislocation must be used.
- Tell the patient and caregiver about positions and activities that increase the patient's risk for dislocation (>90 degrees of flexion, abduction, or internal rotation). Many daily activities may reproduce these positions, including putting on shoes and socks, crossing legs or feet while seated, assuming the side-lying position incorrectly, standing up or sitting down while the body is flexed more than 90 degrees relative to the chair, and sitting on low seats, especially low toilet seats. Teach the patient to avoid these activities for at least 6 weeks.

If a foam abduction wedge is ordered to prevent joint dislocation, place it between the patient's legs. Apply the top straps above the knee to avoid putting pressure on the peroneal nerve at the lateral tibial tubercle. Some health care providers (HCPs) want the patient to keep the abductor wedge in place except when bathing or walking.

When the hip fracture is accessed during surgery with an *anterior approach* (joint reached from front of body), the hip muscles are left intact. This approach provides a more stable hip in the postoperative period with a lower rate of complications. Patient precautions related to motion and weight bearing are few. They may include instructions to avoid hyperextension.

The patient is usually out of bed the first postoperative day. In collaboration with the physical therapist, monitor the patient's ambulation status for proper crutch walking or use of the walker. For the patient to be discharged home, have the patient demonstrate the proper use of crutches or a walker, the ability to transfer into and from a chair and bed, and the ability to ascend and descend stairs.

- Hospitalization averages 3 or 4 days. Patients frequently require care in a subacute unit, skilled nursing facility, or rehabilitation facility before returning home.

Weight bearing after surgery is generally restricted until x-ray examination indicates adequate healing, usually 6 to 12 weeks. Limited weight bearing is typically the only restriction for the patient who had open reduction and internal fixation (ORIF) of the hip fracture.

There are many areas to teach the patient and caregiver for home care.

- Inform the patient and caregiver about the patient's weight-bearing status after surgery.
- Use pillow between legs for first 6 weeks after surgery when lying on nonoperative side or when supine.
- Keep hip in neutral, straight position when sitting, walking, or lying.
- Sudden severe pain, a lump in the buttock, limb shortening, or extreme external rotation indicate prosthesis dislocation. This requires a closed reduction or open reduction to realign the femoral head in the acetabulum. Teach the patient to notify surgeon immediately if severe pain, deformity, or loss of function occurs.
- Teach the patient to use an elevated toilet seat.
- Place chair inside shower or tub and remain seated while washing.
- Assist the patient and caregiver to adjust to the restrictions and dependence of the hip fracture. Anxiety and depression may occur. Inform the patient and caregivers about community

referral services that can assist in the postdischarge rehabilitation phase.
- Discuss risk factors for prosthetic joint infection with surgeon and dentist before dental work.

FRACTURE, HUMERUS

Fractures involving the shaft of the humerus are common among young and middle-aged adults. Manifestations are obvious displacement of the humeral shaft, shortened extremity, abnormal mobility, and pain.
- Major complications are radial nerve injury and vascular injury to the brachial artery caused by laceration, transection, or muscle spasm.

Treatment depends on the specific location and displacement of the fracture.
- Nonoperative treatment may include use of a hanging arm cast, shoulder immobilizer, or the sling and swathe, which prevents shoulder movement.

When these devices are used, elevate the head of the bed to assist gravity in reducing the fracture. Allow the arm to hang freely when the patient is sitting and standing.

Provide measures to protect the axilla and prevent skin maceration. Carefully place absorbable composite dressing pads in the axilla. Change them twice daily or as needed.
- Skin or skeletal traction may be used for purposes of reduction and immobilization.
- During the rehabilitative phase, an exercise program geared toward improving strength and motion of the injured extremity is extremely important. This program should include assisted motion of the hands and fingers. If the fracture is stable, the shoulder can be exercised to prevent stiffness caused by "frozen shoulder" or fibrosis of the shoulder capsule.

FRACTURE, PELVIS

Pelvic fractures may be relatively minor or life-threatening, depending on the mechanism of injury and associated vascular damage. Although only a small number of all fractures are pelvic fractures, this type of injury is associated with a high mortality rate. Attention to more obvious injuries at the time of a traumatic event may result in pelvic injuries being overlooked.

- Pelvic fractures may cause serious intraabdominal injury, such as paralytic ileus, hemorrhage, and laceration of the urethra, bladder, or colon. Patients may survive the pelvic injury to then die from sepsis, fat embolism syndrome, or venous thromboembolism.
- Pelvic fractures are diagnosed by x-ray and CT.
- Physical examination of the abdomen demonstrates local swelling, tenderness, deformity, unusual pelvic movement, and bruising.

Treatment depends on the severity of the injury.

- Stable, nondisplaced fractures require little intervention. Ambulation with weight bearing as tolerated is typically encouraged.
- Complex or displaced fractures (e.g., open book fracture) are often done emergently with external fixation alone or combined with open reduction and internal fixation (ORIF) surgery. Use extreme care in handling or moving the patient to prevent further injury. Only turn the patient when approved by the health care provider (HCP). Because a pelvic fracture can damage other organs, assess bowel and urinary tract function, as well as distal neurovascular status.
- Provide back care with adequate help to turn the patient or while the patient is raised from the bed with use of the trapeze.

GASTRITIS

Description

Gastritis, an inflammation of the stomach mucosa, is a common problem. Gastritis may be acute or chronic, and diffuse or localized.

Pathophysiology

Gastritis occurs when breakdown in the normal gastric mucosal barrier allows hydrochloric acid (HCl) acid and pepsin to diffuse back into the mucosa. This back diffusion results in stomach tissue edema, disruption of capillary walls with plasma lost into the gastric lumen, and possible hemorrhage.

Drugs contribute to the development of acute and chronic gastritis. Corticosteroids and nonsteroidal antiinflammatory drugs (NSAIDs), including aspirin, inhibit the synthesis of prostaglandins that protect the gastric mucosa, making the mucosa more susceptible to injury. Factors that increase the risk for NSAID-induced gastritis include being female; being over age 60 years; having a history of ulcer disease; taking anticoagulants, other NSAIDs, or corticosteroids; and having a chronic debilitating disorder, such as cardiovascular disease. Some drugs, such as digitalis (digoxin) and alendronate (Fosamax), have direct irritating effects on the gastric mucosa.

There are a number of other causes of chronic gastritis.

- Eating large quantities of spicy, irritating foods can cause acute gastritis.
- A key cause of chronic gastritis is *Helicobacter pylori*. Other bacterial, viral, and fungal infections are also associated with chronic gastritis.
- Smoking, radiation exposure, and numerous chronic diseases also cause gastritis.
- After an alcoholic drinking binge, acute damage to the gastric mucosa can range from localized injury of superficial epithelial cells to destruction of the mucosa with mucosal congestion, edema, and hemorrhage. Prolonged damage induced by repeated alcohol use results in chronic gastritis.

Autoimmune metaplastic atrophic gastritis is an inherited condition. An immune response directed against parietal cells leads malabsorption and pernicious anemia. Atrophic gastritis is associated with an increased risk of stomach cancer.

Clinical Manifestations

- *Acute gastritis* symptoms include anorexia, nausea and vomiting, epigastric tenderness, and a feeling of fullness. Acute gastritis is self-limiting, lasting from a few hours to a few days.
- *Chronic gastritis* symptoms are similar to those of acute gastritis. Some patients are asymptomatic. However, when parietal cells are lost as a result of atrophy, the source of intrinsic factor is lost. Intrinsic factor is essential for cobalamin absorption. The lack of cobalamin results in pernicious anemia.

Diagnostic Studies

Diagnosis of acute gastritis is most often based on the patient's symptoms and history.

- Endoscopic examination with biopsy is used to obtain a definitive diagnosis.
- Breath, urine, serum, stool, and gastric tissue biopsy tests can help determine *H. pylori* infection.
- Complete blood count (CBC) may demonstrate anemia from blood loss or lack of intrinsic factor.
- Stools are tested for occult blood.
- Serum tests for antibodies to parietal cells and intrinsic factor are done.

Nursing and Interprofessional Management

Treatment of acute gastritis focuses on eliminating the cause and preventing or avoiding it in the future. The plan of care is supportive (see Nausea and Vomiting, p. 415).

- If vomiting accompanies acute gastritis, rest, NPO status, and IV fluids may be prescribed. Antiemetics are given for nausea and vomiting. In severe cases, a nasogastric (NG) tube may be used to monitor for bleeding, lavage the precipitating agent from the stomach, or keep the stomach empty and free of noxious stimuli.
- Monitor for dehydration. It can occur rapidly in acute gastritis with vomiting.
- Resume clear liquids when acute symptoms subside. Gradually reintroduce solid, bland foods.
- Management strategies for upper gastrointestinal (GI) bleeding apply to the patient with severe gastritis (see Gastrointestinal Bleeding, Upper, p. 237).

Drug therapy focuses on reducing irritation of the gastric mucosa and providing symptomatic relief. Histamine (H2)-receptor blockers (e.g., ranitidine, cimetidine) or proton pump inhibitors (PPIs) (e.g., omeprazole, lansoprazole) reduce gastric HCl acid secretion.

- Antibiotic combinations are used to eradicate *H. pylori*.
- The patient with pernicious anemia needs lifelong administration of cobalamin.

Treatment of chronic gastritis focuses on evaluating and eliminating the specific cause. The patient may have to adapt to lifestyle changes and strictly adhere to a drug regimen. A team approach in which the health care provider (HCP), nurse, dietitian, and pharmacist provide consistent information and support may help patients make these alterations.

GASTROESOPHAGEAL REFLUX DISEASE

Description

Gastroesophageal reflux disease (GERD) results from mucosal damage caused by chronic reflux of stomach acid into the lower esophagus. GERD is not a disease but a syndrome. GERD is the most common upper gastrointestinal (GI) problem. Approximately 15 million Americans have GERD symptoms (heartburn or regurgitation) each day.

Pathophysiology

GERD results when the reflux of acidic gastric contents into the esophagus overwhelms the esophageal defenses (Fig. 10). One of

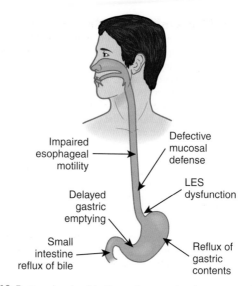

Fig. 10 Factors involved in the pathogenesis of gastroesophageal reflux disease. *LES,* Lower esophageal sphincter.

the primary factors in GERD is an incompetent lower esophageal sphincter (LES). Normally, the LES prevents reflux. An incompetent LES lets gastric contents move from the stomach to the esophagus when the patient is supine or has an increase in intraabdominal pressure. Gastric hydrochloric acid (HCl) acid and pepsin secretions that reflux cause esophageal irritation and inflammation *(esophagitis).*
- Decreased LES pressure can be caused by certain foods and drugs.
- Obesity is a risk factor. In an obese person, the intraabdominal pressure is increased, which can worsen GERD.
- Cigarette and cigar smoking can contribute to GERD.
- Hiatal hernia (see p. 299) often causes GERD.

Clinical Manifestations
Persistent mild symptoms or moderate to severe symptoms that occur at least once a week indicate GERD.
- Heartburn *(pyrosis),* caused by irritation of the esophagus by secretions, is the most common manifestation. Heartburn is a burning, tight sensation that is felt intermittently beneath the lower sternum and spreads upward to the throat or jaw.

- Patients may report dyspepsia, which is pain or discomfort centered in the upper abdomen (in or around the midline).
- Regurgitation is common and often described as a hot, bitter, or sour liquid in the throat or mouth.

GERD-related chest pain can mimic angina. It is described as burning, squeezing, or radiating. Chest pain is more common in older adults with GERD. Unlike angina, GERD-related chest pain is relieved with antacids.

Complications

Complications are related to the effects of gastric acid secretion on the esophageal mucosa. Esophagitis (inflammation of the esophagus) is a common complication of GERD. Repeated esophagitis may cause scar tissue formation, stricture, and ultimately dysphagia. Barrett's esophagus, a precancerous lesion, increases the patient's risk for esophageal cancer.

- Gastric secretions irritating the upper airway cause cough, bronchospasm, laryngospasm, asthma, and chronic bronchitis.
- Acid reflux into the mouth may cause dental erosion.

Diagnostic Studies

Diagnostic studies help determine the cause of the GERD.

- Barium swallow determines if there is protrusion of the upper part of the stomach into the esophagus.
- Endoscopy is useful to assess LES competence, inflammation, potential scarring, and strictures.
- Biopsy and cytologic specimens can differentiate stomach and esophageal cancer from Barrett's esophagus (see Esophageal Cancer, p. 215).
- Radionuclide tests can detect gastric reflux and the rate of esophageal clearance.

Nursing and Interprofessional Management

Most patients with GERD can successfully manage the condition through lifestyle modifications, nutrition therapy, and drug therapy. Encourage the patient to incorporate lifestyle changes (Table 35), including smoking cessation.

Teach patients to avoid foods that aggravate their symptoms, such as chocolate, peppermint, tomatoes, fatty foods, coffee, and tea. Small, frequent meals help prevent overdistention of the stomach. Late evening meals and nocturnal snacking should be avoided. Weight reduction is recommended if the patient is obese.

Drug Therapy

Drug therapy for GERD focuses on decreasing the volume and acidity of reflux, improving LES function, increasing esophageal

TABLE 35   Patient and Caregiver Teaching

Gastroesophageal Reflux Disease (GERD)

Include the following instructions when teaching the patient and caregivers about management of GERD.

1. Explain the reason for a low-fat diet.
2. Encourage the patient to eat small, frequent meals to prevent gastric distention.
3. Explain the reason for avoiding alcohol, smoking (causes an almost immediate, marked decrease in lower esophageal sphincter pressure), and beverages that contain caffeine.
4. Advise the patient to not lie down for 2 to 3 hours after eating, wear tight clothing around the waist, or bend over (especially after eating).
5. Have the patient avoid eating within 3 hours of bedtime.
6. Encourage the patient to sleep with head of bed elevated on 4- to 6-inch blocks or 30-degree angle (gravity fosters esophageal emptying).
7. Provide information about drugs, including reasons for their use and common side effects.
8. Discuss strategies for weight reduction if appropriate.
9. Encourage patient and caregiver to share concerns about lifestyle changes and living with a chronic problem.

clearance, and protecting the esophageal mucosa. Proton pump inhibitors (PPIs) and histamine (H2)-receptor blockers are the most common and effective treatments for symptomatic GERD. The goal of HCl acid suppression treatment is to reduce the acidity of the gastric refluxate. Patients who are symptomatic with GERD but do not have esophagitis (nonerosive GERD) achieve symptom relief with PPIs and H2-receptor blockers.

- PPIs include omeprazole, esomeprazole, lansoprazole, and rabeprazole.
- H_2-receptor blockers, such as cimetidine, ranitidine, famotidine, and nizatidine, reduce symptoms and promote esophageal healing in 50% of patients.

Antacids with or without alginic acid may be useful in patients with mild, intermittent heartburn.

Surgical and Endoscopic Therapy

Surgical therapy is reserved for patients with complications of reflux, including esophagitis, intolerance of medications, stricture, Barrett's esophagus, and persistence of severe symptoms. Most surgical procedures are performed laparoscopically. Alternatives to surgical therapy include endoscopic mucosal resection (EMR) and radiofrequency ablation.

GASTROINTESTINAL BLEEDING, UPPER

Description

In the United States, approximately 250,000 hospital admissions occur each year for upper gastrointestinal (GI) bleeding. About 60% are adults over 65 years of age. Though the mortality rate is still around 2.5%, this rate has decreased over the past few decades because of advances in the prevention and treatment of upper GI bleeding.

Pathophysiology

Although the most serious loss of blood from the upper GI tract is characterized by a sudden onset, insidious occult bleeding can be a major problem. Bleeding severity depends on whether the origin is venous, capillary, or arterial. Bleeding from an arterial source is profuse and bright red. By contrast, "coffee ground" vomitus means that the blood has been in the stomach for some time. *Melena* (black, tarry stools) occur with slow bleeding from an upper GI source.

The most common sites of GI bleeding are the esophagus, stomach, and duodenum. Table 36 lists common causes of upper GI bleeding.

TABLE 36　Common Causes of Upper Gastrointestinal Bleeding

Stomach and Duodenum
- Drug-induced
  - Corticosteroids
  - Nonsteroidal antiinflammatory drugs
  - Salicylates
- Erosive gastritis
- Peptic ulcer disease
- Polyps
- Stress-related mucosal disease
- Stomach cancer

Esophagus
- Esophageal varices
- Esophagitis
- Mallory-Weiss tear

Systemic Diseases
- Blood dyscrasias (e.g., leukemia, aplastic anemia)
- Renal failure

G

- Peptic ulcers, caused by *Helicobacter pylori* infection and the use of nonsteroidal antiinflammatory drugs (NSAIDs), are the most common causes of upper GI bleeding. Aspirin and other NSAIDs and corticosteroids can cause disruption of the gastroduodenal mucosa and upper GI bleeding.
- Stress-related mucosal disease (SRMD), also called *physiologic stress ulcers*, describes mucosal damage in the GI tract ranging from small single lesions to multiple gastric ulcers and major bleeding. SRMD is most commonly seen in critically ill patients who have had severe burns, trauma, or major surgery.
- Bleeding from the esophagus is most likely caused by chronic esophagitis, Mallory-Weiss tear, or esophageal varices. Chronic esophagitis can be caused by GERD, smoking, alcohol use, and ingestion of drugs that irritate the mucosa. Esophageal varices most often occur from cirrhosis of the liver (see Cirrhosis, p. 134).

Diagnostic Studies

- Endoscopy is used to diagnose the source (e.g., peptic ulcer, esophageal varices, gastritis) of upper GI bleeding.
- Angiography is used to diagnose upper GI bleeding when endoscopy cannot be done or when bleeding persists.
- Laboratory studies include complete blood count (CBC), blood urea nitrogen (BUN), serum electrolytes, prothrombin time, partial thromboplastin time, liver enzymes, and arterial blood gases (ABGs).

Interprofessional Management

Endoscopy performed within the first 24 hours of bleeding is important for diagnosis, determining the need for surgical intervention, and providing treatment. The goal of endoscopic hemostasis is to coagulate or thrombose the bleeding vessel. Mechanical therapy, injection therapy with epinephrine, or thermal cautery are used to achieve acute hemostasis.

Surgical intervention is indicated when bleeding continues from an identified site. The site of the hemorrhage determines the choice of operation.

During the acute phase, drugs are used to decrease bleeding, decrease HCl secretion, and neutralize the HCl acid.

- Efforts are made to reduce acid secretion because the acidic environment can alter platelet function and interfere with clot stabilization. Proton pump inhibitors (PPIs) or H_2-receptor blockers are administered IV to decrease acid secretion (see Table 41.10 in Harding et al., *Lewis' Medical-Surgical Nursing,* ed 11).

Octreotide (Sandostatin) or vasopressin may be given when upper GI bleeding is from esophageal or gastric varices.

Nursing Management

Goals

The overall goals are that the patient with upper GI bleeding will have no further GI bleeding, have the cause of the bleeding identified and treated, return to a normal hemodynamic state, and have minimal or no symptoms of pain or anxiety.

Nursing Interventions

The patient with a history of chronic gastritis or peptic ulcer disease is at high risk for upper GI bleeding. Teach the at-risk patient to avoid known gastric irritants, such as alcohol and smoking, and to take only prescribed medications. Over-the-counter (OTC) drugs may contain ingredients (e.g., aspirin) that increase the risk of bleeding.

During acute GI bleeding, monitor for shock. Assess for complications of gut perforation and peritonitis indicated by a tense, rigid, boardlike abdomen.

- IV lines, preferably 2, with a 16- or 18-gauge needle are placed for fluid and blood replacement.
- Whole blood, packed red blood cells (RBCs), and fresh frozen plasma may be used for volume replacement in massive hemorrhage. When bleeding is less profuse, infusion of isotonic saline solution followed by packed RBCs restores the hematocrit more quickly.
- An indwelling urinary catheter may also be inserted so that output can be accurately assessed hourly.
- Supplemental O_2 delivered by face mask or nasal cannula may help increase blood oxygen saturation.

Although room-temperature, cool, or iced gastric lavage is used in some institutions, its effectiveness as a treatment for upper GI bleeding is questionable. When lavage is used, approximately 50 to 100 mL of fluid is instilled at a time into the stomach.

- Monitor vital signs, especially in patients with cardiovascular disease, because dysrhythmias may occur.
- Keep the head of the bed elevated to provide comfort and prevent aspiration.
- Assess stools for blood. Black, tarry stools indicate prolonged upper GI bleeding.
- Monitor the patient's laboratory studies. The hemoglobin and hematocrit are usually evaluated about every 4 to 6 hours if the patient is actively bleeding.
- When oral nourishment is begun, observe the patient for symptoms of nausea and vomiting and a recurrence of bleeding.

G

Feedings initially consist of hourly clear fluids. Gradually introduce food if the patient has no discomfort.

- When hemorrhage is the result of chronic alcohol abuse, closely observe the patient for the delirium tremens of alcohol withdrawal.

▼ **Patient and Caregiver Teaching**

- Teach the patient and caregivers how to avoid future bleeding episodes. Emphasize adhering to prescribed drug therapy and avoiding aspirin and other NSAIDs.
- Encourage elimination of smoking and alcohol because they are sources of gastric irritation.
- Teach the patient and family what to do if an acute hemorrhage occurs.

GLAUCOMA

Description

Glaucoma is a group of disorders characterized by increased intraocular pressure (IOP) and the consequences of increased pressure, optic nerve atrophy, and peripheral visual field loss. Many people with glaucoma are unaware of their condition.

- Glaucoma is the second leading cause of permanent blindness in the United States and the leading cause of blindness among blacks.
- Blindness from glaucoma is largely preventable with early detection and treatment.

Pathophysiology

Increased IOP results when the rate of aqueous production (inflow) is greater than aqueous reabsorption (outflow). If the pressure remains elevated, permanent vision loss may occur.

- *Primary open-angle glaucoma* (POAG) is the most common type of primary glaucoma. In POAG, the aqueous outflow is decreased in the trabecular meshwork. The drainage channels become clogged, like a clogged kitchen sink. Damage to the optic nerve can result.
- *Primary angle-closure glaucoma* (PACG) is caused by reduced outflow of aqueous humor that results from angle closure. Usually this is caused by the lens bulging forward in the aging process. Angle closure may also occur because of pupil dilation in the patient with anatomically narrow angles. An acute attack may occur because of drug-induced mydriasis, emotional excitement, or darkness. Check drug records and documentation before

giving medications to the patient with angle-closure glaucoma. Teach the patient not to take any mydriatic medications.

Clinical Manifestations

- POAG develops slowly without symptoms of pain or pressure. The patient usually does not notice gradual visual field loss until peripheral vision is severely compromised (tunnel vision).
- Acute angle-closure glaucoma causes symptoms of sudden, severe pain in or around the eye that is often accompanied by nausea and vomiting. Visual symptoms include seeing colored halos around lights, blurred vision, and ocular redness.
- Manifestations of subacute or chronic angle-closure glaucoma appear gradually. The patient may report a history of blurred vision, colored halos around lights, ocular redness, or eye or brow pain.

Diagnostic Studies

- IOP measurement with tonometry
- Visual acuity measurement and visual field perimetry
- Slit-lamp microscopy
- Ophthalmoscopy (direct and indirect)

Interprofessional Management

The primary focus of therapy is to keep the IOP low enough to prevent the patient from developing optic nerve damage. Therapy varies with the type of glaucoma.

- In chronic open-angle glaucoma, initial drug therapy can include β-adrenergic receptor blocking agents, α-adrenergic agents, cholinergic agents (miotics), and carbonic anhydrase inhibitors (hyperosmotic agents).
- When prescribed medications are not effective or are not used as recommended, surgical options include argon laser trabeculoplasty (ALT) and trabeculectomy.
- Acute angle-closure glaucoma is an ocular emergency that requires immediate interventions, including miotics and oral or IV hyperosmotic agents. Laser peripheral iridotomy or surgical iridectomy are definitive treatment.

Nursing Management

Because glaucoma requires long-term management, assess the patient's ability to adhere to the plan. Also assess the patient's reaction to a potentially sight-threatening chronic disorder.

Goals

The patient with glaucoma will: (1) have no progression of visual impairment, (2) comply with all aspects of therapy (including medication administration and follow-up care), and (3) have no postoperative complications.

Nursing Interventions

- Encourage adherence by helping the patient set up a medication schedule. Advocate for a change in therapy if the patient reports unacceptable side effects.

▼ **Patient and Caregiver Teaching**

See Table 22, Patient and Caregiver Teaching: After Eye Surgery, p. 114.

Provide accurate information about the disease process and treatment options, including the rationale for each option. Teach about the purpose, frequency, and technique for administration of antiglaucoma drugs.

GLOMERULONEPHRITIS

Glomerulonephritis is an inflammation of the glomeruli, and is the third leading cause of end-stage renal disease. It is described in a number of ways including extent of damage (diffuse or local), cause, and if acute or chronic.

- A variety of conditions can cause glomerulonephritis, ranging from kidney infections to systemic diseases. Glomerulonephritis can be acute or chronic. In *acute glomerulonephritis*, symptoms come on suddenly and may be temporary or reversible. By contrast, *chronic glomerulonephritis* is slowly progressive and generally leads to irreversible renal failure.
- Clinical manifestations of glomerulonephritis include varying degrees of hematuria and urinary excretion of various formed elements, including red blood cells (RBCs), white blood cells (WBCs), proteins, and casts.

Acute Poststreptococcal Glomerulonephritis

- *Acute poststreptococcal glomerulonephritis* (APSGN) develops 1 to 2 weeks after an infection of the tonsils, pharynx, or skin by nephrotoxic strains of group A β-hemolytic streptococci.
- Manifestations include generalized body edema, hypertension, oliguria, hematuria with a smoky or rusty appearance, and proteinuria.
- APSGN management focuses on symptomatic relief. This includes rest, edema and hypertension management, and dietary protein restriction when an increase in nitrogenous wastes (e.g., increased blood urea nitrogen [BUN] value) is present.

Nursing and Interprofessional Management

Management of APSGN focuses on symptomatic relief. Rest is recommended until the signs of glomerular inflammation (proteinuria, hematuria) and hypertension subside. Edema is treated by restricting sodium and fluid intake and administering diuretics.

- Severe hypertension is treated with antihypertensive drugs.
- Dietary protein intake may be restricted if there is evidence of an increase in nitrogenous wastes (e.g., elevated BUN).
- Antibiotics are given if streptococcal infection is still present. Corticosteroids and cytotoxic drugs have not been shown to be of value.

One of the most important ways to prevent APSGN is to encourage early diagnosis and treatment of sore throats and skin lesions. If streptococci are found in the culture, encourage the patient to take the full course of antibiotics to ensure that the bacteria have been eradicated.

- Good personal hygiene is an important factor in preventing the spread of cutaneous streptococcal infections.

Chronic Glomerulonephritis

Chronic glomerulonephritis is a syndrome that reflects the end stage of glomerular inflammatory disease. Most types of glomerulonephritis and nephrotic syndrome can eventually lead to chronic glomerulonephritis. Treatment is supportive and symptomatic (see Kidney Disease, Chronic, p. 358).

GONORRHEA

G

Description and Pathophysiology

Gonorrhea is the second most frequently occurring reportable sexually transmitted infection (STI) in the United States.

Gonorrhea is caused by *Neisseria gonorrhoeae,* a gram-negative diplococcus bacterium. Gonorrhea can be transmitted by exposure to sexual fluids during vaginal, anal, or oral sex. The incubation period is 1 to 14 days. The most common site of infection for men is the urethra and for women, the cervix. Both men and women can get gonorrhea of the rectum from anal sex or of the oropharynx from oral sex. Prior infection does not provide protection from reinfection.

- Gonococcal infection elicits an inflammatory response, which, if left untreated, leads to formation of fibrous tissue and adhesions. This fibrous scarring is responsible for complications, such as strictures and tubal abnormalities, which can lead to tubal pregnancy, chronic pelvic pain, and infertility.

Clinical Manifestations

- Most men will be symptomatic within a few days. The most common symptoms are dysuria, purulent urethral discharge, and epididymitis.
- Most women who contract gonorrhea are asymptomatic or have symptoms that they overlook. For women, common symptoms are increased vaginal discharge, dysuria, frequency of urination, and bleeding after sex. Redness and swelling can occur at the cervix or urethra along with a purulent exudate.
- Symptoms and signs of rectal gonorrhea may include mucopurulent rectal discharge or bleeding, anorectal pain, pruritus, tenesmus, mucus-coated stools, and painful bowel movements.
- Most patients with gonorrheal infections in the throat have few if any symptoms. Some may have of a sore throat within days of performing oral sex.

Complications

Because men often seek treatment early, they are less likely to develop complications, such as prostatitis, urethral strictures, and sterility from orchitis or epididymitis.

Because women who are asymptomatic seldom seek treatment, complications are more common. In women, pelvic inflammatory disease (PID), Bartholin's or Skene's glands abscess, ectopic pregnancy, and infertility are the main complications.

Neonates can develop *gonococcal conjunctivitis* (ophthalmia neonatorum) from exposure to an infected mother during delivery, which can result in permanent blindness. Almost all states have a law or health department regulation requiring prophylactic eye treatment of all newborns.

Diagnostic Studies

- For men, a presumptive diagnosis of gonorrhea is made if there is a history of sexual contact with a new or infected partner followed within a few days by a urethral discharge. Typical clinical manifestations combined with a positive finding in a Gram-stained smear of discharge from the penis give an almost certain diagnosis.
- For women, making a diagnosis of gonorrhea on the basis of symptoms is difficult. Most women are asymptomatic or have complaints that may be confused with other conditions, such as chlamydial infection or a urinary tract infection. A culture must be performed to confirm the diagnosis.

Interprofessional and Nursing Management

Because of a short incubation period and high infectivity, treatment is generally instituted without waiting for culture results. The first-line treatment for gonorrhea is dual therapy with IM ceftriaxone and oral azithromycin (Zithromax). Because of the increasing rate of drug resistance, all patients with gonococcal infection must receive treatment with at least 2 antibiotics.

- All sexual contacts within 60 days should be evaluated and treated to prevent reinfection and further transmission. Teach patients to abstain from sexual contact for 7 days after treatment, or until all partners have been treated and have also abstained from sexual contact for 7 days. Review the ways to reduce risk of acquiring a repeat or new STI in the future.

See Nursing Management: Sexually Transmitted Infections, pp. 547.

GOUT

Description

Gout is a type of acute arthritis characterized by elevation of uric acid (hyperuricemia) and the deposit of uric acid crystals in 1 or more joints. Sodium urate crystals may be found in articular, periarticular, and subcutaneous tissues. Unlike chronic forms of arthritis, gout is marked by painful flares lasting days to weeks followed by long periods without symptoms. More than 8 million Americans are affected by gout, with men affected 3 times as often as women. Black men and women are at increased risk of developing gout in middle and old age compared to whites. In particular, middle-aged black men have higher urate levels.

Hyperuricemia may be classified as primary or secondary. In *primary hyperuricemia*, a hereditary error of purine metabolism leads to the overproduction or retention of uric acid. *Secondary hyperuricemia* may be related to another acquired disorder or may be caused by drugs known to inhibit uric acid excretion (e.g., thiazide diuretics, β-adrenergic blockers, angiotensin-converting enzyme inhibitors). Postmenopausal women and organ transplant recipients taking immunosuppressive agents are also at risk for hyperuricemia.

Pathophysiology

Uric acid is the major end product of purine catabolism and is primarily excreted by the kidneys. Gout is caused by an increase in uric acid production, reduced excretion of uric acid by the kidneys (the

G

most common cause), or increased intake of foods containing purines (e.g., red and organ meat, shellfish, fructose drinks), which are metabolized to uric acid by the body. Increased uric acid production is most commonly linked to obesity. Excessive alcohol consumption is also a risk factor.

- High dietary intake of purine alone has relatively little effect on uric acid levels. Hyperuricemia may result from prolonged fasting or excessive alcohol drinking because of the increased production of keto acids, which then inhibit uric acid excretion. Reduced uric acid excretion can occur with chronic kidney disease or metabolic syndrome.

Clinical Manifestations

Gouty arthritis may occur acutely in 1 or more joints. Affected joints may appear dusky or cyanotic and are extremely tender. Inflammation of the great toe *(podagra)* is the most common initial problem. Other joints affected may include the midfoot, ankle, knee, wrist, and olecranon bursa.

- Acute gouty arthritis is usually triggered by events such as trauma, surgery, alcohol ingestion, or systemic infection. Symptom onset is usually rapid. Swelling and pain peak within several hours, often accompanied by a low-grade fever.
- Individual attacks usually subside in 2 to 10 days. The affected joint returns to normal and patients have no symptoms between attacks.

Chronic gout is characterized by multiple joint involvement and visible deposits of sodium urate crystals *(tophi)*. These are typically seen in the synovium, subchondral bone, olecranon bursa, and vertebrae; along tendons; and in the skin and cartilage. Tophi are generally noted many years after the onset of the disease.

Chronic inflammation may cause joint deformity, and cartilage destruction may predispose the joint to secondary osteoarthritis. Large urate crystal deposits may pierce overlying skin, producing draining sinuses that often become infected. Excessive uric acid excretion may lead to urinary tract stone formation. Pyelonephritis related to intrarenal sodium urate deposits and obstruction may contribute to kidney disease.

The severity of gouty arthritis is variable. The clinical course may consist of infrequent mild attacks or multiple severe episodes and slowly progressive disability.

Diagnostic Studies

- Serum uric acid levels are usually elevated above 6 mg/dL.
- Specimens may be obtained for 24-hour urine uric acid levels to determine if the disease is caused by decreased renal excretion or overproduction of uric acid.

- X-rays appear normal in the early stages of gout, with tophi, an indicator of chronic disease, appearing as eroded areas in the bone.
- Synovial fluid aspiration helps distinguish gout from septic arthritis and *pseudogout* (in which calcium phosphate crystals are formed). Affected fluid characteristically contains needlelike crystals of sodium urate.

Interprofessional Management

Goals for care include ending an acute attack with an antiinflammatory agent, such as colchicine. Drug therapy is the primary way to treat acute and chronic gout. Weight reduction (as needed) and possibly avoiding alcohol and foods high in purine (red and organ meats) are recommended.

Drug Therapy

Acute gouty arthritis is treated with colchicine and nonsteroidal antiinflammatory drugs (NSAIDs). Because colchicine has antiinflammatory effects but is not an analgesic, an NSAID is added to the treatment regimen for pain management. Future attacks are prevented in part by combining colchicine with a xanthine oxidase inhibitor (allopurinol [Zyloprim]), or a drug that increases the excretion of uric acid in the urine (uricosuric) (probenecid [Probalan]). Febuxostat (Uloric), a selective inhibitor of xanthine oxidase, is used for long-term management of hyperuricemia in people with chronic gout.

- Aspirin inactivates the effect of uricosurics, resulting in urate retention, and should be avoided while patients are taking uricosuric drugs (e.g., probenecid). Acetaminophen can be used safely if analgesia is needed.

Patients who cannot take or do not respond to drugs that lower uric acid in the blood may be given pegloticase (Krystexxa). This drug metabolizes uric acid into a harmless chemical excreted in the urine.

- Corticosteroids, either orally or by intraarticular injection, can be helpful in treating acute attacks.
- Adequate urine volume with normal renal function (2 to 3 L/day) must be maintained to prevent precipitation of uric acid in the renal tubules. Allopurinol, which blocks production of uric acid, is particularly useful in patients with uric acid stones or renal impairment, in whom uricosuric drugs may be ineffective or dangerous.

Regardless of which drugs are used to treat gout, serum uric acid levels must be checked regularly to monitor treatment effectiveness.

Nutritional Therapy
Dietary restrictions that limit alcohol and foods high in purine help minimize uric acid production. Instruct obese patients in a carefully planned weight-reduction program.

Nursing Management
Nursing intervention is directed at supportive care of the inflamed joints.

- Bed rest may be appropriate, with affected joints properly immobilized. Use a bed cradle or footboard to protect a painful lower extremity from the weight of bed clothes.
- Assess the limitation of motion and degree of pain. Document treatment response.

▼ **Patient and Caregiver Teaching**
Hyperuricemia and gouty arthritis are chronic problems that can be controlled with careful adherence to a treatment program.

- Explain the importance of drug therapy and the need for periodic determination of serum uric acid levels.
- Teach the patient about triggers for an attack, including purine-containing foods and alcohol, starvation (fasting), medication use (e.g., diuretics), and major medical events (e.g., surgery, heart attack).

GUILLAIN-BARRÉ SYNDROME

Description
Guillain-Barré syndrome (GBS) is an autoimmune process that occurs a few days or weeks after a viral or bacterial infection. GBS is rare, affecting about 1 person in every 100,000. It can occur at any age, but those over age 50 years are at greatest risk. The most common type of GBS is acute inflammatory demyelinating polyneuropathy (AIDP). Other types include acute motor axonal neuropathy (AMAN) and acute motor sensory axonal neuropathy (AMSAN). AMAN is more common in children.

The main features of GBS include acute, ascending, rapidly progressive, symmetric weakness of the limbs. Maximal weakness is reached in 4 weeks. Reflexes in the affected limbs are weak or absent. Respiratory muscles may also be affected. Some patients require mechanical ventilation.

- Although 80% of patients almost completely recover, the process may take months or years.

Pathophysiology

Following an infection, immune responses cause injury to either the myelin sheath (AIDP) or the nerve axon itself (AMAN). There is edema and inflammation of affected nerves. The result is segmental loss of the myelin sheath with exposed nerve membranes in nerve terminals and the nodes of Ranvier. Transmission of nerve impulses is stopped or slowed down. This leads to flaccid paralysis with muscle denervation and atrophy. In the recovery phase, remyelination occurs slowly. Neurologic function returns in a proximal-to-distal pattern. Most cases of GBS follow a viral or bacterial infection of the gastrointestinal or upper respiratory tract. Cytomegalovirus is the most common viral cause. *Campylobacter jejuni* gastroenteritis is the most common bacterial cause.

Clinical Manifestations

GBS symptoms range from mild to severe.

- The first symptoms are pain, paresthesia (numbness and tingling), and hypotonia (reduced muscle tone) of the limbs.
- Areflexia (lack of reflexes) and weakness or paralysis of the limbs usually peak within 4 weeks.
- Autonomic nervous system dysfunction manifests with orthostatic hypotension, hypertension, and abnormal vagal responses (bradycardia, heart block, asystole). Other autonomic dysfunctions include bowel and bladder dysfunction, facial flushing, and diaphoresis.
- Cranial nerve involvement is manifested as facial weakness and paresthesia, extraocular eye movement difficulties, and dysphagia.
- Pain is a common symptom including paresthesias, muscular aches and cramps, and hyperesthesias. Pain appears to be worse at night. Pain may lead to a decrease in appetite and interfere with sleep.

The most serious complication of GBS is respiratory failure, which occurs as paralysis progresses to the nerves that innervate the thoracic area.

Diagnostic Studies

Diagnosis is based primarily on patient history and clinical signs. Clinical features required for the diagnosis include progressive weakness of more than 1 limb and diminished or absent reflexes.

- Cerebrospinal fluid (CSF) analysis is helpful in excluding other causes. In GBS, the CSF has more protein than normal.
- Results of electromyography (EMG) and nerve conduction studies are used to confirm the diagnosis.

G

Nursing and Interprofessional Management

Management of GBS is supportive. Ventilator support is critical during the acute phase. Immunomodulating treatments, such as plasma exchange (plasmapheresis) or high-dose IV immunoglobulin (IVIG), are most effective if used within the first 2 weeks of symptom onset.

- Plasmapheresis removes antibodies and other immune factors. It is used 5 times either daily or every other day in the first 2 weeks.
- IVIG interferes with antigen presentation and is given over 5 days. Because it is readily available, IVIG therapy has replaced plasmapheresis as the preferred treatment in many centers.
- Assess the respiratory system frequently by checking respiratory rate and depth to determine the need for immediate intervention, including intubation and mechanical ventilation (see Tracheostomy, p. 714, and Artificial Airways: Endotracheal Tubes, p. 663). Monitor arterial blood gases (ABGs) and vital capacity.
- Evaluate motor and sensory function. Report changes in motor function (e.g., ascending paralysis), deep tendon reflexes, cranial nerve functions (e.g., swallowing, gag reflex, corneal reflex), and level of consciousness.
- Closely monitor BP and cardiac rate and rhythm during the acute phase because dysrhythmias, orthostatic hypotension, and increased or decreased BP and heart rate may occur. Vasopressors and volume expanders may be needed.
- If fever develops, obtain sputum cultures to identify the pathogen. Appropriate antibiotic therapy is then started initiated.
- Respiratory infection or urinary tract infection (UTI) may occur. Immobility from paralysis can cause paralytic ileus, muscle atrophy, venous thromboembolism (VTE), pressure ulcers, orthostatic hypotension, and nutritional deficiencies.

Nutritional needs must be met in spite of possible problems associated with gastric dilation, paralytic ileus, and aspiration potential if the gag reflex is lost.

- Enteral feedings or parenteral nutrition may be used to ensure adequate caloric intake.

HEAD AND NECK CANCER

Description

Most head and neck cancers arise from squamous cells that line the mucosal surfaces of the head and neck. These cancers may involve the nasal cavity and paranasal sinuses, nasopharynx, oropharynx, larynx, oral cavity, and/or salivary glands. Most patients present with locally advanced disease. Disability from the disease and treatment is great because of the potential loss of voice, disfigurement, and social consequences.

- Head and neck cancer occurs most often in patients over age 50 years. Men are affected twice as often as women.
- Tobacco use causes most head and neck cancers. Excess alcohol consumption is also a major risk factor.
- Cancers in patients younger than 50 years have been associated with human papillomavirus (HPV) infection. Other risk factors include exposure to the sun, asbestos, industrial carcinogens, marijuana use, radiation therapy, and poor oral hygiene.

Clinical Manifestations

Early signs of head and neck cancer vary with tumor location.

- Pharyngeal cancer may first be seen as a red or white patch in the mouth, an ulcer that does not heal, or a change in the fit of dentures.
- Hoarseness that lasts more than 2 weeks may be a symptom of early laryngeal cancer. Some patients have a change in voice quality or what feels like a lump in the throat.
- Other clinical manifestations may include a sore throat that does not get better, unilateral ear pain or ringing in the ears, swelling or lumps in the neck, constant coughing, and coughing up blood.
- Difficulties with chewing, swallowing, moving the tongue, and breathing are typically late symptoms.

Diagnostic Studies

- The health care provider (HCP) may examine upper airways using indirect laryngoscopy or with a flexible nasopharyngoscope.
- A CT scan or MRI may show local and regional spread.
- Multiple biopsy specimens are obtained to determine the extent of the disease.

Interprofessional Management

Staging is slightly different for each type of cancer. In general, Stage 0 is in situ, or confined to where it began, through Stage 4, with more advanced disease. Oral cancer staging considers a patient's HPV status. (TNM staging is discussed on p. 761, Part Three).

- Stage I and II cancers are potentially curable with radiation therapy or larynx-sparing surgery.
- Patients with advanced disease (stages III and IV) are treated with combinations of surgery, radiation, chemotherapy, and targeted therapy. Radiation can be delivered by either external-beam therapy or internal implants (brachytherapy).

H

- In a total laryngectomy, the entire larynx and preepiglottic region are removed and a permanent tracheostomy is created (see Tracheostomy, p. 714, in Part Two). Radical neck dissection frequently accompanies total laryngectomy. Extensive dissection and reconstruction may be performed.
- Changes after a total laryngectomy include loss of speech, loss of the ability to taste and smell, inability to produce audible sounds (including laughing and crying), and a permanent tracheal stoma.
- Some patients refuse surgical intervention for advanced lesions because of the extent of the procedure and the potential risk. In this situation, external radiation therapy is used as the sole treatment or in combination with chemotherapy.
- Chemotherapy (e.g., cisplatin) and targeted therapy (e.g., cetuximab [Erbitux]) are used in combination with radiation therapy for patients with stage III or IV cancers.

Nutritional Therapy

After radical neck surgery, the patient may be unable to consume nutrients through the mouth. Parenteral fluids are given for the first 24 to 48 hours.

- Because of swelling and difficulty swallowing postoperatively, enteral nutrition is usually given through a nasogastric, nasointestinal, or gastrostomy tube that was placed during surgery.

When the patient can successfully swallow with low or no risk of aspiration, small amounts of thickened liquids or pureed foods may be given with the patient in high Fowler's position. Avoid thin, watery fluids because they are hard to swallow, increasing the risk of aspiration. Closely observe for choking. Oral suctioning may be needed.

Nursing Management

Goals

The patient with head or neck cancer will have a patent airway, no complications related to therapy, adequate nutritional intake, minimal to no pain, the ability to communicate, and an acceptable body image.

Nursing Interventions

Include information about risk factors in health teaching. Tobacco and alcohol cessation is still important after a cancer has been diagnosed because continued use of those substances diminishes the likelihood of a cure. Encourage good oral hygiene. Teach patients about safe sex practices to prevent HPV infection.

- Interventions to reduce side effects of radiation therapy include teaching the patient oral care measures to reduce dry mouth and encouraging regular exercise to reduce fatigue.

For procedures that involve a laryngectomy, teaching should include information about expected changes in speech. Establish a means of communication to use postoperatively.

After surgery, a laryngectomy (tracheostomy) tube will be in place. Keeping the airway patent is essential. Immediately after surgery, frequent suctioning is usually needed via the tracheostomy tube.

Position the patient in semi-Fowler's position to decrease edema and tension on the suture lines. Monitor vital signs frequently because of the risk of hemorrhage and respiratory compromise.

- Encourage deep breathing and coughing and provide tracheostomy care as needed.
- Depression, changes in sexuality patterns, and altered body image are common after radical neck dissection. Help the patient regain an acceptable self-concept.
- Schedule a speech therapist to meet with the patient who had a total laryngectomy to discuss voice restoration options.

▼ **Patient and Caregiver Teaching**
- Monitor patency of wound drainage tubes every hour in the first few hours after surgery, then every 4 hours to ensure proper functioning. After drainage tubes are removed, closely monitor the area for swelling. If fluid accumulates, aspiration may be necessary.
- Teach the patient and caregivers how to manage tubes and whom to call if there are problems.
- Provide pictorial instructions for tracheostomy care, suctioning, stoma care, and tube feedings as appropriate.
- Teach the patient to cover the stoma before performing activities such as shaving and applying makeup, to avoid inhaling foreign materials.
- Encourage adequate humidity at home using a bedside humidifier and high oral fluid intake.
- Encourage preparation of food that is colorful, attractive, and nutritious. Taste may be diminished with loss of the sense of smell after surgery or radiation therapy.

H

HEAD INJURY

Description

Head injury includes any trauma to the scalp, skull, or brain. A serious form of head injury is *traumatic brain injury* (TBI). In U.S. emergency departments, an estimated 2.5 million people are treated and released with TBI.

- Falls and motor vehicle crashes are the most common causes of head injury. Other causes of head injury include firearms, assaults, sports-related trauma, recreational injuries, and war-related injuries.
- Men are twice as likely to sustain a TBI as women.
- Deaths from head trauma occur at 3 time points after injury: immediately after injury, within 2 hours of injury, and about 3 weeks after injury.
- Most deaths occur immediately after the injury, either from the direct head trauma or massive hemorrhage and shock.
- Deaths occurring within a few hours of the trauma are caused by worsening of the head injury or internal bleeding. Immediately recognizing changes in neurologic status and rapid surgical intervention are critical in the prevention of deaths.
- Deaths occurring 3 weeks or more after the injury result from multisystem failure.

Types of Head Injuries

Scalp Laceration

Because the scalp contains many blood vessels with poor constrictive abilities, even relatively small wounds can bleed profusely. The major complications of scalp lesions are blood loss and infection.

Skull Fracture

Fractures often occur with head trauma. Fractures may be closed or open, depending on the presence of a scalp laceration or extension of the fracture into the air sinuses or dura.

- The type and severity of a skull fracture depend on the velocity, momentum, direction and shape of the injuring agent, and the site of impact. Specific manifestations of a skull fracture are generally associated with the location of the injury (see Table 56.7, Harding et al., *Lewis' Medical-Surgical Nursing*, ed 11).

Major complications of skull fracture are intracranial infections and hematoma, as well as meningeal and brain tissue damage.

Head Trauma

Brain injuries are categorized as *diffuse* (generalized) or *focal* (localized). In *diffuse injury* (i.e., concussion, diffuse axonal), damage to the brain cannot be localized to 1 particular area, whereas a *focal injury* (e.g., contusion, hematoma) can be localized to a specific area.

Diffuse Injury. Concussion is a minor and diffuse head injury associated with a disruption in neural activity and a change in the level of consciousness (LOC). The patient may not lose total consciousness. A brief disruption in LOC, amnesia for the event (retrograde amnesia), and headache are generally of short duration.

- *Postconcussion syndrome* may develop in some patients and is usually seen from 2 weeks to 2 months after the injury. Manifestations include persistent headache, lethargy, behavior changes, decreased short-term memory, and changes in intellectual ability.

Although concussion is generally considered benign and usually resolves spontaneously, the signs and symptoms may be the beginning of a more serious, progressive problem. At the time of discharge, it is important to give the patient and caregiver instructions for observation and accurate reporting of symptoms or changes in neurologic status.

Diffuse axonal injury (DAI) is widespread axonal damage occurring after a mild, moderate, or severe TBI.

- Clinical signs of DAI include decreased LOC, increased intracranial pressure (ICP), decortication or decerebration, and global cerebral edema. About 90% of patients with DAI remain in a persistent vegetative state.
- Patients are rapidly triaged to an intensive care unit (ICU), where they will be vigilantly watched for signs of increased ICP and treated (see Increased Intracranial Pressure, p. 331).

Focal Injury. Focal injury can be minor to severe and localized to an area of injury. Focal injury consists of lacerations, contusions, hematomas, and cranial nerve injuries.

Lacerations involve tearing of brain tissue and often occur with compound fractures and penetrating injuries. Tissue damage is severe, and surgical repair of the laceration is impossible. If bleeding is deep into the brain parenchyma, focal and generalized signs develop. Prognosis is generally poor for the patient with a large intracerebral hemorrhage.

A *contusion* is bruising of brain tissue within a focal area. It is usually associated with a closed head injury. A contusion may contain areas of hemorrhage, infarction, necrosis, and edema.

- Contusions or lacerations may occur both at the site of the direct impact of the brain on the skull *(coup)* and at a secondary area of damage on the opposite side away from injury *(contrecoup)*, leading to multiple contused areas. Contrecoup injuries tend to be more severe.
- Neurologic assessment may reveal focal and generalized findings, depending on the size and location of the contusion. Seizures can occur.

Complications
Epidural Hematoma

An *epidural hematoma* results from bleeding between the dura and inner surface of the skull. An epidural hematoma is a neurologic emergency. It is usually associated with a linear fracture crossing a major artery in the dura, causing a tear. It can have a venous or an arterial origin.

- Venous epidural hematomas are associated with a tear of the dural venous sinus and develop slowly.
- With arterial hematomas, the middle meningeal artery lying under the temporal bone is often torn. Because this is an arterial hemorrhage, the hematoma develops rapidly.

Manifestations typically include an initial period of unconsciousness at the scene, with a brief lucid interval followed by a decrease in LOC. Other symptoms may be headache, nausea and vomiting, or focal manifestations. Rapid surgical intervention to evacuate the hematoma and prevent cerebral herniation, along with treatment to decrease ICP, can dramatically improve outcomes.

Subdural Hematoma

A *subdural hematoma* occurs from bleeding between the dura mater and arachnoid layer of the meninges. The hematoma usually results from injury to the brain tissue and its blood vessels. A subdural hematoma is usually venous in origin and develops slowly. However, an arterial hemorrhage can cause a subdural hematoma, in which case it develops more rapidly. Subdural hematomas may be acute, subacute, or chronic (Table 37).

- An *acute subdural hematoma* manifests within 24 to 48 hours of the injury. Manifestations are similar to those associated with brain tissue compression in increased ICP (see Increased Intracranial Pressure, p. 331). They include decreasing LOC and headache. The patient may be drowsy, confused, or unconscious. The ipsilateral pupil dilates and becomes fixed if ICP is significantly elevated.
- A *subacute subdural hematoma* usually occurs within 2 to 14 days of the injury. After the initial bleeding, this hematoma may appear to enlarge over time as the breakdown products of the blood draw fluid into the subdural space.
- A *chronic subdural hematoma* develops over weeks or months after a seemingly minor head injury. The presenting symptoms are focal rather than signs of increased ICP. Chronic subdural hematomas are more common in older adults because of a potentially larger subdural space secondary to brain atrophy.

Intracerebral Hematoma

An *intracerebral hematoma* occurs from bleeding in the brain tissue. It usually occurs in the frontal and temporal lobes, possibly from the rupture of intracerebral vessels at the time of injury.

Diagnostic Studies

- CT scan is the best diagnostic test to evaluate for craniocerebral trauma.

TABLE 37	Types of Subdural Hematomas	
Occurrence After Injury	**Progression of Symptoms**	**Treatment**
Acute		
24–48 hr after severe trauma	Immediate deterioration	Craniotomy, evacuation and decompression
Subacute		
48 hr–2 wk after severe trauma	Decline in mental status as hematoma develops. Progression dependent on size and location of hematoma	Evacuation and decompression
Chronic		
Weeks or months, usually >20 days after injury Often injury seemed trivial or was forgotten by patient	Nonspecific, nonlocalizing progression. Progressive change in level of consciousness	Evacuation and decompression, membranectomy

- MRI, positron emission tomography (PET), and evoked potential studies assist in diagnosis and differentiation of head injuries.
- Transcranial Doppler studies are used to measure cerebral blood flow velocity.
- Cervical spine x-ray series, CT scan, or MRI of the spine may be done to check for cervical spine trauma.

Interprofessional Management

Emergency management of the patient with head injury includes measures to prevent secondary injury by treating cerebral edema and managing increased ICP (see Table 56.9, Harding et al., *Lewis' Medical-Surgical Nursing*, ed 11). The principal treatment of head injuries is timely diagnosis and surgery, if needed. For the patient with a concussion or contusion, observation for and management of increased ICP are the main strategies.

- The treatment of skull fractures is usually conservative. For depressed fractures and fractures with loose fragments, a craniotomy is done to elevate depressed bone and remove free fragments. If large amounts of bone are destroyed, the bone may be removed (craniectomy) and a cranioplasty will be needed at a later time (see the section on cranial surgery in Chapter 56 of Harding et al., *Lewis' Medical-Surgical Nursing,* ed 11).

- In cases of large acute subdural and epidural hematomas or those associated with significant neurologic impairment, the blood must be removed. A craniotomy is generally done to see and control the bleeding vessels. Burr-hole openings may be used in an extreme emergency for more rapid decompression, followed by a craniotomy. A drain may be placed postoperatively for several days to prevent blood from reaccumulating.

Nursing Management
Goals
The patient with an acute head injury will maintain adequate cerebral oxygenation and perfusion; stay afebrile; be free of discomfort; be free from infection; have adequate nutrition; and attain maximal cognitive, motor, and sensory function.
Nursing Interventions
One of the best ways to prevent head injuries is to prevent car and motorcycle crashes.

- Be active in campaigns that promote driving safety, and speak to driver education classes regarding the dangers of unsafe driving and driving after drinking alcohol and using drugs.
- Teach community members that using seat belts in cars and helmets for riding on motorcycles are the most effective measures for increasing survival after crashes.
- Protective helmets should also be worn by lumberjacks, construction workers, athletes who play contact sports, miners, horseback riders, bicycle riders, snowboarders, skiers, and skydivers.

Acute Care. The general goal of nursing management of the head-injured patient is to maintain cerebral oxygenation and perfusion and prevent secondary cerebral ischemia. Monitoring for changes in neurologic status is critically important because the patient's condition may deteriorate rapidly, requiring emergency surgery.

- Explain the need for frequent neurologic assessments to both patient and caregiver.
- Behavioral manifestations associated with head injury can result in a frightened, disoriented patient who is combative and resists help.

The Glasgow Coma Scale (GCS) is useful in assessing the LOC (see Glasgow Coma Scale, p. 746). Signs of a deteriorating neurologic state, such as decreasing LOC or motor strength, should be reported promptly to the health care provider (HCP).

The major focus of nursing care for the brain-injured patient relates to increased ICP (see Increased Intracranial Pressure: Nursing Management, p. 335).

- Loss of the corneal reflex may require administering lubricating eye drops or taping the eyes shut to prevent abrasion.
- Periorbital ecchymosis and edema disappear spontaneously, but cold and, later, warm compresses provide comfort and hasten the process.
- Diplopia can be relieved by use of an eye patch.
- Hyperthermia can result in increased metabolism, cerebral blood flow, cerebral blood volume, and ICP. Increased metabolic waste also produces further cerebral vasodilation. Avoid hyperthermia, with a goal of maintaining a body temperature of 36°C to 37°C.
- If cerebrospinal fluid (CSF) rhinorrhea or otorrhea occurs, inform the HCP at once. The head of the bed may be elevated to decrease the CSF pressure so that a tear can seal. A loose collection pad may be placed under the nose or over the ear. Tell the patient not to sneeze or blow the nose. Do not insert a gastric tube or suction catheter through the nose.
- Nausea and vomiting can be alleviated by antiemetic drugs.
- Headache can usually be controlled with acetaminophen or small doses of codeine.

If the patient's condition deteriorates, intracranial surgery may be needed. A burr-hole opening or craniotomy may be done, depending on the underlying injury. The patient is often unconscious before surgery, making it necessary for a family member to sign the consent form for surgery. This is a frightening time for the patient's caregiver and family and requires sensitive nursing management. The suddenness of the situation makes it especially hard for the family to cope.

Rehabilitation. Once the condition has stabilized, the patient is usually transferred for acute rehabilitation. There may be chronic problems related to motor and sensory deficits, communication, memory, and intellectual functioning.

H

- The patient's outward appearance is not a good indicator of how well the patient will function in the home or work environment, given recovery time and rehabilitation.
- The mental and emotional sequelae are often the most incapacitating problems. Many patients who have been comatose for more than 6 hours undergo some personality change. The patient's behavior may indicate a loss of social restraint, judgment, tact, and emotional control.

Progressive recovery may continue for 6 months or more before a plateau is reached and a prognosis for recovery can be made.

Nursing management depends on specific residual deficits. The family needs to understand what is happening and be taught appropriate interaction patterns.

- The family often has unrealistic expectations for the patient's full return to pretrauma status as the coma begins to recede. In reality, the patient usually has reduced awareness and ability to interpret stimuli.
- Prepare the family for the emergence of the patient from coma and explain that the process of awakening often takes several weeks. Arrange for social work and chaplain consultations for the family, in addition to providing open visitation and frequent status updates.
- Family members, particularly spouses, go through role transition from that of spouse to that of caregiver.

HEADACHE

Description

Headache is probably the most common type of pain that people have. Most people have functional headaches, such as migraine or tension-type headaches. Others have organic headaches caused by intracranial or extracranial disease. Headaches tend to occur more often in women than in men.

- *Primary headaches* include tension-type, migraine, and cluster headaches. Primary headaches are not caused by a disease or another medical condition. Characteristics and management of tension-type, migraine, and cluster headaches are shown in Table 38.
- *Secondary headaches* are caused by another condition or disorder, such as sinus infection, neck injury, or brain tumor.

The examination of a person with a headache is often normal. Unexplained abnormal findings require further diagnostic studies to identify the underlying cause.

Nursing Management
Goals

The patient with a headache will have reduced or no pain, understand triggering events and treatments, use positive coping strategies to deal with pain, and have increased quality of life and decreased disability.

Nursing Interventions

An inability to cope with daily stresses can cause headaches. Thus effective treatment may involve helping the patient examine the

TABLE 38 Interprofessional Care

Headaches

Tension-Type Headaches	Migraine Headache	Cluster Headache
Location		
Bilateral, band-like pressure at base of skull	Unilateral in 60%, may switch sides; commonly anterior location	Unilateral, radiating up or down from 1 eye
Quality		
Constant, squeezing tightness	Throbbing, synchronous with pulse	Severe, bone crushing
Frequency		
Cycles for many years	Periodic, cycles of several months and years	May have months or years between attacks Attacks occur in clusters over a period of 2–12 wk
Duration		
30 min–7 days	4–72 hr	5 min–3 hr
Time and Mode of Onset		
Not related to time	May be preceded by premonitory symptoms or aura Onset after awakening Improves with sleep	Nocturnal, often awakens person from sleep

Continued

H

TABLE 38 Interprofessional Care—cont'd

Headaches

Tension-Type Headaches	Migraine Headache	Cluster Headache
Associated Symptoms		
Palpable neck and shoulder muscle tension	Irritability, sweating	Facial flushing or pallor
Stiff neck	Nausea, vomiting	Unilateral lacrimation, ptosis, rhinitis
Tenderness	Photophobia	
	Phonophobia	
	Premonitory symptoms: sensory, motor, or psychic phenomena	
Treatment: Abortive and Symptomatic Drugs		
Nonopioid analgesics: aspirin, acetaminophen, NSAIDs	Nonopioid analgesics: aspirin, NSAIDs	α-Adrenergic blockers
Analgesic combinations	Serotonin receptor agonists	ergotamine tartrate
• butalbital/acetaminophen/caffeine	• almotriptan (Axert)	Serotonin receptor agonists
• butalbital/aspirin/caffeine (Fiorinal)	• eletriptan (Relpax)	• almotriptan
• dichloralphenazone/acetaminophen/ isomethepetene	• frovatriptan (Frova)	• eletriptan
Muscle relaxants	• naratriptan (Amerge)	• frovatriptan
	• rizatriptan (Maxalt)	• naratriptan
	• sumatriptan (Imitrex)	• rizatriptan
	• zolmitriptan (Zomig)	• sumatriptan
		• zolmitriptan

Combination
- sumatriptan/naproxen (Treximet)

α-Adrenergic blockers
- ergotamine tartrate (Ergomar)
- dihydroergotamine nasal spray (Migranal)

Analgesic combinations
- acetaminophen/caffeine/aspirin

Corticosteroids
- dexamethasone

O₂ 100% inhalation via mask

α-Adrenergic blockers
- ergotamine tartrate

Corticosteroid
- prednisone

β-Adrenergic blocker
- propranolol (Inderal)

Antidepressants
- amitriptyline (Elavil)
- imipramine (Tofranil)

Treatment: Preventive

Tricyclic antidepressants
- amitriptyline
- nortriptyline (Pamelor)
- doxepin

Continued

H

TABLE 38 Interprofessional Care—cont'd

Headaches

Tension-Type Headaches	Migraine Headache	Cluster Headache
Selective serotonin reuptake inhibitors	Antiseizure drugs	Calcium-channel blocker
• fluoxetine (Prozac)	• divalproex	• verapamil
• paroxetine (Paxil)	• gabapentin	Lithium
β-Adrenergic blocker:	• topiramate	Biofeedback
• propranolol (Inderal)	• valproic acid (Depakene)	
Antiseizure drugs	Botulinum toxin A	
• topiramate (Topamax)	Calcium-channel blocker	
• divalproex (Depakote)	• nifedipine (Procardia)	
Other drugs	• verapamil	
• mirtazapine (Remeron)	Biofeedback	
Biofeedback	Relaxation therapy	
Psychotherapy	Cognitive-behavioral therapy	
Muscle relaxation training		

NSAIDs, Nonsteroidal antiinflammatory drugs.

daily routine, recognize stressful situations, and develop more effective coping strategies. Help the patient identify precipitating factors
and develop ways to avoid or minimize them.

- Encourage daily exercise, relaxation periods, and socialization as
  ways to decrease headaches. Suggest relaxation, meditation,
  yoga, and other ways to address headache pain.
- Massage and moist hot packs to the neck and head can help a
  patient with tension-type headaches.
- The patient should learn about drugs prescribed for prophylactic
  and symptomatic treatment of headache and should be able to
  describe the purpose, action, dosage, and side effects.
- Active challenge and provocative testing (designed specifically
  to provoke symptoms) with suspect foods may help determine
  specific causes. However, teach the patient that food triggers
  may change over time. Encourage the patient to eliminate foods
  and substances that may provoke headaches (e.g., chocolate,
  alcohol, excessive caffeine, cheese, fermented foods, monoso-
  dium glutamate).
- Cluster headache attacks may occur at high altitudes with low O_2
  levels during air travel. Ergotamine, taken before the plane takes
  off, may decrease the risk.

▼ **Patient and Caregiver Teaching**

A teaching guide for the patient with a headache is provided in
Table 39.

TABLE 39   Patient and Caregiver Teaching

Headaches

*Include the following instructions when teaching the patient with a
headache and the patient's caregiver.*

1. Keep a diary or calendar of headaches and possible precipitating
   events.
2. Avoid possible triggers for a headache:
   - foods containing amines (cheese, chocolate), nitrites (meats
     such as hot dogs), vinegar, onions, monosodium glutamate
   - fermented or marinated foods
   - caffeine
   - oranges
   - tomatoes
   - aspartame
   - nicotine
   - ice cream
   - alcohol (especially red wine)

H

Continued

TABLE 39   Patient and Caregiver Teaching

Headaches—cont'd

- emotional stress
- fatigue
- drugs, such as ergot-containing preparations (ergotamine tartrate) and monoamine oxidase inhibitors (e.g., rasagiline [Azilect])

3. Learn the purpose, action, dosage, and side effects of drugs taken.
4. Self-administer sumatriptan subcutaneously, if prescribed.
5. Use stress management techniques.
6. Take part in regular exercise.
7. Contact health care provider (HCP) if any of the following occur:
   - symptoms become more severe, last longer than usual, or are resistant to medication;
   - nausea and vomiting (if severe or not typical), change in vision, or fever occurs with the headache;
   - problems occur with any drugs.

HEART FAILURE

Description

Heart failure (HF) is a complex clinical syndrome that develops in response to myocardial insult and results in the inability of the heart to provide sufficient blood to meet the oxygen (O_2) needs of tissues and organs. The decreased cardiac output (CO) leads to decreased tissue perfusion, impaired gas exchange, fluid volume imbalance, and decreased functional ability.

The percentage of the total blood volume in the left ventricle (LV) at the end of diastole that is pumped out of the LV with the next systole is called *the left ventricular ejection fraction* (LVEF). Normal LVEF is 55% to 65%. HF manifestations occur because of a defect in either ventricular systolic function/LV contraction (*heart failure with reduced ejection fraction* [HFrEF]) and/or a defect in ventricular diastolic function/filling (*heart failure with preserved ejection fraction* [HFpEF]).

HF is associated with many cardiovascular diseases (CVDs), particularly long-standing hypertension (HTN), coronary artery disease (CAD), and myocardial infarction (MI). HF is increasing in incidence and prevalence, partially because of better survival after cardiac events and the aging population. HF is primarily a disease of older adults. The incidence is similar in men and women.

- HTN and CAD are the primary risk factors for HF. HTN is a modifiable risk factor that should be aggressively treated and managed. Long-term treatment of HTN reduces the incidence of HF by 50%.
- Co-morbidities, such as diabetes, metabolic syndrome, advanced age, tobacco use, and vascular disease, contribute to the development of HF.

Blacks and Hispanic Americans develop HF at an earlier age, are admitted to the hospital more often, and have higher mortality rates related to HF as compared to whites.∎

Pathophysiology

Any interference with the normal mechanisms regulating CO may cause HF. CO depends on: (1) preload, (2) afterload, (3) myocardial contractility, and (4) heart rate (HR). These factors affect stroke volume (SV), which is the amount of blood pumped per heartbeat. Thus the equation: $CO = SV \times HR$. Any changes in these factors can lead to decreased ventricular function and HF.

The major causes of HF are divided into 2 subgroups: primary causes and precipitating causes. Precipitating causes often increase the workload of the heart, resulting in an acute condition and decreased heart function. See the complete listing of causes in Tables 34.1 and 34.2, Harding et al., *Lewis' Medical-Surgical Nursing,* ed. 11.

Left-Sided Heart Failure

The most common form of HF, left-sided HF, results either from the inability of the LV to empty adequately during systole or fill adequately during diastole. Left-sided HF can be further classified as HFrEF (systolic HF), HFpEF (diastolic HF), or a combination of the two.

Heart Failure With Reduced Ejection Fraction (Systolic Failure). HFrEF results from an inability of the heart to pump blood effectively. Patients with HFrEF generally have an LVEF < 40%. It can be as low as 5% to 10%.

- HFrEF is caused by impaired contractile function (e.g., MI), increased afterload (e.g., HTN), cardiomyopathy, and mechanical abnormalities (e.g., valvular heart disorders).

The LV in HFrEF loses the ability to generate enough pressure to eject blood forward through the aorta. Over time, the LV becomes dilated and hypertrophied. The weakened heart muscle cannot generate adequate stroke volume which impairs CO. Because the LV cannot effectively push blood forward, end diastolic volumes and pressures in the LV increase. When the LV fails, blood backs up into the left atrium (LA). This causes fluid accumulation in the lungs. The increased pulmonary hydrostatic pressure causes fluid leakage

H

from the pulmonary capillary bed into the interstitium and then the alveoli. This results in pulmonary congestion and edema.

Heart Failure With Preserved Ejection Fraction (Diastolic Failure).
HFpEF results from the inability of the ventricles to relax and fill during diastole. About 50% of patients with HF have HFpEF. In HFpEF, the LV is generally stiff and noncompliant, resulting in high filling pressures. Decreased filling of the ventricles results in decreased SV. The eventual result of HFpEF is the same as that of HFrEF, a reduced CO leading to fluid congestion.

- HTN is the primary cause of HFpEF. Other risk factors include older age, female gender, diabetes, and obesity.
- The diagnosis of HFpEF is based on: (1) signs and symptoms of HF, (2) normal LVEF, and (3) evidence of LV diastolic dysfunction by echocardiography or cardiac catheterization.

Right-Sided Heart Failure

Right-sided HF occurs when the right ventricle (RV) does not pump effectively. When the RV fails, fluid backs up into the venous system. This causes movement of fluid into the tissues and organs (e.g., peripheral edema, abdominal ascites, hepatomegaly, jugular venous distention [JVD]).

The most common cause of right-sided HF is left-sided HF. As the LV fails, fluid backs up into the pulmonary system, causing increased pressures in the lungs. The RV must work harder to push blood to the pulmonary system. Over time, this increased workload weakens the RV and gradually it fails. Other causes of right-sided HF (independent of the function of the LV) include RV infarction, pulmonary embolism, and cor pulmonale (RV dilation and hypertrophy caused by pulmonary disease).

Biventricular Failure

Biventricular failure includes both right and left ventricular dysfunction, the inability of both ventricles to pump effectively. Because of decreased contractility, fluid build-up and systemic venous engorgement are seen. Inadequate CO results in decreased perfusion to vital organs.

Clinical Manifestations

Acute Decompensated Heart Failure

Acute decompensated HF (ADHF) is an increase (usually sudden) in symptoms of HF with a decrease in functional status, often requiring rapid escalation of therapy and hospital admission. ADHF is the most common cause of hospitalization for older Americans.

The clinical presentation of ADHF typically includes symptoms and signs related to pulmonary congestion and volume overload. ADHF can manifest as *pulmonary edema.* This is an acute, life-threatening situation in which the lung alveoli become filled with serosanguineous fluid. The most common cause of pulmonary edema is acute LV failure secondary to CAD.

- Manifestations of pulmonary edema include acute manifestations of left HF, such as dyspnea, respiratory rate > 30 breaths/min, orthopnea, and paroxysmal nocturnal dyspnea (PND).
- JVD is the most sensitive and specific sign for elevated LV filling pressures.
- Auscultation of the lungs may reveal bubbling, crackles, and wheezes. Wheezing and coughing with production of frothy, blood-tinged sputum may also occur.
- The patient's HR is often rapid, and an abnormal S3 or S4 heart sound may be heard.
- BP may be high or low. Hypotension indicates severe LV systolic dysfunction and the chance of cardiogenic shock.

Chronic Heart Failure

Chronic HF is a progressive syndrome characterized by reduced CO and increased venous pressure, associated with underlying molecular changes that result in the death of cardiac muscle cells. The compensatory mechanisms in response to this reduced CO include neurohormonal and hemodynamic reactions to maintain major organ perfusion through vasoconstriction and sympathetic nervous system (SNS) stimulation, an inflammatory response involving cytokines, and ventricular remodeling. These physiologic responses are responsible for the clinical manifestations of chronic HF. Table 40 lists manifestations of left-sided and right-sided chronic HF. The patient with chronic HF usually has manifestations of biventricular failure.

- Fatigue after usual daily activities is one of the earliest symptoms.
- Dyspnea is common. Shortness of breath occurs when lying down (orthopnea).
- PND occurs when the patient is asleep. The patient awakens in a panic, has feelings of suffocation, and has a strong desire to sit or stand up.
- A dry, nonproductive cough may be the first clinical symptom.
- Other common signs include tachycardia; edema in the legs, liver, abdominal cavity, and lungs; nocturia; dusky skin; restlessness and confusion; angina; and weight changes.

Complications

- Pleural effusion results from increasing pressure in the pleural capillaries.
- Atrial fibrillation or ventricular dysrhythmias form enlargement of the heart chambers in chronic HF.

H

	Right-Sided Failure	**Left-Sided Failure**
Signs	• RV heaves • ↑ HR • Murmurs • Jugular venous distention • Edema (e.g., pedal, scrotum, sacrum) • Weight gain • Ascites • Anasarca (massive generalized body edema) • Hepatomegaly (liver enlargement)	• LV heaves • ↑ HR • Pulsus alternans (alternating pulses: strong, weak) • PMI displaced inferiorly and posteriorly (LV hypertrophy) • ↓ PaO_2, slight ↑ $PaCO_2$ (poor O_2 exchange) • Crackles (pulmonary edema) • S_3 and S_4 heart sounds • Pleural effusion • Changes in mental status • Restlessness, confusion • Shallow, rapid respirations • Dry, hacking cough • Frothy, pink-tinged sputum (advanced pulmonary edema)
Symptoms	• Fatigue • Anxiety, depression • Right upper quadrant pain • Anorexia and GI bloating • Nausea	• Weakness, fatigue • Anxiety, depression • Dyspnea • Paroxysmal nocturnal dyspnea • Orthopnea • Nocturia

TABLE 40 Manifestations of Heart Failure

GI, Gastrointestinal; *HR*, heart rate; *LV*, left ventricular; *PaCO_2*, partial pressure of CO_2 in arterial blood; *PaO_2*, partial pressure of O_2 in arterial blood; *PMI*, point of maximal impulse; *RV*, right ventricular.

- Hepatomegaly may result as the liver becomes congested with venous blood. Hepatic congestion leads to impaired liver function; eventually liver cells die, and cirrhosis can develop.

- The decreased CO that accompanies chronic HF also results in decreased perfusion to the kidneys and can lead to anemia, renal insufficiency or renal failure.

Diagnostic Studies

Diagnosing HF is often difficult because signs and symptoms are not highly specific and may mimic other medical conditions (e.g., anemia, lung disease). Diagnostic tests for ADHF and chronic HF are presented in Table 41.

A primary diagnostic goal is to determine the etiology. An endo-myocardial biopsy (EMB) may be done in patients who develop unexplained, new-onset HF that is unresponsive to usual care. An echocardiogram provides information on the EF, which helps distinguish between HFpEF and HFrEF. In general, b-type natriuretic peptide (BNP) and N-terminal prohormone of BNP (NT-proBNP) levels correlate positively with the degree of left ventricular dysfunction.

Nursing and Interprofessional Management: Acute Decompensated Heart Failure

Patients with ADHF need continuous monitoring and assessment. Stable patients may be managed in an emergency department or telemetry unit. If unstable, these patients are managed in an intensive care unit (ICU). In addition to continual heart rhythm and O_2 saturation monitoring, vital signs and urine output are assessed at least hourly. The patient may have continuous hemodynamic monitoring. Supplemental O_2 helps increase the percentage of O_2 in inspired air. In severe pulmonary edema, the patient may need non-invasive ventilatory support or intubation and mechanical ventilation. Table 41 summarizes interprofessional care of the patient with ADHF.

- Position the patient who has dyspnea in a high Fowler's position with the feet horizontal in the bed or dangling at the bedside. This position helps decrease venous return because of the pooling of blood in the extremities and increases the thoracic capacity, allowing for improved breathing.
- Ultrafiltration can rapidly remove intravascular fluid volume while maintaining hemodynamic stability.
- Circulatory assist devices are used to manage patients with worsening HF. The intraaortic balloon pump (IABP) increases coronary blood flow to the heart muscle and decreases the heart's workload. Ventricular assist devices (VADs) can be used to maintain the pumping action of the heart.

TABLE 41 Interprofessional Care

Heart Failure

Both ADHF and Chronic HF	ADHF	Chronic HF
Diagnostic Assessment		
• History and physical examination • Determine underlying cause • Serum chemistry panel, cardiac markers, BNP or NT-proBNP level (see Table 31.6 in Harding et al., *Lewis' Medical-Surgical Nursing*, ed 11), liver function tests, thyroid function tests, CBC, lipid profile, kidney function tests, urinalysis • Chest x-ray • 12-lead ECG • Two-dimensional echocardiogram • Nuclear imaging • Cardiac catheterization	• Measure LV function • Hemodynamic monitoring • Endomyocardial biopsy in select patients	• Cardiopulmonary exercise stress test • 6-minute walk test • Sleep studies in select patients
Management		
• Treatment of underlying cause • Drug therapy • Circulatory assist devices (e.g., ventricular assist device) • Daily weights	• High Fowler's position • Noninvasive positive pressure ventilation	• Cardiac resynchronization therapy with biventricular pacing and implantable cardioverter-defibrillator (ICD) • Heart transplantation • Rest-activity periods

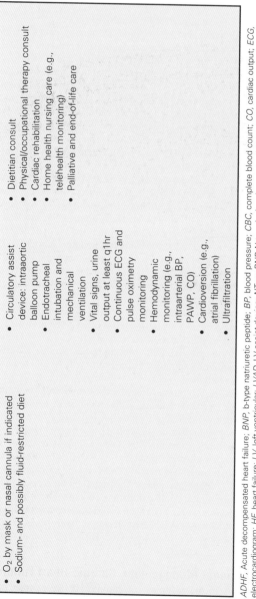

- O₂ by mask or nasal cannula if indicated
- Sodium- and possibly fluid-restricted diet

- Circulatory assist device: intraaortic balloon pump
- Endotracheal intubation and mechanical ventilation
- Vital signs, urine output at least q1hr
- Continuous ECG and pulse oximetry monitoring
- Hemodynamic monitoring (e.g., intraarterial BP, PAWP, CO)
- Cardioversion (e.g., atrial fibrillation)
- Ultrafiltration

- Dietitian consult
- Physical/occupational therapy consult
- Cardiac rehabilitation
- Home health nursing care (e.g., telehealth monitoring)
- Palliative and end-of-life care

ADHF, Acute decompensated heart failure; *BNP,* b-type natriuretic peptide; *CBC,* complete blood count; *CO,* cardiac output; *ECG,* electrocardiogram; *HF,* heart failure; *LV,* left ventricular; *LVAD,* LV assist device; *NT-proBNP,* N-terminal prohormone of BNP; *PAWP,* pulmonary artery wedge pressure.

H

Drug Therapy

Drug therapy is essential in treating acute HF.

- *Diuretics.* Diuretics are the first line for treating patients with volume overload. They decrease sodium reabsorption at various sites within the kidneys, enhancing sodium and water loss. Decreasing intravascular volume with diuretics reduces volume returning to the LV (preload). This allows for more efficient LV pumping, decreased pulmonary vascular pressures, and improved alveolar gas exchange. IV administration of loop diuretics (e.g., furosemide) by bolus or infusion is preferred. We evaluate effectiveness by increased urine output, decreased symptoms, and fluid weight loss. Serum potassium and magnesium levels are continually monitored.

- *Vasodilators.* Vasodilators are used to treat ADHF in the absence of hypotension. IV nitroglycerin is a primary venodilator that reduces circulating blood volume. It also improves coronary artery blood flow by dilating the coronary arteries. So, nitroglycerin reduces preload, slightly reduces afterload (in high doses), and increases myocardial O_2 supply. Sodium nitroprusside reduces both preload and afterload, thereby improving myocardial contraction, increasing CO, and reducing pulmonary congestion. IV nesiritide, a recombinant form of BNP, causes both arterial and venous dilation.

- *Morphine.* Morphine dilates pulmonary and systemic blood vessels, reducing preload and afterload. It is often given in small IV boluses for the dyspnea associated with ADHF. Cautious use and close monitoring are advised. Morphine has serious adverse effects, including respiratory depression, which can require mechanical ventilation.

- *Positive inotropics.* Inotropic drugs increase myocardial contractility and are used for patients with evidence of cardiogenic shock or with low CO. Drugs include β-agonists (e.g., dopamine, dobutamine, norepinephrine [Levophed]) and phosphodiesterase inhibitors (milrinone) and digitalis. The β-agonists are appropriately used as a short-term treatment of ADHF. In addition to increasing myocardial contractility and systemic vascular resistance (SVR), dopamine dilates the renal blood vessels and enhances urine output. Unlike dopamine, dobutamine is a selective β-agonist that works mainly on the β1-receptors in the heart and does not increase SVR. Effectiveness of inotropes is evaluated by assessing for improved CO, BP, urine output, and reduced filling pressures.

Interprofessional Management: Chronic Heart Failure

The main goals in the treatment of chronic HF are to treat the underlying cause and contributing factors, maximize CO, reduce symptoms, improve ventricular function, improve quality of life, preserve target organ function, and improve mortality and morbidity. The treatment of causes, such as dysrhythmias, hypertension, valvular disorders, and CAD, is discussed elsewhere in this book. Chronic HF therapies are tailored to the individual patient based on comorbid conditions. The goals of chronic HF therapies include optimal symptom management; mortality and morbidity benefit; minimizing side effects; and monitoring responses to therapies. Specifically, these therapies treat the underlying cause and contributing factors, maximize CO, improve ventricular function, improve quality of life, and preserve target organ function.

Nondrug Therapy

Supplemental O_2 improves saturation and helps meet tissue O_2 needs. This helps relieve patient dyspnea and fatigue. Physical and emotional rest conserves energy and decreases the need for additional O_2. A patient with severe HF may be on bed rest with limited activity. A patient with mild to moderate HF can be ambulatory with a restriction of strenuous activity.

Patients with a LVEF < 35% may be candidates for an *implantable cardioverter-defibrillator* (ICD), recommended for primary prevention of sudden cardiac death. *Cardiac resynchronization therapy* (CRT) may be used to coordinate right and left ventricular contractility through biventricular pacing. The ability to have normal simultaneous electrical conduction (synchrony) in the right and left ventricles increases left ventricular function and CO. Implanted ICD and CRT devices can also be used for remotely monitoring HF patients. Other mechanical assist devices are available to sustain HF patients with deteriorating function and those awaiting cardiac transplant.

Drug Therapy

The cornerstone of drug therapy in chronic HF is neurohormonal blockade. The result of neurohormonal blockade is decreased plasma aldosterone levels, decreased SNS activity, vasodilation, and sodium and water excretion.

- *Angiotensin-converting enzyme (ACE) inhibitors.* ACE inhibitors (e.g., captopril, enalapril) are first-line drugs for chronic HFrEF. They decrease mortality, morbidity, hospitalizations, and symptoms in patients with HFrEF. ACE inhibitors block the renin-angiotensin-aldosterone system (RAAS) by inhibiting the conversion of angiotensin I to angiotensin II. They reduce afterload and SVR and inhibit the development of ventricular remodeling by inhibiting ventricular hypertrophy.
- *Angiotensin II Receptor Blockers* (ARBs). For patients who are unable to tolerate ACE inhibitors, ARBs are recommended. They prevent the vasoconstrictor and aldosterone-secreting

effects of angiotensin II by binding to the angiotensin II receptor sites. ARBs promote afterload reduction and vasodilation.

- *Neprilysin-Angiotensin Receptor Inhibitors.* Sacubitril/valsartan (Entresto) is a combination of a neprilysin inhibitor (sacubitril) and an ARB (valsartan). This drug provides dual blockade of the RAAS and the natriuretic peptide system. Sacubitril, a recombinant form of BNP, inhibits neprilysin, an enzyme that degrades natriuretic peptides. Sacubitril inhibition allows for more available circulating BNP. This results in decreased SVR, afterload, and central venous pressure (CVP), and increased natriuresis and diuresis. This drug is an alternative to ACE inhibitors and ARBs in patients meeting criteria with symptomatic HFrEF.

- *Aldosterone Antagonists.* Spironolactone (Aldactone) and eplerenone (Inspra) are potassium-sparing diuretics that inhibit aldosterone activation. These drugs work by binding to receptors at the aldosterone-dependent sodium-potassium exchange site in the distal renal tubule where they have a mild diuretic effect. It is critical to carefully monitor serum potassium levels and renal function in patients taking aldosterone antagonists.

- *Nitrates.* Nitrates (e.g., nitroglycerin) cause vasodilation by acting directly on the smooth muscle of the vessel wall. Nitrates are of particular benefit in the management of myocardial ischemia related to HF because they promote vasodilation of the coronary arteries.

- *β-Adrenergic blockers.* β-Blockers directly block the negative effects of the SNS (e.g., increased HR) on the failing heart. Three β-blockers have been shown to decrease mortality in patients with HFrEF: metoprolol succinate (Toprol XL), bisoprolol (Zebeta), and carvedilol (Coreg). These β-blockers may also increase LVEF. However, because β-blockers can reduce myocardial contractility, care must be taken in patients with volume overload. They are usually started at low dose. Major side effects include worsening of HF symptoms, hypotension, fatigue, and bradycardia.

- *Hydralazine/Isosorbide Dinitrate Combination (Bidil).* A fixed combination of the vasodilators hydralazine and isosorbide dinitrate can reduce mortality and improve LVEF and exercise tolerance. The drug is specifically effective in blacks with HFrEF already receiving optimal doses of other medications.

- *Digitalis.* Digitalis (digoxin), a weak positive inotrope, acts primarily as a neurohormonal modulator that reduces the effects of the SNS and suppresses renin secretion from the kidneys. Better outcomes occur with digoxin serum levels of < 0.9 ng/mL.

Higher serum doses are associated with increased mortality rate and digoxin toxicity. Monitor renal function and serum potassium levels of all patients taking digitalis.

- *Diuretics.* Diuretics reduce edema, pulmonary venous pressure, and preload. Thiazide diuretics (e.g., hydrochlorothiazide) inhibit sodium reabsorption in the distal tubule, thus promoting excretion of sodium and water. Loop diuretics, such as furosemide (Lasix), bumetanide (Bumex), and torsemide (Demadex), are potent but can cause hypokalemia and ototoxicity. In chronic HF, the lowest effective dose of diuretic should be used.

Nutritional Therapy

Diet teaching and weight management are essential to the patient's control of chronic HF. Take a detailed diet history to determine what foods the patient eats and also when, where, and how often the person dines out.

- HF guidelines vary with regards to sodium restriction in the management of HF. Excess sodium may worsen HF symptoms and facilitate an exacerbation. The degree of sodium restriction depends on the severity of the HF and the effectiveness of diuretic therapy.
- In general, the dietary recommendation for sodium intake is restricted to 2 gms per day. Teach the patient what foods are low and high in sodium content and how to read labels. Teach ways to enhance food flavors without the use of salt (e.g., substituting lemon juice, various spices).

Fluid restrictions are not often prescribed for the patient with mild to moderate HF. However, fluid restrictions may be needed for stage D HF patients with persistent fluid retention despite appropriate sodium restriction.

- Teach patients to weigh themselves at the same time each day, preferably before breakfast, while wearing the same type of clothing. Tell patients to call the health care provider (HCP) about a weight gain of 3 lb (1.4 kg) over 2 days or a 3- to 5-lb (2.3-kg) gain over a week.

Nursing Management: Chronic Heart Failure

Goals

Nursing care focuses on the priority problems of decreased CO, impaired oxygenation, fluid overload, intolerance of physical activity and managing a complex medication regimen. The overall goals for the patient with HF include: (1) decrease in symptoms (e.g., shortness of breath, fatigue), (2) decrease in peripheral edema,

H

(3) increase in exercise tolerance, (4) adherence with the treatment plan, including appropriate evidence-based medication and device therapies, and (5) no complications related to HF.

See care of the patient with HF in the eNursing Care Plan 34-1 on the website.

Nursing Interventions

Help aggressively identify and treat risk factors for HF to prevent or slow the disease progression. Recommended lifestyle modifications begin with weight management, diet, and regular exercise. Often, medications are needed. For example, teach the patient with HTN or hyperlipidemia measures to manage BP or cholesterol with medication, diet, and exercise. Patients with valvular disease should have valve replacement planned before lung congestion develops.

Acute Care. Many people with HF will experience 1 or more episodes of ADHF. Successful HF care depends on several important principles: (1) HF is a progressive disease, (2) treatment plans are established with QOL goals, (3) symptom management depends to a significant degree on adherence to self-management protocols (e.g., daily weights, diet, exercise, recognizing signs and symptoms of decompensation), and evidence-based therapy (EBT) regimens (drug and device therapies), (4) precipitating factors, etiologies, and contributing comorbid conditions must be addressed, (5) complex care needs often require care in multiple settings, increasing risk for fragmented care, and (6) support systems are essential to the success of the entire treatment plan.

Ambulatory Care. HF is a chronic and progressive condition that will require lifelong therapies. Goals of ambulatory HF care include symptom management, QOL maintenance, morbidity and mortality benefit from EBT, identifying and mitigating factors precipitating ADHF and hospitalization, and closely monitoring responses to and potential side effects of therapies.

- Assess patients with HF for depression and anxiety. Anxiety may increase the SNS response and increase myocardial workload. Reducing anxiety may be facilitated by a variety of nursing interventions and the use of sedatives (e.g., benzodiazepines, morphine sulfate).
- Exercise training, such as in a cardiac rehabilitation program, can improve symptoms of chronic HF. Exercise for patients with HF has been found to be safe, to improve overall sense of well-being, and has been associated with reduced mortality.

A patient and caregiver teaching guide for HF is presented in Table 42.

TABLE 42 Patient and Caregiver Teaching

Heart Failure

Include the following instructions when teaching the patient and caregiver about the management of heart failure.

Dietary Therapy

- Consult the diet plan and list of permitted and restricted foods.
- Adhere to specific sodium restriction guidelines outlined by your health care provider (HCP).
- Examine labels to determine sodium content. Also examine the labels of over-the-counter drugs, such as laxatives, cough medicines, and antacids for sodium content.
- Avoid using salt when preparing foods or adding salt to foods.
- Weigh yourself at the same time each day, preferably in the morning, using the same scale and wearing similar clothes.
- Eat small, frequent meals.

Activity Program

- Increase walking and other activities gradually, provided that they do not cause fatigue or dyspnea.
- Consider a cardiac rehabilitation program.
- Avoid extremes of heat and cold.

Ongoing Monitoring

- Know the signs and symptoms of worsening heart failure including increasing dyspnea, cough, orthopnea, PND, weight gain, edema, fluid retention, fatigue, and tiredness with physical activity.
- Recall the symptoms when illness began. Reappearance of previous symptoms may indicate a recurrence.
- Report any of the following to the HCP at once:
  - weight gain of 3 lb (1.4 kg) in 2 days, or 3–5 lb (1.4–2.3 kg) in a week
  - difficulty breathing, especially with activity or when lying flat
  - waking up breathless at night
  - frequent dry, hacking cough, especially when lying down
  - fatigue, weakness
  - swelling of ankles, feet, or abdomen. Swelling of face or difficulty breathing (if taking ACE inhibitors)
  - nausea with abdominal swelling, pain, and tenderness
  - dizziness or fainting
- Follow up with HCP on regular basis.
- Consider joining a local support group with your family members and caregivers.

H

Continued

TABLE 42   Patient and Caregiver Teaching

Heart Failure—cont'd

Health Promotion

- Obtain annual influenza vaccination.
- Obtain pneumococcal vaccination
- Develop plan to reduce risk factors (e.g., BP control, tobacco cessation, blood sugar/ HGA1C control, weight reduction).

Rest

- Plan a regular daily rest and activity program.
- After exertion, such as exercise and ADLs, plan a rest period.
- Shorten working hours, or schedule rest period during working hours.
- Avoid emotional upsets. Share any concerns, fears, feelings of depression, etc., with HCP.

Drug Therapy

- Take each drug as prescribed.
- Develop a system (e.g., daily chart, weekly pillbox) to ensure that drugs have been taken.
- Count heart rate each day before taking drugs (if appropriate). Know the limits that your HCP wants for your heart rate.
- Take BP at determined intervals (if appropriate). Know your target BP limits.
- Know signs and symptoms of orthostatic hypotension and how to prevent them (see Table 32.12 in Harding et al., *Lewis' Medical-Surgical Nursing*, ed 11).
- If taking anticoagulants, know signs and symptoms of internal bleeding (bleeding gums, increased bruises, blood in stool or urine) and actions to take.
- If taking warfarin (Coumadin), know INR results, target INR level, and how often to have INR checked.

ACE, Angiotensin-converting enzyme; *ADLS,* activities of daily living; *INR,* international normalized ratio; *PND,* paroxysmal nocturnal dyspnea.

HEMOPHILIA AND VON WILLEBRAND DISEASE

Description

Hemophilia is an X-linked recessive genetic disorder caused by a defective or deficient coagulation factor. The 2 major types of hemophilia that can occur in mild to severe forms are *hemophilia A* (classic hemophilia, factor VIII deficiency) and *hemophilia B* (Christmas disease, factor IX deficiency). *von Willebrand disease* is a related disorder involving a deficiency of the von Willebrand coagulation protein.

Hemophilia A is 4 times as common as hemophilia B. There are rare cases of acquired hemophilia A, which is caused by the development of antibodies against the body's own factor VIII. von Willebrand disease is the most common congenital bleeding disorder in humans.

Deficiency and inheritance patterns of these 3 forms of inherited coagulopathy are compared in Table 43.

Clinical Manifestations and Complications

Clinical manifestations and complications related to hemophilia include: (1) slow, persistent, prolonged bleeding from minor trauma and small cuts; (2) delayed bleeding after minor injuries (the delay may be several hours or days); (3) uncontrollable hemorrhage after dental extractions or irritation of the gingiva with a hard-bristle toothbrush; (4) prolonged epistaxis, especially after a blow to the face; (5) gastrointestinal (GI) bleeding from ulcers and gastritis; (6) hematuria from genitourinary (GU) trauma and splenic rupture resulting from falls or abdominal trauma; (7) ecchymoses, subcutaneous hematomas, and possible compartment syndrome; (8) neurologic signs, such as pain, anesthesia, and paralysis, that may develop from nerve compression caused by hematoma formation; and (9) hemarthrosis (bleeding into the joints), which may lead to joint

TABLE 43	Types of Hemophilia	
Type	**Defect/Deficiency**	**Inheritance Pattern**
Hemophilia A	Factor VIII deficiency	Recessive sex-linked (transmitted by female carriers, displayed almost exclusively in men)
Hemophilia B	Factor IX deficiency	Recessive sex-linked (transmitted by female carriers, displayed almost exclusively in men)
von Willebrand disease	vWF, variable factor VIII deficiencies; platelet dysfunction	Autosomal dominant, seen in both genders Recessive (in severe forms of the disease)

vWF, von Willebrand factor.

deformity severe enough to cause crippling (often in knees, elbows, shoulders, hips, and ankles).

Diagnostic Studies

Laboratory studies are done to determine the type of hemophilia. A factor deficiency within the intrinsic system (factor VIII, IX, XI, or XII or von Willebrand factor [vWF]) will yield the laboratory results presented in Table 30.17, Harding et al., *Lewis' Medical-Surgical Nursing,* ed 11.

Interprofessional Management

The goal of care is to prevent and treat bleeding. People with hemophilia or von Willebrand disease require preventive care, the use of replacement therapy during acute bleeding episodes and for prophylaxis, and treatment of complications of the disease and its therapy.

- Replacement of deficient clotting factors is the primary means of supporting patients with hemophilia. In addition to treating acute crises, replacement therapy may be given before surgery and dental care as a prophylactic measure.
- For mild hemophilia A or certain subtypes of von Willebrand disease, desmopressin acetate (DDAVP), a synthetic analog of vasopressin, may stimulate an increase in factor VIII.

Complications of treatment of hemophilia include development of inhibitors to factor VIII or IX, transfusion-transmitted infectious disorders, allergic reactions, and thrombotic complications with the use of factor IX because it contains activated coagulation factors.

The most common problem with acute management is starting factor replacement therapy too late and stopping it too soon. Minor bleeding episodes should be treated for at least 72 hours. Surgery and traumatic injuries may need longer therapy. Eventually, a patient's development of inhibitors to the factor products requires individualized expert patient management.

Nursing Management

Because of the hereditary nature of hemophilia, referral of affected people for genetic counseling before reproduction is important.

Acute interventions are related primarily to controlling the bleeding and include the following:

1. Stop the topical bleeding as quickly as possible. Apply direct pressure or ice, pack the area with Gelfoam or fibrin foam, and apply topical hemostatic agents, like thrombin.
2. Give the specific coagulation factor to raise the patient's level of the deficient coagulation factor. Monitor the patient for signs and symptoms, such as hypersensitivity.

3. When joint bleeding occurs, in addition to giving replacement factors, it is important to use the "RICE" protocol. Rest the involved joint to prevent crippling deformities from hemarthrosis, ice the joint for 20 minutes every 3 to 4 hours, compress/wrap the joint, and elevate. Give analgesics to reduce severe pain. Do not use aspirin and aspirin-containing compounds. As soon as bleeding ceases, encourage mobilization of the affected area through range-of-motion exercises and physical therapy. Avoid weight bearing until all swelling has resolved and muscle strength has returned. Orthotics may be prescribed.
4. Manage life-threatening complications that may develop because of hemorrhage. Examples are prevention or treatment of airway obstruction from hemorrhage into the neck and pharynx and early assessment and treatment of intracranial bleeding.

▼ **Patient and Caregiver Teaching**

Quality of life and survival may be significantly affected by the patient's knowledge of the illness and how to live with it. Provide ongoing assessment of the patient's adaptation to the illness.

- Teach the patient with hemophilia that immediate medical attention is required for severe pain or swelling of a muscle or joint that restricts movement or inhibits sleep and for a head injury, swelling in the neck or mouth, abdominal pain, hematuria, melena, and skin wounds with continued bleeding.
- Teach the patient to perform daily oral hygiene without causing trauma.
- Advise the patient to only participate in noncontact sports (e.g., golf) and to wear gloves when doing household chores, to prevent cuts or abrasions from knives, hammers, and other tools.
- The patient should wear a medical identification (Medic Alert) tag to ensure that health care providers (HCPs) know about the hemophilia in case of an accident.
- Refer the patient and caregiver to a local chapter of the National Hemophilia Foundation for additional information and support.
- Many patients or their caregivers can be taught to self-administer the factor replacement therapies at home.

H

HEMORRHOIDS

Description

Hemorrhoids are dilated veins that may be internal (occurring above the internal sphincter) or external (occurring outside the external sphincter).

Pathophysiology

Hemorrhoids develop because of increased anal pressure and weakening of the connective tissue that supports the hemorrhoidal veins. Weakened supporting tissue allows for downward displacement of the hemorrhoidal veins, causing them to dilate. An intravascular clot in the venule results in a *thrombosed* external hemorrhoid.

Hemorrhoids are the most common reason for bleeding with defecation. Hemorrhoids may be precipitated by many factors, including pregnancy, obesity, constipation, diarrhea, straining to defecate, heavy lifting, prolonged standing and sitting, and ascites.

Clinical Manifestations

Classic manifestations of hemorrhoids include bleeding, anal pruritus, prolapse, and pain.

- *Internal hemorrhoids* cause pain if they become constricted. Internal hemorrhoids can prolapse into the anal canal or externally, causing a sense of pressure with defecation and a protruding mass.
- *External hemorrhoids* are reddish blue and seldom bleed. There may be itching, burning, and edema. They usually do not cause pain and inflammation unless a thrombosis (blood clot) is present. Thrombosed hemorrhoids are bluish purple masses palpable at the anal orifice. The clot can erode through the overlying stretched skin, causing bleeding with defecation. Constipation or diarrhea can worsen the symptoms.

Diagnostic Studies

- *Internal hemorrhoids* are diagnosed by digital examination, anoscopy, and sigmoidoscopy.
- *External hemorrhoids* can be diagnosed by visual inspection and digital examination.

Interprofessional Management

Therapy is directed toward the causes of the condition and the patient's symptoms. A high-fiber diet and increased fluid intake prevent constipation and reduce straining. Ointments, creams, suppositories, and pads that contain antiinflammatory agents (e.g., hydrocortisone) or astringents and anesthetics (e.g., witch hazel, benzocaine) may shrink mucous membranes and relieve discomfort. Topical corticosteroids, such as hydrocortisone agents, should be limited to 1 week or less to prevent side effects such as contact dermatitis and mucosal atrophy. Stool softeners may ease defecation. Sitz baths help relieve pain.

- External hemorrhoids are usually managed by conservative therapy unless they become thrombosed. For internal hemorrhoids, nonsurgical approaches (band ligation, infrared coagulation, cryotherapy, laser treatment) can be used.
- Hemorrhoidectomy (surgical excision of hemorrhoids) is used for patients with severe symptoms related to multiple thrombosed hemorrhoids or marked protrusion.

Nursing Management

Nursing care includes teaching measures to prevent constipation, avoiding prolonged standing or sitting, proper use of over-the-counter preparations, and instructions on when to seek medical care (e.g., excessive pain and bleeding, prolapsed hemorrhoids).

- Severe pain caused by sphincter spasm is common after a hemorrhoidectomy. Most patients initially receive an opioid and nonsteroidal antiinflammatory drug (NSAID) in conjunction with topical preparations that provide anesthesia or reduce internal sphincter spasms, such as such as topical lidocaine, 2% diltiazem, and glyceryl trinitrate.
- Packing inserted into the rectum to absorb drainage is usually removed the first or second postoperative day. Provide privacy. Assess for rectal bleeding.
- Sitz baths are started 1 or 2 days after surgery. Initially, do not leave the patient alone because of the possibility of weakness or fainting. A sponge ring in the bath helps relieve pressure on the area.
- A stool softener, such as docusate sodium (Colace), may be ordered. If the patient does not have a bowel movement within 2 or 3 days, an oil retention enema is given.
- The patient usually dreads the first bowel movement and often resists the urge to defecate. Give pain medication before the bowel movement to reduce discomfort.
- Teach the importance of diet, sitz baths, symptoms of complications (especially bleeding), and avoiding constipation and straining.

HEPATITIS, VIRAL

Description

Hepatitis, an inflammation of the liver, is most often caused by viruses. The types of viral hepatitis are A, B, C, D, E, and G. They differ in their modes of transmission and disease course (Table 44). Other viruses known to damage the liver include cytomegalovirus, Epstein-Barr virus, herpesvirus, coxsackievirus, and rubella virus.

TABLE 44 Characteristics of Hepatitis Viruses

Incubation Period and Mode of Transmission	Sources of Infection	Infectivity
Hepatitis A Virus (HAV)		
Incubation: 15–50 days (average 28)	• Contaminated food, milk, water, shellfish	• Most infectious during 2 wk before onset of symptoms
• Fecal-oral (primarily fecal contamination and oral ingestion)	• Crowded conditions (e.g., day care, nursing home)	• Infectious until 1–2 wk after the start of symptoms
	• Persons with subclinical infections, infected food handlers, sexual contact, IV drug users	
	• Poor personal hygiene	
	• Poor sanitation	
Hepatitis B Virus (HBV)		
Incubation: 115–180 days (average 56–96 days)	• Contaminated needles, syringes, and blood products	• Before and after symptoms appear
• Percutaneous (parenteral) or mucosal exposure to blood or blood products	• HBV-infected mother (perinatal transmission)	• Infectious for months
• Sexual contact	• Sexual activity with infected partners. Asymptomatic carriers	• Carriers continue to be infectious for life
• Perinatal transmission	• Tattoos or body piercing with contaminated needles	

Hepatitis C Virus (HCV)

Incubation: 14–180 days (average 56 days)

- Percutaneous (parenteral) or mucosal exposure to blood or blood products
- High-risk sexual contact
- Perinatal contact

- Blood and blood products
- Needles and syringes
- Sexual activity with infected partners, low risk

- 1–2 wk before symptoms appear
- Continues during clinical course
- 75%–85% go on to develop chronic hepatitis C and remain infectious

Hepatitis D Virus (HDV)

Incubation: 2–26 wk

- HBV must precede HDV
- Chronic carriers of HBV always at risk

- Same as HBV
- Can cause infection only when HBV is present

- Blood infectious at all stages of HDV infection

Hepatitis E Virus (HEV)

Incubation: 15–64 days (average 26–42 days)

- Fecal-oral route
- Outbreaks associated with contaminated water supply in developing countries

- Contaminated water, poor sanitation
- Found in Asia, Africa, and Mexico
- Not common in United States but is increasing in some areas

- Not known
- May be similar to HAV

H

Hepatitis A

Hepatitis A viral infection can cause a mild flu-like illness with jaundice. It can also cause acute liver failure, but does not result in chronic (long-term) infection.

Hepatitis A virus (HAV) is a ribonucleic acid (RNA) virus transmitted primarily through fecal contamination of food or drinking water. Transmission occurs in food handling and among family members, institutionalized persons, and children in day care centers.

- Detection of hepatitis A immunoglobulin (Ig)M indicates acute hepatitis. Anti-HAV (antibody to HAV) IgM appears in the serum as the stool becomes negative for the virus. Hepatitis A IgG indicates past infection.
- Hepatitis A vaccination and thorough hand washing are the best measures to prevent outbreaks.

Hepatitis B

Hepatitis B virus (HBV) is a blood-borne pathogen that can cause either acute or chronic disease. The incidence of HBV infection has decreased where there is widespread use of the HBV vaccine.

- HBV is a deoxyribonucleic acid (DNA) virus. It can be transmitted in several ways, including: (1) perinatally to infants by mothers infected with HBV to their infants, (2) percutaneously (e.g., IV drug use, accidental needlestick punctures), and (3) via small cuts on mucosal surfaces and exposure to infectious blood, blood products, or other body fluids (e.g., semen, vaginal secretions, saliva).

Hepatitis C

Infection with the hepatitis C virus (HCV) can result in both acute and chronic illness.

- HCV is an RNA virus that is blood-borne and primarily transmitted percutaneously. The most common mode of transmission is the sharing of contaminated needles and equipment among injection drug users. High-risk sexual behavior (e.g., unprotected sex, multiple partners), especially among men who have sex with men (MSM), is associated with increased risk of transmission.
- Acute HCV, which is usually asymptomatic, can be hard to detect unless diagnosed with laboratory tests.
- Chronic HCV results in a potentially progressive liver disease, with 20% to 30% of the patients developing cirrhosis and eventually liver failure and/or liver cancer. Hepatitis C is the most common cause of chronic liver disease and the most common indication for liver transplantation in the United States.

Hepatitis D

Hepatitis D virus (HDV), also called *delta virus,* cannot survive on its own and requires HBV to replicate. It can be acquired at the same time as HBV, or a person with HBV can be infected with HDV at a later time. HDV is transmitted percutaneously.

- HDV can cause a spectrum of illness ranging from an asymptomatic chronic carrier state to acute liver failure. There is no vaccine for HDV. However, vaccination against HBV reduces the risk of HDV co-infection.

Hepatitis E

Like hepatitis A, hepatitis E virus (HEV) is an RNA virus transmitted by the fecal-oral route. The usual mode of transmission is drinking contaminated water. Hepatitis E infection occurs primarily in developing countries, with epidemics reported in India, Asia, Mexico, and Africa.

For a more complete description of each hepatitis virus, see Chapter 43 in Harding et al., *Lewis' Medical-Surgical Nursing,* ed 11.

Pathophysiology

In viral hepatitis, hepatocytes become targets of the virus in 1 of 2 ways: through direct action of the virus (as in HCV infection) or through a cell-mediated immune response to the virus (as in HBV and HCV infection). The destruction of hepatocytes leads to liver-related dysfunction in bile production, coagulation, blood glucose, and protein metabolism. Detoxification and processing of drugs, hormones, and metabolites may also be disrupted.

- Liver cells can regenerate and, if no complications occur, resume their normal appearance and function.
- Antigen-antibody complexes may form circulating immune complexes in the early phases of hepatitis and activate the complement system. Manifestations of this activation are rash, angioedema, arthritis, fever, and malaise.
- Chronic viral hepatitis can be insidious and silent, causing persistent and continual destruction of infected hepatocytes. Over time, scar tissue can develop, which leads to fibrosis, cirrhosis and liver failure.

Clinical Manifestations

A large number of patients with acute hepatitis have no symptoms. Manifestations of viral hepatitis may be classified into acute and chronic phases.

The *acute phase* usually lasts 1 to 6 months.

- During the incubation period, symptoms may include intermittent or ongoing anorexia, lethargy, nausea, vomiting, skin rashes, diarrhea or constipation, malaise, fatigue, myalgias,

H

arthralgias, other flu-like symptoms, and right upper quadrant tenderness.

- Physical examination may reveal hepatomegaly, lymphadenopathy, and sometimes splenomegaly. This is the period of maximal infectivity for hepatitis A.
- The acute phase may be *icteric* (jaundice) or anicteric. Jaundice, a yellowish discoloration of body tissues, results from a change in bilirubin metabolism or disrupted flow of bile into the hepatic or biliary duct systems. The urine may darken because of excess bilirubin excreted by the kidneys. If conjugated bilirubin cannot flow out of the liver because of bile duct obstruction, stools will be clay-colored. Pruritus, caused by bile salts beneath the skin, may result from cholestasis.
- Convalescence following the acute phase begins as jaundice is disappearing and lasts an average of 2 to 4 months. During this period patients have malaise and fatigue.

In the *chronic phase,* patients may have intermittent or ongoing malaise, fatigue, myalgias, arthralgias, and hepatomegaly.

Complications
Most patients with acute viral hepatitis recover with no complications. The overall mortality rate for acute hepatitis is < 1%. Complications include acute liver failure, chronic hepatitis, cirrhosis of the liver (see Cirrhosis, p. 134), and hepatocellular carcinoma (see Liver Cancer, p. 379).

The disappearance of jaundice does not mean the patient has totally recovered. Some HBV infections and the majority of HCV infections result in chronic (lifelong) viral infection.

Diagnostic Studies
The only definitive way to distinguish among the various types of viral hepatitis is by testing the patient's blood for the specific antigen or antibody. Table 45 presents the serologic tests for the different types of viral hepatitis. Liver function tests show significant abnormalities. Physical assessment may reveal hepatic tenderness, hepatomegaly, and splenomegaly.

Interprofessional Management
There is no specific treatment for acute viral hepatitis. Most patients are managed at home. Emphasis is on providing adequate nutrition and measures to rest the body while the liver cells regenerate. The degree of rest ordered depends on symptom severity.

Drug Therapy
There are no specific drug therapies for the treatment of acute hepatitis A infection. Supportive drug therapy may include antiemetics

TABLE 45 Diagnostic Tests for Viral Hepatitis

Virus	Tests	Significance
A	Anti-HAV immunoglobulin M (IgM)	Acute infection
	Anti-HAV immunoglobulin G (IgG)	Previous infection or immunization
		Not routinely done in clinical practice
B	HBsAg (hepatitis B surface antigen)	Marker of infectivity
		Present in acute or chronic infection
		Positive in chronic carriers
	Anti-HBs (hepatitis B surface antibody)	Indicates previous infection with HBV or immunization
	HBeAg (hepatitis B e antigen)	Indicates high infectivity
		Used to determine the clinical management of patients with chronic hepatitis B
	Anti-HBe (hepatitis B e antibody)	Indicates previous infection
		In chronic hepatitis B, indicates a low viral load and low degree of infectivity
	Anti-HBc (antibody to hepatitis B core antigen) IgM	Indicates acute infection
		Does not appear after vaccination
	Anti-HBc IgG	Indicates previous infection or ongoing infection with hepatitis B
		Does not appear after vaccination
	HBV DNA quantitation	Indicates active ongoing viral replication
		Best indicator of viral replication and effectiveness of therapy in patient with chronic hepatitis B
	HBV genotyping	Indicates the genotype of HBV

H

Continued

TABLE 45	Diagnostic Tests for Viral Hepatitis—cont'd	
Virus	**Tests**	**Significance**
C	Anti-HCV (antibody to HCV)	Marker for acute or chronic infection with HCV
	HCV RNA quantitation	Indicates active ongoing viral replication
	HCV genotyping	Indicates the genotype of HCV
D	Anti-HDV	Present in past or current infection with HDV
	HDV Ag (hepatitis D antigen)	Present within a few days after infection
E	Anti-HEV IgM and IgG	Present 1 wk–2 mo after illness onset
	HEV RNA quantitation	Indicates active ongoing viral replication

A, Hepatitis A virus (HAV); *B,* hepatitis B virus (HBV); *C,* hepatitis C virus (HCV); *D,* hepatitis D virus (HDV); *DNA,* deoxyribonucleic acid; *E,* hepatitis E virus (HEV); *RNA,* ribonucleic acid.

for nausea, such as prochlorperazine, promethazine, or ondansetron (Zofran).

Treatment of acute hepatitis B is indicated in patients with severe hepatitis and liver failure. Drug therapy for chronic HBV infection is focused on decreasing the hepatitis B viral load and liver enzyme levels and on slowing the rate of disease progression.

- Nucleoside and nucleotide analogs suppress HBV replication by inhibiting viral DNA synthesis. Drugs such as lamivudine (Epivir), adefovir (Hepsera), entecavir (Baraclude), tenofovir (Viread), and telbivudine (Tyzeka) can reduce viral load and liver damage.

Treatment of chronic hepatitis C is based on the genotype of the HCV and the severity of liver disease. Drug therapy is directed at eradicating the virus through the use of direct-acting antivirals (DAAs) and preventing HCV-related complications.

Drug therapy is also used for prevention of HAV and HBV infection.

- Immune globulin (IG) provides temporary (1 to 2 months) passive immunity and is effective for preventing hepatitis A if given within 2 weeks after exposure. Although IG may not prevent infection in all people, it may modify the illness to a subclinical infection.

- IG is recommended for people who do not have anti-HAV anti-bodies and are exposed because of close contact with people who have HAV or foodborne exposure.
- A combined HAV and HBV vaccine available for people older than 18 years of age. The vaccine is given in a series of 3 IM injections in the deltoid muscle.
- For postexposure prophylaxis, the vaccine and hepatitis B IG (HBIG) are used. HBIG contains antibodies to HBV and confers temporary passive immunity. HBIG is recommended for postexposure prophylaxis in cases of needlestick, mucous membrane contact, or sexual exposure and for infants born to mothers who are seropositive for hepatitis B surface antigen (HBsAg).

Nutritional Therapy

No special diet is required in the treatment of viral hepatitis. Stress a well-balanced diet that the patient can tolerate. Vitamin supplements, particularly B-complex vitamins and vitamin K, are frequently used. If anorexia, nausea, and vomiting are severe, IV solutions of glucose or supplemental enteral nutrition therapy may be used.

Nursing Management

Goals

The patient with viral hepatitis will have relief of discomfort, be able to resume normal activities, and return to normal liver function without complications.

Nursing Interventions

A suggested guideline for general practice to prevent you from contracting viral hepatitis from diagnosed and undiagnosed patients and carriers is for you to wear disposable gloves, goggles, and gowns (sometimes) when fecal or blood contamination is likely in handling: (1) soiled bedpans, urinals, and catheters, and (2) when the patient's bed linens are soiled by body excreta or secretions.

During acute intervention, assess for the presence and degree of jaundice. Provide comfort measures to relieve pruritus, headache, and arthralgias.

- Ensuring that the patient receives adequate nutrition is not always easy. Small, frequent meals may be preferable to 3 large ones and may also help prevent nausea. Include measures to stimulate the appetite, such as mouth care, antiemetics, and attractively served meals in pleasant surroundings, in your plan of care.
- Assess the patient's response to rest and activity, and modify plans accordingly.
- Emotional rest is as essential as physical rest. Bed rest may produce anxiety and extreme restlessness in some patients. Diversional activities, such as reading and hobbies, may help.

Viral hepatitis is a community health problem. Your role is important in the prevention and control of this disease.

Hepatitis A. Vaccination is the best protection against HAV infection. Preventive measures include personal and environmental hygiene and health education to promote good sanitation. Hand washing is essential and is probably the most important precaution. Teach about careful hand washing after bowel movements and before eating.

Hepatitis B. The best way to reduce HBV infection is to identify those at risk, screen them for HBV, and vaccinate those who are not infected. Teach those at high risk to reduce risks. Good hygienic practices, including hand washing and using gloves when expecting contact with blood, are important.

- Close contacts and sexual partners of the patient with hepatitis B who are HBsAg-negative and antibody-negative should be vaccinated. A condom is advised for sexual intercourse. Razors, toothbrushes, and other personal items should not be shared.

Hepatitis C. There currently is no hepatitis C vaccine available. Primary measures to prevent HCV transmission include screening of blood, organ, and tissue donors; use of infection control measures; and modification of high-risk sexual behavior.

During acute intervention, assess for the degree of jaundice. Provide comfort measures to relieve pruritus, headache, and arthralgias.

- Small, frequent meals may be preferable to 3 large ones and may also help prevent nausea. Include measures to stimulate the appetite, such as mouth care, antiemetics, and attractively served meals in pleasant surroundings, in your plan of care.
- Assess the patient's response to rest and activity, and modify plans accordingly.
- Emotional rest is as essential as physical rest. Bed rest may produce anxiety and extreme restlessness. Diversional activities, such as reading and hobbies, may help.

▼ **Patient and Caregiver Teaching**

- Teach the patient and caregivers how to prevent transmission.
- Caution the patient about overexertion.
- Assess the patient for manifestations of complications such as bleeding or encephalopathy.
- Teach the patient to have regular follow-up for at least 1 year. Teach the patient the symptoms of recurrent hepatitis B and C and the need for follow-up evaluations. All patients with chronic HBV or HCV infection should avoid alcohol because it can accelerate disease progression.
- Teach the patient who is receiving drug therapy for the treatment of hepatitis B or C about the drug(s).

HERNIA

Description

A *hernia* is a protrusion of the viscus (e.g., the intestine) through an abnormal opening or a weakened area in the wall of the cavity in which it is normally contained. A hernia may occur in any part of the body, but it usually occurs within the abdominal cavity.

- Hernias that easily return to the abdominal cavity are called *reducible*. The hernia can be reduced manually or may reduce spontaneously when the person lies down.
- Irreducible, or incarcerated, hernias cannot be placed back into the abdominal cavity and have abdominal contents trapped in the opening. When the hernia is irreducible and intestinal flow and blood supply are obstructed, the hernia is *strangulated*. See Intestinal Obstruction, p. 351.

Types

Types of hernias include hiatal, inguinal, femoral, umbilical, and ventral (incisional). See Hiatal Hernia, p. 299.

- *Inguinal hernia* is the most common type of hernia and occurs at the point of weakness in the abdominal wall where the spermatic cord in men or the round ligament in women emerges. Inguinal hernia is more common in men.
- *Femoral hernia* occurs when there is a protrusion through the femoral ring into the femoral canal. It easily becomes strangulated and occurs more frequently in women.
- *Umbilical hernia* occurs when the rectus muscle is weak (as with obesity) or the umbilical opening fails to close after birth.
- *Ventral* or *incisional hernia* is caused by a weakness of the abdominal wall at the site of a previous incision or stoma. They occur often in those who are obese, who have had multiple surgical procedures in the area, or who have had inadequate wound healing because of poor nutrition or infection.

Clinical Manifestations and Diagnosis

A hernia is often readily visible, especially with abdominal muscle tension. Pain may worsen with activities that increase intraabdominal pressure, such as lifting, coughing, and straining.

- A strangulated hernia causes severe pain with symptoms of a bowel obstruction, such as vomiting, cramping abdominal pain, and distention.
- Strangulated hernias or painful, inflamed hernias that cannot be reduced require emergency surgery.

H

Diagnosis is based on history and physical examination findings. Ultrasound, CT, and MRI can assist in identifying a hernia and determining the contents.

Nursing and Interprofessional Management

The surgical repair of a hernia, known as a *herniorrhaphy,* is usually an outpatient procedure. Reinforcement of the weakened area with wire, fascia, or mesh is known as a *hernioplasty.* Strangulated hernias are treated immediately with resection of the involved area so that necrosis and gangrene do not occur, and in some cases with a temporary colostomy.

After a hernia repair, the patient may have difficulty voiding. Measure intake and output and observe for a distended bladder.

- Scrotal edema is a painful complication after an inguinal hernia repair. Elevation of the scrotum with a scrotal support and application of an ice bag may help relieve pain and edema.
- Encourage deep breathing, but not coughing. Teach patients to splint the incision and keep the mouth open when coughing or sneezing.
- The patient may be restricted from heavy lifting (>10 lb) for 6 to 8 weeks.

HERPES, GENITAL

Description

Genital herpes is a common, lifelong, incurable infection. Two strains of herpes cause genital infections: herpes simplex virus type 1 (HSV-1) and herpes simplex virus type 2 (HSV-2). Although both forms of HSV may cause genital infection, HSV-1 is usually associated with oral lesions and HSV-2 is more common in the genitals or anus. However, an increasing proportion of anogenital herpes infections are caused by HSV-1.

More than 50 million people in the United States have HSV-2. Most new infections are transmitted by those who are unaware they are infected.

Pathophysiology

The herpes simplex virus (HSV) enters through the mucous membranes or breaks in the skin during contact with an infected person. HSV reproduces inside the cell and spreads to surrounding cells. The virus next enters the peripheral or autonomic nerve endings and ascends to the sensory or autonomic nerve ganglion, where it often becomes dormant. Viral reactivation (recurrence or outbreak) occurs when the virus travels down to the initial site of infection.

The virus usually persists within a person for life. Transmission occurs through direct contact with skin or mucous membranes when an infected person is symptomatic or through asymptomatic viral shedding.

Both HSV-1 and HSV-2 can cause either genital or orolabial infections.

- HSV-1 infections are more common "above the waist," involving the gingivae, dermis, upper respiratory tract, and, rarely the CNS. HSV-2 almost always infects sites "below the waist"—the genital tract, perineum, or anus.

Clinical Manifestations

A *primary (initial) episode* of genital herpes has an incubation of 2 to 12 days. Most people do not have any recognizable symptoms of primary HSV genital infection. If symptoms do occur, they follow a series of stages. During the *prodromal* stage, the period before lesions appear, the patient may have burning, itching, or tingling at the site of inoculation. In the *vesicular* stage, a few to multiple small, often painful vesicles (blisters) may appear on the buttock, inner thigh, penis, scrotum, vulva, perineum, perianal region, vagina, or cervix. The vesicles contain large quantities of infectious viral particles. Urination may be painful from urine touching active lesions. Next, in the *ulcerative* stage, the lesions rupture and form shallow, moist ulcerations. Finally, crusting and epithelialization of the erosions occur.

- Local inflammation and pain, regional (inguinal node) lymphadenopathy, and systemic flu-like symptoms including fever, headache, malaise, and myalgia may occur with the primary episode.

Recurrent genital herpes occurs in many persons during the year after the primary episode. The symptoms of recurrent episodes are less severe, and the lesions usually heal more quickly. HSV-1 genital infections recur less often than HSV-2 genital infections. Over time, both are less frequent.

- Common triggers of recurrence include stress, fatigue, sunburn, general illness, immunosuppression, and menses. Many patients can predict a recurrence by noticing early prodromal symptoms of tingling, burning, and itching at the site where lesions will eventually appear. Symptoms of recurrent episodes are less severe, and the lesions usually heal within 8 to 12 days. With time, the recurrent lesions will generally occur less often.
- The greatest risk for transmitting infection exists when active lesions are present. However, it is possible to transmit the virus

H

when no visible lesions or symptoms are present. HSV transmission occurs most often during asymptomatic periods.

Complications

- HSV-1 and HSV-2 can cause rare but serious complications such as blindness, encephalitis, and aseptic meningitis.
- Autoinoculation can result in the development of lesions in the buttocks, groin, thighs, fingers, and eyes. Genital ulcers form HSV increase the risk of contracting human immunodeficiency virus (HIV).
- Pregnant women with HSV can transmit the virus to the baby if the virus is shed while the infant passes though the birth canal. Women with a primary episode of HSV near the time of delivery have the highest risk of transmitting genital herpes to the neonate. An active genital lesion at the time of delivery is an indication for cesarean delivery.

Diagnostic Studies

- Diagnosis is usually based on the patient's symptoms and history, then confirmed by visual examination.
- Highly accurate blood tests for antibodies are available for HSV-1 and HSV-2, but do not show the location of the infection. These antibodies usually appear by 12 weeks after exposure.
- A viral culture of the active lesion can be used to isolate the virus and distinguish between HSV-1 and HSV-2.

Interprofessional and Nursing Management

Three antiviral agents are available for the treatment of HSV: acyclovir (Zovirax), famciclovir (Famvir), and valaciclovir (Valtrex). These drugs inhibit herpetic viral replication. They are prescribed for both primary and recurrent infections. Taken daily at a lower dose, they can be used as suppressive therapy to decrease frequent anogenital recurrences. IV acyclovir is reserved for severe or life-threatening infections.

The main goal is to keep eruptions clean and dry. Teach patients with active outbreaks to maintain good genital hygiene and wear loose-fitting cotton undergarments.

- Techniques to reduce pain with urination include pouring water onto the perineal area while voiding to dilute the urine or voiding in the shower. Pain may require a local anesthetic such as lidocaine gel or analgesics such as ibuprofen, acetaminophen, acetaminophen with codeine, or aspirin.
- Ice packs to the affected area can provide some relief.
- See Sexually Transmitted Infections, p. 545.

HIATAL HERNIA

Description

Hiatal hernia is herniation of a part of the stomach into the esophagus through an opening, or hiatus, in the diaphragm. It is also referred to as "diaphragmatic hernia" or "esophageal hernia." Hiatal hernias are common among older adults and occur more frequently in women than in men. Hiatal hernias are classified into 2 types (Fig. 11).

- A *sliding hernia* is the most common type. The junction of the stomach and esophagus is above the diaphragm, and a part of the stomach slides through the hiatal opening in the diaphragm. This occurs when the patient is supine, and it usually goes back into the abdominal cavity when the patient is standing upright.
- A *paraesophageal* or *rolling hernia.* The fundus and greater curvature of the stomach roll up through the diaphragm, forming a pocket alongside the esophagus. The esophagogastric junction stays in the normal position. Acute paraesophageal hernia is a medical emergency.

Pathophysiology

Many factors contribute to the development of hiatal hernia. Structural changes, such as weakening of the muscles in the diaphragm around the esophagogastric opening, occur with aging. Factors that increase intraabdominal pressure including obesity, pregnancy, ascites, tumors, intense physical exertion, and frequent heavy lifting predispose patients to development of a hiatal hernia.

Clinical Manifestations

Signs and symptoms of hiatal hernia are similar to those described for gastroesophageal reflux disease (GERD). Some people are asymptomatic.

H

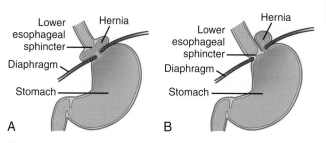

Fig. 11 (A) Sliding hiatal hernia. (B) Rolling or paraesophageal hernia.

- Heartburn is common, especially after a meal or after lying supine. Bending over, large meals, alcohol, and smoking may precipitate pain.
- Nocturnal attacks are common, especially if the person has eaten before lying down.

Complications may include GERD, esophagitis, hemorrhage from erosion, stenosis, ulcerations of the herniated part of the stomach, strangulation of the hernia, and regurgitation with tracheal aspiration.

Diagnostic Studies
- Barium swallow (esophagram) may show gastric mucosa protrusion through the esophageal hiatus. See also tests done for GERD, p. 235.

Nursing and Interprofessional Management
Conservative therapy for hiatal hernia is similar to that for GERD (p. 235). Teach the patient to reduce intraabdominal pressure by eliminating constricting garments and avoiding lifting and straining.

Surgical approaches to hiatal hernias can include reduction of the herniated stomach into the abdomen, *herniotomy* (excision of the hernia sac), *herniorrhaphy* (closure of the hiatal defect), fundoplication, and *gastropexy* (attachment of the stomach below the diaphragm to prevent reherniation).

- Surgery to repair hiatal hernia is often done laparoscopically by Nissen or Toupet techniques.

HODGKIN'S LYMPHOMA

Description
Hodgkin's lymphoma, also called *Hodgkin's disease*, is a cancerous condition characterized by proliferation of abnormal, giant, multinucleated cells called *Reed-Sternberg cells* in the lymph nodes. The disease accounts for 10% of all lymphomas, occurring most often in people 15 to 30 years of age and in those older than 55 years. Long-term survival exceeds 80% for all stages.

Pathophysiology
Several key factors are thought to play a role in the development of Hodgkin's lymphoma. The main interacting factors include infection with the Epstein-Barr virus, genetic predisposition, and exposure to occupational toxins. The incidence is increased in patients who have human immunodeficiency virus (HIV) infection.

The disease is believed to start at a single location (it starts in the cervical lymph nodes in 60%–70% of patients) and then spreads along adjacent lymphatics. It eventually infiltrates the lungs, spleen, and liver.

Clinical Manifestations

The initial sign is most often enlarged cervical, axillary, or inguinal lymph nodes. The enlarged nodes are not painful unless pressure is exerted on adjacent nerves.

- The patient may note weight loss, fatigue, weakness, fever, chills, tachycardia, or night sweats. A group of initial findings, including fever, night sweats, and weight loss (referred to as "B symptoms"), correlate with a worse prognosis.
- Generalized pruritus without skin lesions may develop. Cough, dyspnea, stridor, and dysphagia may all reflect mediastinal node involvement.
- In more advanced disease, there may be hepatomegaly and splenomegaly. Anemia results from increased destruction and decreased production of erythrocytes. Intrathoracic involvement may lead to superior vena cava syndrome. Enlarged retroperitoneal nodes may cause palpable abdominal masses or interfere with renal function.
- Jaundice may result from liver involvement.
- Spinal cord compression leading to paraplegia may occur with extradural involvement.
- Bone involvement may cause bone pain.

Diagnostic Studies

Peripheral blood analysis, excisional lymph node biopsy, bone marrow examination, and radiologic studies are important means of evaluating Hodgkin's lymphoma.

- Microcytic hypochromic anemia, leukopenia, and thrombocytopenia may develop, usually as a consequence of treatment, advanced disease, or hypersplenism (related to the disease process).
- Other blood studies may show increased erythrocyte sedimentation rate, high alkaline phosphatase from liver and bone involvement, hypercalcemia from bone involvement, and hypoalbuminemia from liver involvement.
- Positron emission tomography (PET) scans with or without CT scan are used to stage and then assess response to therapy. The scans may show increased uptake of carbohydrate by cancer cells (by PET) and masses (by CT), such as renal displacement caused

H

by retroperitoneal node enlargement; abdominal or mediastinal lymph node enlargement; and infiltration of the liver, spleen, bone, or brain.

Interprofessional Management

Treatment decisions are made based on the clinical stage of the disease. The standard for chemotherapy is the ABVD regimen: doxorubicin (formerly marketed as Adriamycin), bleomycin, vinblastine, and dacarbazine, given for 2 to 8 cycles of treatment, depending on disease stage and prognosis.

Combination chemotherapy works well because the drugs have an additive antitumor effect without increasing side effects. As with leukemia, therapy must be aggressive. Therefore potentially life-threatening problems are encountered in an attempt to achieve a remission.

A variety of chemotherapy regimens and newer agents, such as brentuximab vedotin, nivolumab, bendamustine, and pembrolizumab, are used to treat patients who have relapsed or refractory disease. Once remission is obtained, a treatment option with the goal of cure may be intensive chemotherapy with the use of autologous or allogeneic hematopoietic stem cell transplantation.

The role of radiation as a supplement to chemotherapy varies depending on site of disease and the presence of resistant disease after chemotherapy.

Nursing Management

Nursing care for patients with Hodgkin's lymphoma is primarily based on managing problems related to the disease, such as pain; and side effects of therapy, such as pancytopenia.

- Because the survival of patients with Hodgkin's lymphoma depends on their response to treatment, support the patient through the consequences of treatment.
- Psychosocial, social, and spiritual considerations are as important as they are with leukemia (see Leukemia, p. 373). However, the prognosis with Hodgkin's lymphoma is better than that with many forms of cancer or leukemia.
- Delayed consequences of the disease and treatment, such as secondary cancers and long-term endocrine, cardiac, and pulmonary toxicities, may not be apparent for many years. The most common secondary cancers are lung and breast cancer. Encourage close follow-up and screening for early detection.

HUMAN IMMUNODEFICIENCY VIRUS INFECTION

Description

Human immunodeficiency virus (HIV) is a retrovirus that causes immunosuppression. Persons with HIV infection are more susceptible to other infections normally controlled through immune responses. With advances in treatment, we view HIV as a chronic disease. The terms *HIV disease* and *HIV infection* are used interchangeably.

Pathophysiology

HIV is a ribonucleic acid (RNA) virus. Like all viruses, HIV cannot replicate unless it is in a living cell. HIV infects human cells that have CD4$^+$ receptors on their surfaces. These include lymphocytes, monocytes/macrophages, astrocytes, and oligodendrocytes. Immune dysfunction in HIV disease is caused predominantly by destruction of *CD4$^+$ cells (CD4 cell),* a type of lymphocyte.

HIV destroys about 1 billion CD4$^+$ cells each day. For many years, the body can produce new CD4$^+$ cells to replace the destroyed cells. Over time, the ability of HIV to destroy CD4$^+$ cells exceeds the body's ability to replace the cells. The decline in the CD4$^+$ cell count impairs immune function. Immune problems begin to occur when the count drops below 500 CD4$^+$ cells/μL. Severe problems develop with fewer than 200 CD4$^+$ cells/μL.

With HIV, eventually so many CD4$^+$ cells have been destroyed that not enough are left to regulate immune responses. This allows opportunistic diseases (infections and cancers that occur in immunosuppressed patients) to develop. Opportunistic diseases are the main cause of disease, disability, and death in patients with HIV infection.

In North America, HIV is most prevalent among men who have sex with men (MSM). HIV can be transmitted through contact with infected blood, semen, vaginal secretions, or breast milk. HIV transmission occurs through sexual intercourse with an infected partner; exposure to HIV-infected blood or blood products; and perinatal transmission during pregnancy, at delivery, or through breastfeeding. HIV is not spread through casual contact.

Clinical Manifestations

The typical course of untreated HIV infection follows the pattern shown in Fig. 12. Disease progression is highly individualized, however, and treatment can alter the pattern. HIV infections have acute and chronic stages.

H

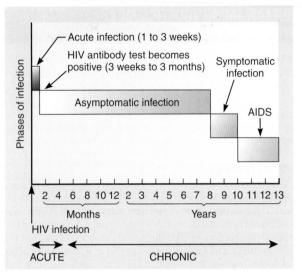

Fig. 12 Timeline for the spectrum of untreated HIV infection. The timeline represents the course of untreated illness from the time of infection to clinical manifestations of disease. *AIDS,* Acquired immunodeficiency syndrome; *HIV,* human immunodeficiency virus.

Acute Infection

During acute HIV infection, HIV-specific antibodies are produced (seroconversion) with a mononucleosis-like syndrome of fever, lymphadenopathy, pharyngitis, headache, malaise, nausea, and/or a diffuse rash.

- Symptoms begin 2 to 4 weeks after initial infection and last for 1 to 3 weeks.
- During this time, a high viral load is noted and $CD4^+$ cell counts fall temporarily but quickly return to baseline. Many people, including health care providers (HCPs), mistake acute HIV symptoms for a bad case of the flu. People are most infectious during the acute infection stage because of the high amounts of circulating HIV.

Chronic Infection

There are 3 stages of chronic infection: asymptomatic infection, symptomatic infection, and acquired immunodeficiency syndrome (AIDS). The interval between untreated HIV infection and a diagnosis of AIDS is about 10 years.

- *Asymptomatic infection*—CD4$^+$ lymphocyte counts remain above 500 cells/μL (normal or slightly decreased) and the viral load in the blood is low. The person has no symptoms or relatively limited signs of infection, so the risk of unknown transmission to others is high.
- *Symptomatic infection* occurs as the CD4$^+$ cell count drops to 200 cells/μL and the viral load increases. Symptoms such as persistent fever, frequent night sweats, chronic diarrhea, recurrent headaches, and severe fatigue may develop.
- *AIDS* is characterized by severe immune system suppression and CD4$^+$ cell counts below 200 cells/μL. A diagnosis of AIDS is made when an HIV-infected patient meets criteria established by the Centers for Disease Control and Prevention (CDC), which include the development of at least 1 of these conditions:
  1. CD4$^+$ lymphocyte count < 200/μL
  2. Development of opportunistic infection (see Table 14.11, Harding et al., *Lewis' Medical-Surgical Nursing,* ed 11)
  3. Development of opportunistic cancer (e.g., Kaposi sarcoma)
  4. *Wasting syndrome* (defined as a loss of 10% or more of ideal body mass)

Diagnostic Studies
Screening
The most useful screening tests detect HIV-specific antibodies. There is a delay of several weeks after infection before antibodies can be detected in blood or saliva.
Progression of Human Immunodeficiency Virus Infection
- CD4$^+$ cell count and viral load monitor progression of infection.
- White blood cell (WBC) count, red blood cell count (RBC) count, and platelets decrease with progression of HIV.

Interprofessional Management
Care focuses on: (1) monitoring HIV disease progression and immune function, (2) initiating and monitoring antiretroviral therapy (ART), (3) preventing the development of opportunistic diseases, (4) detecting and treating opportunistic diseases, (5) managing symptoms, (6) preventing or decreasing complications of treatment, and (7) preventing further transmission of HIV.
Drug Therapy
Combining drugs from different classes can inhibit viral replication in several ways, making it difficult for the virus to recover and decreasing drug resistance.
- Resistance tests can determine if a patient's HIV is resistant to drugs. Genotype and phenotype assays help HCPs know which medications can best control a patient's infection.

- Resistance develops rapidly when ART drugs are used alone or in low doses. The most effective means to suppress HIV replication is using at least 3 ART drugs from different drug classes in optimum schedules and at full dosages (Table 46).
- Many ART agents cause potentially lethal interactions with other commonly used drugs.

Opportunistic diseases associated with HIV infection can be delayed or prevented with adequate ART, vaccines (including hepatitis B, influenza, and pneumococcal), and disease-specific prevention measures.

Nursing Management

Goals

Nursing interventions can the patient with HIV (1) adhere to drug regimens; (2) adopt a healthy lifestyle that includes avoiding exposure to other sexually transmitted infections and blood-borne diseases; (3) protect others from HIV; (4) maintain or develop healthy and supportive relationships; (5) maintain activities and productivity; (6) explore spiritual issues, 7) come to terms with issues related to disease, disability, and death; and (8) cope with symptoms caused by HIV and its treatments.

Nursing Interventions

The complexity of HIV disease is related to its chronic nature. Primary prevention and health promotion are the most effective health care strategies. See Table 14.16 in Harding et al., *Lewis' Medical-Surgical Nursing,* ed 11 for a summary of interventions and strategies throughout the course of HIV infection.

HIV infection is preventable. Avoiding or modifying risky behaviors are the most effective prevention tools. Provide culturally sensitive, language-appropriate, and age-specific teaching and counseling.

Early intervention after detection of HIV infection can promote health and limit disability. Focus on early detection of symptoms, opportunistic diseases, and psychosocial problems.

Interventions for patients with HIV infection include nutritional support; moderation or elimination of alcohol, tobacco, and drug use; keeping recommended vaccines up to date; adequate rest, exercise, and stress reduction; avoiding exposure to new infectious agents; mental health counseling; and attending support groups and community activities.

- Teach patients to recognize symptoms that may indicate disease progression and/or drug side effects and seek prompt medical care.
- Symptomatic care includes teaching and treatment for diarrhea, pneumonia, fatigue, and wasting syndrome.

TABLE 46 Drug Therapy

Human Immunodeficiency Virus (HIV) Infection

Drug Classification	Mechanism of Action	Drug Names
Attachment Inhibitor	Interrupts the ability of HIV to attach to the CD4 cell.	ibalizumab-uiyk (Trogarzo)
Entry Inhibitors	Prevent binding of HIV to cells, thus preventing entry of HIV into cells where replication would occur	enfuvirtide (Fuzeon) maraviroc (Selzentry)
Integrase Inhibitors	Bind with integrase enzyme and prevent HIV from incorporating its genetic material into the host cell	bictegravir[a] elvitegravir[a] dolutegravir (Tivicay) raltegravir (Isentress)
Reverse Transcriptase Inhibitors		
Nucleoside Reverse Transcriptase Inhibitors (NRTIs)	Insert a piece of DNA into the developing HIV DNA chain, blocking further development of the chain and leaving the production of the new strand of HIV DNA incomplete	abacavir (Ziagen) didanosine (Videx, Videx-EC [time-released]) emtricitabine (Emtriva) lamivudine (Epivir) stavudine (Zerit) zidovudine (Retrovir)
Nonnucleoside Reverse Transcriptase Inhibitors (NNRTIs)	Inhibit the action of reverse transcriptase	efavirenz (Sustiva) etravirine (Intelence) delavirdine (Rescriptor) nevirapine (Viramune XR) rilpivirine (Edurant)

Continued

H

TABLE 46 Drug Therapy

Human Immunodeficiency Virus (HIV) Infection—cont'd

Drug Classification	Mechanism of Action	Drug Names
Nucleotide Reverse Transcriptase Inhibitor (NtRTI)	Combines with reverse transcriptase enzyme to block the process needed to convert HIV RNA into HIV DNA	tenofovir (Viread)
Protease Inhibitors (PIs)	Prevent the protease enzyme from cutting HIV proteins into the proper lengths needed to allow viable virions to assemble and bud out from the cell membrane	atazanavir (Reyataz) darunavir (Prezista) fosamprenavir (Lexiva) indinavir (Crixivan) lopinavir + ritonavir (Kaletra) nelfinavir (Viracept) ritonavir (Norvir)[b] saquinavir (Fortovase, Invirase) tipranavir (Aptivus)

[a]Elvitegravir and bictegravir are integrase inhibitors that are only available in fixed-dose combinations with tenofovir AF and emtricitabine.
[b]Most often used in low doses with other PIs to boost effect.
DNA, Deoxyribonucleic acid; *RNA,* ribonucleic acid.

- The focus of end-of-life care is on patient comfort, facilitating emotional and spiritual issues, and helping significant others deal with grief and loss.

▼ **Patient and Caregiver Teaching**

Emphasize prevention and risk reduction. Teach the proper use and placement of male and female condoms and recommend decreasing the number of sex partners. Refer patients to support services for substance use reduction and access to sterile drug equipment.

For an infected patient, teaching is directed toward health promotion, managing the problems caused by HIV infection, and maximizing quality of life.

- Teach about new treatments, including drug therapy, dangers of nonadherence to therapy, how to take each medication, drug interactions to avoid, and side effects that need to be reported to the HCP. Tables 14.17–14.19, Harding et al., *Lewis' Medical-Surgical Nursing,* ed 11, provide guidance for patient teaching.
- Teach patients to conserve energy and maintain safety using assistive devices (e.g., shower chair).
- Discuss infection control measures with the patient, caregivers, family, and visitors.
- Provide information about support groups and community resources.

HUNTINGTON'S DISEASE

Description

Huntington's disease (HD) is a progressive, degenerative brain disorder. It is a genetically transmitted, autosomal dominant disorder. The onset of HD is usually between ages 30 and 50 years. Diagnosis is often made after the affected person has had children. The offspring of a person with HD have a 50% risk of inheriting it.

H

Pathophysiology

As in Parkinson's disease, the pathologic process in HD involves the basal ganglia and extrapyramidal motor system. However, instead of a deficiency of dopamine (DA), HD involves a deficiency of the neurotransmitters acetylcholine (ACh) and γ-aminobutyric acid (GABA). The net effect is an excess of DA, leading to symptoms that are the opposite of those of parkinsonism.

Clinical Manifestations

Manifestations include a movement disorder and cognitive and psychiatric problems. The movement disorder is marked by abnormal and excessive involuntary movements (chorea). These are writhing, twisting movements of the face, limbs, and body. The movements get worse as the disease progresses. Because facial movements involving speech, chewing, and swallowing are affected, aspiration and malnutrition are likely. The gait deteriorates, and ambulation eventually becomes impossible. Eventually all psychomotor processes, including the ability to eat and talk, are impaired.

- Psychiatric symptoms are often present in the early stage of HD, even before the onset of motor symptoms. Depression is common. Other psychiatric symptoms include anxiety, agitation, impulsivity, apathy, social withdrawal, and obsessiveness.
- Cognitive deterioration is more variable. It involves perception, memory, attention, and learning.

Death usually occurs 10 to 30 years after the onset of symptoms. The most common cause of death is pneumonia, followed by suicide. Other causes of death include injuries related to falls and other complications.

Diagnosis

The diagnostic process begins with a review of family history and clinical symptoms. Genetic testing confirms the presence of the disease in a person with symptoms.

People who are asymptomatic but who have a family history must decide if they want genetic testing. If the test result is positive, the person will develop HD, but when and to what extent the disease will develop cannot be determined.

Nursing and Interprofessional Management

Because HD has no cure, interprofessional care is palliative. Drugs are available to control movements and behavioral problems.

- Tetrabenazine (Xenazine) is used to treat chorea. It decreases the amount of DA available at synapses in the brain and thus reducing the involuntary movements of chorea. Deutetrabenzine (Austedo) is related to tetrabenazine. It is also approved for the treatment of chorea.
- Other medications used for the movement disorder include neuroleptics (e.g., haloperidol, risperidone), benzodiazepines, and DA-depleting agents, such as reserpine.
- Cognitive disorders are treated as needed with nondrug therapies (e.g., counseling, memory books). Psychiatric disorders can be treated with selective serotonin reuptake inhibitors, such as sertraline (Zoloft) and paroxetine (Paxil). Antipsychotic medication, such as haloperidol or risperidone, may be needed.

The goal of nursing management is to provide the most comfortable environment possible for the patient and caregiver by maintaining physical safety, treating physical symptoms, and providing emotional and psychologic support.

- Because of the choreic movements, caloric requirements may be as high as 4000 to 5000 cal/day to maintain body weight. As HD progresses, meeting caloric needs becomes a greater challenge when the patient has difficulty swallowing and holding the head still. Depression and mental deterioration can also compromise nutritional intake. Enteral or parenteral nutrition may be indicated as the disease progresses.
- End-of-life issues need to be discussed with the patient and caregiver. These include care in the home or long-term care facility, artificial methods of feeding, advance directives and cardiopulmonary resuscitation (CPR), use of antibiotics to treat infections, and guardianship.

HYPERPARATHYROIDISM

Description

Hyperparathyroidism is a condition involving increased secretion of parathyroid hormone (PTH). PTH helps regulate serum calcium and phosphate levels by stimulating bone resorption, renal tubular reabsorption of calcium, and activation of vitamin D. Oversecretion of PTH is associated with increased serum calcium levels. Hyperparathyroidism is more common in women than in men.

Hyperparathyroidism is classified as primary, secondary, or tertiary.

- *Primary hyperparathyroidism* is caused by increased secretion of PTH leading to disorders of calcium, phosphate, and bone metabolism. The most common cause is a benign tumor (adenoma) in the parathyroid gland. Previous head and neck irradiation may be a risk factor for a parathyroid adenoma.
- *Secondary hyperparathyroidism* is a compensatory response to conditions that induce or cause hypocalcemia, the main stimulus of PTH secretion. These include vitamin D deficiencies, malabsorption, chronic kidney disease, and hyperphosphatemia.
- *Tertiary hyperparathyroidism* occurs when hyperplasia of the parathyroid glands occurs in combination with loss of negative feedback from circulating calcium levels. This causes autonomous secretion of PTH even with normal calcium levels. It is observed in the patient who has had a kidney transplant after a long period of dialysis treatment for chronic kidney disease.

H

Pathophysiology

Excessive levels of circulating PTH usually lead to hypercalcemia and hypophosphatemia, with multiple body systems affected.

- Decreased bone density can occur as a result of the effect of PTH on osteoclastic (bone resorption) and osteoblastic (bone formation) activity.
- In the kidneys, excess calcium cannot be reabsorbed, which leads to hypercalciuria. The excess urinary calcium, along with a large amount of urinary phosphate, can lead to formation of calculi.

Clinical Manifestations

Manifestations are associated with hypercalcemia and range from no symptoms to overt symptoms. Loss of appetite, constipation, fatigue, emotional disorders, shortened attention span, and muscle weakness, particularly in the proximal muscles of the lower extremities, are often noted.

Complications include osteoporosis, renal failure, kidney stones, pancreatitis, cardiac changes, and long bone, rib, and vertebral fractures.

Diagnostic Studies

- PTH levels are increased.
- Serum calcium levels are increased with decreased phosphorus levels.
- Urine calcium, serum chloride, serum uric acid, and serum creatinine are increased.
- Serum amylase (if pancreatitis is present) and alkaline phosphatase (if bone disease is present) are both increased.
- Bone density tests can detect bone loss.
- MRI, CT scan, and ultrasound can be used to localize adenoma.

Interprofessional Management

Treatment objectives are to relieve the symptoms and prevent complications caused by excess PTH. The choice of therapy depends on the urgency of the clinical situation, degree of hypercalcemia, and underlying cause of the disorder.

- The most effective treatment of primary and secondary hyperparathyroidism is partial or complete surgical removal of the parathyroid glands. The procedure most often used involves outpatient endoscopy.
- Severe hypercalcemia is managed with IV sodium chloride solution and loop diuretics, such as furosemide, to increase the urinary excretion of calcium.

A conservative management approach is used in patients who are asymptomatic or have mild symptoms of hyperparathyroidism. This includes an annual examination with tests for serum PTH, calcium, phosphorus, and alkaline phosphatase levels and renal function; x-rays to assess for metabolic bone disease; and measurement of urinary calcium excretion. Dietary measures include high fluid and moderate calcium intake.

- X-rays and dual-energy x-ray absorptiometry (DXA) assess for metabolic bone loss.
- Bisphosphonates (e.g., alendronate [Fosamax]) inhibit osteo-clastic bone resorption and improve bone mineral density. Phosphates are given if the patient has normal renal function and low serum phosphate levels.
- Calcimimetic agents (e.g., cinacalcet [Sensipar]) increase the sensitivity of the calcium receptor on the parathyroid gland, resulting in decreased PTH secretion and calcium blood levels.

Nursing Management

Nursing care after surgery is similar to that for the patient after thyroidectomy (see Hyperthyroidism, p. 321). The major postoperative complications are hemorrhage and fluid and electrolyte problems. Tetany is usually apparent early in the postoperative period or may develop over several days. Mild tetany, characterized by an unpleasant tingling of the hands and around the mouth, may be present but should resolve without problems. IV calcium should be readily available for use if tetany becomes severe (e.g., muscular spasms or laryngospasms).

- Assess calcium, potassium, phosphate, and magnesium levels frequently.
- Monitor intake and output to evaluate fluid status.
- Encourage mobility to promote bone calcification.

▼ **Patient and Caregiver Teaching**

- Assist the patient to adapt the meal plan to their lifestyle. A referral to a dietitian may be useful.
- Because immobility can worsen bone loss, stress the importance of an exercise program.
- Teach the patient the symptoms of hypocalcemia or hypercalcemia and to contact the health care provider (HCP) if they occur.

H

HYPERTENSION

Description

About 46% of adults in the United States meet criteria for the general diagnosis of *hypertension*, or high BP. Hypertension is 1 of the most important modifiable risk factors that can lead to the development of cardiovascular disease (CVD). As BP increases, so does the risk of myocardial infarction (MI), heart failure (HF), stroke, and renal disease.

Normal blood pressure is defined as a systolic BP (SBP) < 120 mm Hg and a diastolic BP (DBP) < 80 mm Hg.

Elevated blood pressure is defined as an SBP between 120–129 mm Hg and a DBP < 80 mm Hg.

Hypertension (Stage 1) is defined as an SBP between 130–139 mm Hg and a DBP between 80–89 mm Hg.

Hypertension (Stage 2) is defined as an SBP > 140 mm Hg and a DBP > 90 mm Hg.

Classification of hypertension for adults according to stages is described in Table 47.

- The classification is based on the average of 2 or more properly measured BP readings on 2 or more office visits.

Hypertension can be classified as primary (essential or idiopathic) or secondary. *Primary hypertension* accounts for 90% to 95% of all cases of hypertension. Although the exact cause of primary hypertension is unknown, there are several contributing factors. These include changes in endothelial function related to vasoconstricting or vasodilating agents, increased sympathetic nervous system (SNS) activity, overproduction of sodium-retaining hormones, increased sodium intake, greater-than-ideal body weight, diabetes, tobacco use, and excess alcohol intake.

Secondary hypertension is elevated BP with a specific cause that can often be identified and corrected. This type of hypertension accounts for 5% to 10% of hypertension in adults. Causes of secondary hypertension include coarctation or congenital narrowing of the aorta, renal artery stenosis, endocrine disorders such as Cushing syndrome, cirrhosis, neurologic disorders such as brain tumors and head injury, sleep apnea, and pregnancy-induced hypertension.

TABLE 47	Classification of Hypertension		
Category	SBP (mm Hg)		DBP (mm Hg)
Normal	<120	and	<80
Elevated	120–129	and	<80
Hypertension, stage 1	130–139	or	80–89
Hypertension, stage 2	≥140	or	≥90

DBP, Diastolic blood pressure; *SBP,* systolic blood pressure.

Whelton PK, Carey RM, Aronow WS, et al. ACC/AHA/AAPA/ABC/ACPM/AGS/APhA/ASH/ASPC/NMA/PCNA Guideline for the Prevention, Detection, Evaluation, and Management of High Blood Pressure in Adults: A Report of the American College of Cardiology/AHA Task Force on Clinical Practice Guidelines. *Hypertension,* 2017.

Treatment of secondary hypertension is directed at removing or treating the underlying cause.

Pathophysiology of Primary Hypertension

The hemodynamic hallmark of hypertension is persistently increased systemic vascular resistance (SVR). Table 48 shows factors that relate to the development of primary hypertension or contribute to its consequences.

TABLE 48	Risk Factors for Primary Hypertension
Risk Factor	**Description**
Age	• SBP rises progressively with age, while DBP may decrease with age • After age 50 years, SBP >140 mm Hg is a more important cardiovascular risk factor than DBP
Alcohol	• Excess alcohol intake is strongly associated with hypertension • Moderate intake of alcohol has cardioprotective properties; males with hypertension should limit their daily intake of alcohol to 2 drinks per day, and 1 drink per day for females with hypertension
Diabetes	• Hypertension is more common in patients with diabetes • When hypertension and diabetes coexist, complications (e.g., target organ disease) are more severe
Elevated serum lipids	• ↑ Levels of cholesterol and triglycerides are primary risk factors for atherosclerosis • Hyperlipidemia is more common in people with hypertension
Ethnicity	• The incidence of hypertension is 2 times higher in blacks than in whites
Excess dietary sodium	• High sodium intake can • Contribute to hypertension in salt-sensitive patients • Decrease the effectiveness of certain antihypertensive drugs
Family history	• History of a close blood relative (e.g., parents, sibling) with hypertension is associated with a ↑ risk of developing hypertension

H

Continued

TABLE 48 Risk Factors for Primary Hypertension—cont'd	
Risk Factor	**Description**
Gender	• Hypertension is more prevalent in men in young adulthood and early middle age • After age 64 years, hypertension is more prevalent in women
Obesity	• Weight gain is associated with ↑ frequency of hypertension • Risk increases with central abdominal obesity
Sedentary lifestyle	• Regular physical activity can help control weight and reduce cardiovascular risk • Physical activity may ↓ BP
Socioeconomic status	• Hypertension is more prevalent in lower socioeconomic groups and among the less educated
Stress	• People exposed to repeated stress may develop hypertension more often than others • People who develop hypertension may respond differently to stress than those who do not develop hypertension
Tobacco use	• Smoking tobacco greatly ↑ risk of cardiovascular disease • People with hypertension who smoke tobacco are at even greater risk for cardiovascular disease

DBP, Diastolic blood pressure; *SBP,* systolic blood pressure.

Clinical Manifestations

Hypertension is called the "silent killer" because it is often asymptomatic until it becomes severe and target organ disease has occurred. A patient with severe hypertension may have a variety of symptoms secondary to effects on blood vessels in the various organs and tissues or to the increased workload of the heart. These secondary symptoms include fatigue, reduced activity tolerance, dizziness, palpitations, angina, and dyspnea.

The most common complications of hypertension are target organ diseases occurring in the heart (hypertensive heart disease), brain (cerebrovascular disease), peripheral vasculature (peripheral vascular disease), kidney (nephrosclerosis), and eyes (retinal damage).

Hypertensive Heart Disease

Hypertension is a major risk factor for coronary artery disease (CAD). The "response-to-injury" theory of atherogenesis suggests that hypertension disrupts the coronary artery endothelium. This results in a stiff arterial wall with a narrowed lumen and accounts for a high rate of CAD, angina, and MI. Sustained high BP also increases the cardiac workload and produces left ventricular hypertrophy (LVH). Progressive LVH, especially in association with CAD, is associated with the development of HF.

Heart failure occurs when the heart's compensatory adaptations are overwhelmed and the heart can no longer pump enough blood to meet the body's demands.

- The patient may have shortness of breath on exertion, paroxysmal nocturnal dyspnea, and fatigue.

Cerebrovascular Disease

Atherosclerosis is the most common cause of cerebrovascular disease. Atherosclerotic plaques are often located at the bifurcation of the common carotid artery. Portions of the atherosclerotic plaque, or the blood clot that forms on the plaque, may break off and travel to intracerebral vessels, producing a thromboembolism. The patient may have transient ischemic attacks or a stroke. Adequate BP control decreases the risk of stroke.

Peripheral Vascular Disease

Hypertension speeds up the process of atherosclerosis in peripheral blood vessels. This leads to aortic aneurysm, aortic dissection, and peripheral vascular disease (PVD). *Intermittent claudication* (ischemic muscle pain precipitated by activity and relieved with rest) is a classic symptom of PVD.

Nephrosclerosis

Hypertension is 1 of the leading risk factors for chronic kidney disease (CKD), especially among blacks. Some degree of renal disease is usually present even with mild hypertension. This disorder is the result of ischemia caused by the narrowing of renal blood vessels. This leads to the destruction of glomeruli, atrophy of tubules, eventual death of nephrons, and renal failure. Nocturia is usually the earliest symptom of renal disease.

Retinal Damage

The appearance of the retina gives important information about the severity and duration of hypertension. We can directly see the blood vessels of the retina with an ophthalmoscope. Damage to the retinal vessels indicates related vessel damage in the heart, brain, and kidneys. Symptoms of severe retinal damage include blurring of vision, retinal hemorrhage, and vision loss.

H

Diagnostic Studies

Accurate measurement of BP is essential in assessing and monitoring hypertension. Basic laboratory studies are performed to evaluate target organ disease, determine overall cardiovascular risk, or establish baseline levels before initiating therapy.

- Routine urinalysis, blood urea nitrogen (BUN), and serum creatinine levels to screen for renal involvement
- Serum electrolytes, especially potassium levels, to detect hyperaldosteronism
- Blood glucose level to assess for diabetes
- Lipid profile to assess for risk factors for atherosclerosis
- Electrocardiogram (ECG) for baseline cardiac status

Interprofessional Management

Treatment goals include achieving and maintaining goal BP and reducing cardiovascular risk and target organ disease. Lifestyle modifications are a part of therapy for all patients with prehypertension and hypertension. The American Heart Association's "Life's Simple 7" steps support ways to modify and improve health. These are: (1) manage blood pressure, (2) control cholesterol, (3) reduce blood sugar, (4) get active, (5) eat better, (6) lose weight, and (7) stop smoking. Other modifications by the taskforce on hypertension address sodium restrictions and alcohol intake.

- Dietary therapy consists of restricting sodium intake to < 2300 mg/day and following the DASH eating plan, which stresses fruits, vegetables, fat-free or low-fat milk and milk products, whole grains, fish, poultry, beans, seeds, and nuts. Compared with the typical American diet, the plan contains less red meat, salt, sweets, added sugars, and sugar-containing beverages. The DASH plan is rich in vegetables, fruit, and nonfat dairy products. Men should limit their intake of alcohol to no more than 2 drinks per day, and women and lighter-weight men to no more than 1 drink per day.
- Adults should perform moderate-intensity aerobic physical activity for at least 30 minutes most days (i.e., more than 5 days per week) or vigorous-intensity aerobic activity for at least 20 minutes 3 days a week.
- Muscle-strengthening activities should also be performed using the major muscles of the body at least twice a week. Flexibility and balance exercises are recommended at least twice a week for older adults, especially for those at risk for falls. Advise sedentary people to increase activity levels gradually.

- Screen for psychosocial risk factors (e.g., depression, social isolation, low socioeconomic status) which can contribute to developing CVD and to a poorer prognosis and clinical course in patients with CVD. Make appropriate referrals (e.g., counseling) when indicated.
- Nicotine in tobacco causes vasoconstriction and increases BP in hypertensive people. Strongly encourage everyone to avoid tobacco use.

Drug Therapy

The following are recommendations for antihypertensive drug therapy from the Eighth Joint National Committee (JNC 8):

- In patients 60 years of age or older, start drug treatment for BP of 130 mm Hg or more systolic or 90 mm Hg or more diastolic, and treat to goal BP less than those thresholds
- In patients younger than 60 years, treatment initiation and goals should be 130/80 mm Hg, the same threshold used in patients 18 years or older with either chronic kidney disease (CKD) or diabetes.
- In all other patients without CVD or other risk factors, a BP of < 130/80 mm Hg may be reasonable.

The drugs currently available for treating hypertension have 2 main actions: reducing SVR and decreasing the volume of circulating blood.

- Drugs used in the treatment of hypertension include diuretics, adrenergic (SNS) inhibitors, direct vasodilators, angiotensin-converting enzyme (ACE) inhibitors, A-II receptor blockers (ARBs), and calcium-channel blockers. (See Tables 32.6–32.8 in Harding et al., *Lewis' Medical-Surgical Nursing*, ed 11, for a description of antihypertensive drug therapy.)
- Most patients who have hypertension require 2 or more antihypertensive drugs to achieve their goal BP.
- Once antihypertensive therapy is started, patients should return for follow-up and adjustment of drug regimens often until the goal BP is reached.

H

Nursing Management

Goals

The overall goals for the patient with hypertension are that the patient will: (1) achieve and maintain the goal BP, (2) have minimal side effects of therapy, and (3) manage and cope with this condition.

Nursing Interventions

You are in an ideal position to assess for the presence of hypertension, identify risk factors for hypertension and CAD, and teach the patient about these conditions.

Initially, take the BP in both arms to note any differences. Atherosclerosis in the subclavian artery can cause a falsely low reading on the side where the narrowing occurs. Use the arm with the highest BP and take at least 2 readings, at least 1 minute apart.

Assess for orthostatic (or postural) changes in BP and pulse in older adults, people taking antihypertensive drugs, and patients who report symptoms consistent with reduced BP on standing (e.g., light-headedness, dizziness, syncope).

Your primary nursing responsibilities for long-term management of hypertension are to assist the patient in reducing BP and adhering to the treatment plan. Your nursing actions include evaluating effectiveness of therapy, detecting and reporting any adverse treatment effects, assessing and enhancing adherence, and teaching patients and caregivers.

▼ Patient and Caregiver Teaching

Help the patient and caregivers understand that hypertension is a chronic illness that cannot be cured. Stress that it can be controlled with drug therapy, diet changes, physical activity, periodic follow-up, and other relevant lifestyle modifications (Table 49).

TABLE 49   Patient and Caregiver Teaching

Hypertension

When teaching the patient and/or caregivers about hypertension, include the following information.

General Instructions

1. Provide patient the BP reading and explain what it means (e.g., high, low, goal, borderline).
2. Encourage patient to monitor BP at home and teach the patient to call the HCP if BP exceeds high or low limits set by HCP.
3. Hypertension is usually asymptomatic, and symptoms (e.g., nosebleeds) do not reliably indicate BP levels.
4. Hypertension means high BP and does not relate to a "hyper" personality.
5. Long-term therapy and follow-up care are necessary to treat hypertension. Therapy involves lifestyle changes (e.g., weight management, sodium reduction, smoking cessation, regular physical activity) and, in most cases, drugs to regulate the blood pressure.
6. Therapy will not cure but should control, hypertension.
7. Controlled hypertension usually results in an excellent prognosis.
8. Explain the potential dangers of uncontrolled hypertension (e.g., stroke, heart attack).

TABLE 49 Patient and Caregiver Teaching

Hypertension—cont'd

Instructions Related to Medication Therapy

1. Be specific about the names, actions, dosages, and side effects of prescribed drugs.
2. Help the patient plan regular and convenient times for taking medications and measuring BP.
3. Do not stop drugs abruptly since withdrawal may cause a severe hypertensive reaction.
4. Do not double up on a dose when a dose is missed.
5. If BP increases or decreases, do not change the dose of the drug without consulting the HCP.
6. Do not take any drugs belonging to someone else.
7. Supplement diet with foods high in potassium (e.g., citrus fruits, green leafy vegetables) if taking potassium-wasting diuretics.
8. Avoid hot baths, excess amounts of alcohol, and strenuous exercise within 3 hours of taking drugs that promote vasodilation.
9. Many drugs cause orthostatic hypotension. Reduce the effects of orthostatic hypotension by rising slowly from the bed, sitting on the side of the bed for a few minutes, standing slowly, and beginning to move if no symptoms develop (e.g., dizziness, lightheadedness). Do not stand still for prolonged periods, do leg exercises to increase venous return, or sleep with the head of the bed raised. Do lie or sit down when dizziness occurs.
10. Some drugs cause sexual problems (e.g., erectile dysfunction, decreased libido). Consult with the HCP about changing drugs or dosages if sexual problems develop.
11. Some side effects may decrease with time (e.g., fatigue, diarrhea).
12. Be careful about taking potentially high-risk over-the-counter drugs such as high-sodium antacids, NSAIDs, appetite suppressants, and cold and sinus medications. Read warning labels and consult with a pharmacist.

HCP, Health care provider; *NSAIDs,* nonsteroidal antiinflammatory drugs.

H

HYPERTHYROIDISM

Description

Hyperthyroidism is hyperactivity of the thyroid gland with a sustained increase in synthesis and release of thyroid hormones. Graves' disease accounts for about 75% of the cases of hyperthyroidism. Other causes include toxic nodular goiter, thyroid-itis, pituitary tumors, and thyroid cancer.

Thyrotoxicosis is hypermetabolism that results from excess circulating levels of thyroxine (T_4), triiodothyronine (T_3), or both. Hyperthyroidism and thyrotoxicosis usually occur together as in Graves' disease. Hyperthyroidism occurs in more women than in men, with the highest frequency in people 20 to 40 years old.

- Since hyperthyroidism may be precipitated by iodinated contrast media used in CT scans and other radiologic studies, monitor those who are at-risk for hyperthyroidism closely after iodinated contrast media exposure.

Pathophysiology

Graves' disease is an autoimmune disease of unknown cause marked by diffuse thyroid enlargement and excess thyroid hormone secretion. The patient develops antibodies to the thyroid-stimulating hormone (TSH) receptor. These antibodies attach to receptors and stimulate the thyroid gland to release T_3, T_4, or both. The excess release of thyroid hormones leads to the manifestations associated with thyrotoxicosis.

- Remissions and exacerbations may progress to thyroid tissue destruction, causing hypothyroidism.
- Precipitating factors, such as insufficient iodine supply, infection, and stressful life events, may interact with genetic factors to cause Graves' disease. Cigarette smoking increases the risk of Graves' disease and the development of eye problems.

Clinical Manifestations

Manifestations are related to the effect of excess thyroid hormones.

- Palpation of the thyroid gland may reveal a goiter. Auscultation of the thyroid gland may reveal bruits, a reflection of increased blood supply.
- *Exophthalmos,* or eyeball protrusion, is caused by impaired venous drainage from the orbit, leading to increased deposits of fat and edema fluid in the orbital tissues. This is a classic finding in Graves' disease. When the eyelids do not close completely, exposed corneal surfaces become dry and irritated. Serious consequences, such as corneal ulcers and eventual loss of vision, can occur. Ocular muscle changes result in muscle weakness, causing diplopia.
- A patient with advanced disease may have many symptoms, whereas a patient in the early stages of hyperthyroidism may only have weight loss and increased nervousness.

Other manifestations are outlined in Table 49.6, Harding et al., *Lewis' Medical-Surgical Nursing,* ed 11.

Complications

Acute thyrotoxicosis (also called *thyrotoxic crisis, thyroid storm*) is a severe and rare condition that occurs when excess amounts of thyroid hormones are released into the circulation. Although this is considered a life-threatening emergency, death is rare when treatment is started early. Thyrotoxicosis is thought to result from stressors (e.g., infection, trauma, surgery) in a patient with preexisting hyperthyroidism. Patients having a thyroidectomy are at risk because manipulation of the hyperactive thyroid gland results in an increase in hormones released.

In acute thyrotoxicosis, symptoms of hyperthyroidism are prominent and severe. Manifestations include severe tachycardia, heart failure, shock, hyperthermia (with temperatures up to 106° F [41.1° C]), agitation, delirium, seizures, abdominal pain, vomiting, diarrhea, and coma.

- Treatment is aimed at reducing circulating thyroid hormone levels by appropriate drug therapy, fever reduction, fluid replacement, and elimination or management of the initiating stressor or stressors.

Diagnostic Studies

- Diagnosis is confirmed with findings of decreased serum TSH levels and elevated free thyroxine (T_4) levels.
- Radioactive iodine uptake (RAIU) differentiates Graves' disease from other forms of thyroiditis.

Interprofessional Management

The goal of management is to block the adverse effects of thyroid hormones, suppress oversecretion of thyroid hormone, and prevent complications. There are several treatment options including antithyroid medications, radioactive iodine therapy, and surgical intervention.

Drug Therapy

Drugs used in the treatment of hyperthyroidism are useful in treating thyrotoxic states, but they are not curative.

Antithyroid Drugs. The first-line antithyroid drugs commonly used are propylthiouracil and methimazole (Tapazole). These drugs inhibit the synthesis of thyroid hormones. Reasons for use include Graves' disease in the young patient, hyperthyroidism during pregnancy, or achieving a euthyroid state before surgery or radiation therapy. Propylthiouracil, which blocks the peripheral conversion of T_4 to T_3, is first-line treatment for thyrotoxic crisis.

Iodine. In large doses, iodine (e.g., Lugol's solution, saturated solution of potassium iodide [SSKI]) inhibits the synthesis of T_3 and T_4

H

and blocks the release of these hormones into circulation. Iodine decreases thyroid vascularity, making surgery safer and easier.

β-Adrenergic Blockers. β-Adrenergic blockers (e.g., propranolol [Inderal]) are used to block the effects of sympathetic nervous stimulation, thereby decreasing tachycardia, nervousness, irritability, and tremors.

Radioactive Iodine. Radioactive iodine (RAI) limits thyroid hormone secretion by damaging thyroid tissue. The maximum effect may not be seen for up to 3 months. Other drug therapy may be used until the effects of radiation become apparent. This treatment results in hypothyroidism for 80% of patients.

Surgical Therapy

Thyroidectomy is done for those who: (1) have a large goiter causing tracheal compression, (2) are unresponsive to antithyroid therapy, or (3) have thyroid cancer. A subtotal thyroidectomy involves the removal of a significant portion (90%) of the thyroid gland. A minimally invasive endoscopic or robotic thyroidectomy can be performed for patients with small nodules (< 3 cm) without evidence of cancer.

Nutritional Therapy

There is a high potential for nutritional deficits when an increased metabolic rate is present. A high-calorie diet (4000–5000 cal/day) may be needed to satisfy hunger and prevent tissue breakdown. This can be achieved with 6 full meals each day and snacks high in protein, carbohydrates, minerals, and vitamins.

- Teach the patient to avoid highly seasoned and high-fiber foods, which can further stimulate the already hyperactive gastrointestinal (GI) tract. Provide substitutes for caffeine-containing liquids such as coffee, tea, and cola, because the stimulating effects of these fluids increase restlessness and sleep problems.
- Refer the patient to a dietitian for help in meeting individual nutritional needs.

Nursing Management

Goals

The patient with hyperthyroidism will have relief of symptoms, have no serious complications related to the disease or treatment, maintain nutritional balance, and cooperate with the therapeutic plan.

Nursing Interventions

Acute thyrotoxicosis requires aggressive treatment, often in an intensive care unit. Give medications (previously discussed) that block thyroid hormone production and the sympathetic nervous system.

Provide supportive therapy to the patient, including monitoring for dysrhythmias and decompensation, ensuring adequate oxygenation, and giving IV fluids to replace fluid and electrolytes. This is especially important in the patient who has fluid losses from vomiting and diarrhea.

Adequate rest may be a challenge because of the patient's irritability and restlessness. Provide a calm, quiet room because increased metabolism and sensitivity of the sympathetic nervous system cause sleep problems.

- Placing the patient in a cool room away from very ill patients and noisy, high-traffic areas; use light bed coverings and change the linen frequently if the patient is diaphoretic
- Encourage and assist with exercise involving large muscle groups (tremors can interfere with small-muscle coordination) to allow the release of nervous tension and restlessness.
- Establish a supportive, trusting relationship to promote coping by a patient who is irritable, restless, and anxious.

If exophthalmos is present, there is a potential for corneal injury. The patient may also have orbital pain. Interventions to relieve eye discomfort and prevent corneal ulceration include applying artificial tears to soothe and moisten conjunctival membranes, elevating the patient's head to reduce periorbital edema, and providing dark glasses to reduce glare and prevent irritation from smoke, air currents, dust, and dirt. If the eyelids cannot be closed, lightly tape them shut for sleep. To maintain flexibility, teach the patient to exercise intraocular muscles several times each day by turning the eyes in the complete range of motion.

Nursing Management: Patient Having Thyroid Surgery

When a subtotal thyroidectomy is the treatment of choice, the patient must be adequately prepared to avoid postoperative complications.

- Preoperative teaching includes showing the patient how to support the head manually while turning in bed to minimize stress on the surgery suture line. The patient should practice neck range-of-motion exercises. Tell the patient that talking is likely to be difficult for a short time after surgery.

Important nursing interventions after a thyroidectomy include the following:

- Assess the patient frequently for signs of hemorrhage or tracheal compression. The patient can expect some hoarseness for 3 or 4 days after surgery because of edema.
- Respiration may become difficult because of excess swelling of the neck, hemorrhage, and hematoma formation.
- Laryngeal stridor (harsh, vibratory sound) may occur during respiration as a result of edema of the laryngeal nerve or because of tetany, which occurs if the parathyroid glands are removed or damaged during surgery.

- Recurrent laryngeal nerve damage is a potential complication that leads to vocal cord paralysis. If both cords are paralyzed, the patient needs an immediate tracheostomy.
- Place the patient in a semi-Fowler's position and support the head with pillows. Avoid flexion of the neck and any tension on the suture lines.
- Monitor vital signs and calcium levels. Check for signs of tetany secondary to hypoparathyroidism (e.g., tingling of toes, fingers, or around the mouth; muscular twitching; apprehension) and by evaluating any difficulty in speaking and hoarseness. To treat tetany, IV calcium salts, such as calcium gluconate, should be available.
- Control postoperative pain by giving medication.
- If postoperative recovery is uneventful, the patient ambulates within hours after surgery and starts a soft diet the next day.

▼ **Patient and Caregiver Teaching**

Follow-up care is important for the patient who has undergone thyroid surgery.

- Thyroid hormone balance should be monitored periodically to ensure that normal function has returned.
- To prevent weight gain, caloric intake must be substantially reduced below the amount that was required before surgery.
- Adequate iodine is needed to promote thyroid function, but excess inhibits the thyroid. Seafood once or twice per week or the normal use of iodized salt should provide enough iodine intake.
- Encourage regular exercise to help stimulate the thyroid gland.
- Teach the patient to avoid high environmental temperatures because they inhibit thyroid regeneration.
- If a complete thyroidectomy has been performed, teach the patient about the need for lifelong thyroid replacement. Teach the patient the signs and symptoms of thyroid failure and to contact the health care provider (HCP) if they develop.

HYPOPARATHYROIDISM

Description

Hypoparathyroidism is an uncommon condition characterized by inadequate circulating parathyroid hormone (PTH) that results in hypocalcemia. PTH resistance at the cellular level may also occur. This is caused by a genetic defect resulting in hypocalcemia in spite of normal or high PTH levels and is often associated with hypothyroidism and hypogonadism.

Pathophysiology

The most common cause of hypoparathyroidism is the accidental removal of parathyroids or damage to the vascular supply of the glands during neck surgery (e.g., thyroidectomy).

- Idiopathic hypoparathyroidism resulting from absence, fatty replacement, or atrophy of the glands is a rare disease that usually occurs early in life and may be associated with other endocrine disorders.
- Severe hypomagnesemia (e.g., malnutrition, renal failure) also leads to suppression of PTH secretion.

Clinical Manifestations

Clinical manifestations of acute hypoparathyroidism are caused by hypocalcemia.

Sudden decreases in calcium concentration cause tetany, characterized by lip tingling and extremity stiffness. Painful tonic spasms of smooth and skeletal muscles can cause dysphagia and laryngospasms that compromise breathing.

Abnormal laboratory findings include decreased serum calcium and PTH levels and increased serum phosphate levels.

Nursing and Interprofessional Management

Treatment goals for the patient with hypoparathyroidism are to treat acute complications such as tetany, maintain normal serum calcium levels, and prevent long-term complications. Emergency treatment of tetany after surgery requires IV calcium administration.

- Give IV calcium slowly. Use electrocardiogram (ECG) monitoring when giving calcium because high serum calcium levels can cause hypotension, serious dysrhythmias, or cardiac arrest.
- Rebreathing may partially relieve acute neuromuscular symptoms associated with hypocalcemia, such as generalized muscle cramps or mild tetany. Have the patient (if able to cooperate) breathe into and out of a paper bag or breathing mask.

▼ Patient and Caregiver Teaching

The patient with hypoparathyroidism needs instruction in long-term nutrition and drug therapy.

- Oral calcium supplements of at least 1.5 to 3 g/day in divided doses, magnesium supplements, and vitamin D are usually prescribed.
- A high-calcium meal plan includes foods such as dark green vegetables, soybeans, and tofu. Tell the patient that foods containing oxalic acid (e.g., spinach, rhubarb), phytic acid (e.g., bran, whole grains), and phosphorus reduce calcium absorption.

H

- Teach the patient about the need for lifelong treatment and follow-up care including monitoring of calcium levels several times a year.

HYPOTHYROIDISM

Description

Hypothyroidism is a deficiency of thyroid hormone that causes a general slowing of the metabolic rate. About 4% of the U.S. population has mild hypothyroidism, with about 0.3% having more severe disease. Hypothyroidism is more common in women than men. Risk factors for hypothyroidism include being female, white ethnicity, advancing age or having type 1 diabetes, Down syndrome, family history of thyroid disease, goiter, previous hyperthyroidism, and external beam radiation in the head and neck area.

Pathophysiology

Hypothyroidism can be *primary* (related to destruction of thyroid tissue or defective hormone synthesis) or *secondary* (related to pituitary disease with decreased thyroid-stimulating hormone [TSH] secretion or hypothalamic dysfunction with decreased thyrotropin-releasing hormone [TRH] secretion). Hypothyroidism can be brief and related to thyroiditis or discontinuing thyroid hormone therapy.

- Iodine deficiency is the most common cause of hypothyroidism worldwide. In the United States, the most common cause of primary hypothyroidism is atrophy of the thyroid gland. This atrophy is the result of Hashimoto's thyroiditis or Graves' disease. These autoimmune diseases destroy the thyroid gland.
- Hypothyroidism can develop after treatment for hyperthyroidism, specifically thyroidectomy or radioactive iodine (RAI) therapy. Drugs such as amiodarone, which contains iodine or lithium that block hormone production, can cause hypothyroidism.
- Hypothyroidism that develops in infancy *(cretinism)* is caused by thyroid hormone deficiencies during fetal or early neonatal life.

Clinical Manifestations

The systemic effects of hypothyroidism are characterized by a slowing of body processes. The patient is often fatigued and lethargic. There may be personality and mental changes including impaired memory, slowed speech, decreased initiative, and somnolence.

Many appear depressed. Weight gain is a result of decreased metabolic rate.

- Hypothyroidism is associated with decreased cardiac output, decreased cardiac contractility, and coronary atherosclerosis. Anemia is a common feature. High serum cholesterol and triglyceride levels and the accumulation of mucopolysaccharides in the intima of small blood vessels can result in coronary atherosclerosis.
- In the older adult, typical manifestations include fatigue, cold and dry skin, hair loss, hoarseness, and cold intolerance. Constipation is common and may progress to obstipation.
- Those with severe long-standing hypothyroidism may display *myxedema*. It alters the skin and subcutaneous tissues with puffiness, facial and periorbital edema, and a masklike affect. Myxedema occurs with the accumulation of hydrophilic mucopolysaccharides in the dermis and other tissues. Persons with hypothyroidism may have an altered self-image.

Complications

The mental sluggishness, drowsiness, and lethargy of hypothyroidism may progress gradually or suddenly to a notable impairment of consciousness or coma. This situation, termed *myxedema coma*, constitutes a medical emergency.

- Myxedema coma can be precipitated by infection, drugs (especially opioids, tranquilizers, and barbiturates), exposure to cold, and trauma. It is characterized by subnormal temperature, hypotension, and hypoventilation.
- For the patient to survive, vital functions must be supported and IV thyroid hormone replacement given.

Diagnostic Studies

- Serum TSH and free thyroxine (FT_4) are the most reliable indicators of thyroid function.
- Serum TSH levels help determine the cause of hypothyroidism. If high, the defect is in the thyroid; if low, it is in the pituitary or hypothalamus.
- The presence of thyroid antibodies suggests an autoimmune origin of the hypothyroidism.
- High cholesterol, triglycerides and creatine kinase can occur, along with anemia.

Interprofessional Management

The treatment goal is the restoration of the euthyroid state as safely and rapidly as possible with hormone therapy. A low-calorie diet can promote weight loss or prevent weight gain.

H

Levothyroxine (Synthroid) is the drug of choice to treat hypothyroidism. In the young, otherwise healthy patient, the maintenance replacement dosage is adjusted according to the patient's response and laboratory findings. The initial dosages are low to avoid increases in resting heart rate and BP. In the patient with compromised cardiac status, careful monitoring is needed when starting and adjusting the dosage because the usual dose may increase myocardial oxygen demand, causing angina and dysrhythmias. Levothyroxine has a peak of action of 1 to 3 weeks. In the patient without side effects the dose is increased at 4- to 6-week intervals.

Liotrix is a synthetic mix of levothyroxine (T_4) and liothyronine (T_3) in a 4:1 combination. Liotrix, with a fast onset of action and a peak of 2 to 3 days, can be used in acutely ill patients with hypothyroidism.

It is important that the patient take replacement medication regularly. Lifelong thyroid therapy is usually required.

Nursing Management

Goals
The patient with hypothyroidism will have relief of symptoms, maintain a euthyroid state, maintain a positive self-image, and adhere to lifelong thyroid therapy.

Nursing Interventions
Most persons with hypothyroidism are treated on an outpatient basis. The patient who develops myxedema coma requires acute nursing care, often in an intensive care unit (ICU) setting. Mechanical respiratory support and cardiac monitoring are often needed. Give thyroid hormone therapy and all other medications IV because severe gastric hypomotility may prevent the absorption of oral agents. Monitor core temperature because the patient with myxedema coma is often hypothermic.

- Use gentle soap and moisturize often to prevent skin breakdown. Frequent changes in patient positioning and a low-pressure mattress help maintain skin integrity.
- Monitor the patient's progress, vital signs, body weight, fluid intake and output, and visible edema. Cardiac assessment is especially important because the cardiovascular response to hormone therapy determines the medication regimen.
- Note energy level and mental alertness, which should increase within 2 to 14 days and continue to rise steadily to normal levels.

▼ Patient and Caregiver Teaching
At first the hypothyroid patient may have a hard time processing complex instructions. Provide written instructions, repeat the information often, and assess the patient's comprehension level.

- Stress the need for receiving lifelong drug therapy and avoiding abruptly stopping the drugs. Teach the patient expected and unexpected side effects. Explain the signs and symptoms that indicate hormone imbalance.
- Teach the patient to contact a health care provider (HCP) right away for signs of overdose, such as orthopnea, dyspnea, rapid pulse, chest pain, palpitations, nervousness, or insomnia.
- The patient with diabetes should test capillary blood glucose at least daily because a return to the euthyroid state often increases insulin requirements.
- Thyroid preparations increase the effects of other common drugs, such as anticoagulants, antidepressants, and digitalis compounds. Teach the patient the toxic signs and symptoms of these medications.
- Medication interactions are an important reason for patients to consult their HCP before switching brands of thyroid replacement medication. Switching brands may change bioavailability of the drug and physiologic response.

INCREASED INTRACRANIAL PRESSURE

Description

Increased intracranial pressure (ICP) is a potentially life-threatening situation that results from an increase in any or all 3 components within the skull: brain tissue, blood, and cerebrospinal fluid (CSF).

Pathophysiology

Common causes of increased ICP include a mass (e.g., hematoma, contusion, abscess, tumor) and cerebral edema (from tumors, hydrocephalus, head injury, or brain inflammation). These cerebral insults, which may result in hypercapnia, cerebral acidosis, impaired autoregulation, and systemic hypertension, worsen the cerebral edema. This edema distorts brain tissue, further increasing the ICP, and leads to even more tissue hypoxia and acidosis. Fig. 13 shows the progression of increased ICP.

There are 3 types of cerebral edema: vasogenic, cytotoxic, and interstitial. More than 1 type may occur in the same patient.

- *Vasogenic cerebral edema,* the most common type of edema, occurs mainly in the white matter and is characterized by leakage of large molecules from capillaries into extracellular space. This edema may produce a continuum of symptoms, ranging from headache to a decrease in consciousness, including coma and focal neurologic deficits.

PATHOPHYSIOLOGY MAP

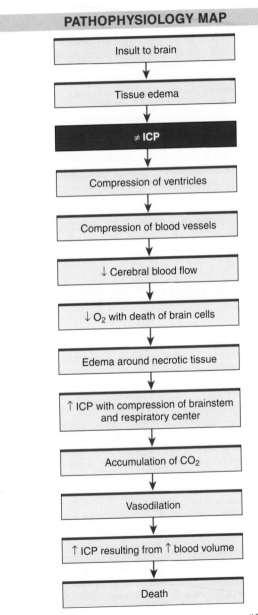

Insult to brain

↓

Tissue edema

↓

≠ ICP

↓

Compression of ventricles

↓

Compression of blood vessels

↓

↓ Cerebral blood flow

↓

↓ O_2 with death of brain cells

↓

Edema around necrotic tissue

↓

↑ ICP with compression of brainstem and respiratory center

↓

Accumulation of CO_2

↓

Vasodilation

↓

↑ ICP resulting from ↑ blood volume

↓

Death

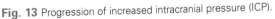

Fig. 13 Progression of increased intracranial pressure (ICP).

- *Cytotoxic cerebral edema* results from disruption of the integrity of the cell membranes. This type of edema develops from destructive lesions or brain trauma resulting in cerebral hypoxia or anoxia and syndrome of inappropriate antidiuretic hormone (SIADH) secretion.
- *Interstitial cerebral edema* is usually a result of hydrocephalus. It is caused by excess CSF production, obstruction of CSF flow, or an inability to reabsorb the CSF.

Clinical Manifestations

Manifestations of increased ICP can take many forms, depending on the cause, location, and rate of increase of ICP.

- *Change in level of consciousness* (LOC). LOC is a sensitive and reliable indicator of the patient's neurologic status. Changes in LOC may be dramatic, as in coma, or subtle, such as a flattening of affect, change in orientation or a decrease in the level of attention.
- *Changes in vital signs.* Manifestations, such as *Cushing's triad* (systolic hypertension with widening pulse pressure, bradycardia with a full and bounding pulse, and irregular respirations), often do not appear until ICP has been increased for some time or is markedly increased (e.g., with head trauma). The effect of increased ICP on the hypothalamus can cause a change in body temperature.
- *Ocular signs.* Compression of the oculomotor nerve (cranial nerve [CN] III) results in dilation of the pupil on the same side (ipsilateral) as the mass lesion, sluggish or no response to light, an inability to adduct and move the eye upward, and ptosis of the eyelid. A fixed, unilaterally dilated pupil is a neurologic emergency that indicates brain herniation. Other cranial nerves may also be affected, with signs of blurred vision, diplopia, and changes in extraocular eye movements.
- *Decrease in motor function.* As ICP continues to rise, the patient shows changes in motor skills. A contralateral (opposite side of the mass lesion) hemiparesis or hemiplegia may develop. If a painful stimulus is used to elicit a motor response, the patient may localize to the stimulus or withdraw from it. *Decorticate* (flexor) and *decerebrate* (extensor) posturing may be elicited by noxious stimuli (see Fig. 56.4, Harding et al., *Lewis' Medical-Surgical Nursing,* ed 11).
- *Headache.* Although the brain is not sensitive to pain, compression of other intracranial structures, such as the walls of arteries and veins and the cranial nerves, can produce headache. A nocturnal headache or a headache in the morning is cause for

concern and may indicate a tumor or other space-occupying lesion that is causing increased ICP. Straining, agitation, or movement may worsen the pain.
- *Vomiting.* Vomiting, usually without nausea, is often a nonspecific sign of increased ICP.

The major complications of uncontrolled increased ICP are inadequate cerebral perfusion and cerebral herniation. *Herniation* occurs as the brain tissue is forcibly shifted from the compartment of greater pressure to a compartment of lesser pressure.

Diagnostic Studies
- MRI, CT scan, and positron emission tomography (PET) can be used to discern the cause of increased ICP.
- Other tests may include cerebral angiography, electroencephalography (EEG), ICP measurement, brain tissue oxygenation measurement via the LICOX catheter, transcranial Doppler studies, and evoked potential studies.

Interprofessional Management
The goals of management of increased ICP are to: (1) identify and treat the underlying cause of increased ICP, and (2) support brain function. The earlier the condition is recognized and treated, the better the patient outcome. A careful history helps direct the search for the underlying cause.

Ensuring adequate oxygenation for brain function is important. Arterial blood gas (ABG) analysis guides the O_2 therapy. To meet the goal of maintaining the partial pressure of O_2 in arterial blood (PaO_2) at 100 mm Hg or greater and to keep the partial pressure of CO_2 in arterial blood ($PaCO_2$) in normal range at 35 to 45 mm Hg, an endotracheal tube or tracheostomy and mechanical ventilation may be needed.
- Surgical removal may be needed if the increased ICP is caused by a mass lesion, such as a tumor or hematoma (see Brain Tumors, p. 82).

Drug Therapy
Drug therapy is an important part of the management of increased ICP.
- IV mannitol (Osmitrol) (25%) is an osmotic diuretic that decreases ICP in 2 ways: plasma expansion and osmotic effect. The immediate plasma-expanding effect reduces the hematocrit and blood viscosity. This increases cerebral blood flow and cerebral oxygenation. The osmotic effect causes fluid to move from the tissue into the blood vessels, which decreases total brain fluid content.

- IV hypertonic saline is used to manage increased ICP. It produces massive movement of water out of swollen brain cells and into the blood vessels.
- Corticosteroids (e.g., dexamethasone) are used to treat vasogenic edema surrounding tumors and abscesses. They are not recommended for traumatic brain injury. Corticosteroids stabilize the cell membrane and inhibit the synthesis of prostaglandins. These drugs also improve cerebral blood flow and restore autoregulation.
- Metabolic demands, such as fever (temperatures above 38°C), agitation/shivering, pain, and seizures, can increase ICP. The interprofessional team should plan to reduce these metabolic demands to lower the ICP.
- High-dose barbiturates (e.g., pentobarbital, thiopental) are used in patients with increased ICP refractory to other treatments. These drugs lower cerebral metabolism to decrease ICP.
- Patients with increased ICP who need mechanical ventilation may receive opiates, sedatives, and neuromuscular blocking agents by continuous infusion.
- Antiseizure prophylaxis against early seizures (within the first 7 days) may be prescribed for patients with severe brain injury.

Nutritional Therapy

The patient with increased ICP is in a hypermetabolic and hypercatabolic state that increases the need for glucose to provide the necessary fuel for metabolism of the injured brain. If the patient cannot maintain an adequate oral intake, other means of meeting the nutritional requirements, such as enteral or parenteral nutrition, should be started. Fluid therapy is directed at keeping patients normovolemic.

Nursing Management
Goals

The overall goals are that the patient with increased ICP will have ICP within normal limits, maintain a patent airway, demonstrate normal fluid and electrolyte balance, and have no complications from immobility and decreased LOC.

Nursing Interventions

Respiratory Function. Maintenance of a patent airway is critical in patients with increased ICP and is a major nursing responsibility. As the LOC decreases, the patient is at increased risk for airway obstruction.

- Be alert to altered breathing patterns. Snoring sounds indicate obstruction and require immediate intervention. An oral airway facilitates breathing and provides an easier suctioning route in the comatose patient.

- In general, any patient with a Glasgow Coma Scale score of 8 or less (see Glasgow Coma Scale, p. 746) or an altered LOC who is unable to maintain a patent airway or effective ventilation needs intubation and mechanical ventilation.
- Careful monitoring is needed for the patient with increased ICP who requires mechanical ventilation and continuous sedation.
- Prevent hypoxia and hypercapnia. Frequently monitor and evaluate the ABG values. Take measures to maintain the levels within prescribed or acceptable parameters. The appropriate ventilatory support can be ordered based on the PaO_2 and $PaCO_2$ values.
- Proper neutral positioning of the head is important. Elevation of the head of the bed by 30 degrees enhances respiratory exchange and aids in decreasing cerebral edema.
- Suctioning and coughing can cause transient increases in ICP and decreases in PaO_2. Remove accumulated secretions by suctioning as needed.
- Try to prevent abdominal distention, which can interfere with respiratory function. Inserting a nasogastric tube to aspirate the stomach contents can prevent distention, vomiting, and possible aspiration. In patients with facial and skull fractures, a nasogastric tube is contraindicated because of risk of inadvertent intracranial placement. Oral insertion of a gastric tube is preferred.

Fluid and Electrolyte Balance. Fluid and electrolyte problems can have an adverse effect on ICP. Closely monitor IV fluids. Intake and output, accounting for insensible losses, and daily weights are important in the assessment of fluid balance.

- Monitor serum electrolytes, especially glucose, sodium, potassium, magnesium, and osmolality.
- Monitor urinary output for problems related to SIADH and diabetes insipidus (DI) (see Diabetes Insipidus, p. 163).

Monitoring Intracranial Pressure. ICP monitoring is used with other parameters to guide care and assess the patient's response to care. (See Intracranial Pressure Monitoring, p. 750). Methods of monitoring ICP are discussed in detail in Chapter 56, Harding et al., *Lewis' Medical-Surgical Nursing,* ed 11.

Body Position. Maintain the patient with increased ICP in the head-up position. Prevent extreme neck flexion, which can cause venous obstruction and increased ICP. Adjust the body position to decrease the ICP maximally and to improve cerebral perfusion pressure (CPP).

- Turn the patient with slow, gentle movements, because rapid changes in position, pain, and agitation may increase ICP. Increased intrathoracic pressure increases ICP by impeding venous return, so coughing, straining, and the Valsalva maneuver should be avoided. Avoid extreme hip flexion to decrease the risk of raising the intraabdominal pressure, which increases ICP.

Protection From Injury. The patient should be in a quiet, calm environment with minimal noise and interruptions. Observe the patient for signs of agitation, irritation, or frustration. Teach the caregiver and family about decreasing stimulation. Coordinate with the interprofessional team to minimize procedures that may cause agitation.

The patient with increased ICP and decreased LOC needs protection from self-injury. Confusion, agitation, and the possibility of seizures increase the risk of injury. Use restraints judiciously in the agitated patient.

Psychologic Considerations. Anxiety over the diagnosis and prognosis can be distressing to the patient, caregiver, family, and nursing staff. Provide support and short, simple explanations. Assess the family members' desire and need to assist in providing patient care and allow for their participation as appropriate.

- Touch and talk to the patient calmly, even the patient who is in a coma and may appear not to hear.

INFLAMMATORY BOWEL DISEASE

Description

Inflammatory bowel disease (IBD) is a chronic inflammation of the gastrointestinal (GI) tract characterized by periods of remission interspersed with periods of exacerbation. IBD is classified as either *Crohn's disease* or *ulcerative colitis* (UC) on the basis of clinical manifestations (Table 50). UC is usually limited to the colon. Crohn's disease can involve any segment of the GI tract from the mouth to the anus.

About 1.3 million Americans have IBD. It often begins during the teenage years and early adulthood and has a second peak in the sixth decade. The highest rates of IBD are in the Northern hemisphere and industrialized nations. The risk of having IBD is greater in urban compared with rural areas and those of white and Ashkenazic Jewish origin than in other racial and ethnic groups. The strongest risk factor is family history.

Pathophysiology

IBD is an autoimmune disease involving an immune reaction to a person's own intestinal tract. An overactive, inappropriate, or sustained immune response causes inflammation and widespread tissue

TABLE 50 Comparison of Ulcerative Colitis and Crohn's Disease

Characteristic	Ulcerative Colitis	Crohn's Disease
Clinical		
Usual age at onset	Teens to mid-30s. After 60 yrs	Teens to mid-30s. After 60 yrs
Abdominal pain	Common, severe constant	Common, cramping
Diarrhea	Common	Common
Fever (intermittent)	During acute attacks	Common
Malabsorption and nutritional deficiencies	Minimal incidence	Common
Rectal bleeding	Common	Sometimes
Tenesmus	Common	Rare
Weight loss	Rare	Common, may be severe
Pathologic		
Location	Usually starts in rectum and spreads in a continuous pattern up the colon	Occurs anywhere along GI tract. Most common site is distal ileum
Cobblestoning of mucosa	Rare	Common
Depth of involvement	Mucosa	Entire thickness of bowel wall (transmural)
Distribution	Continuous areas of inflammation	Healthy tissue interspersed with areas of inflammation (skip lesions)
Pseudopolyps	Common	Rare
Small bowel involvement	Minimal	Common
Complications		
Cancer	Increased incidence of colorectal cancer after 10 yr of disease	Increased incidence of small intestinal cancer Increased incidence of colorectal cancer but less than with ulcerative colitis
Clostridium difficile infection	Increased incidence and severity	Increased incidence and severity

TABLE 50	Comparison of Ulcerative Colitis and Crohn's Disease—cont'd	
Characteristic	Ulcerative Colitis	Crohn's Disease
Perforation	Common (because of toxic megacolon)	Common (because inflammation involves entire bowel wall)
Perianal abscess and fistulas	Rare	Common
Strictures	Occasional	Common
Toxic megacolon	More common	Rare

destruction. The pattern of inflammation differs between Crohn's disease and UC.

Environmental factors, such as diet, smoking, and stress, increase susceptibility by changing the environment of the GI microbial flora. High intake of refined sugar, total fats, polyunsaturated fatty acid (PUFA), and omega-6 fatty acids is associated with an increased risk of IBD. Nonsteroidal antiinflammatory drugs (NSAIDs), antibiotics, and oral contraceptives are associated with increased risk.

Crohn's Disease

The inflammation in *Crohn's disease* involves all layers of the bowel wall and can occur anywhere in the GI tract from the mouth to the anus. It often involves the distal ileum and proximal colon. Segments of normal bowel can occur between diseased portions, the so-called skip lesions.

- Typically, ulcerations are deep and longitudinal and penetrate between islands of inflamed edematous mucosa, causing the classic cobblestone appearance.
- Strictures at the areas of inflammation can cause bowel obstruction.
- Because the inflammation goes through the entire wall, microscopic leaks can allow bowel contents to enter the peritoneal cavity and form abscesses or produce peritonitis.
- Fistulas can develop between adjacent areas of bowel, between bowel and bladder, and between bowel and vagina.

Ulcerative Colitis

UC usually starts in the rectum and moves in progressive fashion toward the cecum. Although mild inflammation sometimes occurs in the terminal ileum, UC is a disease of the colon and rectum.

- Inflammation and ulcerations occur in the mucosal layer, the innermost layer of the bowel wall. Because inflammation does not extend through all of the bowel layers, fistulas and abscesses are rare.
- Areas of inflamed mucosa form pseudopolyps, which are tongue-like projections into the bowel lumen.

Clinical Manifestations

Manifestations are often the same (diarrhea, bloody stools, weight loss, abdominal pain, fever, and fatigue) in both conditions. Bloody stools are more common with UC, and weight loss is more common in Crohn's disease because inflammation of the small intestine impairs nutrient absorption. Both forms of IBD are chronic disorders with mild to severe acute exacerbations that occur at unpredictable intervals over many years.

Crohn's Disease

Diarrhea and colicky abdominal pain are common symptoms of Crohn's disease.

- If the small intestine is inflamed, weight loss occurs from malabsorption.
- Rectal bleeding sometimes occurs with Crohn's disease, although not as often as with UC.

Ulcerative Colitis

The primary symptoms of UC are bloody diarrhea and abdominal pain. Pain may range from the mild, lower abdominal cramping associated with diarrhea to the severe, constant abdominal pain associated with acute perforations.

- With *mild disease*, diarrhea may consist of 1 or 2 semiformed stools daily that contain small amounts of blood. The patient may have no other manifestations.
- In *moderate disease*, there is increased stool output (up to 10 stools/day), increased bleeding, and systemic signs and symptoms (fever, malaise, mild anemia, anorexia).
- In *severe disease*, diarrhea is bloody, with mucus in the stool, and occurs 10 to 20 times a day. In addition, fever, weight loss (more than 10% of total body weight), anemia, tachycardia, and dehydration are present.

Complications

Patients with IBD have both local (confined to the GI tract) and systemic complications.

- GI tract complications include hemorrhage, strictures, perforation (with possible peritonitis), abscesses, fistulas, Clostridium difficile infection, and colonic dilation (toxic megacolon).

- Toxic megacolon is more common with UC, whereas abscesses and perianal fistulas occur more often with Crohn's disease.
- Hemorrhage may lead to anemia and is corrected with blood transfusions and iron supplements.
- People with a history of IBD are at increased risk for colorectal cancer. Those with Crohn's disease are at increased risk for small intestine cancer.

People with IBD may have systemic complications, such as multiple sclerosis and ankylosing spondylitis. Some are related to the inflammatory activity in the bowel and they improve when the IBD improves. Other complications include malabsorption, liver disease (primary sclerosing cholangitis), and osteoporosis. Routine liver function tests are important because primary sclerosing cholangitis can lead to liver failure. Both men and women with IBD are at risk for osteoporosis. They need a bone density scan at baseline and every 2 years.

Diagnostic Studies

Diagnosis of IBD includes ruling out diseases with similar symptoms and then determining whether the patient has Crohn's disease or UC.

- Laboratory studies may indicate electrolyte problems, anemia, leukocytosis, hypoalbuminemia, and a high erythrocyte sedimentation rate.
- Stool is examined for blood, pus, and mucus and cultured to rule out infectious diarrhea.
- Double-contrast barium enema, small bowel series, transabdominal ultrasound, CT scan, and MRI are useful for IBD diagnosis.
- Colonoscopy allows examination of the entire large intestine.

Interprofessional Management

The goals of treatment are to rest the bowel, control inflammation, combat infection, correct malnutrition, provide symptomatic relief, and improve quality of life.

A variety of drugs are available to treat IBD. Hospitalization is indicated if the patient does not respond to drug therapy, the disease is severe, or complications are suspected.

Drug Therapy

Drugs are used to induce and maintain a remission of IBD. Drugs are chosen on the basis of the location and severity of inflammation. Five major classes of medications used to treat IBD are aminosalicylates, antimicrobials, corticosteroids, immunosuppressants, and biologic therapies (Table 51).

TABLE 51 Drug Therapy

Inflammatory Bowel Disease

Class	Action	Examples
5-Aminosalicylates (5-ASA)	Decrease inflammation by suppressing proinflammatory cytokines and other inflammatory mediators	*Systemic:* balsalazide (Colazal), mesalamine (Pentasa), olsalazine (Dipentum), sulfasalazine (Azulfidine) *Topical:* 5-ASA enema (Rowasa), mesalamine suppositories
Antimicrobials	Prevent or treat secondary infection	ciprofloxacin (Cipro), clarithromycin (Biaxin), metronidazole (Flagyl)
Biologic therapies	Inhibit the cytokine tumor necrosis factor (TNF)	adalimumab (Humira), certolizumab pegol (Cimzia), golimumab (Simponi), infliximab (Remicade)
	Prevent migration of leukocytes from bloodstream to inflamed tissue	natalizumab (Tysabri), vedolizumab (Entyvio)
Corticosteroids	Decrease inflammation	*Systemic:* corticosteroids (prednisone, budesonide [Uceris]); hydrocortisone or methylprednisolone (IV for severe IBD) *Topical:* hydrocortisone suppository or foam (budesonide, Cortifoam) or enema (Cortenema)
Immunosuppressants	Suppress immune response	azathioprine, cyclosporine, methotrexate, 6-mercaptopurine

5-ASA, 5-Aminosalicylic acid; IBD, inflammatory bowel disease.

Surgical Therapy

Many patients with Crohn's disease will eventually require surgery for complications such as strictures, bleeding, obstructions, or fistulas.

- The most common surgery involves resecting the diseased segments with reanastomosis of the remaining intestine. Unfortunately, the disease often recurs at the anastomosis site.
- Repeated removal of sections of small intestine can lead to *short bowel syndrome* (SBS). SBS occurs when either surgery or disease leaves too little small intestine surface area to maintain normal nutrition and hydration. Lifetime fluid boluses and parenteral nutrition (PN) may be needed.

In UC, surgical procedures used include total proctocolectomy with ileal pouch/anal anastomosis (IPAA) and total proctocolectomy with permanent ileostomy.

- Since UC affects only the colon, a total proctocolectomy is curative.

For descriptions of these procedures, see Chapter 42 in Harding et al., *Lewis' Medical-Surgical Nursing,* ed 11.

Nutritional Therapy

Diet is an important component of the treatment of IBD. Consult a dietitian regarding dietary recommendations. The goals of diet management are to provide adequate nutrition without exacerbating symptoms, correct and prevent malnutrition, replace fluid and electrolyte losses, and prevent weight loss.

- Nutritional deficiencies are caused by decreased oral intake, blood loss, and, depending on the location of the inflammation, impaired absorption.
- During an acute exacerbation, patients with IBD may not be able to tolerate a regular diet. Liquid enteral feedings are preferred over parenteral nutrition because atrophy of the gut and bacterial overgrowth occur when the GI tract is not used.
- There are no universal food triggers for IBD, but some people may find that certain foods initiate diarrhea. A food diary helps identify problem foods to avoid.

Nursing Management

Goals

The patient with IBD will have a decrease in the number and severity of acute exacerbations, maintain normal fluid and electrolyte balance, be free from pain or discomfort, adhere to medical regimens, maintain nutritional balance, and have an improved quality of life.

Nursing Interventions

During the acute phase, focus your attention on hemodynamic stability, pain control, fluid and electrolyte balance, and nutritional support. Maintain accurate intake and output records and monitor the number and appearance of stools.

- Establish rapport and encourage the patient to talk about self-care strategies. An explanation of all procedures and treatment will help build trust and allay apprehension.
- Many patients have intermittent exacerbations and remissions of symptoms. Given the chronicity and uncertainty related to the frequency and severity of flares, the patient may have frustration, depression, and anxiety. Psychotherapy, behavioral therapies, and support groups may help patients deal with feelings about the disease and help manage their symptoms.
- Severe fatigue limits the patient's energy for physical activity. Nutritional deficiencies and anemia may leave the patient feeling weak and listless.
- Rest is important because patients may lose sleep because of frequent episodes of diarrhea and abdominal pain. Schedule activities around rest periods.
- Help the patient stay clean, dry, and free of odor. Place a deodorizer in the room. Meticulous perianal skin care using plain water (no harsh soap) together with a skin barrier prevents skin breakdown. Dibucaine (Nupercainal), witch hazel, sitz baths, and other soothing compresses or prescribed ointments may reduce perianal irritation.

▼ **Patient and Caregiver Teaching**

The patient and caregivers may need help in setting realistic short- and long-term goals.

- Your teaching should include: (1) the importance of rest and diet management, (2) perianal care, (3) drug action and side effects, (4) symptoms of disease recurrence, (5) when to seek medical care, and (6) use of diversional activities to reduce stress.
- Excellent teaching resources are available from the Crohn's and Colitis Foundation of America (*www.crohnscolitisfoundation .org*).

INTERSTITIAL CYSTITIS/PAINFUL BLADDER SYNDROME

Description

Interstitial cystitis (IC) is a chronic, painful inflammatory disease of the bladder characterized by symptoms of urgency/frequency and pain in the bladder and/or pelvis. IC is often called *bladder pain syndrome* or *painful bladder syndrome* (PBS).

- The term *interstitial cystitis/painful bladder syndrome* (IC/PBS) refers to cases of urinary pain that cannot be attributed to other causes, such as urinary tract infection (UTI) or stones. It is more common in women than in men.

The cause of IC/PBS is unknown. Possible causes including neurogenic hypersensitivity of the lower urinary tract, changes in mast cells in the muscle and/or mucosal layers of the bladder, infection with an unusual organism (e.g., slow-growing virus), and production of a toxic substance in the urine. The bladder wall may be irritated and inflamed and can become scarred.

Clinical Manifestations

Two primary clinical manifestations of IC are pain and bothersome lower urinary tract symptoms (e.g., frequency, urgency).

- The pain is usually in the suprapubic area but may involve the vagina, labia, or entire perineal region. It varies from moderate to severe and can be exacerbated by bladder filling, postponed urination, physical exertion, pressure against the suprapubic area, certain foods, or emotional distress. The pain is temporarily relieved by voiding.
- People with severe cases may void 60 times/day including nighttime urination.
- Women report that pain occurs premenstrually and is aggravated by sexual intercourse or emotional stress. Symptoms may disappear after a period of weeks to months, or persist for years.

Diagnostic Studies

IC/PBS is a diagnosis of exclusion.

- History and physical examination are necessary to rule out other disorders that produce somewhat similar symptoms, such as cancer, UTI, or endometriosis.
- Cystoscopic examination may reveal a small bladder capacity, Hunner lesions (distinct inflammatory areas on the bladder wall), and glomerulations (superficial ulcerations with pinpoint bleeding), but these findings are not always present.

Interprofessional Management

No single treatment consistently reverses or relieves symptoms. People with IC/PBS do not respond to antibiotic therapy. They rarely need surgery.

Various therapies have been effective, including nutritional and drug therapy. Elimination of foods and beverages that are likely to irritate the bladder may provide some relief from symptoms. Typical bladder irritants include caffeine, alcohol, citrus products, carbonated drinks, chocolate, foods containing vinegar, curries, or hot peppers, and foods or beverages likely to lower urinary pH, including fruits such as cranberries.

- An over-the-counter (OTC) dietary supplement, calcium glycerophosphate (Prelief), alkalinizes the urine and can provide relief from the irritating effects of certain foods.
- Because stress can exacerbate IC/PBS, relaxation techniques (e.g., relaxation breathing, imagery) may be helpful.
- Using lubrication or altering positions may decrease pain associated with sexual intercourse.

Two tricyclic antidepressants, amitriptyline and nortriptyline, may reduce the burning and urinary frequency. Pentosan (Elmiron) is used to enhance the protective effects of the glycosaminoglycan layer of the bladder. These drugs provide relief over weeks to months, but immediate relief for an acute exacerbation of symptoms may require a short course of opioid analgesics.

Several agents may be instilled directly into the bladder through a small catheter.

- Dimethyl sulfoxide (DMSO) acts by desensitizing pain receptors in the bladder wall.
- Heparin, lidocaine, or sodium bicarbonate can be instilled into the bladder to relieve acute IC/PBS symptoms.

Surgical procedures, such as urinary diversion with an ileal conduit or fulguration and resection of Hunner lesions, can be used in an attempt to relieve debilitating pain.

Nursing Management

Assess characteristics of the pain associated with IC/PBS. Ask the patient about specific dietary or lifestyle factors that exacerbate or alleviate pain. Teach the patient to keep a bladder log or voiding diary over a period of at least 3 days to determine voiding frequency and patterns of nocturia.

Teach the patient to maintain good nutrition, particularly in light of the dietary restrictions often necessary to control IC-related pain.

- Advise the patient to take a multivitamin containing no more than the recommended dietary allowance for essential vitamins and to avoid high-potency vitamins that may irritate the bladder.
- Advise the patient to avoid clothing that creates suprapubic pressure, including pants with tight belts or restrictive waistlines.
- Written educational materials concerning diet, ways to cope with the need for frequent urination, and strategies for coping with the emotional burden of IC/PBS are available from the Interstitial Cystitis Association (*www.ichelp.org*).

INTERVERTEBRAL DISC DISEASE

Description

Intervertebral disc disease is a condition that involves the deterioration, herniation, or other dysfunction of the intervertebral discs. Disc disorders can affect the cervical, thoracic, and lumbar spine.

Pathophysiology

Intervertebral discs separate the vertebrae of the spinal column and provide shock absorption for the spine. *Degenerative disc disease* (DDD) results from increased wear and tear on the intervertebral discs with aging (Fig. 14). The discs lose their elasticity, flexibility, and shock-absorbing abilities. Unless it is accompanied by pain, this wear-and-tear condition is a normal process.

The discs become thinner as the nucleus pulposus (gelatinous center of the disc) starts to dry out and shrink. This change limits the disc's ability to distribute pressure between vertebrae. The pressure is then transferred to the annulus fibrosus (strong outside part of the disc), causing progressive destruction.

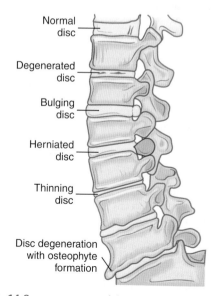

Normal disc

Degenerated disc

Bulging disc

Herniated disc

Thinning disc

Disc degeneration with osteophyte formation

Fig. 14 Common causes of degenerative disc damage.

- When the disc is damaged, the nucleus pulposus may seep through a torn or stretched annulus. This is called a *herniated disc* (slipped disc), a condition in which a spinal disc herniates and bulges outward between the vertebrae.

A herniated disc can result from natural degeneration with age or repeated stress and trauma to the spine. The nucleus pulposus may first bulge and then it can herniate, placing pressure on nearby nerves. The most common sites of rupture are the lumbosacral discs, specifically, L4-5 and L5-S1.

- Disc herniation may result from spinal stenosis, in which narrowing of the spinal canal creates bulging of the intervertebral disc.

Clinical Manifestations
Lumbar Disc Disease
The most common manifestation is low back pain. Radicular pain that radiates down the buttock and below the knee along the distribution of the sciatic nerve generally indicates disc herniation. The straight-leg raising test may be positive, indicating nerve root irritation. Back or leg pain may be reproduced by raising the leg and flexing the foot at 90 degrees.

- Reflexes may be depressed or absent, depending on the spinal nerve root involved. Paresthesia or muscle weakness in the legs, feet, or toes may occur.
- Multiple nerve root (cauda equina) compression may be marked by severe low back pain, progressive weakness, increased pain, or bowel/bladder incontinence. This condition is a medical emergency that requires surgical decompression to reduce pressure on the nerves.

Cervical Disc Disease
Pain often radiates into the arms and hands, following the pattern of the involved nerve. Reflexes may not be present, and the handgrip is often weak.

Diagnostic Studies
- X-rays are done to detect any structural defects.
- A myelogram, MRI, or CT scan is helpful in localizing the damaged site.
- An epidural venogram or diskogram may be necessary if other diagnostic studies are inconclusive.
- Electromyography (EMG) of the extremities can be performed to determine the severity of nerve irritation or to rule out conditions such as peripheral neuropathy.

Interprofessional Management

Conservative Therapy

The patient with suspected disc damage is usually managed first with conservative therapy. This includes limitation of extremes of spinal movement (brace/corset/belt), local heat or ice, ultrasound and massage, traction, and transcutaneous electrical nerve stimulation (TENS). Drug therapy includes nonsteroidal antiinflammatory drugs (NSAIDs), short-term opioids, corticosteroids, antidepressants, and muscle relaxants. Epidural corticosteroid injections may be effective in reducing inflammation and relieving acute pain.

- When symptoms subside, patients begin back-strengthening exercises twice per day, to continue for a lifetime. Teach the patient the principles of good body mechanics, discouraging extreme flexion and torsion.
- Most patients heal with conservative treatment after 6 months.

Surgical Therapy

Surgery for a damaged disc is generally considered when the problem is not responding to conservative treatment and the patient is in consistent pain and/or has a persistent neurologic deficit.

- An *intradiscal electrothermoplasty* (IDET) is a minimally invasive outpatient procedure for treatment of back and sciatica pain. A needle is inserted into the affected disc with x-ray guidance. The heated wire threaded through the needle destroys the small nerve fibers that have grown into the disc.
- A similar outpatient technique is *radiofrequency discal nucleoplasty,* in which a special radiofrequency probe inserted into the disc is used to break up the molecular bonds of the gel in the nucleus.
- A third procedure is the use of an *interspinous process decompression system* (X Stop). This titanium device fits onto a mount that is placed on vertebrae in the lower back. The device works by lifting the vertebrae off the pinched nerve. The X Stop is used in patients with pain caused by lumbar spinal stenosis.
- *Diskectomy* can also be performed to decompress the nerve root. Microsurgical diskectomy is a version of the standard procedure in which the surgeon uses a microscope to better see the disc.
- A *percutaneous diskectomy* is an outpatient surgical procedure that is done by using fluoroscopy and passing a tube through retroperitoneal soft tissues to the lateral border of the disc. A laser is used to destroy the damaged part of the disc.
- A common traditional procedure for lumbar disc disease is a *laminectomy.* Part of the posterior arch of the vertebra (referred to as *the lamina*) is surgically excised to gain access to and

remove all or part of the protruding disc. The procedure may be done as an outpatient or with a short hospital stay.

- A *spinal fusion* may be needed if the spine is unstable. The spine is stabilized by creating an ankylosis (fusion) of adjacent vertebrae with a bone graft from the patient's fibula or iliac crest (autograft) or from donated cadaver bone (allograft). Metal fixation with rods, plates, or screws may be implanted. A posterior lumbar interbody fusion may be performed to give extra support for bone grafting or a prosthetic device. Bone morphogenetic protein (BMP), a genetically engineered protein, may be used to stimulate growth of the bone graft in spinal fusions.
- Artificial disc replacement surgery for patients with DDD includes the use of the Charité disc for lower disc damage and the Prestige cervical disc system.

Nursing Management: Vertebral Disc Surgery

After vertebral disc surgery, a key intervention is maintaining proper alignment of the spine. Depending on the type and extent of surgery and the surgeon's preference, the patient may be able to dangle the legs over the side of the bed, stand, or even ambulate the same day of surgery.

After lumbar fusion, place pillows under the thighs when the patient is supine and between the legs when the patient is in the side-lying position to provide comfort and ensure alignment.

- The patient often fears turning or any movement that increases pain. Offer reassurance to the patient that the proper technique is being used to maintain body alignment. Have the patient logroll when changing position in bed.
- After surgery, most patients will need opioids, such as morphine IV for 24 to 48 hours. Patient-controlled analgesia (PCA) allows for maintaining optimal analgesic levels.
- Once oral fluids are tolerated, the patient may be switched to oral drugs, such as acetaminophen with codeine, hydrocodone, or oxycodone (Percocet). Diazepam (Valium) may be prescribed for muscle relaxation.

Because the spinal canal may be entered during the surgical procedure, there is potential for cerebrospinal fluid (CSF) leakage. Immediately report severe headache or CSF leakage on the dressing.

- Frequently monitor the patient's peripheral neurologic condition. Movement of arms and legs and assessment of sensation should at least equal preoperative status. Paresthesias, such as numbness and tingling, may not be relieved immediately after surgery. Report any new muscle weakness or paresthesias to the surgeon at once and record the finding in the patient's medical record.

Paralytic ileus and interference with bowel function may occur for several days. Assess whether the patient is passing flatus, has bowel sounds in all quadrants, and has a flat, soft abdomen. Stool softeners (e.g., docusate sodium [Colace]) and laxatives may aid in relieving and preventing constipation.

- Emptying the bladder may be hard because of activity restrictions, opioids, or anesthesia. Encourage men to dangle their legs over the side of the bed or stand to urinate if allowed by the surgeon. Urge patients to use a bedside commode or ambulate to the bathroom, when allowed, to promote bladder emptying. Intermittent catheterization or an indwelling urinary catheter may be needed by patients who have problems urinating.

Other nursing actions are required if the patient has had a spinal fusion. Because a bone graft is usually involved, the postoperative healing time is prolonged compared with that for a laminectomy. Activity may be limited for an extended time. A rigid orthosis (thoracic-lumbar-sacral orthosis or chair-back brace) is often used.

After cervical spine surgery, be alert for signs of spinal cord edema, such as respiratory distress and a worsening neurologic status of the upper extremities. The patient's neck may be immobilized in either a soft or a hard cervical collar.

In addition to the primary surgical site, regularly assess the donor site for the bone graft. The donor site usually causes greater postoperative pain than the fused area. A pressure dressing is applied to the donor site to prevent excessive bleeding. If the donor site is the fibula, include neurovascular extremity assessments.

- Teach the patient to avoid sitting or standing for prolonged periods. Encourage activities that include walking, lying down, and shifting weight from 1 foot to the other when standing.
- Teach the patient to think through an activity before starting a task requiring bending or stooping. Any twisting movement of the spine is contraindicated. The thighs and knees, rather than the back, should be used to absorb the shock of activity and movement.
- A firm mattress or bed board is essential.

INTESTINAL OBSTRUCTION

Description

Intestinal obstruction occurs when intestinal contents cannot pass through the gastrointestinal (GI) tract. An obstruction may be a small bowel obstruction (SBO) or large bowel/colon obstruction (LBO). The obstruction can be partial or complete, simple or strangulated. A partial obstruction usually resolves with conservative treatment, whereas a complete obstruction usually requires surgery. A simple obstruction has an intact blood supply, and a strangulated one does not.

Causes of intestinal obstruction are mechanical or nonmechanical (Fig. 15).

- *Mechanical obstruction* is a physical blockage of the intestinal lumen that mostly occurs in the small intestine. Surgical adhesions are the most common cause of SBO. They can develop within days of surgery or years later. Other causes of SBO are hernia, strictures from Crohn's disease, and intussusception after bariatric surgery. The most common cause of LBO is colorectal cancer (malignant obstruction). Other causes include adhesions, ischemia, Crohn's disease and volvulus. A volvulus is a twisting of the bowel that can result in intestinal obstruction.

- *Nonmechanical obstruction* occurs with reduced or absent peristalsis secondary to altered neuromuscular transmission of the parasympathetic innervation to the bowel. It may result from a neuromuscular or vascular disorder. *Paralytic (adynamic) ileus* (lack of intestinal peristalsis and bowel sounds) is the most

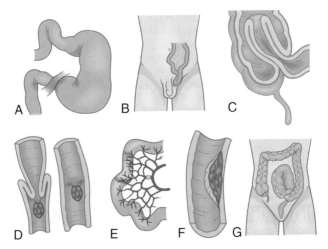

Fig. 15 Bowel obstructions. (A) Adhesions. (B) Strangulated inguinal hernia. (C) Ileocecal intussusception. (D) Intussusception from polyps. (E) Mesenteric occlusion. (F) Neoplasm. (G) Volvulus of the sigmoid colon.

common form of nonmechanical obstruction. It occurs to some degree after any abdominal surgery. Other causes of paralytic ileus include inflammatory reactions (e.g., acute pancreatitis, acute appendicitis), electrolyte abnormalities (especially hypokalemia), and thoracic or lumbar spinal fractures.

- *Vascular obstructions* are rare and are caused by an interference with the blood supply to a portion of the bowel. The most common causes are emboli and atherosclerosis of the mesenteric arteries.
- *Pseudoobstruction* is a GI motility disorder. There are several conditions that are associated with a pseudoobstruction. These include major surgery, electrolyte imbalance, neurologic conditions, medications, sepsis, cancer, trauma, and burns.

Pathophysiology

When fluid, gas, and intestinal contents accumulate proximal to the obstruction, distention occurs and the distal bowel collapses. As the proximal bowel becomes increasingly distended, the intraluminal bowel pressure rises. The high pressure leads to an increase in capillary permeability and extravasation of fluids and electrolytes into the peritoneal cavity. Retention of fluid in the intestine and peritoneal cavity leads to a severe decrease in circulating blood volume and results in hypotension and hypovolemic shock.

- In the most dangerous situation, the bowel becomes so distended that the blood flow is stopped, causing edema, cyanosis, and gangrene of bowel segment. This is called *intestinal strangulation* or *intestinal infarction.* If it is not corrected quickly, the bowel will become necrotic and rupture, leading to infection, septic shock, and death.
- Location of the obstruction determines the extent of fluid, electrolyte, and acid-base imbalances. With a high obstruction (e.g., upper duodenum), metabolic alkalosis may result from the loss of gastric hydrochloric acid (HCl) through vomiting or nasogastric (NG) intubation and suction. In SBO, dehydration occurs rapidly. If the obstruction is below the proximal colon, solid fecal material accumulates until symptoms of discomfort appear.

Clinical Manifestations

- Manifestations vary depending on the location of the obstruction. The most important early manifestations of an SBO are colicky abdominal pain, nausea, vomiting, and abdominal distention.
- Patients with obstructions in the proximal small intestine rapidly develop nausea and vomiting, which is sometimes projectile and contains bile. Vomiting usually relieves pain in higher intestinal

obstructions. Vomiting from more distal obstructions of the small intestine is gradual in onset and more fecal- and foul-smelling.

- Persistent, colicky abdominal pain, abdominal distention, constipation (new-onset), and lack of flatus are signs of lower intestinal obstruction.
- With mechanical obstruction, pain comes and goes in waves. By contrast, paralytic ileus produces a more constant, generalized discomfort. Strangulation causes rapid, severe, constant pain.
- Abdominal distention is usually minimally in proximal SBO and markedly increased in LBO. Abdominal tenderness and rigidity are usually absent unless strangulation or peritonitis has occurred.
- Bowel sounds are high-pitched above the area of obstruction. Bowel sounds may also be absent. *Borborygmi* (audible abdominal sounds caused by hyperactive intestinal motility) are often noted.

Diagnostic Studies

- CT scans and abdominal x-rays are used.
- Sigmoidoscopy or colonoscopy may provide direct visualization of an LBO.
- An elevated white blood cell (WBC) count may indicate strangulation or perforation.
- High hematocrit (Hct) values may reflect hemoconcentration.
- Low hemoglobin (Hgb) and Hct values may indicate bleeding from a neoplasm or strangulation with necrosis.
- Serum electrolytes, blood urea nitrogen (BUN), and serum creatinine are monitored frequently to assess the degree of dehydration.

Interprofessional Management

Treatment of a bowel obstruction depends on the cause. If a strangulated obstruction or perforation is present, the patient will need emergency surgery to relieve the obstruction and survive. In some, especially those resulting from surgical adhesions, an obstruction may resolve without surgery.

Surgery may involve simply resecting the obstructed segment of bowel and anastomosing the remaining healthy bowel back together. Partial or total colectomy, colostomy, or ileostomy may be done when extensive obstruction or necrosis is present. Sometimes, an obstruction can be removed nonsurgically. Colonoscopy offers a means to remove polyps, dilate strictures, and remove and destroy tumors with a laser.

The initial treatment includes placing the patient on NPO status, providing IV fluid therapy with either normal saline or lactated Ringer's solution, and giving IV antiemetics. If needed, insert an

NG tube for decompression and give ordered electrolyte replacement. Obtain blood cultures and start IV antibiotic therapy. Some patients need parenteral nutrition to allow bowel rest and improve nutritional status before surgery.

The treatment goal for a patient with a malignant obstruction is to regain patency and resolve the obstruction. Stents can be placed via endoscopic or fluoroscopic procedures. They are used for palliative purposes or as "a bridge to surgery," allowing a patient to avoid emergency surgery. This gives the interprofessional team time to correct fluid volume problems and treat other problems, thus improving surgical outcomes. Corticosteroids with antiemetic properties that decrease edema and inflammation may be used with stent placement.

Nursing Management
Goals
The patient with an intestinal obstruction will have relief and a return to normal bowel function, minimal to no discomfort, and normal fluid and electrolyte and acid-base status.
Nursing Interventions
Assess the patient regularly and notify the surgeon of changes in vital signs, changes in bowel sounds, decreased urine output, increased abdominal distention, and pain.

- Maintain a strict intake and output record including emesis and tube drainage.
- Monitor the patient closely for signs of dehydration and electrolyte imbalances. A patient with an SBO is more likely to have metabolic alkalosis. A patient with an LBO is at greater risk for metabolic acidosis.
- The patient is often restless, changing position to relieve the pain. Provide comfort measures and promote a restful environment.
- Vomiting leaves an unpleasant taste in the patient's mouth, and fecal odor may be present. With an NG tube in place, the patient will breathe through the mouth. Provide frequent oral care.
- Nursing care of the patient after surgery for an intestinal obstruction is similar to the care of the patient after a laparotomy (see Abdominal Pain, Acute, p. 3).

I

IRRITABLE BOWEL SYNDROME

Description
Irritable bowel syndrome (IBS) is a disorder characterized by chronic abdominal pain or discomfort and alteration of bowel patterns. Patients may have diarrhea or constipation, alternating periods of both.

IBS has no known organic cause. Psychologic stressors (e.g., depression, anxiety, panic disorders, posttraumatic stress disorder) are associated with the development and exacerbation of IBS. Patients often report a history of gastrointestinal (GI) infections and adverse reactions to food. Dietary intolerances that may contribute to symptoms include gluten and fermentable oligo-, di-, and monosaccharides and polyols (FODMAPs).

- Examples of oligosaccharides are wheat and rye products, some fruits and vegetables, onions, garlic, legumes, and nuts. The disaccharide lactose is found in milk and milk products. Fructose is a monosaccharide found in honey, apples, pears, and high-fructose corn syrup. Polyols are found in apples, pears, stone fruits, cauliflower, mushrooms, and artificial sweeteners, like sorbitol.

IBS is diagnosed solely on symptoms. The Rome IV criteria for diagnosing IBS require the presence of abdominal pain and/or discomfort at least 1 day per week for 3 months that is associated with 2 or more of the following: related to defecation, change in stool frequency, or change in the stool form. Depending on the stool patterns, IBS is categorized as IBS with constipation (IBS-C), IBS with diarrhea (IBS-D), IBS mixed, and IBS unsubtyped.

- Other common symptoms include abdominal distention, nausea, flatulence, bloating, urgency, mucus in the stool, and sensation of incomplete evacuation. Non-GI symptoms may include fatigue, headache, and sleep problems.

Ask patients to describe symptoms, health history (including psychosocial factors such as stress and anxiety), family history, and drug and diet history. Determine if and how IBS symptoms interfere with school, work, or recreational activities. Diagnostic tests are used to rule out other disorders, such as colorectal cancer, IBD, endometriosis, and malabsorption disorders (lactose intolerance, celiac disease).

Nursing and Interprofessional Management

No single therapy is effective for all patients with IBS. Treatment may include dealing with psychologic factors, dietary changes, and drugs to regulate stool output and reduce discomfort.

- Patients may benefit from keeping a diary of symptoms, diet, and episodes of stress to help identify any factors that trigger the IBS symptoms. Cognitive behavior therapy and stress management techniques may help a patient cope.
- Participating in regular exercise reduces bloating and constipation and reduces stress related symptoms.

Drug therapy focuses on the dominant bowel symptom and pain. The opioid agonist eluxadoline (Viberzi) decreases colonic contractions, to reduce diarrhea and pain. It is contraindicated in those without a gall bladder.

- An option for women with IBS-D is alosetron (Lotronex). Because of serious side effects (e.g., severe constipation, ischemic colitis), it is available only in a restricted access program.
- Other treatments for IBS-D include loperamide, antidepressants, and antispasmodic medications (hyoscyamine, dicyclomine). Antispasmodics decrease GI motility and smooth muscle spasms, reducing pain and diarrhea.

Women with IBS-C may benefit from lubiprostone (Amitiza). Men or women with IBS-C can take linaclotide (Linzess). It is contraindicated in patients with a history of mechanical obstruction or prior bowel surgery.

Review with the patient foods that are high in FODMAPs and teach them to follow a low FODMAP diet.

- If dairy products tend to cause symptoms, yogurt may be the best option because of the lactobacillus bacteria it contains. Probiotics can improve symptoms.
- Tell the patient with flatulence to avoid common gas-producing foods, such as broccoli and cabbage.
- For those with constipation, encourage an intake of enough dietary fiber to produce soft, painless bowel movements.

KIDNEY CANCER

Kidney cancer arises from the renal cortex or pelvis and calyces. Adenocarcinoma (renal cell carcinoma), the most common type, is twice as frequent in men as in women.

The most significant risk factor is cigarette smoking. Other risk factors include acquired cystic kidney disease, obesity, hypertension, and exposure to cadmium, asbestos, and gasoline.

Early-stage kidney cancer usually has no symptoms. The most common later manifestations are hematuria, flank pain, and a palpable mass in the flank or abdomen. Other signs include weight loss, fever, hypertension, and anemia. Local extension of kidney cancer into the renal vein and vena cava is common. The most common sites of metastases are lungs, liver, and long bones.

- Diagnosis is based on CT scan and ultrasound. Angiography, biopsy, and MRI are also used. Radionuclide scanning is used to detect metastases.

Nursing and Interprofessional Management

Preventive measures, including quitting smoking, maintaining a healthy weight, controlling BP, and reducing or avoiding exposure to toxins, can help reduce the incidence of kidney cancer. Patients in high-risk groups should be aware of their increased risk for kidney cancer. Teach them about symptoms (e.g., hematuria, hypertension).

- Partial nephrectomy or *simple total nephrectomy* (for smaller tumors) or a radical nephrectomy (for larger tumors) is the treatment for some renal cancers. *Radical nephrectomy* involves removal of the kidney, adrenal gland, surrounding fascia, part of the ureter, and draining lymph nodes. Nephrectomy can be performed by a conventional (open) approach or laparoscopically.
- Kidney cancer is resistant to most chemotherapy drug and radiation therapy.
- Immunotherapy, with agents including α-interferon and interleukin-2 (IL-2), is an option in metastatic disease.
- Targeted therapy is another treatment for metastatic kidney cancer. Kinase inhibitors include sunitinib (Sutent), sorafenib (Nexavar), cabozantinib (Cabometyx), and axitinib (Inlyta). Bevacizumab (Avastin), sunitinib (Sutent), and pazopanib (Votrient) inhibit the formation of new blood vessel growth to the tumor. Temsirolimus (Torisel) and everolimus (Afinitor) inhibit a specific protein known as the *mechanistic target of rapamycin* (mTOR).

KIDNEY DISEASE, CHRONIC

Description

Chronic kidney disease (CKD) involves progressive, irreversible loss of kidney function. CKD can be defined as either the presence of kidney damage or a decreased glomerular filtration rate (GFR) to < 60 mL/min/1.73 m^2 for more than 3 months. The classification of CKD is presented in Table 52. The last stage of kidney failure, termed *end-stage renal disease* (ESRD), occurs when the GFR is < 15 mL/min. At this point, renal replacement therapy (dialysis or transplantation) is required.

CKD has many different causes. The leading ones are diabetes (about 50%) and hypertension (about 25%). Less common causes include glomerulonephritis, cystic diseases, and urologic diseases. One of every 9 Americans has CKD. Over half a million Americans are receiving treatment (dialysis, transplantation).

Because the kidneys are highly adaptive, kidney disease is often not recognized until there is considerable nephron loss. CKD is underdiagnosed and undertreated because patients are often

TABLE 52 Stages of Chronic Kidney Disease

Description	GFR (mL/min/1.73 m²)	Clinical Action Plan
Stage 1		
Kidney damage with normal or ↑ GFR	≥90	Diagnosis and treatment CVD risk reduction Slow progression
Stage 2		
Kidney damage with mild ↓ GFR	60–89	Estimation of progression
Stage 3A		
Moderate ↓ GFR	45–59	Evaluation and treatment of complications
Stage 3B		
Moderate ↓ GFR	30–44	More aggressive treatment of complications
Stage 4		
Severe ↓ GFR	15–29	Preparation for renal replacement therapy (dialysis, kidney transplantation)
Stage 5		
Kidney failure	<15 (or dialysis)	Renal replacement therapy (if uremia is present and patient desires treatment)

CVD, Cardiovascular disease; *GFR,* glomerular filtration rate.
Source: Alseiari M, Meyer KB, Wong JB: Evidence underlying KDIGO (Kidney Disease: Improving Global Outcomes) guideline recommendations: A systematic review Am J Kid Dis 67:417, 2016.

asymptomatic. It is believed that about 70% of people with CKD are unaware they have the disease.

Prognosis and course of CKD are highly variable depending on the cause, patient's condition and age, and adequacy of health care. Some people live normal, active lives with compensated renal failure, while others rapidly progress to ESRD.

Clinical Manifestations

As kidney function deteriorates, every body system is affected. Manifestations are a result of retained substances including urea, creatinine, phenols, hormones, water, and electrolytes (see Fig. 46.2 in Harding et al., *Lewis' Medical-Surgical Nursing,* ed 11). *Uremia* is a syndrome in which kidney function declines and symptoms develop in multiple body systems. It often occurs when the GFR is < 10 mL/min. Manifestations of uremia vary among patients depending on the cause of kidney disease, comorbid conditions, age, and degree of adherence to the prescribed medical regimen.

- *Urinary system.* As CKD progresses, patients have increasing fluid retention and need diuretic therapy. After a period on dialysis, patients may develop anuria.
- *Metabolic disturbances.* As GFR decreases, blood urea nitrogen (BUN) and serum creatinine levels increase. Serum creatinine and creatinine clearance determinations (calculated GFR) are considered more accurate indicators of kidney function. As BUN increases, patients have nausea, vomiting, lethargy, fatigue, impaired thought processes, and headaches.
- *Electrolyte and acid-base imbalances.* Hyperkalemia results from decreased renal excretion, breakdown of cellular protein, bleeding, and metabolic acidosis. Sodium may be high, normal, or low in kidney failure. Sodium retention contributes to edema, hypertension, and heart failure. Metabolic acidosis results from the kidneys' impaired ability to excrete excess acid and from the defective reabsorption and regeneration of bicarbonate.
- *Altered carbohydrate metabolism and elevated triglycerides.* Mild to moderate hyperglycemia and hyperinsulinemia occur. Insulin and glucose metabolism may improve after the initiation of dialysis. Patients with diabetes who develop uremia may require less insulin than before the onset of CKD. Insulin, which depends on the kidneys for excretion, remains in circulation longer.
- *Hematologic system.* Anemia results from a lack of erythropoietin. Bleeding tendencies occur because of a defect in platelet function. Cellular and humoral immune responses are suppressed, resulting in increased susceptibility to infection.
- *Cardiovascular system.* The most common cause of death in patients with CKD is cardiovascular disease (CVD). Vascular calcification and arterial stiffness are major contributors to CVD in CKD. Hypertension is highly prevalent among patients with CKD because hypertension is both a cause and a consequence of CKD. Hypertension is worsened by sodium retention and increased extracellular fluid volume.
- *Musculoskeletal system.* CKD mineral and bone disorder results in skeletal complications, such as *osteomalacia* (bone

demineralization from slow bone turnover and defective mineralization of newly formed bone) and *osteitis fibrosa* (decalcification of the bone and replacement of bone tissue with fibrous
tissue).

Additional systemic signs include pulmonary edema, constipation, peripheral neuropathy, pruritus, infertility, and personality
and behavior changes.

Diagnostic Studies

- Urinalysis detects red blood cells (RBCs), white blood cells
  (WBCs), casts, protein, and glucose.
- BUN and serum creatinine are elevated.
- GFR, obtained from 24-hour urine creatinine clearance mea-
  sures, is decreased.
- Hematocrit (Hct) and hemoglobin (Hgb) levels are decreased.
- Ultrasound can be used to detect obstructions and kidney size.
- Kidney biopsy provides a definitive diagnosis.

Interprofessional Management

The focus in CKD is to preserve existing kidney function, reduce the
risks of CVD, prevent complications, and provide for the patient's
comfort. It is important that patients with CKD receive appropriate
follow-up care with referral to a nephrologist early in the course of
the disease. The focus during stages 1 through 4 (see Table 52) before
the need for dialysis (stage 5) includes the control of hypertension,
hyperparathyroid disease, anemia, hyperglycemia, and dyslipidemia.

- Acute hyperkalemia may require treatment with IV glucose and
  insulin to move potassium into the cells, or IV 10% calcium gluconate. Sodium polystyrene sulfonate, a cation-exchange resin
  or patiromer (Veltassa), an oral suspension that binds potassium
  in the GI tract, are used to lower potassium levels in stage 4
  CKD. Dialysis may be required to decrease potassium if dysrhythmias are present.
- Control and treatment of hypertension is discussed in Hypertension, p. 318. Treatment of hypertension includes weight loss (if
  obese), therapeutic lifestyle changes (e.g., exercise, avoiding
  alcohol, smoking cessation), diet recommendations, and administration of antihypertensive agents. Drugs most commonly used
  include diuretics, β-adrenergic blockers, calcium-channel
  blockers, angiotensin-converting enzyme (ACE) inhibitors,
  and angiotensin receptor blockers.
- Phosphate binders such as calcium carbonate (e.g., Caltrate)
  and calcium acetate are used to bind phosphate in the bowel, which
  is then excreted in the stool. Phosphate binders that do not contain
  calcium include sevelamer (Renagel) and lanthanum (Fosrenol) or

the iron-based, calcium-free phosphate binders, such as sucroferric oxyhydroxide (Velphoro) and ferric citrate (Auryxia).

- Exogenous erythropoietin (epoetin alfa [Epogen, Procrit]) is used to treat the anemia of CKD.

The kidneys partially or totally excrete many drugs. CKD causes decreased elimination, leading to drug accumulation and the potential for drug toxicity. Drugs of particular concern include digoxin, diabetic agents (metformin, glyburide), antibiotics (e.g., vancomycin, gentamicin), and opioids.

Nutritional Therapy

The diet for CKD is designed to maintain good nutrition (see Table 46.10 for specific recommended restrictions in Harding et al., *Lewis' Medical-Surgical Nursing*, ed 11). Refer patients with CKD to a dietitian for nutritional teaching. For CKD stages 1 to 4, many health care providers (HCPs) encourage a normal protein intake. However, teach patients to avoid high-protein diets and supplements, because they may overstress the diseased kidneys. Nutritional therapy also includes the restriction of fluid, sodium, potassium, and phosphate.

Nursing Management

Goals

The overall goals are that the patient with CKD will show knowledge of and ability to adhere to the therapeutic plan, take part in decision making for the plan of care and future treatment modality, have effective coping strategies, and continue with activities of daily living within physiologic limitations.

Additional information on nursing diagnoses for the patient with CKD is presented in eNursing Care Plan 46-1 (available on the website).

Nursing Interventions

Identify people at risk for CKD including those diagnosed with diabetes or hypertension and those with a history (or a family history) of kidney disease or repeated urinary tract infections. These persons should have regular checkups that include routine urinalysis and calculation of GFR.

- Those at risk need to take measures to prevent or delay the progression of CKD, including glycemic control for patients with diabetes; BP control; and lifestyle modifications, including smoking cessation.
- Because patients with CKD take many drugs, a pillbox organizer or a list of the drugs and the times of administration may be helpful. Teach the patient to avoid over-the-counter drugs such as nonsteroidal antiinflammatory drugs (NSAIDs) and magnesium-based laxatives and antacids.

- When potentially nephrotoxic drugs are prescribed, monitor the patient's renal function with serum creatinine, BUN, and GFR.
- Advise patients with diabetes to report any changes in urine appearance (color, odor), frequency, or volume to the HCP.
- Inform the patient that if dialysis is chosen, transplantation is still an option. If a transplanted organ fails, the patient can return to dialysis.

Even though transplantation offers the best therapeutic management for patients with kidney failure, the critical shortage of donor organs limits this option.

Patients may initiate a conversation about palliative care. Respect the patient's choice to decline treatment. Listen to the patient and caregivers, allowing them to do most of the talking, and pay special attention to their hopes and fears.

▼ Patient and Caregiver Teaching
Teach the patient and family about the diet, drugs, and follow-up medical care (Table 53).

TABLE 53   Patient and Caregiver Teaching

Chronic Kidney Disease

Include the following information in the teaching plan for the patient and caregiver.

1. Dietary (sodium, potassium, phosphate) and fluid restrictions.
2. Common problems patient will encounter in modifying diet and fluid intake.
3. Signs and symptoms of electrolyte imbalance, especially high potassium.
4. Alternative ways of reducing thirst, such as sucking on ice cubes, lemon, or hard candy.
5. Reasons for prescribed drugs and common side effects. Examples:
   - Phosphate binders (including calcium supplements used as phosphate barriers) should be taken with meals.
   - Take calcium supplements prescribed to treat hypocalcemia on an empty stomach, but not at the same time as iron supplements.
   - Iron supplements should be taken between meals.
6. The importance of reporting any of the following: Weight gain >4 lb (2 kg), increasing BP, shortness of breath, edema, increasing fatigue or weakness, or confusion or lethargy
7. Need for support and encouragement. Share concerns about lifestyle changes, living with a chronic illness, and decisions about type of dialysis or transplantation.

KIDNEY INJURY, ACUTE

Description

Acute kidney injury (AKI) is the term used to encompass the entire range of the syndrome ranging from a slight deterioration in kidney function to severe impairment. Evidence of severity can range from a small increase in serum creatinine or reduction in urine output to the development of azotemia (an accumulation of nitrogenous waste products [urea nitrogen, creatinine] in the blood). AKI can develop over hours or days with progressive elevations of blood urea nitrogen (BUN), creatinine, and potassium with or without a reduction in urine output.

Although AKI is potentially reversible, it has a high mortality rate. AKI usually affects people with other life-threatening conditions. It often follows severe, prolonged hypotension or hypovolemia or exposure to a nephrotoxic agent.

Pathophysiology

AKI is categorized as prerenal, intrarenal (or intrinsic), or postrenal (Fig. 16).

- *Prerenal* causes of AKI involve factors external to the kidneys that reduce renal blood flow and lead to decreased glomerular perfusion and filtration. In prerenal oliguria, there is no damage to the kidney tissue (parenchyma). The oliguria is caused by a decrease in circulating blood volume (e.g., severe dehydration, decreased cardiac output) and is reversible with treatment. Prerenal conditions can lead to intrarenal disease if renal ischemia is prolonged.
- *Intrarenal* causes include conditions that cause direct damage to the kidney tissue, resulting in impaired nephron function. Intrarenal AKI is usually caused by prolonged ischemia, nephrotoxins (e.g., antibiotics), myoglobin released from necrotic muscle cells, or hemoglobin released from hemolyzed red blood cells (RBCs). Kidney diseases such as systemic lupus erythematosus and glomerulonephritis may also cause AKI. *Acute tubular necrosis* (ATN) is the most common cause of intrarenal AKI in hospitalized patients and is primarily the result of ischemia, nephrotoxins, or sepsis.
- *Postrenal* causes involve mechanical obstruction of urinary outflow. As the flow of urine is obstructed, urine refluxes into the renal pelvis, impairing kidney function. The most common causes are prostate cancer, benign prostatic hyperplasia (BPH), urinary tract calculi, trauma, and extrarenal tumors. Bilateral ureteral obstruction leads to *hydronephrosis* (kidney dilation),

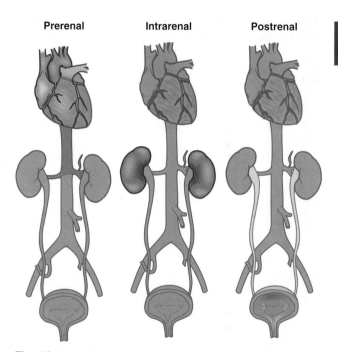

Fig. 16 Prerenal, intrarenal, and postrenal causes of acute kidney injury (AKI).

increase in hydrostatic pressure, and tubular blockage, resulting in a progressive decline in kidney function. If bilateral obstruction is relieved within 48 hours of onset, complete recovery is likely. After 12 weeks, recovery is unlikely.

Clinical Manifestations

Clinically, AKI may progress through 3 phases: oliguric, diuretic, and recovery. In some situations, the patient does not recover from AKI, and chronic kidney disease (CKD) results (see Kidney Disease, Chronic, p. 358).

The RIFLE classification describes the stages of AKI (Table 54): *R*isk, the first stage of AKI, is followed by *i*njury, the second stage; AKI then increases in severity to the final or third stage, *f*ailure. The 2 outcome variables are *l*oss and *e*nd-stage kidney disease.

Oliguric Phase

The most common initial manifestation of AKI is oliguria, a reduction in urine output to < 400 mL/day. Oliguria usually occurs

TABLE 54   RIFLE Classification for Staging Acute Kidney Injury

	GFR Criteria	Urine Output Criteria	Clinical Example
Risk	Serum creatinine increased × 1.5 OR GFR decreased by 25%	Urine output <0.5 mL/kg/hr for 6 hr	• 68-yr-old black woman with type 2 diabetes, hypertension, CAD, and CKD • Scheduled to undergo emergency coronary artery bypass graft • Serum creatinine is 1.8 mg/dL (increased), weight 60 kg • Calculated GFR is 35 mL/min/1.73 m^2 • Has Stage 3b CKD
Injury	Serum creatinine increased × 2 OR GFR decreased by 50%	Urine output <0.5 mL/kg/hr for 12 hr	• During surgery, she is hypotensive for a sustained period • Diagnosed with acute tubular necrosis • After surgery: Serum creatinine is 3.6 mg/dL, urine output reduced to 28 mL/hr
Failure	Serum creatinine increased × 3 OR GFR decreased by 75% OR Serum creatinine >4 mg/dL with acute rise of ≥0.5 mg/dL	Urine output <0.3 mL/kg/hr for 24 hr (oliguria) OR Anuria for 12 hr	• 72 hours after surgery, develops ventilator-associated pneumonia and sepsis while in ICU • Serum creatinine rises to 5.2 mg/dL, urine output drops to 10 mL/hr • BP remains low despite dopamine therapy

K

Loss	Persistent acute kidney failure Complete loss of kidney function for >4 wk	—	• Starts on continuous venovenous hemodialysis
End-stage renal disease	Complete loss of kidney function for >3 mo	—	• After 3 wk of therapy she has a cardiopulmonary arrest and does not survive
			—

CAD, Coronary artery disease; *CKD,* chronic kidney disease; *GFR,* glomerular filtration rate; *ICU,* intensive care unit.

within 1 to 7 days of injury to the kidneys. If the cause is ischemia, oliguria often occurs within 24 hours. By contrast, when nephrotoxic drugs are involved, onset may be delayed for up to a week. The oliguric phase lasts on average about 10 to 14 days but can last for months. The longer this phase lasts, the poorer the prognosis for complete recovery of renal function.

Nonoliguric AKI has a urine output > 400 mL/day. About 50% of patients will be nonoliguric, making the initial diagnosis more difficult.

While changes in urine output generally do not correspond to changes in glomerular filtration rate (GFR), they can be helpful in distinguishing the cause of AKI. For example, anuria (no urine output) is usually seen with urinary tract obstruction. Oliguria is often seen with prerenal causes. Nonoliguric AKI is seen with acute interstitial nephritis and ATN.

- A urinalysis may show casts, red blood cells (RBCs), white blood cells (WBCs), a specific gravity fixed at around 1.010, and urine osmolality around 300 mOsm/kg (300 mmol/kg). This is the same specific gravity and osmolality as for plasma.
- Fluid retention occurs as urinary output decreases. Neck veins may be distended with a bounding pulse, and edema and hypertension may develop. Fluid overload can lead to heart failure, pulmonary edema, and pericardial and pleural effusions.
- Metabolic acidosis results when the kidneys cannot synthesize ammonia (needed for hydrogen ion excretion) or excrete acid products of metabolism. The serum bicarbonate level decreases because bicarbonate is depleted in buffering hydrogen ions. The patient may develop Kussmaul (rapid, deep) respirations to excrete more carbon dioxide.
- Damaged tubules cannot conserve sodium. Urinary excretion of sodium may increase, resulting in normal or below-normal levels of serum sodium.
- In AKI, the serum potassium level increases because the kidney's normal ability to excrete potassium is impaired. Acute or rapid development of hyperkalemia may result in clinical signs that are apparent on electrocardiogram (ECG). These changes include peaked T waves, widening of the QRS complex, and ST segment depression. Because cardiac muscle is intolerant of acute increases in potassium, treatment is essential when hyperkalemia develops.
- Leukocytosis is often present. The most common cause of death in AKI is infection.
- BUN and serum creatinine levels are elevated in kidney failure.
- Neurologic changes can occur as nitrogenous waste products accumulate in the brain and other nervous tissue. Manifestations

can be as mild as fatigue and difficulty concentrating and can escalate to seizures, stupor, and coma.

Diuretic Phase

During the diuretic phase, daily urine output is 1 to 3 L/day but may reach 5 L/day or more. The kidneys have recovered the ability to excrete wastes but not to concentrate urine.

- The diuretic phase may last 1 to 3 weeks, with the patient's acid-base, electrolyte, and waste product values beginning to normalize. Because of large losses of fluid and electrolytes, monitor the patient for hyponatremia, hypokalemia, and dehydration.

Recovery Phase

The recovery phase begins when the GFR increases, allowing the BUN and serum creatinine levels to decrease. Kidney function may take up to 12 months to stabilize.

- The patient's overall health, severity of renal failure, and number and type of complications influence the outcome of AKI. Some patients progress to end-stage renal disease (ESRD). Patients who recover may achieve clinically normal kidney function but remain in an early stage of CKD.

Diagnostic Studies

- History is essential to determine the cause.
- Urine output and serum creatinine help make the diagnosis.
- Urinalysis is done to assess sediment, casts, hematuria, pyuria, and crystals.
- Urine osmolality, sodium content, and specific gravity help in differentiating the cause.
- Ultrasound and renal scan are used to assess renal blood flow, tubular function, and the collecting system.
- CT scan can identify lesions, masses, obstructions, and vascular abnormalities.

Interprofessional Management

Because AKI is potentially reversible, the primary goals of treatment are to eliminate the cause, manage the signs and symptoms, and prevent complications while the kidneys recover. The first step is to determine if there is adequate intravascular volume and cardiac output (CO) to ensure adequate perfusion of the kidneys.

- Diuretic therapy usually includes loop diuretics (e.g., furosemide [Lasix], bumetanide [Bumex]) or an osmotic diuretic (e.g., mannitol). If AKI is already established, forcing fluids and diuretics will not be effective.
- Closely monitor fluid intake during the oliguric phase.
- Hyperkalemia can cause dysrhythmias. Both insulin and sodium bicarbonate temporarily shift potassium into the cells, but it

eventually shifts back out. Calcium gluconate raises the threshold at which dysrhythmias occur. Only sodium polystyrene sulfonate (Kayexalate), patiromer (Veltassa), or dialysis actually remove potassium from the body.

If conservative therapy is not effective in treating AKI, renal replacement therapy (RRT) is used. The most common indications for RRT in AKI are: (1) volume overload, resulting in compromised cardiac and/or pulmonary status; (2) high serum potassium level; (3) metabolic acidosis (serum bicarbonate level < 15 mEq/L [15 mmol/L]); (4) BUN level > 120 mg/dL (43 mmol/L); (5) significant change in mental status; and (6) pericarditis, pericardial effusion, or cardiac tamponade.

- Peritoneal dialysis is an option for renal replacement, but not often used.
- Intermittent hemodialysis (HD) (4 hours daily, every other day, or 3 or 4 times per week) and continuous renal replacement therapy (CRRT) have both been used effectively. CRRT is provided continuously over 24 hours through cannulation of an artery and a vein, or of 2 veins.

Nutritional Therapy

The goal of nutritional management is to provide adequate calories to prevent catabolism despite the restrictions that prevent electrolyte and fluid problems and azotemia. Adequate energy should primarily be from carbohydrate and fat sources to prevent ketosis from endogenous fat breakdown and gluconeogenesis from muscle protein breakdown.

- 30 to 35 kcal/kg and 0.8 to 1.0 g protein/kg is recommended to prevent the further breakdown of body protein for energy purposes. Essential amino acid supplements can be given.
- Fat emulsion IV infusions provide a good source of nonprotein calories.
- Potassium and sodium are regulated per plasma levels. Sodium is restricted as needed to prevent edema, hypertension, and heart failure.

If a patient cannot maintain adequate oral intake, enteral nutrition is the preferred route for nutritional support (see Enteral Nutrition, p. 685). When the gastrointestinal tract is not functional, parenteral nutrition is needed (see Parenteral Nutrition, p. 710).

Nursing Management

Goals

The overall goals for the patient with AKI are to recover without any loss of kidney function, maintain normal fluid and electrolyte balance, have decreased anxiety, and adhere to and understand the need for follow-up care.

Nursing Interventions

Prevention and early recognition of AKI are essential because of the high mortality rate. Focus on: (1) identifying and monitoring high-risk populations, (2) controlling exposure to industrial chemicals and nephrotoxic drugs, and (3) preventing prolonged episodes of hypotension and hypovolemia. In the hospital, the factors that increase the risk for developing AKI are advanced age, massive trauma, extensive burns, heart failure, obstetric complications, and preexisting CKD.

- Carefully monitor intake and output and electrolyte balance. Record extrarenal losses of fluid from vomiting, diarrhea, and hemorrhage.
- Prompt replacement of significant fluid losses helps prevent ischemic tubular damage associated with trauma, burns, and extensive surgery. Intake and output records and the patient's weight provide valuable indicators of fluid volume status.
- Monitor renal function in persons taking potentially nephrotoxic drugs. Caution the patient about the use of over-the-counter analgesics (especially nonsteroidal antiinflammatory drugs [NSAIDs]), because these may worsen kidney function in the patient with mild CKD.
- Angiotensin-converting enzyme (ACE) inhibitors can decrease perfusion pressure and cause hyperkalemia. If other measures, such as diet modification and diuretics, cannot control hyperkalemia, the ACE inhibitor may need to be reduced or stopped.

You have a key role in managing fluid and electrolyte balance during the oliguric and diuretic phases. Observe and record accurate intake and output.

- Assess for common signs and symptoms of hypervolemia (in the oliguric phase) or hypovolemia (in the diuretic phase), potassium and sodium changes, and other electrolyte imbalances that may occur in AKI.
- Because infection is the leading cause of death in AKI, meticulous aseptic technique is critical. A patient with renal failure who has an infection may not have an elevated temperature. Teach patients to avoid crowds and those with infections.
- If antibiotics are used to treat infection, the type, frequency, and dosage must be carefully considered. The kidneys are the primary route of excretion for many antibiotics.
- Perform skin care and take measures to prevent pressure injuries, because mobility may be impaired. Mouth care is important to prevent stomatitis.
- The long-term convalescence of 3 to 12 months may cause psychosocial and financial hardships for both the patient and family. Make appropriate referrals for counseling.

Encourage the patient to schedule regular follow-up and evaluation of kidney function.

LACTASE DEFICIENCY

Description

Lactase deficiency is a condition in which the lactase enzyme that breaks down lactose into 2 simple sugars (glucose and galactose) is deficient or absent.

Primary lactase insufficiency is most often a result of genetic factors. People in certain ethnic or racial groups, especially those with Asian or African ancestry, develop low lactase levels in childhood. Other causes include low lactase levels resulting from premature birth and congenital lactase deficiency, a rare genetic disorder. Lactose malabsorption can also occur when bacterial overgrowth promotes lactose fermentation in the small bowel, and when intestinal mucosal damage interferes with absorption (e.g., inflammatory bowel disease, celiac disease).

Clinical Manifestations

Manifestations of lactose intolerance include bloating, flatulence, crampy abdominal pain, and diarrhea. Diarrhea results from the excess undigested lactose in the small intestine. The lactose attracts water molecules, which prevents water being properly absorbed. Symptoms generally occur within 30 minutes to several hours after drinking a glass of milk or ingesting a milk product.

Diagnostic Studies

Many lactose-intolerant people are aware of their milk intolerance and avoid milk products. Lactose intolerance is diagnosed by a lactose tolerance test, lactose hydrogen breath test, or genetic testing.

Nursing and Interprofessional Management

Treatment consists of eliminating lactose from the diet by avoiding milk and milk products and/or replacing lactase with commercially available preparations. Teach the patient the importance of adherence to the diet.

- A lactose-free diet may be gradually advanced to a low-lactose diet.
- Many lactose-intolerant people can tolerate small amounts of lactose.
- Avoiding milk and milk products can lead to calcium deficiency. Supplements may be necessary to prevent osteoporosis.

- Lactase enzyme (Lactaid), available as an over-the-counter product, is mixed with milk and breaks down lactose before the milk is ingested. A number of milk products pretreated with lactase enzyme are available.

LEIOMYOMAS

Leiomyomas (uterine fibroids) are common benign smooth muscle tumors in the uterus. The cause of leiomyomas is unknown. They appear to depend on estrogen and progesterone, because they grow slowly during the reproductive years and undergo atrophy after menopause.

Most women with leiomyomas do not have symptoms. Those who develop symptoms present with abnormal uterine bleeding, pain, or symptoms associated with pelvic pressure. Pain is associated with infection or twisting of the pedicle from which the tumor is growing. Pressure on surrounding organs may result in rectal, bladder, and lower abdominal discomfort.

Diagnosis is based on pelvic examination findings of an enlarged uterus distorted by nodular masses. Treatment depends on the patient's symptoms, age, and desire to bear children, and the location and size of the tumor or tumors. Ultrasound can confirm the diagnosis.

- The most common treatment is hormonal therapy using oral contraceptives to slow tumor growth and manage abnormal uterine bleeding.
- Persistent heavy menstrual bleeding causing anemia and large tumors are indications for surgery. Leiomyomas are removed by hysterectomy or myomectomy. A myomectomy (removal of only the fibroid tumor) is performed for women who wish to preserve the uterus.
- Uterine artery embolization is an alternative treatment for uterine fibroids. Embolic material (small plastic or gelatin beads) injected into the uterine artery blocks blood flow to shrink the fibroid.

LEUKEMIA

Description

Leukemia is a general term used to describe a group of cancers affecting the blood and blood-forming tissues of the bone marrow, lymph system, and spleen. It results in an accumulation of dysfunctional cells secondary to loss of regulation in cell division.

Leukemia has no single cause. Most types of leukemia result from a combination of factors including genetic and environmental influences.

Classification

Leukemia can be classified as acute or chronic and by the type of white blood cell (WBC) involved. By combining the acute and chronic categories with the cell type involved, one can identify 4 major types of leukemia. Table 55 summarizes the relative incidence and features of the 4 types of leukemia.

Acute myelogenous leukemia (AML) represents only one-third of all leukemias, but it makes up about 80% of the acute leukemias in adults. Its onset is often abrupt and dramatic. A patient may have serious infections and abnormal bleeding from onset of the disease. AML is characterized by uncontrolled proliferation of myeloblasts, the precursors of granulocytes. There is bone marrow hyperplasia. Clinical manifestations are related to replacement of normal cells in the marrow by leukemic myeloblasts and to infiltration of other organs and tissue.

Acute lymphocytic leukemia (ALL) is the most common type of leukemia in children and accounts for about 20% of acute leukemias in adults. In ALL, immature lymphocytes proliferate in the bone marrow. Most are of B cell origin. Most patients have fever at time of diagnosis. Signs and symptoms may appear abruptly with bleeding or fever, or their onset may be insidious, with progressive weakness, fatigue, and bleeding tendencies. Central nervous system (CNS) manifestations are especially common in ALL.

Chronic myelogenous leukemia (CML) is caused by excessive development of neoplastic granulocytes in the bone marrow. CML usually has a chronic stable phase that lasts for several years, followed by development of an acute aggressive phase (blastic phase).

- The Philadelphia chromosome, which is present in 90% to 95% of patients with CML, is a diagnostic hallmark of CML. In addition, its presence is an important indicator of residual disease or relapse after treatment.

Chronic lymphocytic leukemia (CLL) is the most common leukemia in adults in Western countries. It is characterized by the production and accumulation of functionally inactive but long-lived, small, mature-appearing lymphocytes. The B lymphocyte is usually involved. Lymph node enlargement (lymphadenopathy) is present throughout the body. Because CLL is usually a disease of older adults, treatment decisions should consider disease progression and side effects. Many patients in the early stages of CLL require

L

TABLE 55 Types of Leukemia

Type	Age at Onset	Clinical Manifestations	Diagnostic Findings
Acute myelogenous leukemia (AML)	Accounts for 15%–20% of acute leukemia in children and 80% in adults Increase in incidence with advancing age after 60 yr	Fatigue and weakness, headache, mouth sores, anemia, bleeding, fever, infection, sternal tenderness, gingival hyperplasia, mild hepatosplenomegaly (in one-third of patients)	Low RBC count, Hgb, Hct, platelet count Low to high WBC count with myeloblasts High LDH Hypercellular bone marrow with myeloblasts
Acute lymphocytic leukemia (ALL)	Median diagnosis is 15 years with 57.2% diagnosed at younger than 20 years. About 27% of cases are diagnosed at age 4 yr or older and only 11% at age 65 yr or older	Fever, pallor, bleeding, anorexia, fatigue and weakness. Bone, joint, and abdominal pain. Generalized lymphadenopathy, infections, weight loss, hepatosplenomegaly, headache, mouth sores, neurologic manifestations: CNS involvement, increased intracranial pressure (nausea, vomiting, lethargy, cranial nerve dysfunction) from meningeal infiltration. Men may have painless enlargement of the scrotum	Low RBC, Hgb, Hct, platelet count. Low, normal, or high WBC count. High LDH. Hypercellular bone marrow with lymphoblasts. Lymphoblasts may be in cerebrospinal fluid. Presence of Philadelphia chromosome (up to 30% of patients). Up to 15% may have a mediastinal mass

Continued

TABLE 55　Types of Leukemia—cont'd

Type	Age at Onset	Clinical Manifestations	Diagnostic Findings
Chronic myelogenous leukemia (CML)	Increase in incidence with advancing age with median age at diagnosis of 67 yr Rare in children	No symptoms early in disease Fatigue and weakness, fever, sternal tenderness, weight loss, joint pain, bone pain, massive splenomegaly, increase in sweating	Low RBC count, Hgb, Hct High platelet count early, lower count later ↑ banded neutrophils and myeloblasts and often basophils, normal number of lymphocytes, and normal or low number of monocytes Nucleated red cells are common Low leukocyte alkaline phosphatase Presence of Philadelphia chromosome in 90% or more of patients
Chronic lymphocytic leukemia (CLL)	Increase in incidence with advancing age after 65 yr, with predominance in men	Frequently no symptoms Detection of disease often during examination for unrelated condition, chronic fatigue, anorexia, splenomegaly and lymphadenopathy, hepatomegaly May progress to fever, night sweats, weight loss, fatigue, and frequent infections	Mild anemia and thrombocytopenia with disease progression Total WBC count >100,000/μL Increase in peripheral lymphocytes and lymphocytes in bone marrow May have autoimmune hemolytic anemia, idiopathic thrombocytopenic purpura, and hypogammaglobulinemia

CNS, Central nervous system; *Hct,* hematocrit; *Hgb,* hemoglobin; *LDH,* lactate dehydrogenase; *RBC,* red blood cell; *WBC,* white blood cell.

no treatment, but 30% require immediate intervention at time of diagnosis.

Clinical Manifestations

Although the manifestations of leukemia are varied, they relate to problems caused by bone marrow failure and the formation of leukemic infiltrates (see Table 55). The patient is predisposed to development of anemia, thrombocytopenia, and decreased number and function of WBCs.

- WBC infiltration into the organs leads to problems such as splenomegaly, hepatomegaly, lymphadenopathy, bone pain, meningeal irritation, and oral lesions.

Diagnostic Studies

- Peripheral blood evaluation and bone marrow examination are the primary methods of diagnosing and classifying the types of leukemia.
- Morphologic, histochemical, immunologic, and cytogenetic methods are all used to identify leukemic cell types, stage of development and significant genetic mutations.
- Studies such as lumbar puncture and positron emission tomography (PET) or CT scans can detect leukemic cells outside the blood and bone marrow.

Interprofessional Management

Care first focuses on the goal of attaining remission.

- In some cases, such as nonsymptomatic patients with CLL, watchful waiting with active supportive care may be appropriate.
- Because cytotoxic chemotherapy is the mainstay of treatment for some patients, you must understand the principles of cancer chemotherapy, including cellular kinetics, the use of multiple drugs rather than single agents, and the cell cycle (see Chemotherapy, p. 674).
- Corticosteroids and radiation therapy may have a role in therapy for the patient with leukemia. Total body radiation may be used to prepare a patient for bone marrow transplantation, or radiation may be restricted to certain areas (fields), such as the liver, spleen, or other organs affected by infiltrates.
- In ALL, prophylactic intrathecal methotrexate or cytarabine is given to decrease CNS involvement. When CNS leukemia occurs, cranial radiation may be used. Immunotherapy and targeted therapy are indicated for specific types of leukemia (see Chapter 30 in Harding et al., *Lewis' Medical-Surgical Nursing,* ed 11).

Combination chemotherapy is the mainstay of treatment for leukemia. The 3 purposes for using multiple drugs are to: (1) decrease drug resistance, (2) minimize drug toxicity to the patient by using multiple drugs with varying toxicities, and (3) interrupt cell growth at multiple points in the cell cycle.

Hematopoietic stem cell transplantation (HSCT) is another type of therapy used for patients with different forms of leukemia. The goal of HSCT is to totally eliminate leukemia cells from the body using combinations of chemotherapy with or without total body radiation. This treatment also eradicates the patient's hematopoietic stem cells, which are then replaced with those of a human leukocyte antigen (HLA)-matched sibling, with those of a volunteer donor (allogeneic) or an identical twin (syngeneic), or with the patient's own (autologous) stem cells that were removed (harvested) before the intensive therapy. (See content on HSCT in Chapter 30 of Harding et al., *Lewis' Medical-Surgical Nursing,* ed 11.)

The primary complications of patients with allogeneic HSCT are graft-versus-host disease (GVHD), relapse of leukemia, and infection or sepsis. The patient must weigh the significant risks of treatment-related death or treatment failure (relapse) against the hope of cure.

Nursing Management
Goals
The patient with leukemia will understand and cooperate with the treatment plan, have minimal side effects and complications associated with both the disease and its treatment, and feel hopeful and supported during periods of treatment, relapse, or remission.

See nursing care plans available on the website for anemia (eNursing Care Plan 30-1), thrombocytopenia (eNursing Care Plan 30-2), and neutropenia (eNursing Care Plan 30-3).

Nursing Interventions
The nursing role during acute phases of leukemia is extremely challenging because the patient has many physical and psychosocial needs. The diagnosis of leukemia can evoke great fear and be equated with death.

- Help the patient realize that although the future may be uncertain, one can have a meaningful quality of life while in remission or with disease control.
- Families also need help in adjusting to the stress of the abrupt onset of serious illness and losses imposed by the sick role. The diagnosis of leukemia often brings with it the need to make difficult decisions at a time of profound stress for the patient and family.
- You are an important advocate in helping the patient and family understand the complexities of treatment decisions and manage the side effects and toxicities. A patient may require protective

isolation or may need to temporarily geographically relocate to an appropriate treatment center. This situation can lead a patient to feel deserted and isolated at a time when support is most needed.

From a physical care perspective, you are challenged to make assessments and plan care to help the patient deal with the severe side effects of chemotherapy. The life-threatening results of bone marrow suppression (anemia, thrombocytopenia, neutropenia) require aggressive nursing interventions.

Review all drugs being administered. Assess laboratory data reflecting the effects of the drugs. Quality nursing care significantly affects patient survival and comfort during aggressive chemotherapy.

▼ Patient and Caregiver Teaching

Teach the patient and caregivers the importance of continued diligence in disease management and the need for follow-up care.

Involving the patient in survivor networks, support groups, or services may help the patient adapt to living with a life-threatening illness. Exploring community resources (e.g., American Cancer Society, Leukemia Society) may reduce the financial burden and feelings of dependence. Also provide resources for spiritual support.

LIVER CANCER

Description

Primary *liver cancer* (hepatocellular carcinoma [HCC]) is the fifth most common cancer in the world and the second most common cause of cancer death worldwide. It is the most common cause of death in patients with cirrhosis.

The incidence of HCC is rising in the United States because of the large number of patients infected with chronic hepatitis C. Cirrhosis caused by hepatitis C is the most common cause of HCC in the United States. Other primary liver tumors are cholangiomas or bile duct cancers. Primary liver tumors often metastasize to the lung.

Metastatic carcinoma of the liver is more common than primary carcinoma. The liver is a common site of metastatic cancer growth because of its high rate of blood flow and extensive capillary network.

- Liver cancer grows rapidly. Death may occur within 6 to 12 months as a result of hepatic encephalopathy or massive gastrointestinal (GI) bleeding.

Clinical Manifestations

Liver cancer can be difficult to distinguish from cirrhosis because of similar clinical manifestations (e.g., hepatomegaly, splenomegaly, fatigue, jaundice, weight loss, peripheral edema, ascites, portal hypertension).

- Other common manifestations include dull abdominal pain in the epigastric or right upper quadrant region, anorexia, nausea and vomiting, and increased abdominal girth.

Diagnostic Studies

- Ultrasound, CT, and MRI are used to screen and diagnose liver cancer.
- A percutaneous biopsy is performed if the results of diagnostic imaging studies are inconclusive.
- Serum α-fetoprotein (AFP) is often elevated.

Nursing and Interprofessional Management

Treatment depends on the size and number of tumors, metastasis beyond the liver, and the patient's age and overall health. In general, management is similar to that for cirrhosis (see Cirrhosis, p. 134). Surgical liver resection (partial hepatectomy) offers the best chance for a cure. However, only about 15% of patients have sufficient healthy liver tissue for this option.

- For those who have early-stage liver cancer, liver transplantation offers a good prognosis.
- Other options are radiofrequency ablation, chemoembolization, and alcohol injection.
- In patients with advanced HCC, sorafenib (Nexavar) is typically the first-line treatment. This kinase inhibitor is a type of targeted therapy agent which blocks proteins (kinases) that play a role in tumor growth and cancer progression.

Nursing interventions focus on keeping the patient as comfortable as possible. Because liver cancer manifests the same problems as advanced liver disease, the nursing interventions discussed for the patient with cirrhosis of the liver apply (see Cirrhosis, pp. 134).

LOW BACK PAIN, ACUTE

Description

Low back pain is common and has affected 80% of adults in the United States at least once during their lifetime. Risk factors associated with low back pain include smoking, stress, poor posture, lack of muscle tone, excess weight, pregnancy, prior compression fracture of the spine, spinal problems since birth, and a family history of back pain. Jobs that require repetitive heavy lifting, vibration (e.g., jackhammer operator), and extended periods of sitting are also associated with low back pain. Low back pain is most often caused by a musculoskeletal problem.

L

- Health care personnel who engage in direct patient care activities are at high risk for low back pain. Lifting and moving patients, excessive bending or leaning forward, and frequent twisting can result in low back pain.

Pathophysiology

Low back pain is a common problem because the lumbar region: (1) bears most of the weight of the body, (2) is the most flexible region of the spinal column, (3) has nerve roots that are at risk for injury or disease, and (4) has a naturally unstable biomechanical structure. The causes of low back pain of musculoskeletal origin include acute lumbosacral strain, instability of lumbosacral bony mechanism, osteoarthritis of the lumbosacral vertebrae, degenerative disc disease, and herniation of the intervertebral disc.

Acute low back pain lasts 4 weeks or less. It is caused by trauma or activity that causes undue stress on the lower back. Often symptoms develop later because of swelling or a gradual increase in pressure on the nerve by an intervertebral disc.

- Symptoms may range from muscle ache to shooting or stabbing pain, limited flexibility or range of motion, or inability to stand upright.
- Few definitive diagnostic abnormalities are present with nerve irritation and muscle strain. One test is the straight-leg-raising test. MRI and CT scans are generally not done unless trauma or systemic disease (e.g., cancer, spinal infection) is suspected.

Nursing and Interprofessional Management

If the acute muscle spasms and accompanying pain are not severe and unbearable, the patient may be treated on an outpatient basis with nonsteroidal antiinflammatory drugs (NSAIDs), muscle relaxants, massage and back manipulation, acupuncture, and use of alternating heat and cold compresses. Severe pain may require a brief course of corticosteroids or opioid analgesics.

Some people may need a brief period (1 to 2 days) of rest at home, but prolonged bed rest should be avoided. Most patients do better if they continue their regular activities. Patients should refrain from activities that increase the pain, including lifting, bending, twisting, and prolonged sitting. Most symptoms subside within 2 weeks.

■ As a role model, use proper body mechanics at all times. This includes increasing the patient's bed height, bending at the knees, asking for help in lifting and moving patients, and using lifting devices.

Primary nursing responsibilities in acute low back pain are to assist the patient to maintain activity limitations, promote comfort, and teach the patient about the health problem and appropriate exercises.

■ Referral to a physical therapist or personal trainer to address posture and core and abdomen strength may be appropriate. Ensure that the patient understands the type and frequency of exercise prescribed, as well as the rationale.

▼ Patient and Caregiver Teaching

Assess the patient's use of body mechanics and offer advice when the person does activities that could produce back strain (Table 56).

TABLE 56 Patient and Caregiver Teaching

Low Back Problems

Include the following instructions when teaching the patient and caregivers how to manage low back problems.

Do

- Maintain healthy body weight.
- Maintain a neutral pelvic position if standing. Place one foot on a low stool if standing for long periods.
- Choose a seat with good lower back support, armrests, and a swivel base. Place a pillow at the lumbar spine to maintain normal curvature. Keep knees and hips level.
- Sleep in a side-lying position with knees and hips bent, and a pillow between the knees for support.
- Sleep on back with a lift under knees and legs or on back with 10-inch-high pillow under knees to flex hips and knees.
- Use proper body mechanics when lifting heavy objects. Bend at the knees, not at the waist, and stand up slowly while holding object close to your body.
- Take part in regular strength and flexibility training and low-impact aerobic exercise.
- Use local heat and cold application to relieve muscle tension.

TABLE 56 Patient and Caregiver Teaching

Low Back Problems—cont'd

Do Not
- Lean forward without bending knees.
- Lift anything above level of elbows.
- Stand unmoving for prolonged time.
- Sleep on abdomen or on back or side with legs out straight.
- Exercise without consulting health care provider (HCP) if having severe pain.
- Exceed prescribed amount and type of exercises without consulting HCP.
- Smoke or use tobacco products.

LOW BACK PAIN, CHRONIC

Description

Chronic low back pain lasts more than 3 months or involves repeated incapacitating episodes. It is often progressive.

Causes, which can be hard to determine, include: (1) degenerative conditions such as arthritis or disc disease; (2) osteoporosis or other metabssolic bone diseases; (3) weakness from the scar tissue of prior injury; (4) chronic strain on lower back muscles from obesity, pregnancy, or stressful postures on the job; and (5) congenital spine problems.

Spinal stenosis is a narrowing of the spinal canal. When it occurs in the lumbar area of the spine, it is a common cause of chronic low back pain. Spinal stenosis can be acquired or inherited.

- A common acquired cause is osteoarthritis in the spine. Arthritic changes (bone spurs, calcification of spinal ligaments, degeneration of discs) narrow the space around the spinal canal and nerve roots, eventually leading to compression. Inflammation caused by the compression results in pain, weakness, and numbness.
- Inherited conditions that lead to spinal stenosis include congenital spinal stenosis and scoliosis.

The pain associated with lumbar spinal stenosis often starts in the low back and radiates to the buttock and leg. It is worse with walking and prolonged standing. Numbness, tingling, weakness, and sensation of heaviness in the legs and buttocks may be present. Decreased pain when the patient bends forward or sits down is often a sign of spinal stenosis.

- Spinal stenosis usually progresses slowly and does not cause paralysis.

Nursing and Interprofessional Management

Treatment regimens are similar to those recommended for acute low back pain. Pain and stiffness are managed with mild analgesics, such as nonsteroidal antiinflammatory drugs (NSAIDs). Antidepressants, such as duloxetine (Cymbalta), may help with pain management and sleep problems. The antiseizure drug gabapentin (Neurontin) may improve walking and relieve leg symptoms.

Weight management, sufficient rest periods, local heat/cold application, and exercise and activity throughout the day help keep the muscles and joints mobilized.

- Therapies such as biofeedback, acupuncture, and yoga may help reduce the pain.
- Minimally invasive treatments, such as epidural corticosteroid injections and implanted devices that deliver pain medication, are options.
- Surgery may be indicated for patients with severe chronic low back pain who do not respond to conservative care or have continued neurologic deficits. (See the Surgical Therapy section in Intervertebral Disc Disease, pp. 349.)

LUNG CANCER

Description

Lung cancer is the leading cause of cancer-related death in the United States and accounts for 28% of all cancer deaths. Smoking is responsible for approximately 80% to 90% of all lung cancers.

- There is no safe form of tobacco or tobacco product. Tobacco smoke contains over 7000 chemicals, of which 250 are harmful. Exposure to tobacco smoke causes changes in the bronchial epithelium, which usually returns to normal when smoking is discontinued.

Assessment of lung cancer risk is based on smoking exposure, with patients assigned to 1 of 3 categories: (1) smokers, people who are currently smoking; (2) nonsmokers, people who formerly smoked; and (3) never-smokers. The risk of developing lung cancer is directly related to total exposure to tobacco smoke, measured by total number of cigarettes smoked in a lifetime, age at smoking onset, depth of inhalation, tar and nicotine content, and the use of unfiltered cigarettes. Sidestream smoke (smoke from burning cigarettes, cigars) has the same carcinogens found in mainstream smoke (smoke inhaled and exhaled by the smoker). This exposure to secondhand smoke creates a health risk for nonsmoking adults and children.

- Other causes of lung cancer include high levels of pollution, radiation (especially radon exposure), and asbestos. Heavy or prolonged exposure to industrial agents, such as ionizing radiation, coal dust, uranium, formaldehyde, and arsenic, can increase the risk of lung cancer.
- Genetic, hormonal, and molecular influences may contribute to differences in lung cancer incidence, risk factors, and survival.

Pathophysiology

Most primary lung tumors are believed to arise from mutated epithelial cells. The growth of mutations that are caused by carcinogens is influenced by various genetic factors. Once started, tumor development is promoted by epidermal growth factor. These cells grow slowly, taking 8 to 10 years for a tumor to reach 1 cm in size, the smallest lesion detectable on an x-ray. Lung cancers occur primarily in the segmental bronchi or beyond and have a preference for the upper lobes of the lungs.

Primary lung cancers are categorized into 2 broad types: *non–small cell lung cancer* (NSCLC) (85%) and *small cell lung cancer* (SCLC) (15%). Lung cancers metastasize primarily by direct extension and through the blood and lymph system. Common sites for metastasis are the liver, brain, bones, and adrenal glands.

Clinical Manifestations

Manifestations are usually nonspecific, appear late in the disease process, and depend on the type of primary lung cancer, its location, and extent of metastatic spread.

- Often the first sign is a persistent cough. Blood-tinged sputum may be present because of bleeding caused by the tumor.
- The patient may report dyspnea or wheezing. Chest pain, if present, may be localized or unilateral, ranging from mild to severe.

Later manifestations include nonspecific symptoms and signs, such as anorexia, nausea and vomiting, fatigue, and weight loss. Hoarseness may be present because of laryngeal nerve involvement. Dysphagia, unilateral paralysis of the diaphragm, and superior vena cava obstruction may occur because of intrathoracic spread of the cancer. Lymph nodes are often palpable in the neck or axillae. Mediastinal involvement may lead to pericardial effusion, cardiac tamponade, and dysrhythmias.

Paraneoplastic syndrome is caused by *humoral* factors *(hormones, cytokines)* excreted by tumor cells or by an *immune response* against the tumor. SCLCs are most often associated with the paraneoplastic syndrome. Symptoms of paraneoplastic syndrome may manifest before the diagnosis of the cancer.

- Examples of paraneoplastic syndrome are hypercalcemia, syndrome of inappropriate antidiuretic hormone (SIADH) secretion, hematologic disorders, and neurologic syndromes. These conditions may stabilize with treatment of the cancer.

Diagnostic Studies

- Chest x-ray is used for diagnosis and assessing for metastasis.
- Biopsy is needed for a definitive diagnosis. If thoracentesis is done to relieve a pleural effusion, the fluid is also analyzed for cancer cells.
- Additional tests include bone scans, CT scans, MRI, positron emission tomography (PET), blood tests, renal function tests, and pulmonary function tests.

Staging of NSCLC is performed according to the tumor-node-metastasis (TNM) staging system (see TNM Classification System, p. 761).

Interprofessional Management

Surgical resection is the treatment of choice in NSCLC stages I and IIIA without mediastinal involvement, because resection gives the best chance for a cure. For other NSCLC stages, patients may have surgery along with radiation therapy and/or chemotherapy and targeted therapy. Many NSCLCs are not resectable at the time of diagnosis. Surgical procedures that may be performed include segmental or wedge resection, lobectomy (removal of 1 or more lung lobes), and pneumonectomy (removal of 1 entire lung) procedures.

Radiation therapy may be used for both NSCLC and SCLC (see Radiation Therapy, p. 712).

- Radiation relieves symptoms of dyspnea and hemoptysis from bronchial obstruction tumors and treats superior vena cava syndrome.
- Radiation can be used to treat the pain of metastatic bone lesions or cerebral metastasis, to reduce tumor mass preoperatively, or as an adjuvant measure postoperatively.

Stereotactic body radiotherapy (SBRT) uses high doses of radiation delivered accurately to the tumor. SBRT is an option for patients with early-stage lung cancers who are not surgical candidates for other reasons.

Chemotherapy is the main treatment for SCLC. It is used for nonresectable tumors or as an adjuvant therapy to surgery in NSCLC. A variety of chemotherapy drugs and multidrug protocols have been used (see Chemotherapy, p. 674).

One type of targeted therapy for patients with NSCLC is erlotinib (Tarceva), which blocks signals for growth in cancer cells. Other drugs, such as bevacizumab (Avastin), inhibit new blood vessel growth (angiogenesis). Drugs such as crizotinib (Xalkori), brigatinib (Alunbrig), and ceritinib (Zykadia) directly inhibit the kinase protein made by the *ALK* gene responsible for cancer development and growth.

Immunotherapy with nivolumab (Opdivo), atezolizumab (Tecentriq), or pembrolizumab (Keytruda) may be used to boost the immune response and can shrink some tumors or slow their growth.

Nursing Management

Goals

The patient with lung cancer will have adequate airway clearance, effective breathing patterns, adequate oxygenation of tissues, minimal to no pain, and a realistic outlook about treatment and prognosis.

Nursing Interventions

The best way to halt the epidemic of lung cancer is to prevent people from smoking, help smokers stop smoking, and decrease exposure to environmental pollutants. Modeling healthy behavior by not smoking, promoting smoking cessation programs, and actively supporting education and policy changes related to smoking are important nursing activities. A wealth of material is available to the smoker who is interested in smoking cessation. See Chapter 10 in Harding et al., *Lewis' Medical-Surgical Nursing,* ed 11.

You have a role in early detection of lung cancer. Encourage adults ages 55 to 77 years with a history of smoking (30-pack year smoking history or currently smoke) or who quit smoking < 15 years ago to consider annual screening for lung cancer using low-dose CT.

Care of the patient with lung cancer involves support and reassurance during the diagnostic evaluation. Individualized care depends on the plan for treatment.

- For many patients who have lung cancer, little can be done to prolong their lives. Assessment and symptom management are pivotal.
- Radiation therapy and chemotherapy can provide palliative relief from distressing symptoms. Constant pain may become a major problem.
- Provide patient comfort, monitor for side effects of prescribed medications, foster appropriate coping strategies, assess smoking cessation readiness, and help patients access resources.

▼ Patient and Caregiver Teaching

- Encourage the patient and family to provide a smoke-free environment. This may include smoking cessation for family members. If the treatment plan includes home oxygen, teach the patient and family about safe use.
- Teach the patient to recognize signs and symptoms that indicate cancer progression or recurrence.

LYME DISEASE

Description

Lyme disease is an infection caused by the spirochete *Borrelia burgdorferi* and transmitted through the bite of an infected deer tick. The tick typically feeds on mice, dogs, cats, cows, horses, deer, and humans. It is the most common vector-borne disease in the United States with an infection rate of 7.9 cases per 100,000 persons. Wild animals do not exhibit the illness, but clinical Lyme disease does occur in domestic animals. Person-to-person transmission does not occur.

The summer months are the peak season for human infection. Most U.S. cases occur in 3 areas: along the northeastern states from Maryland to northern Massachusetts, in the midwestern states of Wisconsin and Minnesota, and along the northwestern coast of California and Oregon. Reinfection is not uncommon.

Clinical Manifestations

The most characteristic sign is erythema migrans (EM), a skin lesion that occurs at the site of the tick bite within 1 month of exposure.

- The EM lesion begins as a central red macule or papule that slowly expands to include a red outer ring of up to 12 inches, resembling a bull's-eye. It may be warm to the touch but is not itchy or painful. The rash is often accompanied by flu-like symptoms, such as low-grade fever, headache, neck stiffness, fatigue, loss of appetite, and migratory joint and muscle pain. Flu-like symptoms generally resolve over weeks or months, even if untreated.
- If not treated, the spirochete can disseminate within several weeks or months to the heart, joints, and central nervous system (CNS). Bell's palsy is the most common neurologic effect.
- Other complaints include short-term memory loss, cognitive impairment, shooting pains, and numbness and tingling in the feet.
- Cardiac symptoms such as heart block and pericarditis may require hospitalization.
- About 60% of persons with untreated infection develop chronic arthritic pain and swelling in the large joints, primarily the knee. Arthritis remains the second most common manifestation of Lyme disease.

Diagnostic Studies

Diagnosis is often based on clinical manifestations, in particular the EM lesion, and a history of exposure in an endemic area.

- Complete blood count (CBC) and erythrocyte sedimentation rate (ESR) are usually normal.
- A 2-step laboratory testing process is recommended to confirm the diagnosis. The first step is the enzyme immunoassay (EIA), a test that will have positive results for most people with Lyme disease. If the EIA is positive or inconclusive, a Western blot test can confirm the infection.
- In those with neurologic involvement, cerebrospinal fluid should also be examined.

Nursing and Interprofessional Management

Active lesions can be treated with oral antibiotics. Doxycycline (Vibramycin), cefuroxime (Ceftin), and amoxicillin are often effective in early-stage infection and in preventing disease progression. Doxycycline is preferred because it treats both Lyme disease and human granulocytic anaplasmosis, which can be transmitted as a co-infection with a single tick bite. Doxycycline is effective in preventing Lyme disease when given within 3 days after the bite of a deer tick.

- A small percentage of people treated with antibiotics for Lyme disease may have lingering fatigue or joint and muscle pain. The International Lyme and Associated Diseases Society supports a diagnosis of chronic Lyme disease in these cases. Antibiotic treatment should be extended as needed because the risks of untreated Lyme disease outweigh those of long-term antibiotic therapy.
- Patient and caregiver teaching for the prevention of Lyme disease in endemic areas focuses on strategies for avoiding tick bites, as outlined in Table 64.13, Harding et al., *Lewis' Medical-Surgical Nursing*, ed 11.

MACULAR DEGENERATION

Description

Age-related *macular degeneration* (AMD) is the most common cause of irreversible central vision loss in people over age 60 years in the United States. AMD is divided into 2 classic forms: *dry* (atrophic), which is more common, and *wet* (exudative), which is more severe. Wet AMD accounts for most cases of AMD-related blindness.

Pathophysiology

AMD is related to retinal aging. Risk factors for AMD include family history of AMD, light-colored irises, high levels of C-reactive protein, smoking, and hypertension.

- In *dry AMD*, yellowish extracellular deposits called *drusen* accumulate in the retinal pigment epithelium. Atrophy and degeneration of macular cells then lead to slowly progressive and painless vision loss.
- *Wet AMD* is characterized by the growth of new blood vessels in an abnormal location in the retinal epithelium. As the new blood vessels leak, scar tissue gradually forms.

Clinical Manifestations

The patient may have blurred and darkened vision, *scotomas* (blind spots in the visual fields), or *metamorphopsia* (distortion of vision). Acute vision loss may occur from either form of AMD.

Diagnostic Studies

- Visual acuity measurement
- Ophthalmoscopic examination to look for drusen and other changes in the fundus
- Amsler grid test to define the involved area and provide a baseline for future comparison
- Fundus photography and IV fluorescein angiography to define the extent and type of AMD
- Optical coherence tomography (OCT) or scanning laser ophthalmoscopy to image retinal anatomy.

Nursing and Interprofessional Management

Visual prognosis varies greatly for people with AMD. Limited treatment options for patients with wet AMD include several medications (i.e., ranibizumab [Lucentis], bevacizumab [Avastin], aflibercept [Eylea], and pegaptanib [Macugen]) injected directly into the vitreous cavity. These drugs inhibit endothelial growth factor and help slow vision loss.

- Photodynamic therapy is used in wet AMD to destroy abnormal blood vessels without permanent damage to the retinal pigment epithelium and photoreceptor cells.
- Patients who have or are at risk for AMD (in consultation with their health care provider [HCP]) should consider supplements of vitamins and minerals. Those with AMD should eat dark green, leafy vegetables containing lutein (e.g., kale and spinach) and fatty fish at least twice a week.
- Smoking cessation may help in halting the progression of dry AMD.

- Many patients with low-vision assistive devices can continue reading and keep a license to drive during the daytime at low speeds.

The permanent loss of central vision associated with AMD has significant psychosocial implications for nursing care. Nursing management of the patient with uncorrectable visual impairment is discussed in Chapter 20 of Harding et al., *Lewis's Medical-Surgical Nursing*, ed 11. Avoid giving patients the impression that "nothing can be done" about the problem. Although therapy will not recover lost vision, much can be done to augment the remaining vision.

MALIGNANT MELANOMA

Description

Malignant melanoma is a tumor arising in cells producing melanin, usually the melanocytes of the skin. Melanoma, the deadliest form of skin cancer, can metastasize to any organ, including the brain and heart. Unlike most cancers whose incidence is stable or decreasing, the incidence of melanoma is steadily rising.

Melanoma is nearly 100% curable by excision if diagnosed early. However, the 5-year survival rate with advanced disease is < 10%, so early detection is critical.

The exact cause of melanoma is unknown. Ultraviolet (UV) radiation from the sun is the main cause of melanoma, but artificial sources of UV radiation such as sunlamps and tanning booths can play a role. UV radiation damages the deoxyribonucleic acid (DNA) in skin cells, causing mutations in the genetic code. People with fair skin and eyes, a prior diagnosis of melanoma, or a first-degree relative diagnosed with melanoma have an increased risk. Immunosuppression and dysplastic nevi also increase the risk.

Clinical Manifestations

About 25% of melanomas occur in existing nevi or moles; about 20% occur in dysplastic nevi. Melanoma frequently occurs on the lower legs in women and on the trunk, head, and neck in men. Because most melanoma cells continue to produce melanin, melanoma tumors are often brown or black.

- Persons should consult a health care provider (HCP) immediately if a mole or lesion shows any sudden or progressive increase in the size, color, or shape of a mole. melanoma (See Figures in Chapter 23 of Harding et al., *Lewis's Medical-Surgical Nursing*, ed 11.) These ABCDE signs include *a*symmetry, *b*order irregularity, *c*olor varied from one area of the lesion to another, *d*iameter > 6 mm, and *e*volving, changing appearance.

Interprofessional Management

Suspicious pigmented lesions are biopsied using an excisional biopsy technique. The most important prognostic factor is tumor thickness at the time of diagnosis.

- Two methods are used to determine tumor thickness: the *Breslow measurement,* which indicates tumor depth in millimeters, and the *Clark level,* which indicates the depth of invasion of the tumor. The higher the number, the deeper the melanoma.

Treatment depends on the site of the original tumor and stage of the cancer. Initial treatment is wide surgical excision. Melanoma that has spread to the lymph nodes or nearby sites requires combinations of chemotherapy, immunotherapy, targeted therapy, and/or radiation therapy.

Immunotherapy can include cytokines (α-interferon, interleukin-2), programmed cell death protein 1 (PD-1) inhibitors, and cytotoxic T lymphocyte antigen 4 (CTLA-4) inhibitors. Cytokines enhance the production of many immune system cells, including T cells and B cells. PD-1 inhibitors include nivolumab (Opdivo) and pembrolizumab (Keytruda). These drugs block PD-1, a protein on T cells that keeps T cells from attacking other cells in the body. Ipilimumab (Yervoy) also helps the immune system. It blocks the action of CTLA-4, another protein that normally suppresses the action of T cells. Drugs blocking PD-1 and CTLA-4 boost the immune response against melanoma cells.

Targeted therapy for melanoma includes BRAF and MEK inhibitors. About half of all melanomas have mutations in the *BRAF* gene, which makes an altered BRAF protein that signals melanoma cells to proliferate. Vemurafenib (Zelboraf), dabrafenib (Tafinlar), trametinib (Mekinist), and cobimetinib (Cotellic) are drugs that target BRAF mutations.

Chemotherapy is not as effective for melanoma as it is for most other cancers. It is usually given only for advanced disease. Drugs used include dacarbazine, temozolomide, cisplatin, paclitaxel, carboplatin, and vincristine. Radiation therapy has a role in treating lymph node and brain metastases.

▼ **Patient and Caregiver Teaching**

Stress the importance of protection from the damaging effects of the sun, such as wearing a large-brimmed hat, sunglasses, and a long-sleeved shirt of a lightly woven fabric.

- Inform patients that the rays of the sun are most dangerous at midday. Recommend that patients use a broad-spectrum

sunscreen with a minimum sun protection factor (SPF) of 15 daily. Sunscreen should be reapplied every 2 hours.
- Teach patients to self-examine their skin at least monthly to detect new or persistent skin lesions.

MALNUTRITION

Description

Malnutrition is an excess, deficit, or imbalance of essential nutrients. Malnutrition is also described as undernutrition or overnutrition. *Undernutrition* occurs when nutritional reserves are depleted, and nutrient and energy intake are not sufficient to meet daily needs or added metabolic stress. *Overnutrition* refers to the ingestion of more food than is required for body needs, as in obesity.
- The incidence of hospitalized patients who are malnourished or at nutritional risk is 30% to 50%. The prevalence of malnutrition in older adults ranges from 3% (community-dwelling older adults) to 30% (rehabilitation settings).

The following terms indicate the interaction and importance of inflammation on nutritional status:
- *Starvation-related malnutrition*, or *primary protein-calorie malnutrition (PCM)*, occurs when nutritional needs are not met. It is a clinical state in which there is chronic starvation without inflammation (e.g., anorexia nervosa).
- *Chronic disease–related malnutrition*, or *secondary PCM*, is related to conditions that impose sustained inflammation of a mild to moderate degree. This occurs when tissue needs are not met, although the dietary intake would be satisfactory under normal conditions. Conditions associated with this type of malnutrition include organ failure, cancer, rheumatoid arthritis, and obesity.
- *Acute disease- or injury-related malnutrition* is related to a marked inflammatory response after major infection, burn, trauma, or surgery.

Many factors contribute to the development of malnutrition, including socioeconomic factors, physical illnesses, incomplete diets, and drug-nutrient interactions.

Pathophysiology of Starvation

Initially, the body selectively uses carbohydrates (glycogen), rather than fat and protein, to meet metabolic needs. This may deplete glycogen stores in the liver and muscles within 18 hours.
- When carbohydrate stores are depleted, skeletal protein begins to be converted to glucose for energy, resulting in a negative

nitrogen balance. Within 5 to 9 days, the body mobilizes fat to supply energy.

- In prolonged starvation, fat provides up to 97% of calories, conserving protein. Depletion of fat stores depends on the amount available. Fat stores are generally used up in 4 to 6 weeks. Once fat stores are used, body proteins, including those in internal organs and plasma, are the only remaining source of energy.

The liver is the body organ that loses the most mass during protein deprivation. It gradually becomes infiltrated with fat secondary to decreased synthesis of lipoproteins. If dietary protein and other necessary constituents are not given, death will rapidly ensue.

Clinical Manifestations

Manifestations of malnutrition range from mild to emaciation and death. The most obvious clinical manifestations on physical examination are apparent in the skin (dry and scaly skin, brittle nails, rashes, hair loss), mouth (crusting and ulceration, changes in tongue), muscles (decreased mass and weakness), and CNS (mental changes such as confusion, irritability).

- The person is more susceptible to infection. Both humoral and cell-mediated immunity are deficient. Leukocytes decrease in the peripheral blood. Phagocytosis is impaired as a result of the lack of energy necessary to drive the process. Many malnourished persons are also anemic.

Diagnostic Studies

- Serum albumin and prealbumin levels are decreased.
- C-reactive protein (CRP) and serum potassium are often elevated.
- Red blood cell (RBC) count and hemoglobin (Hgb) levels indicate the presence and degree of anemia.
- White blood cell (WBC) count and total lymphocyte count are decreased.
- Liver enzyme studies may be elevated.
- Waist circumference and waist-to-hip ratio help evaluate the response to therapy.

Nursing and Interprofessional Management
Goals
The patient with malnutrition will gain weight, consume a specified number of calories per day, and have no adverse consequences related to malnutrition or nutritional therapies.
Nursing Interventions
It is part of your role to teach and reinforce healthy eating habits. Use MyPlate, the Dietary Guidelines for Americans, and Nutrition Facts

food labels to promote healthy nutrition. The MyPlate approach is a visual guide for sensible meal planning. It helps Americans eat healthfully and make good food choices. MyPlate focuses on the proportions of 5 food groups (grains, protein, fruits, vegetables, and dairy) that you should eat at each meal. At the health professionals' link at *www.choosemyplate.gov*, you can download daily food plans, sample menus, and tips for how to be physically active. These materials are valuable to use in patient teaching. MyPlate materials for older adults are available at *https://hnrca.tufts.edu/myplate/*.

Collaborate with the health care provider (HCP) and dietitian to identify patients with malnutrition and implement appropriate interventions to meet the patient's nutritional needs. Assess nutritional state during your assessment of the patient's other physical problems. Identify risk factors for malnutrition and why they exist. Hospital-specific screening tools are based on common admission assessment criteria that typically include history of weight loss, intake before admission, use of nutritional support, chewing or swallowing issues, and skin breakdown.

Obtaining an accurate measure of body weight and height and recording this information are critical components of nutritional assessment. *Body mass index* (BMI) is a measure of weight in proportion to height. BMIs outside the normal weight range are associated with increased morbidity and mortality.

- Daily weights provide an ongoing record of body weight change. To obtain an accurate weight, weigh the patient at the same time each day, using the same scale, with the patient wearing the same type or amount of clothing.
- You and the dietitian can assist the patient and caregiver in the selection of high-calorie and high-protein foods.
- If the patient is unable to consume enough nutrition with a high-calorie, high-protein diet, oral liquid nutritional supplements can be added.
- Encourage the family to bring the patient's favorite food while the patient is hospitalized.

Some patients may benefit from appetite stimulants, such as megestrol acetate or dronabinol (Marinol), to improve intake. If the patient is still unable to take in enough calories, enteral feedings may be considered (see Enteral Nutrition, p. 685). Parenteral nutrition (PN) might be initiated if enteral feedings are not feasible (see Parenteral Nutrition, p. 710).

▼ **Patient and Caregiver Teaching**
- Teach the patient and caregivers the importance of good nutrition and the rationale for recording the daily weight, intake, and output.

- Assess the ability of the patient and caregiver to follow dietary instructions related to past eating habits, religious and ethnic preferences, age, income, other resources, and state of health.
- Ensure proper follow-up care, such as visits by the home health nurse and outpatient dietitian referrals.

MÉNIÈRE'S DISEASE

Description
Ménière's disease is an inner ear problem characterized by episodic vertigo, tinnitus, sensation of aural fullness, and progressive hearing loss. Sudden, severe attacks of vertigo with nausea and vomiting are incapacitating. Symptoms usually begin between the ages of 30 and 60 years.

Pathophysiology
An accumulation of endolymph in the membranous labyrinth leads to hearing and balance problems.

Clinical Manifestations
- Attacks may occur without warning or be preceded by a sense of ear fullness, increasing tinnitus, and muffled hearing.
- The patient may report a whirling sensation and the feeling of being pulled to the ground ("drop attack").
- Autonomic signs and symptoms include pallor, sweating, nausea, and vomiting.
- An attack may last hours or days, and may occur several times per year. The clinical course is highly variable.
- Low-pitched tinnitus may be present continuously or intensify during an attack.
- Hearing loss fluctuates, with the risk of progression to permanent hearing loss.

Diagnostic Studies
- Audiogram results demonstrate mild, low-frequency hearing loss.
- Vestibular tests may isolate the cause of vertigo.
- Glycerol test: may show hearing improvement after oral glycerol dose.

Nursing and Interprofessional Management
During an acute attack, corticosteroids, antihistamines, anticholinergics, and benzodiazepines can decrease the abnormal sensation and lessen symptoms such as nausea and vomiting. Acute vertigo is

treated symptomatically with bed rest, sedation, and antiemetics or antivertigo drugs for motion sickness. Diazepam (Valium), meclizine, and fentanyl with droperidol may reduce the vertigo. Most patients respond to the medications drugs but must learn to live with the unpredictability of the attacks and the loss of hearing.

- During an acute attack, reassure the patient that the condition is not life-threatening.
- Place the patient in a quiet, darkened room. Teach the patient to avoid sudden head movements or and position changes and to close the eyes until vertigo stops.
- Keep side rails up and the bed in low position. Avoid lights and television, which worsen symptoms. Have an emesis basin available because vomiting is common. Help the patient with ambulation because unsteadiness remains after an attack.

Careful management can decrease the possibility of progressive sensorineural loss in many patients. Management between attacks may include calcium-channel blockers, diuretics, antihistamines, and a low-sodium diet. Teach the patient to sit or lie down at the onset of dizziness to prevent falls.

With frequent incapacitating attacks and reduced quality of life, surgical therapy is indicated. Surgical options include endolymphatic shunt, vestibular nerve resection, and labyrinth ablation.

MENINGITIS, BACTERIAL

Description

Meningitis is an acute inflammation of the meningeal tissues surrounding the brain and spinal cord. Older adults and people who are debilitated are more often affected than the general population. College students living in dormitories and persons living in institutions (e.g., prisoners) are also at a high risk for contracting meningitis.

Bacterial meningitis is considered a medical emergency. If untreated, the mortality rate is 50% to 100%. See Table 34, p. 207, for a comparison of meningitis and encephalitis.

Pathophysiology

Organisms usually gain entry to the central nervous system (CNS) through the upper respiratory tract or bloodstream, but they may enter by direct extension from penetrating wounds of the skull or through fractured sinuses in basal skull fractures. *Streptococcus pneumoniae* and *Neisseria meningitidis* are the leading causes of bacterial meningitis. *N. meningitidis* has at least 13 different subtypes (serogroups), with 5 of them (A, B, C, Y, W) causing most cases. The use of *Haemophilus influenzae* vaccine has resulted in a significant decrease in meningitis from *H. influenzae*.

The inflammatory response to the infection tends to increase cerebrospinal fluid (CSF) production with a moderate increase in intracranial pressure (ICP). The purulent secretion produced by bacteria quickly spreads to other areas of the brain through the CSF.

- Observe patients with meningitis closely for signs of increased ICP, which is thought to result from swelling around the dura and increased CSF volume (see Increased Intracranial Pressure, p. 331).

Clinical Manifestations

Fever, severe headache, nausea, vomiting, and *nuchal rigidity* (resistance to flexion of the neck) are key signs.

- Photophobia, a decreased level of consciousness (LOC), and signs of increased ICP may be present.
- If the infecting organism is the meningococcus, a skin rash is common and petechiae may be seen on the trunk, lower extremities, and mucous membranes.
- Seizures occur in one-third of all cases of meningitis.
- Coma is associated with a poor prognosis. It occurs in 5% to 10% of patients with bacterial meningitis.

Complications

The most common acute complication of bacterial meningitis is increased ICP. Another complication is residual neurologic dysfunction of 1 or more cranial nerves.

- The optic nerve (CN II) is compressed by increased ICP. Papilledema is often present, and blindness may occur.
- When the oculomotor (CN III), trochlear (CN IV), and abducens (CN VI) nerves are irritated, ocular movements are affected. Ptosis, unequal pupils, and diplopia are common.
- Irritation of the trigeminal nerve (CN V) results in sensory losses and loss of the corneal reflex. Irritation of the facial nerve (CN VII) may produce facial paresis. Irritation of the vestibulocochlear nerve (CN VIII) causes tinnitus, vertigo, and deafness.
- Hemiparesis, dysphasia, and hemianopsia usually resolve over time.
- Acute cerebral edema may cause seizures, optic nerve palsy, bradycardia, hypertensive coma, and death.
- Headaches may occur for months until the irritation and inflammation have completely resolved.
- A noncommunicating hydrocephalus may occur if the exudate causes adhesions that prevent the normal flow of the CSF from

the ventricles. CSF reabsorption by the arachnoid villi may be obstructed by the exudate. Surgical implantation of a shunt is the only treatment.

- A complication of meningococcal meningitis is *Waterhouse-Friderichsen syndrome*. The syndrome is manifested by petechiae, disseminated intravascular coagulation (DIC), and adrenal hemorrhage.

Diagnostic Studies

When a patient has manifestations suggesting bacterial meningitis, a blood culture and CT scan should be done. Diagnosis is usually verified by lumbar puncture with analysis of the CSF.

- CSF, sputum, and nasopharyngeal secretions are used to identify the causative organism.
- Skull x-rays may detect infected sinuses.
- CT scans may reveal increased ICP or hydrocephalus.

Interprofessional Management

Rapid diagnosis based on a history and physical examination is crucial because the patient is usually in a critical state when health care is sought. When meningitis is suspected, antibiotic therapy is instituted after collection of culture specimens, even before the diagnosis is confirmed. Penicillin, ampicillin, vancomycin, cefuroxime, cefotaxime, ceftriaxone, ceftizoxime, and ceftazidime are some commonly prescribed drugs for treating bacterial meningitis. Dexamethasone may also be prescribed before or with the first dose of antibiotics.

Nursing Management

Goals

The patient with meningitis will have a return to maximal neurologic functioning, resolution of infection, and control of pain and discomfort.

Nursing Interventions

Prevention of respiratory infections through vaccination programs for pneumococcal pneumonia and influenza is important. Early and vigorous treatment of respiratory and ear infections that could spread to meningitis is important. People who have had close contact with someone who has meningitis should be given prophylactic antibiotics.

The patient with meningitis is acutely ill. The fever is high, and head pain is severe. Irritation of the cerebral cortex may result in seizures with changes in mental status and level of consciousness

(LOC). The severity of manifestations is dependent on the level of ICP.

- Assess and record vital signs, neurologic status, fluid intake and output, skin, and lung fields regularly based on the patient's condition.
- Head and neck pain with movement require attention. Codeine provides some pain relief without undue sedation for most patients. A darkened room and cool cloth over the eyes relieve the discomfort of photophobia. For the delirious patient, additional low lighting may help decrease hallucinations.
- All patients have some degree of mental distortion and hypersensitivity. They may be frightened and misinterpret the environment. Try to minimize environmental stimuli and prevent injury.

If seizures occur, take protective measures. Administer antiseizure medications as ordered. Manage problems associated with increased ICP (see Increased Intracranial Pressure, p. 331).

Treat fever vigorously because it increases cerebral edema and the risk of seizures. Aspirin or acetaminophen may reduce fever. If the fever is resistant to aspirin or acetaminophen, more vigorous means are needed, such as use of a cooling blanket. High fever greatly increases the metabolic rate, so assess the patient for dehydration and adequacy of intake. Supplemental feeding (e.g., enteral nutrition) may be needed.

- Meningitis generally requires respiratory isolation until the cultures are negative. Meningococcal meningitis is highly contagious, while other causes of meningitis may pose minimal to no infection risk with patient contact.
- After the acute period has passed, stress the importance of good nutrition with an emphasis on a high-protein, high-caloric diet in small, frequent feedings.
- Muscle rigidity may persist in the neck and backs of the legs. Progressive range-of-motion (ROM) exercises and warm baths are useful. Have the patient gradually increase activity as tolerated but encourage adequate rest and sleep.
- Residual effects can result in sequelae, such as dementia, seizures, deafness, hemiplegia, and hydrocephalus. Assess vision, hearing, cognitive skills, and motor and sensory abilities after recovery with appropriate referrals as indicated.
- Throughout the acute and convalescent periods, be aware of the anxiety and stress felt by the caregiver and other family members.

METABOLIC SYNDROME

Description

Metabolic syndrome is a group of metabolic risk factors that increase a person's chance of developing cardiovascular disease, stroke, and diabetes. About 1 in 3 adults have metabolic syndrome. The syndrome is more prevalent in those 60 years of age and older.

Metabolic syndrome is a cluster of health problems, including obesity, hypertension, abnormal lipid levels, and high blood glucose.

M

Pathophysiology

The main underlying risk factor for metabolic syndrome is insulin resistance related to excessive visceral fat (Fig. 17). Insulin resistance is the body's cells decreased ability to respond to the action

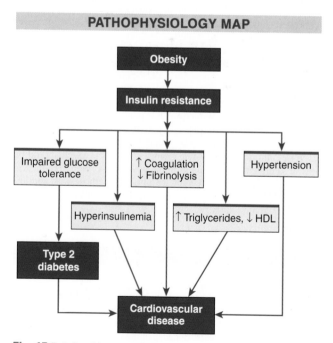

PATHOPHYSIOLOGY MAP

Fig. 17 Relationship among insulin resistance, obesity, diabetes and cardiovascular disease. *HDL,* High-density lipoprotein.

of insulin. The pancreas compensates by secreting more insulin, resulting in hyperinsulinemia. Other characteristics of metabolic syndrome include hypertension, increased risk for clotting, and abnormalities in cholesterol levels. Persons with this syndrome are at a higher risk of heart disease, stroke, diabetes, renal disease, and polycystic ovary syndrome. Those who have metabolic syndrome and smoke are at an even higher risk.

Clinical Manifestations

The signs of metabolic syndrome are impaired fasting blood glucose, hypertension, abnormal cholesterol levels, and obesity. Medical problems develop over time if the condition is not addressed.

Nursing and Interprofessional Management

There is no specific management of metabolic syndrome. Interventions focus on reducing the major risk factors of cardiovascular disease and type 2 diabetes: reducing low-density lipoprotein (LDL) cholesterol, stopping smoking, lowering BP, losing weight, and reducing glucose levels.

There are no specific medications for metabolic syndrome. Patients receive cholesterol-lowering and antihypertensive drugs as needed.

- Metformin (Glucophage) can lower glucose levels and enhance the cells' sensitivity to insulin.

For long-term risk reduction, the person needs to maintain a healthy weight, increase physical activity, and follow healthy diet habits. You can help patients by giving information on healthy diets, exercise, and positive lifestyle changes. The diet, which should be low in saturated fats, should promote weight loss. Weight reduction and maintaining a lower weight are a priority in those with abdominal obesity and metabolic syndrome. Obese patients may be candidates for bariatric surgery.

MULTIPLE MYELOMA

Description

Multiple myeloma, or plasma cell myeloma, is a condition in which cancerous plasma cells proliferate and destroy bone. The disease is more common in men than in women and usually develops between the ages of 65 and 74 years. Because of the variety of treatments that can be provided, over 40% of patients have more than a 10-year survival rate.

Pathophysiology

The cause of multiple myeloma is unknown. Exposure to organic chemicals (such as benzene), herbicides, and insecticides may play a role. Viral infections, such as human immunodeficiency virus (HIV), may influence the risk of developing multiple myeloma.

Instead of plasma cells producing antibodies to fight different infections, myeloma tumors produce monoclonal antibodies (immunoglobulins). *Monoclonal* means they are all of one kind, making them ineffective and harmful. They do not fight infections and they infiltrate the bone marrow. These monoclonal proteins (called *M proteins*) are made up of 2 light chains and 2 heavy chains. *Bence Jones proteins* show up in the urine of many patients with multiple myeloma.

The body's normal immune response is compromised by the reduction in number of normal plasma cells. Excessive amounts of interleukins (IL-4, IL-5, IL-6) contribute to the bone destruction.

- Ultimately the end-organ effects of myeloma are seen in the bones and kidneys and possibly the spleen, lymph nodes, and liver.

Clinical Manifestations

Multiple myeloma develops slowly and insidiously.

- The patient often does not manifest symptoms until the disease is advanced. Skeletal pain is the major symptom. Pain in the pelvis, spine, and ribs is common.
- Diffuse osteoporosis develops as the myeloma protein destroys bone. Osteolytic lesions are seen on x-rays in the skull, vertebrae, long bones, and ribs. Loss of bone integrity can lead to the development of pathologic fractures, including vertebral collapse and with spinal cord compression.
- Degeneration causes calcium loss from bones, resulting in hypercalcemia. Hypercalcemia may cause renal, gastrointestinal (GI), or neurologic changes, such as polyuria, anorexia, confusion, and ultimately seizures, coma, and heart problems.
- The high levels of M protein can result in renal failure from renal tubular obstruction and interstitial nephritis.
- The patient may have anemia, thrombocytopenia, and granulocytopenia related to the replacement of normal bone marrow with plasma cells.

Diagnostic Studies

- Pancytopenia, hyperuricemia, hypercalcemia, and elevated creatinine may be found.
- Excessive production and secretion of monoclonal (M) protein is found in blood and urine.

- The light-chain part of the M protein (called *Bence Jones protein*) can be detected in the urine.
- Skeletal bone surveys, MRI, and/or positron emission tomography (PET) and CT scans show distinct areas of bone erosions; generalized thinning of the bones or fractures, especially in the vertebrae, ribs, pelvis, and bones of the thigh and upper arms.
- The simplest measure of prognosis is based on blood levels of 2 markers: β_2-microglobulin and albumin. Higher levels of these 2 markers are associated with a poorer prognosis.
- Bone marrow examination shows significantly increased numbers of plasma cells. Cytogenetic studies of the bone marrow plays a role in prognostic stratification. For example, deletion of chromosome 17p13 is considered a high risk (poor prognostic) feature.

Interprofessional Management

The therapeutic approach involves managing both the disease and its symptoms. Multiple myeloma is seldom cured, but treatment can relieve symptoms, produce remission, and prolong life. Current treatment options include "watchful waiting" (for early multiple myeloma), chemotherapy, immunotherapy and targeted therapy, and hematopoietic stem cell transplantation (HSCT).

Chemotherapy includes a corticosteroid (dexamethasone or prednisone) plus 2 chemotherapy agents, such as bortezomib and lenalidomide or bortezomib and cyclophosphamide (see Chemotherapy, p. 674). High-dose chemotherapy followed by HSCT has evolved as the standard of care in eligible patients.

Immunotherapy and targeted therapy are options. Immunomodulator drugs include thalidomide, lenalidomide, and pomalidomide. Proteosome inhibitors include bortezomib, carfilzomib, and ixazomib. Panobinostat is a drug that affects enzymes that promote cancer cell growth. Daratumumab is a monoclonal antibody against CD38, a protein which is found on the surface of myeloma cells.

Drugs may be used to treat the complications of multiple myeloma. For example, allopurinol may be given to reduce hyperuricemia, and IV furosemide promotes renal excretion of calcium. Radiation therapy is another component of treatment, primarily because of its effect on localized lesions.

Control of pain and prevention of pathologic fractures are other goals of interprofessional care. Analgesics, orthopedic supports, and localized radiation help reduce skeletal pain. Surgical procedures, such as vertebroplasty, may be done to support degenerative vertebrae.

Nursing Management

Ambulation and adequate hydration are used to treat hypercalcemia, dehydration, and potential renal damage. Weight bearing helps the bones reabsorb some calcium, and fluids dilute calcium and prevent protein precipitates from causing renal tubular obstruction. Fluids are administered to achieve a urine output of 1.5 to 2 L/day if the patient does not already have renal compromise. Because of the myeloma proteins, the patient is at additional risk for renal problems. Monitor electrolytes and fluid balance closely.Because of the potential for pathologic fractures, use caution when moving and ambulating the patient. A slight twist or strain on a weakened bone may cause a fracture.

Pain management requires innovative and knowledgeable nursing interventions. Analgesics, such as nonsteroidal antiinflammatory drugs (NSAIDs), acetaminophen, or acetaminophen with codeine, may be more effective than opioids alone in diminishing bone pain. Braces, especially for the spine, may also help prevent pain.

- Assessment and prompt treatment of infection are important.
- The patient's psychosocial needs require sensitive, skilled management. Help the patient and significant others adapt to changes fostered by chronic sickness and adjust to the losses related to the disease process, while helping maximize functioning and quality of life.

MULTIPLE SCLEROSIS

Description

Multiple sclerosis (MS) is a chronic, progressive, degenerative disorder of the central nervous system (CNS) characterized by demyelination of the nerve fibers of the brain and spinal cord. The onset of MS is usually between 20 and 50 years of age, with symptoms first appearing at an average of 30 to 35 years of age. People diagnosed at 50 years of age or older generally have more progressive disease. MS affects women 2 to 3 times more often than men.

- MS is more prevalent in temperate climates (between 45 and 65 degrees of latitude), such as those found in the northern United States, Canada, and Europe.

Pathophysiology

While the cause of MS is unknown, it is unlikely due to a single cause. We think MS develops in a genetically susceptible person after an environmental exposure, such as an infection. Multiple genes are believed to be involved in the inherited susceptibility to MS. Having a first-degree relative with MS increases a person's risk of developing the disease. Common genetic factors have been found in families with more than 1 affected member. Possible precipitating factors include infection, smoking, physical injury, emotional stress, excessive fatigue, pregnancy, and a poor state of health.

MS is marked by 3 processes: chronic inflammation, demyelination, and gliosis in the CNS. The primary condition is an autoimmune process driven by activated T cells. An unknown trigger in a genetically susceptible person may initiate this process. The activated T cells in the systemic circulation go to the CNS and disrupt the blood-brain barrier. This may be the first event in the development of MS. Subsequent antigen-antibody reaction within the CNS activates the inflammatory response and leads to axon demyelination.

- Attacks on the myelin sheaths of the neurons in the brain and spinal cord first cause damage to the myelin sheath. The nerve fiber is not affected. Transmission of nerve impulses still occurs, but it is slowed. The patient may have a noticeable impairment of function (e.g., weakness). However, myelin can still regenerate. When it does, symptoms disappear. At that point, the patient has a remission.
- As inflammation continues, nearby oligodendrocytes are affected. Myelin loses the ability to regenerate. Eventually damage occurs to the underlying axon. Nerve impulse transmission is disrupted, and nerve function is lost permanently.
- As inflammation subsides, glial scar tissue replaces damaged tissue. This leads to the formation of hard, rigid plaques. These plaques are found throughout the white matter of the CNS.

Clinical Manifestations

The onset is often insidious and gradual, with vague, intermittent symptoms. The disease may not be diagnosed until years after the onset of the first symptom.

- For some patients, MS is marked by rapid, progressive deterioration. Others have remissions and exacerbations. With repeated exacerbations, the overall trend is progressive deterioration in neurologic function. Clinical manifestations vary according to areas of the CNS involved. A classification scheme with 4 primary patterns of MS has been developed (Table 57).
- Blurred or double vision, red-green color distortion, or even blindness in 1 eye may be the first symptom experienced by a person with MS.

TABLE 57 Patterns of Multiple Sclerosis

MS Category	Characteristics
Relapsing-remitting	• Clearly defined attacks of worsening neurologic function *(relapses)* with partial or complete recovery *(remission)*. • 85% of people first diagnosed with this type of multiple sclerosis (MS).
Primary-progressive	• Steadily worsening neurologic function from the beginning with minor improvements but no distinct relapses or remissions. • 10% of people first diagnosed with this type of MS.
Secondary-progressive	• A relapsing-remitting initial course, followed by progression with or without occasional relapses, minor remissions, and plateaus. • New treatments may slow progression. • Most people initially diagnosed with relapsing-remitting MS eventually transition to this type.
Progressive-relapsing	• Progressive disease from onset, with clear acute relapses, with or without full recovery. Periods between relapses are characterized by continuing progression. • 5% of people with MS.

M

- Many patients describe extremity muscle weakness and problems with coordination and balance. Those symptoms may affect walking or standing. MS can cause partial or complete paralysis.
- Sensory symptoms include numbness and tingling, vertigo, tinnitus, decreased hearing, and chronic neuropathic pain.
- Other frequent problems include speech impairments, hearing loss, tremors, and dizziness.
- Cerebellar signs include nystagmus, ataxia, dysarthria, and dysphagia.
- Severe fatigue is aggravated by heat, humidity, deconditioning, and drug side effects.

- Bowel and bladder function can be affected if the sclerotic plaque is located in the areas of the CNS that control elimination. Problems usually include constipation and a spastic (uninhibited) bladder.
- Sexual problems occur in many people. Physiologic erectile dysfunction may result from spinal cord involvement in men. Women may have decreased desire for sexual activity (libido), difficulty with orgasm, painful intercourse, and decreased vaginal lubrication.
- About half of people with MS will have some problems with cognitive function, including difficulties with short-term memory, attention, information processing, and word finding. General intellect remains unchanged and intact, including long-term memory, conversational skills, and reading comprehension.

The average life expectancy after the onset of symptoms is more than 25 years. Death usually occurs because of the infectious complications (e.g., pneumonia) of immobility or because of unrelated disease.

Diagnostic Studies

Because there is no definitive diagnostic test for MS, the history, clinical manifestations, and results of diagnostic testing are important.

- MRI of the brain and spinal cord may show the presence of plaques, inflammation, atrophy, and tissue breakdown and destruction.
- Cerebrospinal fluid (CSF) analysis may show an increase in immunoglobulin G (IgG) or the presence of oligoclonal banding.
- Evoked potentials are often delayed as a result of decreased nerve conduction from the eye and ear to the brain.

To be diagnosed with MS, the patient must have: 1) evidence of at least 2 inflammatory demyelinating lesions in at least 2 different locations within the CNS, 2) damage or an attack occurring at different times (usually 1 month or more apart), and 3) all other possible diagnoses ruled out.

Interprofessional Management

Because there is currently no cure for MS, interprofessional care is aimed at treating the disease process and providing symptomatic relief.

Drug Therapy

Disease-modifying therapy is more effective early in the course of MS. The initial treatment of MS is the use of immunomodulator drugs to modify the disease progression and prevent relapses. These drugs include interferon β-1a (Rebif, Plegridy, Avonex), interferon β-1b (Betaseron, Extavia), and glatiramer acetate (Copaxone, Glatopa).

- Teriflunomide (Aubagio) is an immunomodulatory agent with antiinflammatory properties.
- Fingolimod (Gilenya) reduces MS disease activity by preventing lymphocytes from reaching the CNS and causing damage.
- For more active and aggressive forms of MS, natalizumab (Tysabri), alemtuzumab (Lemtrada), mitoxantrone, ocrelizumab (Ocrevus), and dimethyl fumarate (Tecfidera) may be used. Natalizumab is given when patients have had an inadequate response to other drugs.
- Corticosteroids (e.g., methylprednisolone, prednisone) are most helpful to treat acute exacerbations of MS by reducing edema and acute inflammation at the site of demyelination. However, these drugs do not affect the ultimate outcome or degree of residual neurologic impairment from the exacerbation. Therapeutic plasma exchange (plasmapheresis) and IV immunoglobulin G may be considered for a short time when treatment with corticosteroids alone does not achieve symptom improvement.

M

Many other drugs are used to treat the various symptoms of MS. These may include drugs for spasticity, fatigue, tremor, vertigo or dizziness, depression, pain, bowel problems, bladder problems, sexual problems, and cognitive changes. For example, amantadine, modafinil (Provigil), and fluoxetine (Prozac) are used to treat fatigue. Anticholinergics are used to treat bladder symptoms. Tricyclic antidepressants and antiseizure drugs are used for chronic pain syndromes.

Other Therapy
Surgical intervention (e.g., neurectomy, rhizotomy, cordotomy), dorsal-column electrical stimulation, or intrathecal baclofen (Lioresal) delivered by pump may be required if spasticity is not controlled with drugs. Tremors that become unmanageable with pharmacologic therapy are sometimes treated by thalamotomy or deep brain stimulation.

Neurologic function sometimes improves with physical therapy and speech therapy. Exercise decreases spasticity, increases coordination, and retrains unaffected muscles to act for impaired ones. An especially beneficial type of physical therapy is water exercise.

Nursing Management
Goals
The patient with MS will maximize neuromuscular function, maintain independence in activities of daily living for as long as possible, manage disabling fatigue, optimize psychosocial well-being, adjust to the illness, and reduce factors that precipitate exacerbations.

Nursing Interventions
The patient with MS should be aware of triggers that may cause exacerbations or worsening of the disease. Exacerbations of MS

are triggered by infection (especially upper respiratory and urinary tract infections), trauma, childbirth, stress, fatigue, and climatic changes. Assist the patient to identify particular triggers and develop ways to avoid them or minimize their effects.

- During the diagnostic phase, the patient needs reassurance that even though there is a tentative diagnosis of MS, certain diagnostic studies must be made to rule out other neurologic disorders. The patient with recently diagnosed MS may need assistance with the grieving process.
- During an acute exacerbation, the patient may be immobile. The focus of nursing intervention at this phase is to prevent complications of immobility.

▼ **Patient and Caregiver Teaching**

- Teach about building a general resistance to illness. This includes avoiding fatigue, extremes of heat and cold, and exposure to infection.
- Teach the patient to achieve a good balance of exercise and rest, eat nutritious and well-balanced meals, and minimize caffeine intake.
- Patients should know their treatment regimens, the side effects of drugs, and drug interactions with over-the-counter preparations.
- Bladder control is a major problem for many patients. Although anticholinergics may be beneficial for some patients to decrease spasticity, you may need to teach others self-catheterization.
- Increasing dietary fiber may help some patients avoid constipation.

The National Multiple Sclerosis Society and its local chapters can offer a variety of services to meet the needs of MS patients and their families.

MYASTHENIA GRAVIS

Description

Myasthenia gravis (MG) is an autoimmune disease of the neuromuscular junction marked by fluctuating weakness of certain skeletal muscle groups. The mean age at onset in women is 28 years, with a mean age at onset in men of 42 years.

Pathophysiology

MG is caused by an autoimmune process in which antibodies attack acetylcholine (ACh) receptors. A reduction in the number of ACh receptor sites at the neuromuscular junction prevents ACh molecules from attaching to receptors and stimulating muscle contraction. Anti-ACh antibodies are found in the serum of most patients with MG. Thymic hyperplasia and tumors are common in patients with MG, suggesting that autoantibody production occurs in the thymus.

Clinical Manifestations

The key feature of MG is fluctuating weakness of skeletal muscle. Muscles are generally strongest in the morning and become exhausted with continued activity. Muscle weakness is prominent by the end of the day. A period of rest usually restores strength. The muscles most often involved are those used to move the eyes and eyelids, chew, swallow, speak, and breathe.

M

- In more than half of patients, the first muscles involved are the ocular muscles, causing ptosis (drooping of the eyelids) in 1 or both eyes and double vision.
- Facial mobility and expression can be impaired. There may be difficulty in chewing and swallowing food. Speech is affected, and the voice often fades during conversations.
- No other signs of neural disorder accompany MG. There is no sensory loss. Reflexes are normal and muscle atrophy is rare.
- The course of the disease is highly variable. Some patients have short-term remissions and others stabilize. Still others may have severe progressive involvement.
- Fatigue, pregnancy, illness, trauma, temperature extremes, stress, and hypokalemia can exacerbate MG. Certain drugs, including β-adrenergic blockers, quinidine, phenytoin (Dilantin), certain anesthetics, and aminoglycoside antibiotics, can worsen MG.
- The major complications of MG result from muscle weakness affecting swallowing and breathing. An acute exacerbation of MG that results in aspiration, respiratory infection, and respiratory insufficiency is known as a "myasthenic crisis."

Diagnostic Studies

The diagnosis of MG can be made on the basis of history and physical examination.

- Electromyography (EMG) may show a decreased response to repeated stimulation of the hand muscles, indicating muscle fatigue.
- The Tensilon test reveals improved muscle contractility after an IV injection of the anticholinesterase agent edrophonium chloride.
- If MG is confirmed, a chest CT scan may be done to evaluate the thymus.

Interprofessional Management

Drug Therapy

Drug therapy for MG includes anticholinesterase drugs, alternate-day corticosteroids, and immunosuppressants.

- Acetylcholinesterase inhibitors prolong the action of ACh and facilitate transmission of impulses at the neuromuscular junction. Pyridostigmine (Mestinon) is the most successful drug in this group.
- Corticosteroids (prednisone) are used to suppress the immune response. Drugs such as azathioprine (Imuran), mycophenolate (CellCept), and cyclosporine (Sandimmune) may also be used for immunosuppression.

Other Therapies

Because the presence of the thymus gland in the patient with MG appears to enhance the production of ACh receptor antibodies, removal of the thymus gland results in improvement in a majority of patients.

- Plasmapheresis and IV immunoglobulin G can provide a short-term improvement in symptoms. They are indicated for patients in crisis or in preparation for surgery when corticosteroids must be avoided.

Nursing Management

Goals

The patient with MG will have a return of normal muscle endurance, manage fatigue, avoid complications, and maintain a quality of life appropriate to disease course.

Nursing Interventions

The patient with MG who is admitted to the hospital usually has a respiratory tract infection or is in acute myasthenic crisis. Nursing care is aimed at maintaining adequate ventilation, continuing drug therapy, and watching for side effects of therapy. Be able to distinguish cholinergic from myasthenic crisis, because the causes and treatment of the 2 differ greatly (Table 58).

- Care focuses on reducing the impact of MG on activities of daily living.
- Scheduling doses of medication so that peak action is reached at mealtime may make eating easier. Teach the patient about a balanced diet of foods that can be chewed and swallowed. Semisolid foods may be easier to eat than solids or liquids.
- Arrange diversional activities that require little physical effort and match the patient's interests.

▼ Patient and Caregiver Teaching

Focus teaching on adherence to the treatment plan, complications, potential adverse reactions to specific drugs, complications of therapy (crisis conditions), and what to do about them.

- Explore community resources, such as the Myasthenia Gravis Society and MG support groups.

TABLE 58 Comparison of Myasthenic and Cholinergic Crises	
Myasthenic Crisis	**Cholinergic Crisis**
Causes	
Exacerbation of myasthenia after precipitating factors or failure to take drug as prescribed or drug dose too low	Overdose of anticholinesterase drugs resulting in increased ACh at the receptor sites, remission (spontaneous or after thymectomy)
Differential Diagnosis	
Improved strength after IV administration of anticholinesterase drugs	Weakness within 1 hr after ingestion of anticholinesterase drugs
Increased weakness of skeletal muscles manifesting as ptosis, bulbar signs (e.g., difficulty swallowing, difficulty articulating words), or dyspnea	Increased weakness of skeletal muscles manifesting as ptosis, bulbar signs, dyspnea
	Effects on smooth muscle include pupillary miosis, salivation, diarrhea, nausea or vomiting, abdominal cramps, increased bronchial secretions, sweating, or lacrimation

ACh, Acetylcholine.

M

MYOCARDIAL INFARCTION

Myocardial infarction is part of the spectrum referred to as "acute coronary syndrome." See Acute Coronary Syndrome, p. 5, for the discussion of this disorder.

MYOCARDITIS

Description

Myocarditis is a focal or diffuse inflammation of the myocardium associated with viral, bacterial, and fungal infections and with radiation therapy, pharmacologic and chemical factors, and autoimmune disorders. Coxsackieviruses A and B are the most common etiologic agents.

Pathophysiology

When the myocardium becomes infected, the causative agent invades the myocytes and causes cellular damage and necrosis. The immune response is activated, cytokines and oxygen free radicals are released, and an autoimmune response occurs, resulting in further destruction of myocytes. Myocarditis results in cardiac dysfunction and possibly dilated cardiomyopathy (see Cardiomyopathy, p. 106).

Clinical Manifestations

The clinical features of myocarditis vary from a benign course without overt symptoms to progressive heart failure (HF), dysrhythmias, or sudden cardiac death (SCD). Fever, fatigue, malaise, myalgias, pharyngitis, dyspnea, lymphadenopathy, and nausea and vomiting are early manifestations of the viral illness.

- *Early:* Cardiac signs appear 7 to 10 days after viral infection and include pericardial chest pain with a pericardial friction rub and effusion.
- *Late:* Cardiac signs relate to the development of HF and include S_3, crackles, jugular venous distention, syncope, peripheral edema, and angina.

Diagnostic Studies

- Electrocardiography (ECG) changes are often nonspecific but reflect pericardial involvement, including diffuse ST-segment abnormalities. Dysrhythmias and conduction problems may be present.
- Laboratory findings are often inconclusive, with mild to moderate leukocytosis and atypical lymphocytes, elevated viral titers, increased erythrocyte sedimentation rate (ESR), C-reactive protein (CRP), and cardiac biomarkers such as troponin, and elevated viral titers. (Virus is generally present in tissue and fluid samples during the first 8 to 10 days of illness.)
- Endomyocardial biopsy provides histologic confirmation. A biopsy is most diagnostic during the first 6 weeks of acute illness, when lymphocytic infiltration and myocyte damage are present.
- Echocardiography, radionuclide scans, and MRI are used to assess heart function.

Interprofessional Management

The treatment for myocarditis consists of managing symptoms.

- Angiotensin-converting enzyme (ACE) inhibitors and β-adrenergic blockers are used if the heart is enlarged or to treat HF.
- Diuretics reduce fluid volume and decrease preload. If the patient is not hypotensive, nitroprusside and milrinone may reduce afterload and improve cardiac output by decreasing systemic vascular resistance.
- Anticoagulation reduces the risk of clot formation from blood stasis in patients with a low ejection fraction (EF).
- Digoxin (Lanoxin) improves heart contractility and reduces heart rate. However, it is used cautiously in patients with myocarditis because of increased sensitivity to the adverse effects (e.g., dysrhythmias) and the potential toxicity.

Myocarditis with an autoimmune basis is treated with immunosuppressive agents to reduce heart inflammation and damage. However, the use of these drugs for the treatment of myocarditis is controversial because they may lead to recurrence. Antivirals may be used as adjunct therapy to treat myocarditis.

General supportive measures for management of myocarditis include O_2 therapy, bed rest, and restricted activity. In cases of severe HF, intraaortic balloon pump therapy and ventricular assist devices (VAD) may be needed

Nursing Management

Focus your interventions on improving cardiac output (CO) and managing the signs and symptoms of HF. Select nursing measures to decrease cardiac workload (e.g., semi-Fowler's position, spaced activity and rest, a quiet environment). Carefully monitor medications that increase the heart's contractility and decrease the preload or afterload.

The patient may be anxious about the diagnosis of myocarditis. Assess the level of anxiety an institute measures to decrease anxiety. Keep the patient and caregivers informed about the therapeutic plan.

The patient who receives immunosuppressive therapy is at an increased risk for infection. Monitor for complications and provide the patient with proper infection control procedures.

NAUSEA AND VOMITING

Description

Nausea and vomiting are the most common manifestations of gastrointestinal (GI) diseases. Although each manifestation can occur independently, they are closely related and usually treated as one problem. Nausea and vomiting occur in a wide variety of GI disorders and in conditions unrelated to GI disease, including pregnancy, infection, central nervous system (CNS) disorders (e.g., meningitis), cardiovascular problems (e.g., myocardial infarction [MI], heart failure [HF]), metabolic disorders (e.g., diabetes), side effects of drugs (e.g., chemotherapy, digitalis), and psychologic factors (e.g., stress, fear).

Nausea is a feeling of discomfort in the epigastrium with a conscious desire to vomit. Anorexia usually accompanies nausea.

Regurgitation is an effortless process in which partially digested food slowly comes up from the stomach.

Vomiting (emesis) is the forceful ejection of partially digested food and secretions from the upper GI tract. *Projectile vomiting* is a forceful expulsion of stomach contents without nausea.

Pathophysiology

A vomiting center in the medulla coordinates the components involved in vomiting. Neural impulses reach the vomiting center by way of afferent pathways through branches of the autonomic nervous system. Receptors for these afferent fibers are in the GI tract, kidneys, heart, and uterus. When stimulated, these receptors relay information to the vomiting center, which initiates the vomiting reflex. In addition, the chemoreceptor trigger zone (CTZ) located in the brain responds to chemical stimuli of drugs and toxins. Once stimulated (e.g., in motion sickness), the CTZ transmits impulses directly to the vomiting center.

The simultaneous closure of the glottis, deep inspiration with contraction of the diaphragm in the inspiratory position, closure of the pylorus, relaxation of the stomach and lower esophageal sphincter, and contraction of the abdominal muscles with increasing intraabdominal pressure, force stomach contents up and out of the mouth.

- Early morning vomiting is common in pregnancy.
- Emotional stressors may elicit vomiting during or immediately after eating.
- Cyclic vomiting syndrome consists of recurring episodes of nausea, vomiting, and fatigue that last from a few hours up to 10 days.

Clinical Manifestations

When nausea and vomiting occur over a long period, dehydration can develop rapidly. Water and essential electrolytes (e.g., potassium, sodium, chloride, hydrogen) are lost. As vomiting persists, the patient may have severe electrolyte imbalances, extracellular fluid volume loss, decreased plasma volume, and eventually circulatory failure.

- Metabolic alkalosis may result from loss of gastric hydrochloric acid (HCl). Less frequently, metabolic acidosis can occur when vomiting the contents of the small intestine.
- Weight loss from fluid loss may occur in a short time with severe vomiting.

The threat of pulmonary aspiration is a concern when vomiting occurs in older or unconscious patients or those with an impaired gag reflex. To prevent aspiration, put the patient who cannot adequately manage self-care in a semi-Fowler's or side-lying position.

Nursing and Interprofessional Management

The goals of management are that the patient will experience minimal or no nausea and vomiting, have normal electrolyte levels and hydration status, and return to a normal pattern of fluid balance and nutrient intake.

Assess the patient for precipitating factors and describe the contents of the emesis. The use of drugs in the treatment of nausea and vomiting depends on the cause of the problem. Using antiemetics before determining the cause can mask the underlying disease process and delay diagnosis and treatment. Many antiemetic drugs act in the CNS via the CTZ to block the neurochemicals that trigger nausea and vomiting.

- Drugs may include anticholinergics (e.g., scopolamine), antihistamines (e.g., promethazine), phenothiazines (e.g., prochlorperazine), and butyrophenones (e.g., droperidol). Other drugs with antiemetic effects include benzamides (metoclopramide [Reglan]), 5-hydroxytryptamine [5-HT] (serotonin) receptor antagonists (e.g., ondansetron [Zofran]), and neurokinin-1 receptor antagonists (e.g., aprepitant [Emend]). A comprehensive list of drugs used for nausea and vomiting is included in Table 41.1, Harding et al., *Lewis' Medical-Surgical Nursing,* ed 11.

The patient with severe vomiting requires IV fluid therapy with electrolyte and glucose replacement until able to tolerate oral intake. Some patients may need a nasogastric (NG) tube and suction to decompress the stomach. Secure the NG tube to prevent tube movement in the nose and throat that can stimulate nausea and vomiting. Record intake and output, position the patient to prevent aspiration, and monitor vital signs.

- Assess for signs of dehydration, and observe for changes in the patient's physical comfort and mentation. Provide physical and emotional support and maintain a quiet, odor-free environment.

Once symptoms have subsided, oral nutrition begins with clear liquids. Water is the initial fluid of choice for oral rehydration. Have the patient sip small amounts of fluid (5 to 15 mL) every 15 to 20 minutes. Other options include carbonated beverages with the carbonation removed at room temperature and warm tea. As the patient's condition improves, provide a diet high in carbohydrates and low in fat.

Alternative therapies such as acupressure or acupuncture have been effective in reducing postoperative nausea and vomiting. Patients may use herbs, such as ginger and peppermint oil. Relaxation breathing exercises, changes in body position, or exercise may help some patients. An oral cannabinoid (e.g., dronabinol) may be part of the regimen to manage chemotherapy-induced nausea when other therapies are not effective.

▼ **Patient and Caregiver Teaching**

- Provide explanations for diagnostic tests and procedures.
- Teach the patient and caregiver how to manage the unpleasant sensations of nausea, methods to prevent nausea and vomiting, and strategies to maintain fluid and nutritional intake.
- Use of relaxation techniques, frequent rest periods, effective pain management strategies, and diversional tactics can prevent or reduce nausea and vomiting.
- Cleansing the face and hands with a cool washcloth and providing mouth care between episodes provide comfort.
- When food is identified as the precipitating cause of nausea and vomiting, help the patient identify the specific food and when it was eaten, prior history with that food, and whether anyone else who ate the food is sick.

A patient may be reluctant to resume fluid intake because of fear of nausea recurring. Suggest clear liquids, cola beverages, sports drinks, tea or broth, dry crackers or toast, and then plain gelatin. Bland foods, such as pasta, rice, cereal, baked potato, or cooked chicken, are generally well tolerated in small amounts.

NEPHROTIC SYNDROME

Description

Nephrotic syndrome results when the glomerulus of the kidney is excessively permeable to plasma protein, causing proteinuria and leading to low plasma albumin and tissue edema. Common causes include primary glomerular disease, infections (e.g., hepatitis, streptococcal), neoplasms (e.g., Hodgkin's lymphoma), allergens (e.g., bee sting), drugs (e.g., nonsteroidal antiinflammatory drugs [NSAIDs]), and multisystem diseases (e.g., diabetes, systemic lupus erythematosus [SLE]).

Pathophysiology and Clinical Manifestations

The increased glomerular membrane permeability found in nephrotic syndrome is responsible for massive excretion of protein in the urine. This results in decreased total serum protein and subsequent edema formation, including ascites and anasarca.

- Diminished plasma oncotic pressure from the decrease in serum proteins stimulates hepatic lipoprotein synthesis, which results in hyperlipidemia. Fat bodies (fatty casts) in the urine cause urine to appear foamy.
- Immune responses are altered. As a result, infection is a major cause of morbidity and mortality.
- Calcium and skeletal abnormalities may occur, including hypocalcemia, blunted calcemic response to parathyroid hormone, hyperparathyroidism, and osteomalacia.
- Hypercoagulability from the urinary loss of anticoagulant proteins increases the risk for arterial and venous thromboembolism, including pulmonary embolism and deep vein or renal thrombus.

Characteristic manifestations of nephrotic syndrome include peripheral edema, massive proteinuria, hypertension, hyperlipidemia, hypoalbuminemia, and foamy urine.

Interprofessional Management

The goals are to relieve the symptoms and cure or control the primary disease. Corticosteroids and cyclophosphamide may be used. Prednisone is effective to varying degrees for some causes of nephrotic syndrome (e.g., membranous glomerulonephritis, lupus nephritis). Management of diabetes and treatment of edema are important.

Angiotensin-converting enzyme inhibitor or angiotensin receptor blocker drugs are used to try to reduce urine protein losses. Management of edema includes low sodium intake (2 to 3 g/day), and a moderate-protein diet (1 to 2 g/kg per day). Diuretics (typically loop diuretics) can improve edema. The treatment of hyperlipidemia includes lipid-lowering agents.

Nursing Management

The major focus of care is related to edema. Assess the edema by weighing the patient daily, accurately recording intake and output, and measuring abdominal girth or extremity size. Monitor effectiveness of diuretic therapy. Clean edematous areas carefully to avoid trauma to the skin.

Patients have the potential to become malnourished from anorexia and the loss of protein in the urine. Serve small, frequent meals in a pleasant setting to encourage better dietary intake.

- Teach the patient to avoid exposure to people with known infections.
- Support the patient in coping with an altered body image because embarrassment may be associated with the edematous appearance.

NON-HODGKIN'S LYMPHOMAS

Description

Non-Hodgkin's lymphomas (NHLs) are a broad group of cancers of primarily B-, T-, natural killer (NK), histiocytic and dendritic cells. They affect persons of all ages. There are over 75 types categorized by the level of differentiation (maturity), cell of origin, immunophenotype (cell surface markers), genetic, and clinical features. NHL is the most commonly occurring hematologic cancer.

Pathophysiology

The cause of NHL is usually unknown. NHLs may result from chromosomal translocations, infections, environmental factors, and immunodeficiency states. Chromosomal translocations have a key role in the pathogenesis of many NHLs. Viruses and bacteria implicated in NHL include *HTLV-1, EBV, human herpesvirus 8, hepatitis B* and *C, Helicobacter pylori, Chlamydophila psittaci, Campylobacter jejuni,* and *Borrelia burgdorferi.*

Environmental factors linked to the development of NHL include chemicals (e.g., pesticides, herbicides, solvents, organic chemicals, wood preservatives). NHL is more common in those with inherited immunodeficiency syndromes, have used immunosuppressive agents, (e.g., to prevent rejection after organ transplantation or to treat autoimmune disorders), or received chemotherapy or radiation therapy.

All NHLs involve lymphocytes arrested in various stages of development and may mimic a leukemia. *Diffuse large B cell lymphoma,* the most common aggressive lymphoma, starts in the lymph nodes, usually in the neck or abdomen. *Burkitt's lymphoma* is the most aggressive type of NHL.

Clinical Manifestations

The method of spread can be unpredictable and most patients have widespread disease at the time of diagnosis. The primary clinical manifestation is painless lymph node enlargement. The lymphadenopathy can wax and wane in indolent disease. NHLs can originate outside the lymph nodes and the method of spread can be unpredictable. The majority of patients have widely disseminated disease at the time of diagnosis.

- The primary manifestation is painless lymph node enlargement.
- Because the disease has usually spread, other symptoms are present depending on where the disease is present (e.g., hepatomegaly with liver involvement, neurologic symptoms with central nervous system [CNS] disease).
- NHL can manifest in nonspecific ways, such as an airway obstruction, hyperuricemia and renal failure from tumor lysis syndrome, pericardial tamponade, and gastrointestinal (GI) symptoms.
- Patients with high-grade lymphomas may have lymphadenopathy and B symptoms such as fever, night sweats, and weight loss.

Diagnostic Studies

Diagnostic studies for NHL resemble those used for Hodgkin's lymphoma. However, because NHL is more often found in extranodal sites, more diagnostic studies may be done. These include MRI or lumbar puncture to rule out CNS disease, a bone marrow biopsy to determine bone marrow infiltration, or a barium enema, upper endoscopy, or CT to look for GI involvement.

Nursing and Interprofessional Management

Treatment for NHL involves chemotherapy, biotherapy, radiation, and sometimes phototherapy and topical therapy (see Chemotherapy, p. 674; Radiation Therapy, p. 712). Ironically, more aggressive lymphomas (diffuse large B cell) are generally more responsive to treatment. In contrast, indolent lymphomas (e.g., follicular lymphomas) have a naturally long course but are hard to effectively treat.

- Rituximab, a monoclonal antibody against the CD20 antigen on the surface of normal and malignant B lymphocytes, is used to treat NHL in combination with other agents (see Table 30.29, Harding et al., *Lewis' Medical-Surgical Nursing*, ed 11).
- Numerous chemotherapy combinations have been used to try to overcome the resistant nature of this disease.
- Hematopoietic stem cell transplantation may be of benefit in certain subtypes of NHL.
- Other therapies for some types of NHL include the monoclonal antibody ibritumomab tiuxetan (Zevalin).
- For more diffuse disease, treatment may include methotrexate, α-interferon, brentuximab vedotin, or other drugs.

Nursing care for patients with NHL is similar to that for patients with Hodgkin's lymphoma. It is largely based on managing problems related to the disease (pain, spinal cord compression, tumor lysis syndrome), pancytopenia, and effects of therapy.

- The patient undergoing external beam radiation therapy needs special care Concepts related to safety with radiation therapy are important in the plan of care (see Chapter 15, Harding et al., *Lewis' Medical-Surgical Nursing,* ed 11).
- Psychosocial considerations are important. Help the patient and family understand the disease, treatment, and expected and potential side effects.
- Evaluation of patients with NHL for long-term effects of therapy is important because the consequences of disease and treatment may not become apparent for many years.

OBESITY

Description

Obesity is an excessively high amount of body fat or adipose tissue. Obesity is a global problem because it is a major risk factor for leading causes of death, including type 2 diabetes, heart disease, and certain cancers. Overweight persons often have problems with mobility and sleeping that affect their health.

The consequences of obesity extend beyond the physical changes. Social stigma can take an emotional toll on a person's psychologic well-being. Many have problems related to altered body image, depression, and low self-esteem, and withdraw from social interaction.

The obesity problem is a public health crisis. After decades of rising obesity rates among adults, the rate of increase is beginning to slow, but rates are still far too high. Currently, about 37% of adults in the United States are obese. Significant geographic, racial and ethnic, and income disparities exist. Obesity rates are highest in the South and among blacks, Hispanics, and lower-income, less-educated Americans.

- Attitudes about obesity can create biases and discrimination against people who are obese. Obesity must be viewed and treated as a chronic disease similar to other chronic diseases such as diabetes and hypertension.
- Obesity in adulthood is often a problem that begins in childhood or adolescence. One in 10 children becomes obese as early as age 2 to 5 years. Reversing the childhood obesity crisis is key to addressing the overall obesity epidemic.

The most common measure of obesity is the *body mass index* (BMI). BMI is calculated by dividing a person's weight (in kilograms) by the square of the height in meters.

- Persons with a BMI < 18.5 kg/m^2 are considered underweight, whereas a BMI between 18.5 and 24.9 kg/m^2 reflects a normal body weight. A BMI of 25 to 29.9 kg/m^2 is classified as being *overweight* and people with values at 30 kg/m^2 or above are considered *obese*. The term *extreme obesity* (morbid or severe obesity) is used for those with a BMI > 40 kg/m^2.
- The waist-to-hip ratio (WHR) is another method used to assess obesity. This ratio describes the distribution of both subcutaneous and visceral adipose tissue. The ratio is calculated by using the waist measurement divided by the hip measurement. A WHR < 0.8 is best. A WHR > 0.8 indicates more truncal fat, which puts the person at greater risk for health complications.
- Persons with fat located primarily in the abdominal area *(apple-shaped body)* are at greater risk for obesity-related complications than those whose fat is primarily located in the upper legs *(pear-shaped body)*.

Pathophysiology

The cause of obesity involves significant genetic/biologic susceptibility factors that are highly influenced by environmental and psychosocial factors.

Most obese people have *primary obesity*, which is excess calorie intake over energy expenditure for the body's metabolic demands. Others have *secondary obesity* from various congenital anomalies, chromosomal anomalies, metabolic problems, central nervous system lesions and disorders, or drugs (e.g., corticosteroids, antipsychotics).

- Neuropeptide Y, made in the hypothalamus, is a powerful appetite stimulant. When it is imbalanced, it leads to overeating and obesity. Hormones and peptides made in the gut and adipocyte cells affect the hypothalamus and have a critical role in appetite and energy balance.

The 2 major consequences of obesity are caused by the sheer increase in fat mass and the production of adipokines by fat cells. Adipocytes make at least 100 different proteins. These proteins (secreted as enzymes), adipokines, growth factors, and hormones, contribute to the insulin resistance, dyslipidemia, and high BP.

Environmental factors play a key role in obesity. In today's culture, people have greater access to food (particularly prepackaged and fast foods) and soft drinks, which have poor nutritional quality. In addition, eating outside of the home interferes with the ability to control the quality and quantity of food. Portion size of meals has increased dramatically. Underestimating portion sizes and therefore caloric intake is common.

- Lack of physical exercise is another factor that contributes to weight gain and obesity.
- Socioeconomic status is a known risk factor for obesity in a variety of ways. People with low incomes may try to stretch their food dollars by buying less expensive foods that have poor nutritional quality with a greater caloric content.
- The association of food with comfort, reward, pleasure, and fun is a powerful incentive for overeating.

Diagnostic Studies
- History and physical examination are done to assess the extent and duration of obesity.
- Laboratory tests of liver function, fasting glucose level, triglyceride level, and low- and high-density lipoprotein cholesterol levels assist in evaluating the cause and effects of obesity.
- Classifications of body weight and obesity are defined by BMI, standardized height-weight charts, or WHR.

Interprofessional Management
A multifaceted approach needs to be taken with attention to nutritional therapy, exercise, behavior modification, and for some, medication or surgical intervention. Stress healthy eating habits and adequate physical activity as lifestyle patterns to develop and maintain. Restricting dietary intake so that it is below energy requirements is a cornerstone for any weight loss or maintenance program. It is best to recommend a dietary approach in which calorie restriction includes all food groups.
- Setting a realistic and healthy goal, such as losing 1 to 2 lb/wk, should be mutually agreed on at the beginning of a weight loss program.
- During plateau periods, when no weight is lost for days to weeks, patients need encouragement and support.
- Exercise is an essential part of a weight control program. Patients should exercise daily, with a goal of more than 10,000 steps per day. Exercise is especially important in maintaining weight loss.
- People who are in a behavioral therapy program are more successful in maintaining their losses over an extended time than those who do not take part in such training.
- Joining a support or self-help group with others having the same experiences may be useful.

Drug Therapy
Medications, if used, should be part of a comprehensive weight-reduction program that includes reduced-calorie diet, exercise, and behavior modification. Drugs should be reserved for adults with

a BMI of 30 kg/m^2 or greater (obese), or adults with a BMI of 27 kg/m^2 or greater (overweight) who have at least 1 weight-related condition such as hypertension, type 2 diabetes, or dyslipidemia. The drugs currently approved by the U.S. Food and Drug Administration (FDA) for treatment of obesity are presented in Table 59.

Surgical Therapy

Bariatric surgery, surgery on the stomach and/or intestines to help a person lose weight, has become a viable option for treating extreme obesity. Surgery is currently the only treatment that has a lasting impact of sustained weight loss for those with extreme obesity.

- Bariatric surgeries are categorized as restrictive, malabsorptive, or a combination of restrictive and malabsorptive. In restrictive procedures, the stomach is reduced in size (less food eaten). In malabsorptive procedures, the small intestine is shortened or bypassed (less food absorbed). Most procedures are performed laparoscopically.

- Common restrictive surgeries include adjustable gastric banding and sleeve gastrectomy. These surgeries are discussed further in Chapter 40 of Harding et al., *Lewis' Medical-Surgical Nursing,* ed 11.

- An intragastric balloon, placed using an endoscope, can help patients feel full, curb appetite, and reduce food intake.

The Roux-en-Y gastric bypass (RYGB) procedure is a combination of restrictive and malabsorptive surgery. This surgical procedure is the most common bariatric procedure done in the United States and is considered the gold standard among bariatric procedures.

- This procedure involves creating a small gastric pouch and attaching it directly to the small intestine using a Y-shaped limb of the small bowel. After the procedure, food bypasses 90% of the stomach, the duodenum, and a small segment of jejunum.

- A complication of the RYGB is *dumping syndrome,* in which gastric contents empty too rapidly into the small intestine, overwhelming its ability to digest nutrients. Signs and symptoms can include vomiting, nausea, weakness, sweating, faintness, and diarrhea.

An alternative to gastrointestinal restriction or bypass surgery is an implantable gastric stimulation device (e.g., Maestro Rechargeable System). It consists of a pacemaker-like electrical pulse generator, wire leads, and electrodes implanted in the abdomen. Intermittent electrical pulses to the vagus nerve signal to the brain that the stomach feels empty or full.

Cosmetic surgeries may be used to reduce fatty tissue and skinfolds. These procedures include a *lipectomy* (adipectomy) to remove unsightly adipose folds and *liposuction* for cosmetic purposes.

TABLE 59 Drug Therapy

Obesity

Drug	Mechanism of Action	Nursing Considerations
bupropion/naltrexone (Contrave)	*bupropion*: antidepressant *naltrexone*: opioid antagonist	• Common side effects are nausea, constipation, headache, dizziness, insomnia, dry mouth • Suicidal thoughts and behaviors and neuropsychiatric reactions can occur • Can increase BP and heart rate. Should not be used in patients with uncontrolled hypertension • Can cause seizures. Must not be used in patients who have seizure disorder
liraglutide (Saxenda)	• Glucagon-like peptide 1 (GLP-1) agonist • Induces satiety	• Used to treat type 2 diabetes • Injected • Side effects include thyroid tumors and pancreatitis
lorcaserin (Belviq)	• Selective serotonin (5-HT) agonist • Suppresses appetite and creates a sense of satiety	• Side effects include headache, dizziness, fatigue, nausea, dry mouth, constipation
orlistat (Xenical, Alli [low-dose form available over the counter])	• Blocks fat breakdown and absorption in intestine • Inhibits the action of intestinal lipases, resulting in undigested fat excreted in feces	• Associated with leakage of stool, flatulence, diarrhea, abdominal bloating, especially if a high-fat diet is consumed • Severe liver injury may occur • May need fat-soluble vitamin supplements

| phentermine/topiramate ER (Qsymia) | *phentermine:* Sympathomimetic *topiramate:* decreases appetite | • Common side effects include dizziness, insomnia, dry mouth
 • Do not use in patients with glaucoma or hyperthyroidism
 • Must avoid pregnancy
 Can increase heart rate. Should not be used in patients with uncontrolled hypertension or heart disease |

0

Nursing Management

Goals

The overall goals are that the patient with obesity will modify eating patterns, participate in a regular physical activity program, achieve weight loss to a specified level, maintain weight loss at a specified level, and minimize or prevent health problems related to obesity.

Nursing Interventions

Together with other members of the interprofessional team, you have a major role in planning for and managing the care of an obese patient. It is essential that you have a nonjudgmental approach in helping patients manage their problems related to obesity.

- Focusing on the reasons for wanting to lose weight may help patients develop strategies for a weight loss program. Directed the plan of care at 2 different processes: (1) successful weight loss, which requires a short-term energy deficit, and (2) successful weight control, which requires long-term behavior changes.

Preoperative care for gastric surgery includes planning for the special needs of an obese patient, such as the availability of a larger-sized BP cuff, hospital gown, bed, and chair. Consider how the patient will be weighed, transported through the hospital, and turned. Teach the patient the proper coughing technique, deep breathing, use of an incentive spirometer, and methods of turning and positioning to prevent pulmonary complications after surgery.

Postoperative care focuses on careful assessment and immediate intervention for cardiopulmonary complications, deep vein thrombosis, anastomosis leaks, and electrolyte imbalances. Facilitate patient respiratory efforts (elevating the head of the bed, turning, coughing, deep breathing); monitor for wound infection, dehiscence, and delayed healing; and promote early ambulation. Patients have considerable abdominal pain after surgery. Give pain medications as needed during the immediate postoperative period.

- Some patients express guilt feelings that the only way they could lose weight was by surgical means. Be ready to provide support in moving away from such negative feelings.
- Stress the importance of long-term follow-up care to prevent and treat potential complications late in the recovery period. Encourage patients to adhere to the prescribed diet and inform the health care provider (HCP) of changes in their physical or emotional condition.

OBSTRUCTIVE SLEEP APNEA

Description

Obstructive sleep apnea (OSA), also called *obstructive sleep apnea–hypopnea syndrome,* is characterized by partial or complete upper airway obstruction during sleep. *Apnea* is the cessation of spontaneous respirations lasting longer than 10 seconds. *Hypopnea* is a condition characterized by shallow respirations (30% to 50% reduction in airflow).

- Sleep apnea occurs in 2% to 10% of Americans. Risk increases with age > 65 years, craniofacial abnormalities that affect the upper airway, acromegaly, obesity, and tobacco smoking. OSA patients with excessive daytime sleepiness have increased mortality.

Pathophysiology

Airflow obstruction occurs when: (1) narrowing of the air passages with relaxation of muscle tone during sleep leads to apnea and hypopnea, and (2) the tongue and soft palate fall backward and partially or completely obstruct the pharynx.

- Each obstruction may last 10 to 90 seconds. During the apneic period, hypoxemia and hypercapnia may cause the person to arouse briefly and snort or gasp without fully awakening.
- Apnea and arousal cycles occur as many as 200 to 400 times during 6 to 8 hours of sleep.

Clinical Manifestations

Manifestations of sleep apnea include frequent arousals during sleep, insomnia, excessive daytime sleepiness, and witnessed apneic episodes. A bed partner may complain about the person's loud snoring. Other symptoms include morning headaches, personality changes, and irritability.

- Untreated sleep apnea may cause hypertension, right-sided heart failure from pulmonary hypertension, and dysrhythmias. Chronic sleep loss can lead to decreased ability to concentrate, impaired memory, failure to complete daily tasks, and interpersonal difficulties.

Diagnostic Studies

- Sleep and medical history
- Polysomnography. OSA is defined as more than 5 apnea/hypopnea events per hour with a 3% to 4% decrease in O_2 saturation.

Nursing and Interprofessional Management

Conservative Treatment

Conservative home treatment for mild sleep apnea (5 to 10 apnea/hypopnea events per hour) includes sleeping on the side rather than the back, elevating the head of the bed, and avoiding sedatives or alcoholic beverages 3 to 4 hours before sleep. Excessive weight worsens sleep apnea; refer patient to a weight loss program if needed.

- Continuous positive airway pressure (CPAP) is often used for patients with severe symptoms (more than 15 apnea/hypopnea events per hour). A nasal mask, nasal pillows, or full-face mask is worn attached to a high-flow blower (see figures in Chapter 7 of Harding et al., *Lewis's Medical-Surgical Nursing*, ed 11). CPAP reduces apnea episodes, daytime sleepiness, and fatigue.
- Benefits of CPAP are dose-dependent. It must be used at least 4 hours each night to reduce the negative cardiovascular effects of OSA.
- Using a special mouth guard during sleep to prevent airflow obstruction may reduce symptoms.
- Opioid analgesics and sedating medications may worsen OSA symptoms by depressing respiration.
- Teach hospitalized patients with OSA to bring their home devices and continue CPAP use.

Surgery

If conservative measures fail, common surgical procedures are uvulopalatopharyngoplasty and genioglossal advancement and hyoid myotomy. Radiofrequency ablation may be used.

- Postoperative complications include airway obstruction or hemorrhage.
- Snoring may persist until inflammation has subsided.
- Patients are usually discharged within 1 day after surgery. Tell patients to expect a sore throat and to reduce foul breath odor by rinsing with diluted mouthwash and then salt water for several days.

ORAL CANCER

Description

There are 2 types of *oral cancer:* oral cavity cancer, which starts in the mouth, and oropharyngeal cancer, which develops in the part of the throat just behind the mouth (the oropharynx). *Head and neck squamous cell carcinoma* (HNSCC) is a broad term for cancers of the oral cavity, pharynx, and larynx. Most oral cancer lesions occur on the lower lip. Other common sites are the lateral border and undersurface of the tongue, labial commissure, and buccal mucosa.

- Cancer of the lip has a more favorable prognosis because the lesions are visible and are usually diagnosed earlier.
- The 5-year survival rate is 84% for localized cancer and 65% for all stages of cancer of the oral cavity and pharynx combined.

Pathophysiology

Oral cancer has several predisposing factors including prolonged sun exposure, tobacco use (cigar, cigarette, pipe, snuff), and frequent alcohol consumption. Human papillomavirus (HPV) contributes to 25% of oral cancer cases.

Clinical Manifestations

Common manifestations include the following:

- *Leukoplakia,* called *smoker's patch,* is a whitish precancerous lesion on the mucosa of the mouth or tongue that results from chronic irritation, especially from smoking. The patch may become keratinized (hard and leathery) and is then sometimes described as hyperkeratosis.
- *Erythroplakia* is a red velvety patch on the mouth or tongue. More than 50% of cases of erythroplakia progress to squamous cell carcinoma.

Patients may report nonspecific symptoms, such as chronic sore throat, sore mouth, and voice changes. Some patients with oral cancer have an asymptomatic neck mass. Later symptoms of oral cancer are pain, dysphagia (difficulty swallowing), and difficulty moving the jaw.

Cancer of the lip usually appears as an indurated, painless lip ulcer. The first sign of tongue cancer is an ulcer or area of thickening. Soreness or pain of the tongue may occur, especially on eating hot or highly seasoned foods.

- Later symptoms and signs of tongue cancer include increased salivation, slurred speech, dysphagia, toothache, and earache.

Diagnostic Studies

- Biopsy of suspected lesion
- Oral exfoliative cytology and toluidine blue test are used to screen for oral cancer.
- CT scan, MRI, and positron emission tomography (PET) are used in staging cancer.

Interprofessional Management

Management usually consists of surgery, radiation therapy, and/or chemotherapy. Surgery remains the most effective treatment. Some patients with small tumors in the mouth and throat are candidates for minimally invasive robotic-assisted surgery. Many surgeries are radical procedures involving extensive resections. Some examples are hemiglossectomy (removal of one-half of the tongue), glossectomy (removal of the entire tongue), and radical neck dissection (wide excision of the lymph nodes and their lymphatic channels). A tracheostomy (see Tracheostomy, p. 714) is common with radical neck dissection.

Chemotherapy and radiation therapy are used together when there are positive margins, bone erosion, or positive lymph nodes (see Chemotherapy, p. 674, and Radiation Therapy, p. 712). Chemotherapy agents used include fluorouracil, cisplatin, carboplatin, paclitaxel, docetaxel, and hydroxyurea.

Palliative treatment is used when the prognosis is poor, the cancer is inoperable, or the patient decides against surgery. If it becomes difficult for the patient to swallow, placing a gastrostomy will allow for adequate nutritional intake. Frequent oral suctioning may be needed.

Nursing Management

Goals
The patient with carcinoma of the oral cavity will have a patent airway, be able to communicate, have adequate nutritional intake to promote wound healing, and have relief of pain and discomfort.

Nursing Interventions
You have a significant role in early detection and treatment of oral cancer. Identify patients at risk (users of tobacco products, alcoholics, those with poor dental hygiene, pipe smokers) and provide information regarding predisposing factors. Inform the patient who smokes about smoking cessation programs available in the community. Warn adolescents and teenagers about the dangers of using snuff or chewing tobacco.

- Refer any person with an ulcerative lesion that does not heal within 2 to 3 weeks to a health care provider (HCP).
- Teach the patient to report unexplained pain or soreness of the mouth, unusual bleeding, dysphagia, sore throat, voice changes, or swelling or lump in the neck.

See Head and Neck Cancer, p. 250, for care of the preoperative or postoperative patient with a radical neck dissection.

OSTEOARTHRITIS

Description
Osteoarthritis (OA), the most common form of joint disease, is a slowly progressive noninflammatory disorder of the diarthrodial

(synovial) joints. Currently over 30 million adults in the United States are affected by OA. Numbers are expected to rise as the population ages. (See Table 60.)

OA is not considered to be a normal part of the aging process, but aging is 1 risk factor for disease development. OA involves gradual loss of articular cartilage with formation of bony outgrowths (spurs or osteophytes) at the joint margins. Cartilage destruction may begin at ages 20 years, and a majority of adults are affected by age 40 years. Few patients have symptoms until after age 50 or 60 years, but more than half of those over age 65 years have x-ray evidence of the disease in at least 1 joint. After age 50 years, women are more often affected than men.

- Obesity is a modifiable risk factor that contributes to hip and knee OA by increasing the mechanical stress on the joints.
- Anterior cruciate ligament injury from quick stops and pivoting, as in football and soccer, has been linked to an increased risk for knee OA. Occupations that require frequent kneeling and stooping also increase the risk for knee OA.

Pathophysiology

The development of OA is complex. Genetic, metabolic, and local factors interact to cause cartilage deterioration from damage at the level of the chondrocytes. The normally smooth, white, translucent articular cartilage becomes dull, yellow, and granular as the disease progresses. Affected cartilage steadily becomes softer and less elastic. It is less able to resist wear with heavy use.

The body's attempts at cartilage repair cannot keep up with the destruction of OA. As the collagen in the cartilage changes, articular surfaces become cracked and worn. While central cartilage becomes thinner, cartilage at the joint edges becomes thicker, and osteophytes form. Joint surfaces become uneven, affecting the distribution of stress across the joint and causing reduced motion.

Although inflammation is not typical of OA, secondary synovitis may occur when phagocytes try to rid the joint of small pieces of cartilage torn from the joint surface. These changes cause the early pain and stiffness of OA. Pain in later disease occurs when articular cartilage is lost and bony joint surfaces rub on each other.

Clinical Manifestations

Fatigue, fever, and organ involvement are not present in OA. This is an important distinction between OA and inflammatory joint disorders, such as rheumatoid arthritis (Table 60). Manifestations of OA range from mild discomfort to significant disability.

TABLE 60 Comparison of Rheumatoid Arthritis and Osteoarthritis

Parameter	Rheumatoid Arthritis	Osteoarthritis
Age at onset	Young to middle age	Usually >40 yr
Gender	Female:male ratio is 2:1 or 3:1 Fewer marked sex differences after age 60 yr	Female:male ratio 2:1 after age 60 yr; except for traumatic arthritis, men less affected until age 70 or 80 yr
Weight	Lost or maintained weight	Often overweight or obese
Disease	Systemic disease with exacerbations and remissions	Localized disease with variable, progressive course
Affected joints	Small joints typically affected first (PIPs, MCPs, MTPs), wrists, elbows, shoulders, knees Usually bilateral, symmetric joint involvement	Weight-bearing joints of knees and hips, small joints (MCPs, DIPs, PIPs), cervical and lumbar spine Often asymmetric
Pain characteristics	Stiffness lasts 1 hr to all day and may decrease with use. Pain is variable, may disrupt sleep.	Stiffness occurs on arising but usually subsides after 30 min. Pain gradually worsens with joint use and disease progression, relieved with joint rest but may disrupt sleep.
Effusions	Common	Uncommon
Nodules	Present, especially on extensor surfaces	Heberden's (DIPs) and Bouchard's (PIPs) nodes
Synovial fluid	WBC count 3000–25,000/μL with mostly neutrophils; decreased viscosity	WBC count <2000/μL (mild leukocytosis); normal viscosity

X-rays	Joint space narrowing and erosion with bony overgrowths, subluxation with advanced disease	Joint space narrowing, osteophytes, subchondral cysts, sclerosis
	Osteoporosis related to decreased activity, corticosteroid use	
Laboratory findings	RF-positive in 70%–90% of patients; negative titers in early disease for about 25% of patients	RF-negative
	Increase in ANA titer likely.	ANA-negative
	Positive anti-CCP in 60%–80% of patients	Anti-CCP–negative
	Elevated ESR, CRP indicative of active inflammation	Transient elevation in ESR related to synovitis

ANA, Antinuclear antibodies; anti-CCP, anti-citrullinated peptide; CRP, C-reactive protein; DIPs, distal interphalangeals; ESR, erythrocyte sedimentation rate; MCPs, metacarpophalangeals; MTPs, metatarsophalangeals; PIPs, proximal interphalangeals; RF, rheumatoid factor.

Joints

Joint pain is the primary symptom and the typical reason the patient seeks medical attention. Pain generally gets worse with joint use. In early stages of OA, joint pain is relieved by rest. However, the patient with advanced disease may report pain at rest or have trouble sleeping because of increased joint pain. Pain may also worsen as the barometric pressure falls before the onset of severe weather. The pain of OA may be referred to the groin, buttock, or side of the thigh or knee. Sitting down becomes difficult, as does rising from a chair when the hips are lower than the knees. As OA develops in intervertebral joints of the spine, localized pain and stiffness are common.

Unlike pain, which typically worsens with activity, joint stiffness occurs after periods of rest or static position. Early-morning stiffness is common but generally resolves within 30 minutes, a feature that distinguishes OA from inflammatory joint disorders, such as rheumatoid arthritis.

- Overactivity can temporarily increase stiffness. *Crepitation,* a grating sensation caused by loose cartilage particles in the joint cavity, can also contribute to stiffness.
- OA usually affects joints asymmetrically. The most commonly involved joints are the distal interphalangeal (DIP) and proximal interphalangeal (PIP) joints of the fingers, the metacarpophalangeal (MCP) joint of the thumb, the weight-bearing joints (hips, knees), the metatarsophalangeal (MTP) joint of the foot, and the cervical and lower lumbar vertebrae.

Deformity

Deformity or instability associated with OA is specific to the involved joint. For example, *Heberden's nodes* occur on the distal interphalangeal joints because of osteophyte formation and loss of joint space. *Bouchard's nodes* on the proximal interphalangeal joints indicate similar disease involvement. Heberden's and Bouchard's nodes are often red, swollen, and tender. These bony enlargements do not usually cause significant loss of function.

Knee OA often leads to joint deformity as a result of cartilage loss in the medial compartment. For example, the patient becomes bowlegged (varus deformity) in response to medial joint arthritis. Lateral joint arthritis causes a "knock-knee" appearance (valgus deformity). In advanced hip OA, one of the patient's legs may become shorter as the joint space narrows.

Diagnostic Studies

- A bone scan, CT scan, or MRI may be useful to diagnose OA. X-rays also confirm disease and monitor the progression of joint damage. However, these changes do not always reflect the degree of pain the patient experiences.

- No laboratory abnormalities or biomarkers are specific diagnostic indicators. The erythrocyte sedimentation rate (ESR) is normal except for slight elevations during acute inflammation.
- Synovial fluid analysis helps distinguish OA from types of inflammatory arthritis. In OA, fluid remains clear yellow with little or no sign of inflammation.

Interprofessional Management

Care focuses on managing pain and inflammation, preventing disability, and maintaining and improving joint function. Nondrug interventions are the basis of management.

The affected joint should be rested during any periods of acute inflammation and maintained in a functional position with splints or braces if necessary. Immobilization should not exceed 1 week because joint stiffness increases with inactivity. The patient may need to modify activities or use an assistive device to decrease stress on affected joints. Teach the patient with knee OA to avoid prolonged standing, kneeling, or squatting.

- Applications of heat and cold may help reduce pain and stiffness. Heat therapy is helpful for stiffness, including hot packs, whirlpool, ultrasound, and paraffin wax baths.
- If the patient is overweight, weight reduction is critical to the treatment plan. Help the patient evaluate the current diet to make needed changes. Exercise is an important part of OA management. Aerobic conditioning, range-of-motion exercises, and specific programs to strengthen muscles around the affected joint have been beneficial for many patients with knee OA.

Complementary and alternative therapies for OA symptom management are popular with patients who have not found relief through traditional medical care. Teach the patient to carefully research any alternative therapies and avoid replacing conventional OA treatments with unproven approaches. Acupuncture may reduce arthritis pain and improve joint mobility. Massage and Tai Chi may also reduce pain and improve function. These therapies are generally safe when performed by an experienced practitioner.

Some nutritional supplements may have antiinflammatory effects (e.g., fish oil, ginger, Sam-e), but research results have been inconsistent. The U.S. Food and Drug Administration has also warned consumers about tainted supplement with hidden ingredients that may cause unexpected side effects or interact with medications in a harmful way. The American College of Rheumatology conditionally recommends that patients do not use glucosamine or chondroitin sulfate. The American Academy of Orthopaedic Surgeons strongly recommends against their use. Teach patients to discuss any supplement use with their health care providers (HCPs) to identify possible interactions with prescribed medications.

Drug Therapy

Drug therapy is based on the severity of the patient's symptoms. The patient with mild to moderate joint pain may receive relief from acetaminophen (Tylenol). Topical agents, such as capsaicin cream, salicylates, camphor, eucalyptus oil, and menthol, may provide temporary pain relief.

If a patient does not get adequate pain management with acetaminophen or has moderate to severe OA pain or signs of joint inflammation, a nonsteroidal antiinflammatory drug (NSAID) may be more effective.

- NSAID therapy typically is initiated in low-dose over-the-counter (OTC) strengths (e.g., ibuprofen, 200 mg up to 4 times daily). The dose may be increased if needed. If the patient is at risk for or develops gastrointestinal (GI) side effects with an NSAID, additional treatment with a protective agent, such as misoprostol (Cytotec), may be needed. Arthrotec, a combination of misoprostol and the NSAID diclofenac, is also available. Diclofenac gel may be applied to the affected joint. Teach the patient who is taking an oral NSAID to avoid use of a topical NSAID because of increased risk for adverse effects.
- As an alternative to traditional NSAIDs, treatment with the cyclooxygenase (COX)-2 inhibitor celecoxib (Celebrex) may be considered. However, all NSAIDs carry the same risk for GI effects.

Intraarticular injections of corticosteroids may decrease local inflammation and effusion. Systemic use of corticosteroids is not indicated and may actually accelerate the disease process.

Symptoms of OA are often managed conservatively for many years. However, the patient's loss of joint function, unmanaged pain, and decreased independence in self-care may lead to consideration of surgery. Arthroscopy was previously performed for patients with knee OA, often to remove loose bodies from the joint. However, it has been found to provide no additional benefit over physical therapy and medical treatment.

Nursing Management

Goals

The patient with OA will maintain or improve joint function through a balance of rest and activity, use joint protection measures to improve activity tolerance, achieve independence in self-care and maintain optimal role function, and use drug and nondrug strategies to manage pain satisfactorily.

Nursing Interventions

Focus community education on altering modifiable risk factors. For example, encourage the patient to lose weight and reduce occupational or recreational hazards. For athletic instruction and physical fitness programs, include safety measures that protect and reduce trauma to the joints. Traumatic joint injuries should be treated promptly to decrease the risk of developing OA.

The patient with OA is usually treated on an outpatient basis, often by an interprofessional team that includes a rheumatologist, a nurse, an occupational therapist, and a physical therapist.

- Drugs are administered for the treatment of pain and inflammation. Nondrug strategies to decrease pain and disability may include massage, use of heat (thermal packs) or cold (ice packs), meditation, and yoga.
- Home and work environment modification is essential for patient safety, accessibility, and self-care. Teach about removing scatter rugs, providing rails at the stairs and bathtub, using night-lights, and wearing well-fitting supportive shoes. Assistive devices such as canes, walkers, elevated toilet seats, and grab bars reduce joint load and promote safety.
- Sexual counseling may help the patient and their partner enjoy physical closeness by introducing the idea of alternate positions and timing for intercourse.

▼ **Patient and Caregiver Teaching**

Patient and caregiver teaching related to OA is an important nursing responsibility.

- Provide information about the nature and treatment of the disease, pain management, posture and body mechanics, correct use of assistive devices such as a cane or walker, principles of joint protection and energy conservation, and an exercise program.
- Individualize home management goals to meet the patient's needs. Include the patient caregiver, family, and significant others in goal setting and teaching.
- Assure the patient that OA is a localized disease and that severe deforming arthritis is not the usual course. The patient may appreciate community resources, such as the Arthritis Foundation's Self-Help Course (*www.arthritis.org*).

OSTEOMALACIA

Osteomalacia is caused by vitamin D deficiency, which results in bone losing calcium and becoming soft. The disease is uncommon in the United States. It is the same disorder as rickets in children, except that the epiphyseal growth plates are closed in adults.

- Vitamin D is required for absorption of calcium from the intestine. Insufficient vitamin D intake can interfere with the normal bone mineralization; with little or no calcification, bones become soft.
- Causes include limited sun exposure (ultraviolet rays needed for vitamin D synthesis), gastrointestinal (GI) malabsorption (post weight loss surgery, Celiac disease), chronic diarrhea, and pregnancy.

Common manifestations are bone pain and muscle weakness. The pain is often worse at night and affects the lower back, pelvis, hips, legs, and ribs. Muscle weakness and progressive deformity of weight-bearing bones (e.g., spine, extremities) can lead to problems walking and a waddling gait. Fractures are common and slow to heal.

Laboratory findings include decreased serum calcium or phosphorus levels, decreased serum 25-hydroxyvitamin D, and increased serum alkaline phosphatase. X-rays may demonstrate generalized bone demineralization, especially a loss of calcium in the bones of the pelvis, and the presence of associated bone deformity.

- *Looser's transformation zones* (ribbons of decalcification in bone found on x-ray) are diagnostic of osteomalacia. Significant osteomalacia may exist without x-ray changes.

Interprofessional care is directed toward correcting vitamin D deficiency. When vitamin D_3 (cholecalciferol) and vitamin D_2 (ergocalciferol) are used as supplements, the patient often shows a dramatic response. Calcium or phosphorus supplements may also be prescribed.

- Exposure to sunlight and weight-bearing exercise are valuable.
- Encourage consumption of eggs, meat, oily fish, and milk and breakfast cereals fortified with calcium and vitamin D.

OSTEOMYELITIS

Description

Osteomyelitis is a severe infection of the bone, bone marrow, and surrounding soft tissue. Although *Staphylococcus aureus* is the most common cause of infection, a variety of pathogens can cause osteomyelitis (Table 61).

Pathophysiology

Infecting microorganisms can invade by indirect or direct entry. *Indirect entry* (hematogenous) is usually associated with infection

TABLE 61	Organisms Causing Osteomyelitis
Organism	Predisposing Problem(s)
Staphylococcus aureus	Pressure injury, penetrating wound, open fracture, orthopedic surgery, disorders with vascular insufficiency (e.g., diabetes, atherosclerosis)
Staphylococcus epidermidis	Indwelling prosthetic devices (e.g., joint replacements, fracture fixation devices)
Streptococcus viridans	Abscessed tooth, gingival disease
Escherichia coli	Urinary tract infection
Mycobacterium tuberculosis	Tuberculosis
Neisseria gonorrhoeae	Gonorrhea
Pseudomonas	Puncture wounds, IV drug use
Salmonella	Sickle cell disease
Fungi, mycobacteria	Immunocompromised host

with 1 microorganism. Indirect injury accounts for only 20% of all cases. It most often affects children younger than 17 years of age. Risk factors in adults are older age, debilitation, hemodialysis, sickle cell disease, and IV drug use. The vertebrae are the most common site of infection in adults.

Direct entry osteomyelitis most often affects adults. It can occur when an open wound (e.g., penetrating wounds, fractures, surgery) allows microorganisms to enter the body. Osteomyelitis may also be related to a foreign body, such as an implant or an orthopedic prosthetic device (e.g., plate, total joint prosthesis). It may occur in the feet of patients with diabetes or vascular disease–related ulcers or in the hips or sacrum near a pressure injury. More than 1 microorganism is usually involved.

After entering the blood, the microorganisms grow, and pressure increases because of the nonexpanding nature of most bone. This leads to ischemia and vascular compromise of the periosteum.

- The infection spreads through the bone cortex and marrow cavity, ultimately resulting in cortical devascularization and necrosis. Bone death occurs resulting from ischemia.
- The areas of devitalized bone eventually separate from surrounding living bone, forming *sequestra*. The part of the periosteum that continues to have a blood supply forms new bone called *involucrum*. It is difficult for blood-borne

antibiotics or defending white blood cells (WBCs) to reach the sequestra. A sequestrum may become a reservoir for microorganisms that spread to other sites, including the lungs and brain. If the sequestrum does not resolve on its own or is not debrided surgically, a sinus tract may develop with chronic, purulent drainage.

Acute osteomyelitis refers to the initial infection or an infection of < 1 month in duration.

Chronic osteomyelitis refers to a bone infection that persists for longer than 1 month or an infection that did not respond to an initial course of antibiotic therapy. Chronic osteomyelitis may be a continuous, persistent problem (a result of inadequate acute treatment), or a process of exacerbations and remissions. Over time, granulation tissue turns to avascular scar tissue, providing an ideal site for microorganism growth that cannot be penetrated by antibiotics.

Clinical Manifestations
Acute Osteomyelitis
Systemic manifestations include fever, night sweats, restlessness, nausea, and malaise.
- Local manifestations include constant bone pain that is unrelieved by rest and worsens with activity; swelling, tenderness, and warmth at the infection site; and restricted movement of the affected part.
- Later signs include drainage from the sinus tracts to the skin and/or fracture site.
Chronic Osteomyelitis
Local signs of infection become more common, including constant bone pain and swelling and warmth at the infection site. Systemic signs may be less severe than those seen with the acute form.

Diagnostic Studies
- Bone or soft tissue biopsy is definitive for determining the microorganism.
- Blood and/or wound cultures are frequently positive.
- Elevated WBC and erythrocyte sedimentation rate (ESR) may be found.
- MRI and CT scan may be used to help identify the extent of the infection.
- Radionuclide bone scans (gallium and indium) show abnormalities earlier than x-ray.
- X-ray signs suggestive of osteomyelitis usually do not appear until 2 to 4 weeks after the appearance of clinical symptoms. By this time, the disease will have progressed.

Interprofessional Management

Aggressive and prolonged IV antibiotic therapy is the treatment of choice for acute osteomyelitis if bone ischemia has not occurred. Any related soft tissue abscess or ulceration often needs surgical debridement or drainage.

Patients are often discharged to home care with IV antibiotics delivered through a central venous access device (CVAD). IV antibiotic therapy may be started in the hospital then continued at home for 4 to 6 weeks. A few persons need therapy for 3 to 6 months. A variety of antibiotics are used, depending on the culture results and likelihood of resistance. These include oxacillin, nafcillin, clindamycin, vancomycin, ceftriaxone, cefazolin, ceftazidime, gentamicin, and linezolid.

Treatment of chronic osteomyelitis includes: (1) surgical removal of the poorly perfused tissue and dead bone, and (2) extended use of antibiotics.

- In adults with chronic osteomyelitis, oral therapy with a fluoroquinolone (ciprofloxacin [Cipro]) for 6 to 8 weeks may be prescribed instead of IV antibiotics.
- Oral antibiotic therapy may also be given for 4 to 8 weeks after IV therapy is complete.
- Patient response to drug therapy is monitored through bone scans and ESR tests.

Surgical treatment for chronic osteomyelitis includes surgical removal of the poorly vascularized tissue and dead bone. Antibiotic-impregnated acrylic bead chains may be implanted during surgery.

- Intermittent or constant irrigation of the affected bone with antibiotics may be used.
- Hyperbaric oxygen therapy using 100% oxygen may be given as an adjunct therapy in chronic osteomyelitis.

If an orthopedic prosthetic device is a source of chronic infection, it must be removed. Muscle flaps or skin grafting provide wound coverage over the dead space (cavity) in the bone. Bone grafts may help restore blood flow. However, flaps or grafts should never be placed in the presence of active or suspected infection. Amputation of the extremity may be indicated to preserve life or improve quality of life (see Amputation, p. 661).

- Rare complications of osteomyelitis include septicemia, septic arthritis, pathologic fractures, and amyloidosis.

Nursing Management

Goals

The patient with osteomyelitis will have satisfactory pain and fever control, not have any complications associated with osteomyelitis, cooperate with the treatment plan, and maintain a positive outlook on the disease outcome.

Nursing Interventions

Control of other infections (e.g., urinary and respiratory tract, deep pressure injuries) is important in preventing osteomyelitis. Those at risk for osteomyelitis are those who are immunocompromised or have diabetes, orthopedic implants, or vascular insufficiency.

- Teach patients at risk regarding signs of osteomyelitis and to immediately contact the health care provider (HCP) about bone pain, fever, swelling, and restricted limb movement so that treatment can be started.

Some immobilization of the affected limb (e.g., splint, traction) is usually needed to decrease pain. Carefully handle the involved limb to avoid excessive manipulation, which increases pain and may cause a pathologic fracture.

- Assess the patient's pain. Muscle spasms may cause minor to severe pain. Nonsteroidal antiinflammatory drugs (NSAIDs), opioid analgesics, and muscle relaxants may be prescribed to provide patient comfort. Encourage nondrug (e.g., guided imagery, relaxation breathing) approaches to pain.

- Dressings are used to absorb wound drainage and to debride devitalized tissue. Sterile technique is essential when changing the dressing.

The patient is often placed on bed rest in the early stages of acute infection. Good body alignment and position changes prevent complications associated with immobility and promote comfort.

- Peak and trough blood levels of most antibiotics should be monitored to avoid adverse drug effects.

▼ **Patient and Caregiver Teaching**

- Teach the patient the possible adverse and toxic reactions associated with prolonged high-dose antibiotic therapy. These reactions include hearing deficit, impaired renal function, and neurotoxicity (e.g., limb weakness or numbness, cognitive changes, vision changes, headache, behavioral problems). Reactions associated with cephalosporins (e.g., cefazolin) include hives, severe or watery diarrhea, blood in stools, and throat or mouth sores.

- Long-term antibiotic therapy can result in an overgrowth of *Candida albicans* and *Clostridium difficile* in the genitourinary tract and oral cavities. Teach the patient to report any whitish yellow, curdlike lesions to the HCP.

- If at home, teach patient and family about managing the venous access device, administering the antibiotic when scheduled and follow-up laboratory testing. Stress the importance of continuing to take antibiotics after the symptoms have improved.

- Instruct the patient and caregiver in the technique for wound dressing changes and assist them to obtain supplies.
- The patient and caregivers are often anxious and discouraged because of the serious nature of the disease, uncertainty of the outcome, and the long, costly treatment. Continued emotional support is an integral part of nursing management.

OSTEOPOROSIS

Description

Osteoporosis, or porous bone (fragile bone disease), is a chronic, progressive metabolic bone disease marked by low bone mass and structural deterioration of bone tissue, leading to increased bone fragility. Over 5 million people in the United States have decreased bone density or osteoporosis. One in 2 women and 1 in 4 men over the age of 50 years will sustain an osteoporosis-related fracture.

Risk factors for osteoporosis are female gender, advancing age (older than 65 years), white or Asian ethnicity, family history, low body weight, postmenopausal (estrogen deficiency), sedentary lifestyle, and a diet low in calcium or vitamin D deficiency. Low testosterone levels are a major risk factor in men.

- Current guidelines recommend an initial bone density test in all women over age 65 years. Women who are younger than 65 years and at high risk (e.g., low body weight, smoker, prior fractures) should also have a bone density test. If results are normal and the person is at low risk for osteoporosis, another test is not needed for 15 years. Testing should start earlier and be done more frequently if a person is at high risk for fractures.

Pathophysiology

Peak bone mass (maximum bone tissue) is typically achieved before age 20 years. It is largely determined by 4 factors: heredity, nutrition, exercise, and hormone function. Heredity may be responsible for up to 70% of peak bone mass.

- Bone loss from midlife (age 35 to 40 years) onward is inevitable, but the rate of loss varies. Women have rapid bone loss when estrogen production declines at menopause. This rate of loss then slows and eventually matches the rate of bone lost by men aged 65 to 70 years.

Bone is continually deposited by osteoblasts and resorbed by osteoclasts, a process called *remodeling*. Normally, the rates of bone deposition and resorption are equal, and total bone mass remains constant. In osteoporosis, bone resorption exceeds bone deposition.

- Specific diseases associated with osteoporosis include inflammatory bowel disease, intestinal malabsorption, kidney disease, rheumatoid arthritis, hyperthyroidism, chronic alcohol use, cirrhosis, and diabetes.
- Many drugs can interfere with bone metabolism, including corticosteroids, antiseizure drugs (phenytoin [Dilantin]), heparin, aluminum-containing antacids, certain cancer chemotherapy agents, and excess thyroid hormones. Long-term corticosteroid use is a major contributor to osteoporosis.

Clinical Manifestations

Bone loss occurs without symptoms. People may not know they have osteoporosis until a sudden strain, bump, or fall causes a hip, wrist, or vertebral fracture.

- The first indication of osteoporosis is usually back pain or spontaneous fractures. A person who has 1 spinal vertebral fracture because of osteoporosis has an increased risk for a second vertebral fracture within 1 year.
- Over time, wedging and fractures of the vertebrae produce loss of height and a humped back known as "dowager's hump," or *kyphosis.*

Diagnostic Studies

Osteoporosis often goes unnoticed because it cannot be detected by conventional x-ray until 25% to 40% of the calcium in the bone is lost.

- Serum calcium, phosphorus, and alkaline phosphatase levels remain normal, although alkaline phosphatase may be increased after a fracture.
- Bone mineral density (BMD) measurements are used to measure bone density.
  - Quantitative ultrasound (QUS) measures bone density with sound waves in the heel, kneecap, or shin.
  - One of the most common BMD studies is dual-energy x-ray absorptiometry (DEXA), which measures bone density in the spine, hips, and forearm (the most common sites of fractures resulting from osteoporosis). DEXA studies are useful to evaluate changes in bone density over time and to assess the effectiveness of treatment.
  - DEXA results are reported as T-scores: The *T-score* is the number of standard deviations below the average for normal bone density. A T-score of > -1 indicates normal bone density. Osteoporosis is defined as a BMD of < -2.5 (at least 2.5 standard deviations) below the mean BMD of young adults. A T-score between +1 and −1 is considered normal.

A T-score between −1 and −2.5 indicates *osteopenia* (bone loss that is greater than normal, but not yet at the level for a diagnosis of osteoporosis). A T-score of −2.5 or lower indicates osteoporosis. The greater the negative number, the more severe the osteoporosis.

- Sometimes the health care provider (HCP) asks for a *Z-score* instead of a T-score. For this score, a person is compared with someone their own age, gender, and/or ethnic group instead of a healthy 30-year-old. Among older adults, Z-scores can be misleading because decreased bone density is common. If the Z-score is −2 or lower, it may suggest that something other than aging is causing abnormal bone loss.

Nursing and Interprofessional Management

Care of the patient with osteoporosis focuses on proper nutrition, calcium and Vitamin D supplementation, exercise, prevention of falls and fractures, and drugs. Treatment is recommended for postmenopausal women who have: (1) a T-score of < −2.5, (2) a T-score between −1 and −2.5 with additional risk factors, or (3) a prior history of a hip or vertebral fracture.

- A patient's risk of fracture caused by osteoporosis can also be calculated using the Fracture Risk Assessment (FRAX) tool (*www.shef.ac.uk/FRAX*).

The recommended calcium intake is 1000 mg/day for women ages 19 to 50 years and men ages 19 to 70 years and 1200 mg/day in women 51 years or older and men 71 years or older).

- If dietary intake of calcium is inadequate, supplemental calcium may be recommended. The amount of elemental calcium varies in different calcium preparations. Teach the patient to take calcium supplements as divided doses to increase absorption.
- Vitamin D is important in calcium absorption and function. Being in the sun for 20 minutes a day is generally enough. However, supplemental vitamin D (800 to 1000 IU) is recommended for postmenopausal women, older adults, people who are homebound or in long-term care settings, and those in northern climates, because of decreased sun exposure.
- Regular physical activity is important to build up and maintain bone mass. The best exercises are those that are weight bearing and force a person to work against gravity, such as walking, weight training, stair climbing, and dancing. Encourage walking (for 30 minutes 3 times per week) over high-impact aerobics or running, both of which may put too much stress on the bones resulting in fractures.

Vertebroplasty and kyphoplasty are minimally invasive procedures that are used to treat osteoporotic vertebral fractures. In *vertebroplasty,* bone cement is injected into the collapsed vertebra to stabilize it, but it does not correct the deformity. In *kyphoplasty,* an air bladder is inserted into the collapsed vertebra and inflated to restore vertebral body height, and then bone cement is injected.

Drug Therapy

The recommended drug therapies for the prevention and treatment of osteoporosis are the bisphosphonates alendronate, risedronate, and zoledronic acid, or denosumab.

- Bisphosphonates inhibit osteoclast-mediated bone resorption and slow the cycle of bone remodeling. Although a modest increase in BMD is typical, bone remodeling may be suppressed to the extent that normal bone formation is impaired and fracture risk increases. These drugs are widely used in the prevention and treatment of osteoporosis. Common side effects are anorexia, weight loss, and gastritis. Teach the patient to take the medication correctly to improve its absorption and decrease GI side effects (especially esophageal irritation). Alendronate (Fosamax) is available as a daily or weekly oral tablet. The immediate-release form of risedronate (Actonel) is given daily, weekly, or monthly based on the dose. Zoledronic acid (Reclast) is given as a once-yearly or every 2 years IV infusion. Renal function tests and serum calcium must be assessed before administration.
- Denosumab (Prolia) may be given to postmenopausal women with osteoporosis who are at high risk for fractures. It is a monoclonal antibody that binds to a protein (RANKL) involved in the formation and function of osteoclasts. Denosumab is given by a health care professional as a subcutaneous injection every 6 months.
- Another group of drugs used to treat osteoporosis is the selective estrogen receptor modulators, such as raloxifene (Evista). These drugs mimic the effect of estrogen on bone by reducing bone resorption without stimulating the tissues of the breast or uterus.
- Teriparatide (Forteo) is a portion of human parathyroid hormone that is used for the treatment of osteoporosis by increasing the action of osteoblasts. It is the first drug for osteoporosis that stimulates new bone formation rather than just preventing further bone loss.
- Estrogen replacement therapy and estrogen with progesterone are no longer routinely given after menopause to prevent osteoporosis because they are associated with increased risk of heart disease and breast and uterine cancer.

Persons who must take corticosteroids over many years to manage medical conditions are at high risk for osteoporosis. The corticosteroids should be prescribed in the lowest possible dose of the drug for the shortest possible time. Ensure an adequate intake of calcium and vitamin D, including supplementation when osteoporosis drugs are prescribed. If osteopenia is evident on bone densitometry, treatment with bisphosphonates may be considered.

OVARIAN CANCER

Description

Ovarian cancer is a malignant tumor of the ovaries. It is the fifth leading cause of cancer deaths in women in the United States. Most women with ovarian cancer have advanced disease at diagnosis.

Women who have mutations of the *BRCA* genes have an increased susceptibility to ovarian (and breast) cancer. Additional risk factors are presented in Table 62. Protective factors decrease the risk of ovarian cancer by reducing the number of ovulatory cycles and thus reducing exposure to estrogen.

Pathophysiology

The cause of ovarian cancer is unknown. About 90% of ovarian cancers are epithelial carcinomas that arise from malignant transformation of the surface epithelial cells.

Intraperitoneal dissemination is a common characteristic of ovarian cancer. It metastasizes to the uterus, bladder, bowel, and omentum. In advanced disease, ovarian cancer may spread to the stomach, colon, and liver.

TABLE 62 Risk Factors for Ovarian Cancer	
Increased Risk	**Decreased Risk (Protective)**
• Family or personal history of ovarian, breast, or colon cancer • Personal history of hereditary nonpolyposis colorectal cancer • Hormone replacement therapy • Mutant *BRCA* gene • Early menarche and late menopause • Increasing age • Nulliparity • High-fat diet	• Oral contraceptive use for >5 yr • Breastfeeding • Multiple pregnancies • Early age at birth of first baby

Clinical Manifestations

Early ovarian cancer usually has no obvious symptoms. Most manifestations are vague and nonspecific. These include pelvic or abdominal pain, bloating, urinary urgency or frequency, and difficulty eating or feeling full quickly.

- Late-stage disease manifests with abdominal enlargement with ascites (fluid in the abdominal cavity), unexplained weight loss or gain, and menstrual changes.

Diagnostic Studies

No accurate screening test exists for early detection of ovarian cancer.

- Bimanual pelvic examinations may identify an ovarian mass.
- Abdominal or vaginal ultrasound can be used to detect ovarian masses.
- An exploratory laparotomy may be used to establish the diagnosis and disease stage.
- For women at high risk for ovarian cancer, screening using a combination of the tumor marker CA-125 and ultrasound is often recommended in addition to a yearly pelvic examination.

Interprofessional Management

Women identified as high risk based on family and health history may need counseling regarding options such as prophylactic oophorectomy and oral contraceptives.

Most patients with ovarian cancer have widespread disease at presentation. The initial treatment for all stages of ovarian cancer is surgery, which is usually a total abdominal hysterectomy and bilateral salpingo-oophorectomy with removal of the omentum and as much of the tumor as possible (i.e., tumor debulking).

Treatment options include intraperitoneal and systemic chemotherapy, intraperitoneal instillation of radioisotopes, and external abdominal and pelvic radiation therapy.

- The chemotherapy agents most commonly used are taxanes (paclitaxel or docetaxel) and platinum-based agents (carboplatin or cisplatin).
- Targeted therapy agents include bevacizumab (Avastin), rucaparib (Rubraca), and olaparib (Lynparza). Bevacizumab is an angiogenesis inhibitor. Olaparib and rucaparib area polyadenosine diphosphate-ribose polymerase (PARP) inhibitors that block enzymes involved in repairing damaged deoxyribonucleic acid (DNA).

Nursing Management: Cancers of the Female Reproductive Tract
See Cervical Cancer, p. 116.

PAGET'S DISEASE

Description
Paget's disease (osteitis deformans) is a chronic skeletal bone disorder in which there is excessive bone resorption followed by replacement of normal marrow by vascular, fibrous connective tissue and new bone that is larger, more disorganized, and weaker. Areas commonly affected are the pelvis, long bones, spine, ribs, sternum, and skull.

The cause of Paget's disease may be viral or genetic. Up to 40% of all patients with Paget's disease have a relative with the disorder. Men are affected more often than women.

Clinical Manifestations
In mild Paget's disease may not have any symptoms. The disease may be discovered incidentally on x-ray or serum chemistry findings indicating a high alkaline phosphatase (ALP) level.

- Bone pain may develop gradually and progress to severe intractable pain. Other early manifestations include fatigue and progressive development of a waddling gait.
- Headaches, dementia, vision deficits, and loss of hearing can result with an enlarged, thickened skull. Increased bone volume in the spine can cause spinal cord or nerve root compression.

Pathologic fracture is the most common complication and may be the first sign of the disease. Other complications include osteosarcoma, osteoclastoma (giant cell tumor), and fibrosarcoma.

Diagnostic Studies
- Serum ALP levels are markedly increased (indicating rapid bone turnover) in advanced disease.
- X-rays may show curvature of an affected bone and thickened bone cortex, especially in weight-bearing bones and the cranium.
- Bone scans using a radiolabeled bisphosphate show increased uptake in the affected skeletal areas.

Nursing and Interprofessional Management
Care is usually limited to symptomatic and supportive care, with correction of secondary deformities by either surgical intervention or braces.

P

- Bisphosphonate drugs are used to slow bone resorption. Zoledronic acid may also be given as a bone-building drug. Calcium and vitamin D are often given to decrease hypocalcemia, a common side effect with these drugs. Monitor drug effectiveness by regular assessment of serum ALP.
- Calcitonin therapy is an option for patients who cannot tolerate bisphosphonate drugs. Response to calcitonin therapy often ends when therapy stops.
- Pain is usually managed with nonsteroidal antiinflammatory drugs (NSAIDs).
- Orthopedic surgery for fractures, hip and knee replacements, and knee realignment may be necessary.

A firm mattress should be used to provide back support and relieve pain. The patient may need to wear a corset or light brace to relieve back pain and to provide support when in the upright position. Teach the patient correct application of such devices, and how to regularly examine areas of the skin for friction damage.

- Good body mechanics are essential. Discourage activities such as lifting and twisting. Physical therapy may increase muscle strength.
- A healthy diet, especially as it pertains to vitamin D, calcium, and protein, is important for bone formation.
- Teach the patient to use an assistive device and make environmental changes (e.g., do not use throw rugs) to decrease risk for falls and related fractures.

PANCREATIC CANCER

Description

Pancreatic cancer is most often an adenocarcinoma. More than half of the tumors occur in the head of the pancreas. As the tumor grows, the common bile duct becomes obstructed and obstructive jaundice develops. Tumors starting in the body or the tail of the pancreas often remain silent until their growth is advanced.

The median age at diagnosis is around 71 years of age. The majority of cancers have metastasized at the time of diagnosis, with a poor prognosis. Most patients die within 5 to 12 months of the initial diagnosis, and the 5-year survival rate is only 8%.

Pathophysiology

The cause of pancreatic cancer is unknown. Risk factors are cigarette smoking, high-fat diet, diabetes, chronic pancreatitis, family history of pancreatic cancer, and exposure to chemicals, such as benzidine. Black have a higher incidence of pancreatic cancer than whites. Smokers are 2 to 3 times more likely to develop pancreatic cancer than nonsmokers.

Clinical Manifestations

Signs and symptoms of pancreatic cancer are often similar to those of chronic pancreatitis. Manifestations include abdominal pain (dull or aching), anorexia, rapid and progressive weight loss, nausea, and jaundice.

- The most common manifestations when the cancer occurs in the head of the pancreas are pain, jaundice, and weight loss. Weight loss is caused by poor digestion and absorption caused by lack of digestive enzymes from the pancreas.
- Pruritus may accompany obstructive jaundice.
- Pain is related to the location of the cancer. Extreme, unrelenting pain is related to extension of the cancer into the retroperitoneal tissues and nerve plexuses. The pain is often in the upper abdomen or left hypochondrium, radiating to the back. It is often related to eating and also occurs at night.

Diagnostic Studies

- Abdominal ultrasound or endoscopic ultrasound (EUS), spiral CT scan, MRI, and MR cholangiopancreatography (MRCP) are used for diagnosing and staging pancreatic cancer.
- Endoscopic retrograde cholangiography (ERCP) allows for visualization and collection of secretions and tissues from the pancreatic duct and biliary system.
- Carbohydrate antigen (CA)19-9, which is increased in pancreatic cancer, is the most commonly used tumor marker.

Interprofessional Management

Surgery is the most effective treatment, but only 15% to 20% of patients have resectable tumors at the time of diagnosis. The classic surgery is a *radical pancreaticoduodenectomy* or *Whipple procedure*. This procedure is a resection of the proximal pancreas (proximal pancreatectomy), the adjoining duodenum (duodenectomy), the distal part of the stomach (partial gastrectomy), and the distal segment of the common bile duct. An anastomosis of the pancreatic duct, common bile duct, and stomach to the jejunum is done.

- If the pancreatic tumor cannot be removed surgically, palliative measures may include a cholecystojejunostomy to relieve biliary obstruction and/or endoscopic placement of biliary stents.
- Radiation therapy alters survival rates little but is effective for pain relief.

- The role of chemotherapy in pancreatic cancer is limited. Chemotherapy usually consists of fluorouracil (5-FU) and gemcitabine (Gemzar), either alone or in combination with agents such as capecitabine (Xeloda), paclitaxel (Abraxane), or erlotinib (Tarceva). Erlotinib is a targeted therapy agent.

Nursing Management

Because the patient with pancreatic cancer has many of the same problems as the patient with pancreatitis, nursing care includes the same measures (see Pancreatitis, Acute, p. 454).

- Provide symptomatic and supportive nursing care, including comfort measures and medications to relieve pain.
- Psychologic support is essential, especially during times of anxiety or depression.
- Support adequate nutrition with measures to manage anorexia, nausea, and vomiting. Offer frequent and supplemental feedings.
- Because bleeding can result from impaired vitamin K production, assess for bleeding from body orifices and mucous membranes.
- Helping the patient and caregivers through the grieving process is an important aspect of nursing care.

PANCREATITIS, ACUTE

Description

Acute pancreatitis is inflammation of the pancreas, varying from mild edema to severe hemorrhagic necrosis. Pancreatic enzymes spilling into the surrounding pancreatic tissue cause autodigestion and severe pain.

Acute pancreatitis is most common in middle-aged men and women, with the rate 3 times higher in blacks than in whites.

The severity of the disease varies according to the extent of pancreatic destruction. Some patients recover completely, others have recurring attacks, and still others develop chronic pancreatitis. Acute pancreatitis can be life-threatening.

Pathophysiology

Many factors can cause injury to the pancreas. In the United States the most common cause is gallbladder disease (gallstones), which is more common in women. The second most common cause is chronic alcohol intake, which is more common in men. Smoking is an independent risk factor for acute pancreatitis.

Less common causes include drug reactions, pancreatic cancer, and hypertriglyceridemia. Autodigestion of the pancreas is precipitated by injury to pancreatic cells or activation of pancreatic enzymes in the pancreas rather than in the intestine. The pathophysiologic involvement in acute pancreatitis is classified as either *mild pancreatitis* (also known as *edematous* or *interstitial*) or *severe pancreatitis* (also called *necrotizing pancreatitis*). Patients with severe pancreatitis are at high risk for developing pancreatic necrosis, organ failure, and septic complications.

Clinical Manifestations

Abdominal pain is the predominant symptom of acute pancreatitis. The pain is usually in the left upper quadrant but may be in the mid-epigastric area. It often radiates to the back because of the retroperitoneal location of the pancreas.

- The pain has a sudden onset and is described as severe, deep, piercing, and continuous or steady. Eating worsens the pain, which is not relieved by vomiting. Pain frequently begins when the patient is lying down. The pain may be accompanied by flushing, cyanosis, and dyspnea.

Other manifestations include nausea and vomiting, low-grade fever, leukocytosis, hypotension, tachycardia, and jaundice. Abdominal tenderness with muscle guarding is common. Bowel sounds may be decreased or absent. Paralytic ileus may occur and causes marked abdominal distention. The lungs are often involved, with crackles present.

- Shock may occur from hemorrhage into the pancreas, toxemia from the activated pancreatic enzymes, or hypovolemia because of massive fluid shifts into the retroperitoneal space.
- Intravascular damage from circulating trypsin may cause areas of cyanosis or greenish to yellow-brown discoloration of the abdominal wall. Other areas of ecchymoses are the flanks (*Grey Turner's spots* or *sign,* a bluish flank discoloration) and the periumbilical area (*Cullen's sign,* a bluish periumbilical discoloration).

Complications

Local complications of acute pancreatitis are pseudocyst and abscess.

- A *pancreatic pseudocyst* is an accumulation of fluid, pancreatic enzymes, tissue debris, and inflammatory exudates surrounded by a wall. Manifestations of pseudocyst are abdominal pain, palpable epigastric mass, nausea, vomiting, and anorexia. The serum amylase level is often high. CT, MRI, and endoscopic ultrasound (EUS) may be used in the diagnosis. The cysts usually resolve spontaneously within a few weeks but may perforate, causing peritonitis, or rupture into the stomach or the duodenum. Treatment options include surgical drainage, percutaneous catheter placement and drainage, and endoscopic drainage.

- A *pancreatic abscess* is a collection of pus resulting from extensive necrosis in the pancreas. It may perforate into adjacent organs. Manifestations include upper abdominal pain, abdominal mass, high fever, and leukocytosis. Pancreatic abscesses need prompt surgical drainage to prevent sepsis.

Systemic complications of acute pancreatitis include pleural effusion, atelectasis, pneumonia, hyperglycemia, hypotension, and hypocalcemia leading to tetany.

Diagnostic Studies

- High serum amylase and lipase are primary diagnostic findings.
- Liver enzymes, triglycerides, glucose, and bilirubin are high with a decrease in calcium.
- Abdominal ultrasound, x-ray, or contrast-enhanced CT scan can identify pancreatic problems.
- Endoscopic retrograde cholangiopancreatography (ERCP) is used along with EUS, magnetic resonance cholangiopancreatography (MRCP), and angiography to diagnose pancreatic problems.

Interprofessional Management

Goals of management for acute pancreatitis include relief of pain, prevention or alleviation of shock, reduction of pancreatic secretions, correction of fluid and electrolyte imbalances, prevention or treatment of infections, and removal of the precipitating cause, if possible.

Treatment is focused on supportive care, including aggressive hydration, pain management, management of metabolic complications, and minimization of pancreatic stimulation. If shock is present, blood volume replacements, volume expanders, and fluids may be given. Treatment and control of pain are very important. Pain medications may be combined with an antispasmodic.

It is important to reduce or suppress pancreatic enzymes to decrease stimulation of the pancreas. Usually the patient is NPO, and nasogastric (NG) suction is used to reduce vomiting and prevent gastric digestive juices from entering the duodenum. Drugs that neutralize or suppress formation of hydrochloric acid (HCl) in the stomach, such as antacids, histamine H_2-receptor antagonists, and proton pump inhibitors, may help suppress gastric acid secretion.

- As pancreatitis resolves, the patient resumes oral intake. Enteral nutrition support may be needed.

- Inflamed and necrotic pancreatic tissue is a good medium for bacterial growth. Antibiotic therapy should be started early if an infection occurs.

When the acute pancreatitis is related to gallstones, an urgent ERCP with endoscopic sphincterotomy may be performed. This may be followed by laparoscopic cholecystectomy to reduce the potential for recurrence. Surgical intervention may be indicated when the diagnosis is uncertain and in patients who do not respond to therapy. Patients with severe acute pancreatitis may need drainage of necrotic fluid collections performed surgically, under CT guidance, or endoscopically. Percutaneous pseudocyst drainage can be done, and a drainage tube is left in place.

Several drugs are used to prevent and treat problems associated with pancreatitis. These include antacids, antispasmodics, opioids, proton pump inhibitors, insulin, and pancreatic enzyme products.

Nursing Management
Goals
The patient with acute pancreatitis will have relief of pain, normal fluid and electrolyte balance, minimal to no complications, and no recurrent attacks.
Nursing Interventions
Encourage early diagnosis and treatment of biliary tract disease, such as cholelithiasis. Encourage the patient to eliminate alcohol intake, especially if there have been previous episodes of pancreatitis.

During the acute phase, it is important to monitor vital signs. Hypotension, fever, and tachypnea may compromise hemodynamic stability. Monitor the response to IV fluids. Closely monitor fluid and electrolyte balance. Frequent vomiting, along with gastric suction, may result in decreased chloride, sodium, and potassium levels.

Respiratory tract infections are common because the retroperitoneal fluid raises the diaphragm, which causes the patient to take shallow, guarded abdominal breaths. Measures to prevent respiratory tract infections include turning, coughing, deep breathing, and assuming a semi-Fowler's position.

Respiratory failure may develop in the patient with severe acute pancreatitis. Assess respiratory function (e.g., lung sounds, O_2 saturation levels). If acute respiratory distress syndrome (ARDS) develops, the patient may need intubation and mechanical ventilation support.

A major focus of your care is pain relief. Pain and restlessness can increase the metabolic rate and stimulate pancreatic enzymes. Measures such as comfortable positioning, frequent changes in position, and relief of nausea and vomiting assist in reducing the restlessness that usually accompanies the pain.

- A side-lying position with the head elevated 45 degrees decreases tension on the abdomen and may help ease the pain.
- For the patient who is on NPO status or has an NG tube, provide frequent oral and nasal care to relieve dryness of the mouth and nose.

Patients may require follow-up home care. Physical therapy may be needed because of loss of muscle strength.

▼ **Patient and Caregiver Teaching**

- Counseling about abstinence from alcohol is important to prevent future attacks of acute pancreatitis and development of chronic pancreatitis.
- Because nicotine can stimulate the pancreas, smoking should be avoided.
- Dietary teaching should include fat restriction because fats stimulate the secretion of cholecystokinin, which then stimulates the pancreas. Encourage carbohydrates, which are less stimulating to the pancreas. Teach the patient to avoid crash and binge dieting, which can precipitate attacks.
- Teach the patient and caregiver to recognize symptoms of infection, diabetes, or *steatorrhea* (foul-smelling, frothy stools). These changes indicate ongoing destruction of pancreatic tissue and a possible need for exogenous enzyme supplementation.

PANCREATITIS, CHRONIC

Description

Chronic pancreatitis is a continuous, prolonged, inflammatory, and fibrosing process involving the pancreas. The pancreas is progressively destroyed as it is replaced by fibrotic tissue with strictures and calcifications. Chronic pancreatitis may follow acute pancreatitis or occur in the absence of any history of an acute condition.

Chronic pancreatitis can be caused by alcohol abuse; obstruction caused by cholelithiasis (gallstones), tumor, pseudocysts, or trauma; or systemic diseases (e.g., systemic lupus erythematosus), autoimmune pancreatitis, or cystic fibrosis.

Pathophysiology

The most common cause of *obstructive* pancreatitis is inflammation of the sphincter of Oddi associated with gallstones. Cancer of the ampulla of Vater, duodenum, or pancreas can also cause this type of chronic pancreatitis.

The most common cause of *nonobstructive* pancreatitis (the most common type of chronic pancreatitis) is alcohol abuse. In nonobstructive pancreatitis, there is inflammation and sclerosis, mainly in the head of the pancreas and around the pancreatic duct.

Clinical Manifestations

As with acute pancreatitis, a major manifestation of chronic pancreatitis is abdominal pain. The patient may have episodes of acute pain, but it usually is chronic (recurrent attacks at intervals of months or years). The attacks may become more frequent until the pain is almost constant, or they may decrease as the pancreatic fibrosis develops. The pain is in the same areas as in acute pancreatitis but is usually described as a heavy, gnawing feeling or sometimes as burning and cramplike. Food or antacids do not relieve the pain.

- Other manifestations include signs and symptoms of pancreatic insufficiency, including malabsorption with weight loss, constipation, mild jaundice with dark frothy urine, steatorrhea, and diabetes. The steatorrhea may become severe, with voluminous, foul, fatty stools. Abdominal tenderness may be present.
- Complications of chronic pancreatitis may include pseudocyst formation, bile duct or duodenal obstruction, pancreatic ascites or pleural effusion, or pancreatic cancer.

Diagnostic Studies

Confirming the diagnosis of chronic pancreatitis can be challenging and is based on the patient's signs and symptoms, laboratory studies, and imaging.

- Serum amylase and lipase levels may be slightly increased.
- Serum bilirubin and alkaline phosphatase levels may be high.
- Mild leukocytosis and elevated sedimentation rate may be found.
- Endoscopic retrograde cholangiopancreatography (ERCP) is used to visualize the pancreatic and biliary ductal system.
- CT, MRI, MR cholangiopancreatography (MRCP), abdominal ultrasound, and endoscopic ultrasound may be used in the diagnostic workup.
- A secretin test can assess the degree of pancreatic dysfunction.

Nursing and Interprofessional Management

When the patient with chronic pancreatitis has an acute attack, the therapy is similar to that for acute pancreatitis. At other times the focus is on the prevention of further attacks, relief of pain, and control of pancreatic exocrine and endocrine insufficiency. Sometimes large, frequent doses of analgesics are needed to relieve the pain.

- A bland diet low in fat and high in carbohydrates, pancreatic enzyme replacement such as pancrelipase (Pancrease, Zenpep,

Creon, Viokace), and management of diabetes are measures used to control the pancreatic insufficiency.

- Treatment of chronic pancreatitis sometimes requires endoscopic therapy or surgery. When biliary disease is present or obstruction or pseudocyst develops, surgery may divert bile flow or relieve ductal obstruction.

▼ **Patient and Caregiver Teaching**

- Instruct the patient to take measures to prevent further attacks. Explain dietary control, and consistency in taking pancreatic enzymes with meals and snacks.
- Teach the patient and caregiver to observe the stools for steatorrhea to help determine the effectiveness of the enzyme replacement.
- Teach the patient not to consume alcohol and caffeinated beverages. If the patient is dependent on alcohol, refer to other agencies or resources as needed.
- If diabetes has developed, teach the patient regarding blood glucose testing and drug therapy (see Diabetes Mellitus, p. 165).

PARKINSON'S DISEASE

Description

Parkinson's disease (PD) is a chronic, progressive neurodegenerative disorder characterized by slowness in the initiation and execution of movement *(bradykinesia)*, increased muscle tone *(rigidity)*, tremor at rest, and gait disturbance. It is the most common form of *parkinsonism* (a syndrome characterized by similar symptoms).

Up to 1 million Americans will be living with PD by 2020. Sixty thousand persons are diagnosed each year. Incidence of PD increases with age, but about 4% of people with PD are diagnosed before age 50 years. Men are 1.5 times more likely to have PD than women.

Pathophysiology

Although the exact cause of PD is unknown, a complex interplay of environmental and genetic factors is involved. About 15% of PD patients have a family history of the disease, indicating a strong genetic basis for PD. In other people, exposure to toxins or certain viruses may trigger PD.

There are many forms of secondary (atypical) parkinsonism other than PD. Parkinson-like symptoms can occur after intoxication with a variety of chemicals, including carbon monoxide and manganese (among copper miners) and the product of meperidine analog synthesis, MPTP (1-methyl-4-phenyl-1,2,3,6-tetrahydropyridine).

Drug-induced parkinsonism can follow metoclopramide (Reglan), reserpine, methyldopa, lithium, haloperidol (Haldol), and chlorpromazine. It is also seen after use of amphetamine and methamphetamine.

- The pathology of PD involves the degeneration of the dopamine-producing neurons in the substantia nigra of the midbrain, which disrupts the balance between dopamine (DA) and acetylcholine (ACh) in the basal ganglia.
- DA is a neurotransmitter essential for normal functioning of the extrapyramidal motor system, including control of posture, support, and voluntary motion. Symptoms do not occur until 80% of neurons in the substantia nigra are lost.
- *Lewy bodies,* unusual clumps of protein, are found in the brains of patients with PD. It is not known what causes these bodies to form, but their presence indicates abnormal functioning of the brain.

Clinical Manifestations

Onset of PD is gradual, with an ongoing progression. Classic manifestations of PD are easily remembered using the mnemonic *TRAP* (Tremor, Rigidity, Akinesia, and Postural instability). In the beginning stages, only a mild tremor, slight limp, or decreased arm swing may be evident. Later the patient may have a shuffling, propulsive gait with arms flexed and loss of postural reflexes. Some patients exhibit a slight change in speech patterns.

- *Tremor,* often the first sign, may initially be minimal, so that only the patient notices it. This tremor is more prominent at rest and is aggravated by emotional stress or increased concentration. The hand tremor is described as "pill rolling" because the thumb and forefinger appear to move in a rotary fashion as if rolling a pill, coin, or other small object. Tremor can involve the diaphragm, tongue, lips, and jaw.
- *Rigidity* is increased resistance to passive motion when the limbs are moved through their range of motion. Parkinsonian rigidity is typified by jerky (cogwheel) rigidity, as if there were intermittent catches when the joint is passively moved.
- *Akinesia* is the absence or loss of control of voluntary muscle movements. *Bradykinesia* (slow movement) is particularly evident in the loss of automatic movements, secondary to the physical and chemical alteration of the basal ganglia. A lack of spontaneous activity (blinking of the eyelids, swinging of the arms while walking, swallowing of saliva, self-expression with facial and hand movements, and minor movement of postural adjustment) in PD accounts for the "old man" image with

P

stooped posture, masklike face ("deadpan" expression), drooling of saliva, and shuffling gait.

- *Postural instability* is common, and patients may report being unable to stop themselves from going forward (propulsion) or backward (retropulsion).

Other signs and symptoms include depression, anxiety, apathy, fatigue, pain, urinary retention, erectile dysfunction, and memory changes. Sleep problems are common and include difficulty staying asleep at night, restless sleep, nightmares, and drowsiness or sudden sleep onset during the day.

Complications

- As PD progresses, complications increase. These include motor symptoms (e.g., dyskinesias [spontaneous, involuntary movements], weakness, neurologic problems (e.g., dementia), and neuropsychiatric problems (e.g., depression, hallucinations, psychosis). As PD progresses, dementia often results and is associated with increased mortality. Swallowing becomes more difficult *(dysphagia)*; malnutrition or aspiration may result.
- General debilitation may lead to pneumonia, urinary tract infections, and skin breakdown.
- Orthostatic hypotension along with the loss of postural reflexes may result in fall injuries.

Diagnostic Studies

Because there is no specific diagnostic test for PD, the diagnosis is based on the history and clinical features.

- A definitive diagnosis can be made when TRAP manifestations are present.
- The ultimate confirmation is a positive response to antiparkinsonian drugs.

Interprofessional Management

Because there is no cure, management is aimed at relieving symptoms.

Drug Therapy

Drug therapy for PD is aimed at correcting the imbalance of central nervous system (CNS) neurotransmitters. Antiparkinsonian drugs either enhance the release or supply of DA (dopaminergic) or antagonize or block the effects of overactive cholinergic neurons in the striatum. Levodopa with carbidopa (Sinemet) is the primary treatment for symptomatic patients. Levodopa is a precursor of DA and can cross the blood-brain barrier. It is converted to DA in the basal ganglia. Prolonged use of levodopa can result in dyskinesias and "off/on" periods when the medication will unpredictably start or stop working. See Table 63 for the actions of drugs commonly used to manage PD.

Surgical Therapy

Surgical procedures are aimed at relieving symptoms of PD for patients who are unresponsive to drug therapy or who have developed severe motor complications. Procedures fall into 3 categories: ablation (destruction), deep brain stimulation (DBS), and transplantation.

Nutritional Therapy

Malnutrition and constipation can be serious consequences of inadequate nutrition. Patients who have dysphagia and bradykinesia need appetizing foods that are easily chewed and swallowed, with adequate fiber to avoid constipation. Provide ample time for eating to avoid frustration.

Nursing Management

Goals

The patient with PD will maximize neurologic function, maintain independence in activities of daily living for as long as possible, and optimize psychosocial well-being.

Nursing Interventions

Promotion of physical exercise and a well-balanced diet are major nursing concerns. Exercise can limit the consequences of decreased mobility, such as muscle atrophy, contractures, and constipation. Include exercises for overall muscle tone and to strengthen the muscles involved with speaking and swallowing.

Because PD is a chronic degenerative disorder, focus on teaching and nursing care directed towards maintaining good health, encouraging independence, and avoiding complications such as contractures.

▼ Patient and Caregiver Teaching

- For patients who are at risk for falling and tend to "freeze" while walking, have them think consciously about stepping over imaginary lines, practice stepping over rice kernels, rock from side to side, lift the toes when stepping, or take 1 step backward and 2 steps forward.
- Teach the patient to facilitate getting out of a chair by using an upright chair with arms and placing the back legs on small (2-inch) blocks.
- An elevated toilet seat can facilitate getting on and off the toilet.
- Encourage environmental alterations, such as removing rugs and excess furniture to avoid stumbling.
- Clothing can be simplified by the use of slip-on shoes and hook-and-loop (Velcro) fasteners or zippers on clothing instead of buttons and hooks.

TABLE 63 Drug Therapy

Parkinson's Disease

Drug	Mechanism of Action
Dopaminergics	
Dopamine Precursors	
levodopa (L-dopa) levodopa/carbidopa (Sinemet)	Converted to dopamine in basal ganglia
Dopamine Receptor Agonists	
pramipexole (Mirapex) opinirole (Requip, Requip XL) rotigotine (Neupro [transdermal patch])	Stimulate dopamine receptors
Dopamine Agonists	
amantadine	Blocks NMDA-type glutamate receptors, increases dopamine release, and blocks dopamine reuptake
apomorphine (Apokyn)	Stimulates postsynaptic dopamine receptors
Anticholinergics	
benztropine (Cogentin) trihexyphenidyl	Block cholinergic receptors, thus helping balance cholinergic and dopaminergic activity
Antihistamine	
diphenhydramine	Has anticholinergic effect
Monoamine Oxidase Inhibitors	
rasagiline (Azilect) safinamide (Xadago) selegiline (Eldepryl)	Block breakdown of dopamine
Catechol *O*-Methyltransferase (COMT) Inhibitors	
entacapone (Comtan) tolcapone (Tasmar)	Block COMT and slow the breakdown of levodopa, thus prolonging the action of levodopa

NMDA, N-Methyl-D-aspartic acid.

- As the disease progresses, the impact on the psychologic well-being of the patient increases. Assist the patient through listening, providing education, encouraging social interactions, and referral to the American Parkinson Disease Association (*www.apdaparkinson.org*).

Family members (e.g., spouse, children) provide care for the majority of patients with PD. Their burden increases as the disease progresses. This often occurs while the caregiver's physical and mental health also decline. Help them find appropriate resources.

PELVIC INFLAMMATORY DISEASE

Description

Pelvic inflammatory disease (PID) is an infectious condition of the pelvic cavity that may involve the fallopian tubes (salpingitis), ovaries (oophoritis), and pelvic peritoneum (peritonitis).

Pathophysiology

PID is often the result of untreated cervical infection. The organism infecting the cervix can spread into the uterus, fallopian tubes, ovaries, and peritoneal cavity. The most common causes are *Chlamydia trachomatis* and *Neisseria gonorrhoeae.* These organisms, as well as anaerobes, mycoplasmas, streptococci, and enteric gram-negative rods, gain entrance during sexual intercourse or after pregnancy termination, pelvic surgery, or childbirth.

Clinical Manifestations

Lower abdominal pain is a common manifestation of PID.

- The pain gradually becomes constant, ranging from mild to severe. Movement such as walking and intercourse increases the pain.
- Spotting after intercourse and purulent cervical or vaginal discharge are common.
- Fever and chills may also be present.
- Women who have milder symptoms, such as increased cramping pain with menses, irregular bleeding, and some pain with intercourse, may go untreated because they did not seek care or the HCP does not recognize the symptoms.

Complications

Complications of PID include septic shock, perihepatitis, tubo-ovarian abscess, peritonitis, and embolism. PID can cause adhesions and strictures in the fallopian tubes, which may lead to ectopic pregnancy or infertility.

Diagnostic Studies

A pelvic examination aids in the diagnosis of PID. Women with PID have lower abdominal tenderness, adnexal tenderness, and cervical motion tenderness.

- Diagnostic testing includes examination for *N. gonorrhoeae* and *C. trachomatis.*
- A pregnancy test is done to rule out ectopic pregnancy.
- When pain or obesity compromises the pelvic examination, an ultrasound may be ordered.

Interprofessional and Nursing Management

PID is usually treated on an outpatient basis. With effective combination antibiotic therapy, the pain should subside. The patient should abstain from intercourse for 3 weeks. Her partner(s) must be examined and treated. An important part of care is physical rest and oral fluids. Reevaluation in 48 to 72 hours, even if symptoms are improving, is an essential part of outpatient care.

If a tubo-ovarian abscess is present, or if the patient is acutely ill or in severe pain, hospital admission is indicated. Maximum doses of IV antibiotics are given. Corticosteroids may be added to the regimen to reduce inflammation, allowing for faster recovery and optimizing the chances for subsequent fertility. Analgesics to relieve pain and IV fluids to prevent dehydration are also used.

- Applying heat to the lower abdomen or sitz baths may improve circulation and decrease pain.
- Bed rest in a semi-Fowler's position promotes drainage of the pelvic cavity by gravity; this may prevent the development of abscesses high in the abdomen.

Surgery is indicated for abscesses that fail to resolve with IV antibiotics. An abscess may be drained using a laparoscopic approach or via laparotomy.

Prevention, early recognition, and prompt treatment of vaginal and cervical infections can help prevent PID and its serious complications. Provide information regarding factors that place a woman at increased risk for PID.

- Urge women to seek medical attention for any unusual vaginal discharge or possible infection of their reproductive organs.
- The patient may feel guilty about having PID, especially if it was associated with a sexually transmitted infection. She may be concerned about the complications associated with PID, such as infertility and the increased incidence of ectopic pregnancy. Discuss her feelings and concerns to assist her to cope.

PELVIC PAIN, CHRONIC

Description

Chronic pelvic pain refers to pain in the pelvic region (below the umbilicus and between the hips) that lasts 6 months or longer. The cause of chronic pelvic pain is often hard to find.

- Gynecologic causes include pelvic inflammatory disease (PID), endometriosis, ovarian cysts, uterine fibroids, pelvic adhesions, and ectopic pregnancies.
- Abdominal causes include irritable bowel syndrome, interstitial cystitis, appendicitis, and colitis.
- Psychologic factors (e.g., depression, chronic stress, history of sexual or physical abuse) may increase the risk of developing chronic pelvic pain. Emotional distress makes pain worse, and living with chronic pain contributes to emotional distress.

Clinical Manifestations and Diagnostic Studies

- Manifestations include severe and steady pain, intermittent pain, dull and achy pain, sensation of pelvic pressure or heaviness, and sharp pains or cramping. Pain may occur during intercourse or while having a bowel movement. In addition to a detailed history and physical examination (including a pelvic examination), the patient may be asked to keep a journal of the onset of symptoms and precipitating factors.
- Diagnostic tests may include specimens from cervix or vagina (used to detect sexually transmitted infections [STIs]), and ultrasound, CT scan, or MRI to detect abnormal structures or growths.
- Laparoscopy may be used to see the pelvic organs. This procedure is especially useful in detecting endometriosis and chronic PID.

Interprofessional and Nursing Management

If the cause of chronic pelvic pain is found, treatment focuses on that cause. If no cause can be found, treatment involves managing the pain. Over-the-counter drugs (e.g., aspirin, ibuprofen, acetaminophen) may provide some relief. Sometimes stronger pain drugs may be needed. Birth control pills or other hormonal agents may help relieve cyclic pelvic pain related to menstrual cycles. If an infection is the source of the problem, antibiotics are used.

Laparoscopic surgery may be used to remove pelvic adhesions or endometrial tissue. As a last resort, a hysterectomy may be done.

Tricyclic antidepressants (e.g., amitriptyline, nortriptyline [Pamelor]) have pain-relieving and antidepressant effects. These drugs may help relieve chronic pelvic pain even in women who do not have depression.

PEPTIC ULCER DISEASE

Description

Peptic ulcer disease (PUD) is an erosion of the mucosa resulting from the digestive action of hydrochloric acid (HCl) and pepsin. Any part of the gastrointestinal (GI) tract that comes into contact with gastric secretions is susceptible to ulcer development, including the lower esophagus, stomach, and duodenum, and at the margin of a gastrojejunal anastomosis site after surgical procedures. PUD affects about 4.5 million people in the United States each year.

Peptic ulcers are acute or chronic, depending on the degree and duration of mucosal involvement, and gastric or duodenal, according to the location.

- An *acute ulcer* is associated with superficial erosion and minimal inflammation. It is of short duration and resolves quickly when the cause is identified and removed.
- A *chronic ulcer* is of long duration, eroding through the muscular wall with the formation of fibrous tissue. It is continuously present for many months or recurs intermittently. Chronic ulcers are more common than acute erosions.
- *Gastric* and *duodenal* ulcers, although defined as peptic ulcers, are distinctly different in etiology and incidence (Table 64). Generally, the treatment of all ulcer types is similar.

Pathophysiology

Peptic ulcers develop only in the presence of an acid environment. The back-diffusion of HCl into the gastric mucosa results in cellular destruction and inflammation. Histamine is released from the damaged mucosa. This results in vasodilation and increased capillary permeability and further secretion of acid and pepsin. A variety of agents are known to destroy the mucosal barrier (see Gastritis, p. 231).

Helicobacter pylori is associated with chronic gastritis and peptic ulcer development. Eighty percent of gastric and 90% of duodenal ulcers are related to *H. pylori*. In the United States, *H. pylori* affects 20% of persons younger than 30 years, and 50% of those older than 60 years. The rate is highest in blacks and Hispanic people.

- In 1 patient, *H. pylori* may lead to intestinal metaplasia in the stomach and result in chronic atrophic gastritis, whereas in other

TABLE 64 Comparison of Gastric and Duodenal Ulcers

Gastric Ulcers	Duodenal Ulcers
Lesion	
Superficial, smooth margins. Round, oval, or cone shaped	Penetrating (associated with deformity of duodenal bulb from healing of recurrent ulcers)
Location of Lesion	
Predominantly antrum, also in body and fundus of stomach	First 1–2 cm of duodenum
Gastric Secretion	
Normal to decreased	Increased
Incidence	
Greater in women	Greater in men, but increasing in women (especially postmenopausal)
Peak age 50–60 yr	Peak age 35–45 yr
Increased cancer risk	No increase in cancer risk
H. pylori infection in 80%	*H. pylori* infection in 90%
↑ With incompetent pyloric sphincter and bile reflux	Associated with other diseases (e.g., chronic obstructive pulmonary disease, pancreatic disease, hyperparathyroidism, Zollinger-Ellison syndrome, chronic renal failure)
Clinical Manifestations	
Burning or gaseous pressure in epigastrium	Burning, cramping, pressure-like pain across midepigastrium and upper abdomen. Back pain with posterior ulcers
Pain 1–2 hr after meals. If penetrating ulcer, aggravation of discomfort with food	Pain 2–5 hr after meals and midmorning, midafternoon, middle of night. Periodic and episodic. Pain relief with antacids and food
Recurrence Rate	
High	High

P

patients *H. pylori* may alter gastric secretion and produce tissue damage leading to peptic ulcer disease. Response to *H. pylori* is likely to be influenced by many factors, including genetics, environment, and diet.

The use of nonsteroidal antiinflammatory drugs (NSAIDs) is responsible for most non–*H. pylori* peptic ulcers. NSAID use in the presence of *H. pylori* further increases the risk of PUD. NSAIDs inhibit prostaglandin synthesis, increase gastric acid secretion, and reduce the integrity of the mucosal barrier.

Clinical Manifestations

Discomfort generally associated with gastric ulcer is high in the epigastrium and occurs about 1 to 2 hours after meals. The pain is described as burning or gaseous. If the ulcer has eroded through the gastric mucosa, food tends to worsen the pain.

Duodenal ulcer symptoms occur when gastric acid comes in contact with the ulcer, generally 2 to 5 hours after a meal. The pain is described as "burning" or "cramplike." It is most often located in the midepigastric region beneath the xiphoid process. Duodenal ulcers can also produce back pain. A characteristic of duodenal ulcer is its tendency to occur continuously for a few weeks or months and then disappear for a time, only to recur some months later.

- Not all patients with gastric or duodenal ulcers have pain or discomfort. Silent peptic ulcers are more likely to occur in older adults and those taking NSAIDs. The presence or absence of symptoms is not directly related to the size of the ulcer or the degree of healing.

Diagnostic Studies

- Endoscopy is used to obtain tissue for biopsy, confirm the absence of cancer, obtain specimens to test for *H. pylori,* and determine the degree of ulcer healing after treatment.
- Biopsy of the antral mucosa and testing for urease (rapid urease testing) confirm a diagnosis of *H. pylori* infection. Noninvasive tests include a urea breath test, which can identify active infection.
- Complete blood count (CBC), urinalysis, liver enzyme studies, serum amylase determination, and stool examination may be performed for further diagnostic information.

Interprofessional Management
Conservative Therapy

The aim of treatment is to decrease gastric acidity and enhance mucosal defense mechanisms. The regimen consists of rest, drug therapy, smoking cessation, and long-term follow-up care. Strict adherence to the prescribed regimen of drugs is important because ulcers frequently recur.

Drug therapy includes the use of histamine H₂-receptor antagonists, proton pump inhibitors (PPIs), antisecretory agents, cytoprotective agents, antacids, and anticholinergics. Aspirin and NSAIDs are stopped for 4 to 6 weeks. When aspirin must be continued, co-administration with a PPI, H₂-receptor blocker, or misoprostol may be prescribed. See Table 41.10, Harding et al., *Lewis' Medical-Surgical Nursing,* ed 11.

The patient is given antibiotics and a PPI for 10 to 14 days to eradicate *H. pylori* infection. Because of the development of antibiotic-resistant organisms, patients may not have *H. pylori* eradicated with a single round of therapy.

Healing of a peptic ulcer requires many weeks of therapy. Pain disappears after 3 to 6 days, but complete healing may take 3 to 9 weeks.

An acute exacerbation is frequently accompanied by bleeding, increased pain and discomfort, and nausea and vomiting.

- With hemorrhage, management is similar to that described for upper GI bleeding (see pp. 237).
- With perforation, the focus of therapy is to stop the spillage of gastric contents by nasogastric (NG) tube or surgery. Blood volume is replaced with IV solutions, and packed red blood cells (RBCs) may be necessary. Broad-spectrum antibiotic therapy is started immediately to treat bacterial peritonitis. Pain medication is also given.
- With gastric outlet obstruction, the aim of therapy is to decompress the stomach using an NG tube. IV fluids and electrolytes may be given for dehydration, vomiting, and electrolyte imbalances. Pain relief results from the decompression.

Nutritional Therapy

There are no recommended dietary modifications for peptic ulcer disease. Patients are taught to eat and drink foods and fluids that do not cause distressing symptoms. Foods that may cause gastric irritation include caffeine; hot, spicy foods; pepper; carbonated beverages; and broth (meat extract). Teach the patient to eliminate alcohol consumption because it can delay healing.

Surgical Therapy

With the use of drug therapy and endoscopic therapy, surgery for peptic ulcer disease is used less often. Surgery is done for complications unresponsive to medical management or concerns about stomach cancer.

Surgical procedures include partial gastrectomy, vagotomy, or pyloroplasty. Partial gastrectomy with removal of the distal two-thirds of the stomach and anastomosis of the gastric stump to the duodenum is called a *gastroduodenostomy* or *Billroth I* operation; removal of the distal two-thirds of the stomach with anastomosis of the gastric stump to the jejunum is called a *gastrojejunostomy* or *Billroth II* operation. *Vagotomy* (severing of the vagal nerve) is done to decrease gastric acid secretion. *Pyloroplasty* is the surgical enlargement of the pyloric sphincter to facilitate the passage of contents from the stomach.

Postoperative complications from surgery are dumping syndrome, postprandial hypoglycemia, and bile reflux gastritis.

- *Dumping syndrome* occurs when surgery drastically reduces the reservoir capacity of the stomach and causes loss of control over the amount of gastric chyme entering the small intestine. The large bolus of hypertonic fluid entering the intestine causes a fluid shift into the bowel, creating a decrease in plasma volume along with distention of the bowel lumen and rapid intestinal transit. The patient usually describes feelings of generalized weakness, sweating, palpitations, and dizziness caused by the decrease in plasma volume. The patient may have abdominal cramps, borborygmi, and the urge to defecate. The onset of symptoms occurs within 15 to 30 minutes of eating, and symptoms usually last about 1 hour after eating.
- *Postprandial hypoglycemia* is considered a variant of dumping syndrome, because it is the result of uncontrolled gastric emptying of a bolus of fluid high in carbohydrates, resulting in hyperglycemia and the release of excessive amounts of insulin into the circulation. Symptoms and signs are similar to those of a hypoglycemic reaction, including sweating, weakness, mental confusion, palpitations, and tachycardia. Symptoms generally occur 2 hours after eating.
- Gastric surgery that involves the pylorus can result in reflux of bile into the stomach. The major symptom of *bile reflux gastritis* is continual epigastric distress that increases after meals. Vomiting relieves distress temporarily. The administration of cholestyramine to bind with the bile salts, either before or with meals, successfully treats this problem.

Because of surgical changes, the stomach's reservoir is diminished, and meal size must be reduced accordingly. Advise the patient to limit fluids with meals. Dry foods with a low carbohydrate content and moderate protein and fat content are better tolerated initially. Dietary changes and a short rest period after each meal reduce the likelihood of dumping syndrome.

Nursing Management

Goals

The overall goals are that the patient with PUD will adhere to the prescribed therapeutic regimen, have a reduction in or absence of discomfort, exhibit no signs of GI complications, have complete healing of the peptic ulcer, and make appropriate lifestyle changes to prevent recurrence.

Nursing Interventions

During an acute phase the patient may be NPO, have an NG tube inserted and connected to intermittent suction, and have IV fluid replacement. Explain the rationale for this therapy to the patient and caregiver. The volume of fluid lost, the patient's signs and symptoms, and laboratory test results determine the type and amount of IV fluids administered. When the stomach is kept empty of gastric secretions, the ulcer pain diminishes and ulcer healing begins. The patient's immediate environment should be quiet and restful.

Major complications of peptic ulcers are hemorrhage, perforation, and gastric outlet obstruction. All are considered emergencies and may require surgical intervention. Manifestations of perforation are sudden and dramatic in onset. They include severe upper abdominal pain that quickly spreads throughout the abdomen. Bowel sounds are usually absent.

If the patient has surgery, postoperative care is similar to that after abdominal laparotomy (see Abdominal Pain, Acute, p. 3). Additional considerations for a patient with a partial gastrectomy include:

- It is essential that the NG suction be working and that the tube remain patent so that accumulated gastric secretions do not put a strain on the anastomosis. Observe the gastric aspirate for color, amount, and odor.
- Observe the patient for signs of decreased peristalsis and lower abdominal discomfort that may indicate impending intestinal obstruction.
- Observe the dressing for signs of bleeding or odor and drainage indicative of an infection.
- Keep the patient comfortable and free of pain by administering prescribed drugs and by frequent changes in position.
- Encourage early ambulation.
- While the NG tube is connected to suction, maintain IV therapy. Add potassium and vitamin supplements (as ordered) to the infusion until oral feedings are resumed.
- The patient may require cobalamin therapy.

▼ Patient and Caregiver Teaching

General instructions should cover aspects of the disease process, drugs, possible changes in lifestyle, and regular follow-up evaluation

TABLE 65 Patient and Caregiver Teaching

Peptic Ulcer Disease (PUD)

1. Avoid foods that cause epigastric distress, such as acidic foods.
2. Avoid cigarettes. In addition to promoting ulcer development, smoking delays ulcer healing.
3. Reduce or eliminate alcohol intake.
4. Avoid over-the-counter (OTC) drugs unless approved by the HCP. Many preparations contain ingredients, such as aspirin, which should not be taken unless approved by the HCP. Check with the HCP about the use of nonsteroidal antiinflammatory drugs.
5. Do not interchange brands of PPIs, antacids, or H_2-receptor blockers that can be bought OTC without checking with the HCP. This can lead to harmful side effects.
6. Take all medications as prescribed. This includes both antisecretory and antibiotic drugs. Failing to take medications as prescribed can result in relapse.
7. It is important to report any of the following:
   - increased nausea or vomiting
   - increased epigastric pain
   - bloody emesis or tarry stools
8. Stress can be related to signs and symptoms of PUD. Learn and use stress management strategies.
9. Share concerns about lifestyle changes and living with a chronic illness.

(Table 65). Stress the need for long-term follow-up care. Encourage the patient to seek immediate intervention if symptoms return.

PERICARDITIS, ACUTE

Description

Pericarditis is a condition caused by inflammation of the pericardium, often with fluid accumulation. The pericardium anchors the heart, provides lubrication to decrease friction between heart contractions, and helps prevent excess dilation of the heart during diastole.

Pathophysiology

Acute pericarditis is most often idiopathic (unknown) or viral. Coxsackievirus B group is the most commonly identified virus. Other causes include uremia, bacterial infection, acute myocardial infarction (MI), neoplasm, and trauma.

There are 3 types of pericarditis: acute, subacute, and chronic. *Acute pericarditis* develops rapidly, causing the pericardial sac to become inflamed and leak fluid (pericardial effusion). *Subacute pericarditis* occurs weeks to months after an event. We refer to pericarditis lasting more than 6 months to as *chronic*.

- MI causes 5% to 8% of acute pericarditis cases. Post-MI syndrome (Dressler syndrome) pericarditis can occur 4 to 6 weeks after transmural MI. This syndrome is more common after a large anterior inferior infarct.

An inflammatory response is the characteristic pathologic finding in acute pericarditis. There is an influx of neutrophils, increased pericardial vascularity, and eventual fibrin deposition on the pericardium.

Clinical Manifestations

Clinical symptoms include progressive, severe sharp chest pain. The pain generally worsens with deep inspiration and when lying flat. Sitting up and leaning forward relieves the pain.

- The pain may radiate to the neck, arms, or left shoulder, making it hard to distinguish from angina. One distinction is that pericarditis pain can be referred to the trapezius muscle (shoulder, upper back).
- Dyspnea that accompanies acute pericarditis is related to the patient's breathing in rapid, shallow breaths to avoid chest pain. Pain may be aggravated by fever and anxiety.
- The hallmark finding is a *pericardial friction rub,* which is a scratching, grating, high-pitched sound believed to arise from friction between the roughened pericardial and epicardial surfaces. It is best heard with the stethoscope diaphragm firmly placed at the lower left sternal border of the chest with the patient leaning forward. Because it is hard to tell a pericardial friction rub from a pleural friction rub, ask the patient to hold their breath. If you still hear the rub, then it is cardiac. Pericardial friction rubs may be intermittent.

Complications

Pericardial effusion is buildup of fluid in the pericardium. Large effusions compress nearby structures. Pulmonary tissue compression can cause cough, dyspnea, and tachypnea. Phrenic nerve compression can induce hiccups, and compression of the recurrent laryngeal nerve may cause hoarseness. Heart sounds are distant and muffled. BP is usually maintained.

Cardiac tamponade develops as the pericardial effusion volume increases and compresses the heart. The speed of fluid accumulation affects the severity of clinical signs. Cardiac tamponade can occur acutely (e.g., rupture of heart, trauma) or subacutely (e.g., from renal failure, cancer). The patient may report chest pain and is often confused, anxious, and restless. Heart sounds become muffled, pulse pressure is narrowed, and the patient develops tachypnea, tachycardia, and decreased cardiac output. Neck veins may be markedly distended because of jugular venous pressure elevation. *Pulsus paradoxus* is a decrease in systolic BP with inspiration.

Diagnostic Studies

- Electrocardiogram (ECG) changes (e.g., diffuse ST-segment elevation) are noted in approximately 90% of the cases.
- Echocardiography is used to determine the presence of pericardial effusion or cardiac tamponade.
- Doppler and color M-mode imaging assess diastolic function and help diagnose constrictive pericarditis.
- Laboratory findings include leukocytosis and increased erythrocyte sedimentation rate (ESR) and C-reactive protein (CRP). Troponin levels may be increased in patients with ST-segment elevation and acute pericarditis, indicating myocardial damage.
- CT scan and MRI permit visualization of the pericardium and pericardial space.

Interprofessional Management

Management is directed toward identification and treatment of the underlying problem and symptoms. Antibiotics treat bacterial pericarditis, and nonsteroidal antiinflammatory drugs (NSAIDs) (e.g., salicylates [aspirin], ibuprofen) control the pain and inflammation of acute pericarditis. Corticosteroids are reserved for patients with pericarditis secondary to systemic lupus erythematosus, those already taking corticosteroids for a rheumatologic or other immune system condition, or those who do not respond to NSAIDs. Colchicine, an antiinflammatory drug used to treat gout, can be used in recurrent pericarditis.

- Pericardiocentesis is usually done for pericardial effusion with acute cardiac tamponade, purulent pericarditis, or suspected cancer. Hemodynamic support for the patient undergoing pericardiocentesis may include administering volume expanders and inotropic agents (e.g., dopamine) and discontinuing anticoagulants.
- A *pericardial window* is a surgical procedure for diagnosis or drainage of excess fluid. Cutting a "window," or part of the

pericardium, allows the fluid to drain continuously into the peritoneum or chest.

Nursing Management

Managing the patient's pain and anxiety is your key nursing consideration. Assess to distinguish the pain of myocardial ischemia (angina) from the pain of pericarditis. Pericarditis pain is in the precordium or over the left trapezius ridge and has a sharp quality that increases with inspiration. Relief from this pain is often obtained by sitting or leaning forward and is worse when the patient is lying flat.

- Pain relief measures include maintaining the patient on bed rest with the head of the bed elevated to 45 degrees and providing an overhead table for arm support.
- Antiinflammatory agents help alleviate the patient's pain. Give these drugs with food and tell the patient to avoid alcohol because of the risk of gastrointestinal (GI) bleeding.
- Monitor for the signs and symptoms of tamponade and prepare for possible pericardiocentesis.
- Provide simple, complete explanations of procedures and possible causes of the pain to help reduce anxiety for the patient with acute pericarditis. These explanations are particularly important for the patient whose diagnosis is being established and for the patient who has previously had angina or an MI.

P

PERIPHERAL ARTERY DISEASE

Description

Peripheral artery disease (PAD) involves thickening of artery walls. This results in a progressive narrowing of the arteries of the upper and lower extremities. PAD is strongly related to other types of cardiovascular disease (CVD) and their risk factors. In the United States, about 8.5 million people over age 40 years have PAD, with a higher prevalence in blacks.

Pathophysiology

The leading cause of PAD is atherosclerosis, which is a gradual thickening of the *intima* (the innermost layer of the arterial wall) and *media* (middle layer of the arterial wall). This results from cholesterol and lipids deposited within the vessel walls and leads to narrowing of the artery. Although the exact cause(s) of atherosclerosis are unknown, inflammation and endothelial injury play a major role.

- Risk factors for PAD are tobacco use (most important), atherosclerosis, diabetes, hypertension, high cholesterol, and age over 60 years.
- Atherosclerosis often affects certain segments of the arterial tree. These include the coronary, carotid, and lower extremity arteries. Symptoms occur when vessels are 60% to 75% blocked.

Peripheral Artery Disease: Lower Extremities

Lower extremity PAD may affect the iliac, femoral, popliteal, tibial, or peroneal arteries. The femoral-popliteal area is the most common site in nondiabetic patients. Patients with diabetes tend to develop PAD in the arteries below the knee.

Clinical Manifestations

Severity of the symptoms depends on the site and extent of the obstruction and the amount of collateral circulation.

- The classic symptom of PAD is *intermittent claudication,* which is ischemic muscle pain that is caused by exercise, resolves within 10 minutes or less with resting, and is reproducible.
- Some persons with PAD either have no symptoms or atypical leg symptoms (e.g., burning, hardness, heaviness, knotting, pressure, soreness, tightness, weakness) in atypical locations (e.g., ankle, foot, hamstring, hip, knee, shin).
- *Paresthesia* (numbness or tingling) in the toes or feet, may result from nerve tissue ischemia. Reduced blood flow to neurons causes loss of pressure and deep pain sensation.
- Pallor (blanching) of the foot is noted in response to leg elevation. *Reactive hyperemia* (redness) develops when the limb is allowed to hang in a dependent position *(dependent rubor).* The skin becomes shiny and taut. The lower legs lose their hair. Pedal, popliteal, or femoral pulses are diminished or absent.
- As PAD progresses and involves multiple arterial segments, continuous pain develops at rest. Rest pain most often occurs in the forefoot or toes and is worse with limb elevation.

The most serious complications are nonhealing arterial ulcers and gangrene, which may require lower extremity amputation.

Diagnostic Studies

- Doppler ultrasound and duplex imaging assess blood flow.
- Segmental BPs are obtained (using Doppler ultrasound and a sphygmomanometer) at the thigh, below the knee, and at ankle level while the patient is supine. A drop in segmental BP of > 30 mm Hg suggests PAD.
- Angiography or magnetic resonance angiography (MRA) delineates location and extent of PAD.

Interprofessional Management

The first treatment goal is to reduce cardiovascular risk factors. Tobacco cessation and aggressive management of diabetes, hypertension, and hyperlipidemia are essential. Dietary interventions and drug therapy are needed.

- Statins (e.g., simvastatin [Zocor]) and a fibric acid derivative (gemfibrozil [Lopid]) lower low-density lipoprotein (LDL) and triglyceride levels.
- Antiplatelet agents are critical for reducing the risk of CVD events and death. Oral antiplatelet therapy should include 75 to 325 mg/day of aspirin. Aspirin-intolerant patients may take 75 mg of clopidogrel (Plavix) daily.
- Two drugs are available to treat intermittent claudication: cilostazol and pentoxifylline. Pentoxifylline, a xanthine derivative, improves the flexibility of red blood cells (RBCs) and white blood cells (WBCs) and decreases fibrinogen concentration, platelet adhesiveness, and blood viscosity. Cilostazol is usually stopped within 3 months because of side effects.

A supervised exercise program is recommended for all patients with intermittent claudication. Exercise should be done for 30 to 45 minutes/day, at least 3 times per week, for a minimum of 3 months. Although walking is most commonly prescribed exercise, other modes of exercise (e.g., cycling) also improve walking ability and quality of life.

- Teach patients to adjust caloric intake so that an ideal body weight can be achieved and maintained. Recommend a diet high in fruits, vegetables, and whole grains and low in cholesterol, saturated fat, and salt.
- Patients taking antiplatelet agents, nonsteroidal antiinflammatory drugs (NSAIDs) (e.g., ibuprofen), or anticoagulants (e.g., warfarin) should consult their health care provider (HCP) before taking any dietary or herbal supplements, because of potential interactions and bleeding risks.

Critical limb ischemia is characterized by chronic ischemic rest pain lasting more than 2 weeks, arterial leg ulcers, or gangrene of the leg as a result of PAD. Conservative management goals for critical limb ischemia include protecting the patient's extremity from trauma, decreasing ischemic pain, preventing and controlling infection, and maximizing perfusion. Carefully inspect, cleanse, and lubricate both feet to prevent skin cracking and infection.

Interventional radiology catheter-based procedures are alternatives to open surgery for treatment of lower extremity PAD.

- *Percutaneous transluminal angioplasty* uses a catheter with a balloon at the tip. The end of the catheter is advanced to the stenotic area of the artery. The balloon is inflated, compressing the atherosclerotic intimal lining.

- *Stents,* expandable metallic devices, are positioned to hold the artery open immediately after balloon angioplasty. The stents may be covered with Dacron or a drug-eluting agent (e.g., paclitaxel) to reduce restenosis by limiting the new tissue growth into the stent.
- *Atherectomy* removes the obstructing plaque. A directional atherectomy device uses a high-speed cutting disk that cuts long strips of the atheroma. Laser atherectomy uses ultraviolet energy to break apart the atheroma.
- Various surgical approaches can be used to improve arterial blood flow beyond a blocked artery. The most common is a peripheral arterial bypass operation with autogenous (native) vein or synthetic graft material to bypass or carry blood around the lesion.
- Other surgical options include *endarterectomy* (opening the artery and removing the obstructing plaque) and *patch graft angioplasty* (opening the artery, removing the plaque, and sewing a patch to the opening to widen the lumen).
- Amputation may be needed if tissue necrosis is extensive, gangrene or osteomyelitis develops, or all major arteries are blocked.

Nursing Management
Goals
The patient with lower extremity PAD will have adequate tissue perfusion, relief of pain, increased exercise tolerance, and intact, healthy skin on extremities. Additional information on care for the patient with PAD of the lower extremities is presented in eNursing Care Plan 37-1 on the website.

Nursing Interventions
After surgical or radiologic intervention, check the operative extremity every 15 minutes initially and then hourly for color, temperature, capillary refill, presence of peripheral pulses, and movement and sensation. Immediately notify the HCP of any loss of palpable pulses or a change in the Doppler sound over a pulse.

After the patient leaves the recovery area, continue to monitor extremity perfusion and assess for complications such as bleeding, hematoma, thrombosis, embolization, and compartment syndrome. A dramatic increase in pain, loss of previously palpable pulses, extremity pallor or cyanosis, decreasing ankle-brachial index (ABI) on serial measurements, numbness or tingling, or a cold extremity suggests blockage of the graft or stent. Report these findings to the HCP immediately.

- Do not place the patient in knee-flexed positions except for exercise. Turn the patient frequently and position with pillows to support the incision. Starting on postoperative day 1, assist patient out of bed several times. Walking even short distances is desirable.
- Discourage prolonged sitting with legs lowered because it may cause pain and edema, increase the risk of venous thrombosis, and place stress on the suture lines. Graduated compression stockings may help control leg edema. If edema develops, position the patient supine and elevate the leg above the heart level.

▼ **Patient and Caregiver Teaching**

- Encourage supervised exercise training after revascularization. Explain that exercise decreases CVD risk factors including hypertension, hyperlipidemia, obesity, and glucose levels.
- Teach foot care to all patients with PAD. Meticulous foot care is especially important for the diabetic patient with PAD. Thick or overgrown toenails and calluses are potentially serious and need regular attention by an HCP (e.g., podiatrist).
- Tell patients to inspect their legs and feet daily for changes in skin color or texture. Show patients how to check skin temperature and capillary refill and to palpate pulses. Stress reporting any changes in these findings or the development of ulceration or inflammation to the HCP.
- Encourage patients to wear clean, all-cotton or all-wool socks and comfortable shoes with rounded (not pointed) toes and soft insoles. Tell patients to lace shoes loosely and to break in new shoes gradually.

PERITONITIS

Description

Peritonitis results from a localized or generalized inflammatory process involving the peritoneum. Causes are listed in Table 66. Primary peritonitis occurs when blood-borne organisms enter the peritoneal cavity. For example, the ascites that occurs with cirrhosis of the liver provides an excellent liquid environment for bacteria to flourish. Organisms can also enter the peritoneum during peritoneal dialysis. Secondary peritonitis is more common and occurs when abdominal organs perforate or rupture and release their contents (bile, enzymes, bacteria) into the peritoneal cavity.

Pathophysiology

Intestinal contents irritate the normally sterile peritoneum, producing an initial chemical peritonitis that is followed a few hours later

TABLE 66   **Causes of Peritonitis**
Primary
• Blood-borne organisms
• Cirrhosis with ascites
• Genital tract organisms
Secondary
• Appendicitis with rupture
• Blunt or penetrating trauma to abdominal organs
• Diverticulitis with rupture
• Ischemic bowel disorders
• Pancreatitis
• Perforated intestine
• Perforated peptic ulcer
• Peritoneal dialysis
• Postoperative (breakage of anastomosis)

by bacterial peritonitis. The resulting inflammatory response leads to massive fluid shifts (peritoneal edema) and formation of adhesions as the body tries to wall off the infection.

Clinical Manifestations and Complications

- Abdominal pain is the most common symptom.
- A universal sign of peritonitis is tenderness over the involved area. Rebound tenderness, muscular rigidity, and spasm are other major signs of peritoneum irritation.
- Abdominal distention or ascites, fever, tachycardia, tachypnea, nausea, vomiting, and altered bowel habits may also be present.

Complications include hypovolemic shock, sepsis, intraabdominal abscess, paralytic ileus, and acute respiratory distress syndrome. If treatment is delayed, peritonitis may be fatal.

Diagnostic Studies

- Complete blood count (CBC) will determine elevations in WBC count and hemoconcentration from fluid shifts.
- Peritoneal aspiration and analysis for blood, bile, pus, bacteria, fungi, and amylase content.
- Abdominal x-ray may show dilated loops of bowel consistent with paralytic ileus, free air if perforation has occurred, or air-fluid levels if an obstruction is present.
- CT scan and ultrasound may be useful in identifying ascites or abscesses.
- Peritoneoscopy may be helpful in patients without ascites.

Interprofessional Management

Patients with milder cases of peritonitis or who are poor surgical candidates may be managed conservatively with antibiotics, nasogastric (NG) suction, analgesics, and IV fluid administration. Surgery is indicated to locate the cause, drain purulent fluid, and repair damage (e.g., perforated organs).

Nursing Management

Goals

The patient with peritonitis will have resolution of inflammation, relief of abdominal pain, freedom from complications (especially hypovolemic shock and sepsis), and normal nutritional status.

Nursing Interventions

The patient with peritonitis is extremely ill and needs skilled supportive care. Establish IV access to replace lost fluids and deliver antibiotic therapy. Monitor the patient for pain and response to analgesics. The patient may be positioned with knees flexed to increase comfort. Sedatives may be given to allay anxiety.

- Accurately monitor fluid intake and output and electrolyte status to determine replacement therapy. Monitor vital signs frequently.
- Antiemetics may be given to decrease nausea and vomiting and prevent further fluid and electrolyte losses. The patient is NPO and may have an NG tube in place to decrease gastric distention and further leakage of bowel contents into the peritoneum.
- If the patient has an open surgical procedure, drains are inserted to remove purulent drainage and excess fluid. Postoperative care is similar to that for the patient with an exploratory laparotomy (see Abdominal Pain, Acute, p. 3).

PNEUMONIA

Description

Pneumonia is an infection of the lung parenchyma. Despite new antimicrobial agents to treat pneumonia, it is still associated with significant morbidity and mortality. Pneumonia can be caused by bacteria, viruses, *Mycoplasma* organisms, fungi, parasites, and chemicals.

Pneumonia can be classified as *community-acquired pneumonia* (CAP) or *hospital-acquired pneumonia* (HAP). Classifying pneumonia is important because of the differences in the likely causative organisms (Table 67) and the selection of appropriate treatment.

TABLE 67 Organisms Causing Pneumonia	
Community-Acquired Pneumonia	**Hospital-Acquired Pneumonia**
• *Chlamydophila pneumoniae* • *Chlamydophila psittaci* • *Coxiella burnettii* • Gram-negative bacilli • Fungi • *influenzae* • Influenza A and Influenza B • *Klebsiella pneumoniae* • *Legionella pneumophila*[a] • Methicillin Resistant *Staphylococcus aureus*[a] • *Moraxella catarrhalis* • *Mycobacterium tuberculosis* • *Mycoplasma pneumoniae* • Oral anaerobes (e.g., alcohol use, IV drug use) • *Pseudomonas aeruginosa* • Respiratory viruses • *Streptococcus pneumoniae*[a]	• *Acinetobacter* species[b] • *Enterobacter* species • *Escherichia coli*[b] • *Haemophilus influenzae* • *Klebsiella pneumoniae*[b] • *Proteus* species • *Pseudomonas aeruginosa*[b] • *Staphylococcus aureus* • *Streptococcus pneumoniae*

[a]Most common causes of community-acquired pneumonia (CAP).
[b]Most common causes of hospital-acquired pneumonia (HAP).

- *CAP* is an acute infection of the lung occurring in patients who have not been hospitalized or lived in a long-term care facility within 14 days of the onset of symptoms.
- *HAP* is pneumonia in a nonintubated patient that begins 48 hours or longer after admission to a hospital and was not present at the time of admission.
- *Ventilator-associated pneumonia (VAP)*, a type of HAP, refers to pneumonia that develops more than 48 hours after endotracheal intubation.

Pathophysiology

Normally, various defense mechanisms protect the airway distal to the larynx. Pneumonia is more likely to result when defense mechanisms are incompetent or overwhelmed by infectious agents because of:

- a weak cough or epiglottal reflexes;
- tracheal intubation interfering with the normal cough reflex and the mucociliary escalator mechanism;

- impaired mucociliary mechanism caused by air pollution, cigarette smoking, viral upper respiratory tract infections, and normal aging changes;
- chronic diseases, such as cancer, diabetes and heart disease, which can suppress the immune system's ability to inhibit bacterial growth.

Organisms that cause pneumonia reach the lungs by aspiration from the nasopharynx or oropharynx, inhalation of microbes present in the air, or hematogenous spread from a primary infection elsewhere in the body.

Most organisms trigger an inflammatory response in the lung. Inflammation, characterized by an increase in blood flow and vascular permeability, activates neutrophils to engulf and kill the offending organisms. As a result, the inflammatory process attracts more neutrophils, edema of the airways occurs, and fluid leaks from the capillaries and tissues into alveoli. Normal O_2 transport is affected, leading to clinical manifestations of hypoxia (e.g., tachypnea, dyspnea, tachycardia).

Consolidation, a feature of bacterial pneumonia, occurs when normally air-filled alveoli are filled with fluid and debris. Complete resolution and healing occur if there are no complications. Macrophages lyse and process the debris, normal lung tissue is restored, and gas exchange returns to normal.

Clinical Manifestations and Complications

The most common manifestations of pneumonia are cough, fever, shaking chills, dyspnea, tachypnea, and pleuritic chest pain.

- Cough may or may not be productive. Sputum may be green, yellow, or rust-colored (bloody).
- Viral pneumonia may initially seem to be influenza, with respiratory symptoms appearing and/or worsening 12 to 36 hours after onset.
- In older or debilitated patients, confusion or stupor (possibly related to hypoxia) may be the only finding.

On physical examination, fine or coarse crackles may be auscultated over the affected area. If consolidation is present, bronchial breath sounds, egophony, and increased fremitus may be noted.

Complications include *atelectasis* (collapsed, airless alveoli), *pleurisy* (inflammation of the pleura), pleural effusion, bacteremia, lung abscess, pericarditis, sepsis, and acute respiratory failure.

Diagnostic Studies

- History, physical examination, and chest x-ray often give enough information for making early treatment decisions.

- Chest x-ray often shows a pattern characteristic of the infecting organism.
- Sputum culture, gram stain of sputum, and blood cultures are used to identify the causative organism.
- Arterial blood gases (ABGs) are used to assess for hypoxemia, hypercapnia, and acidosis.
- White blood cell (WBC) count often reveals leukocytosis.

Interprofessional Management

Pneumococcal vaccine is used to prevent *Streptococcus pneumoniae* (pneumococcus) pneumonia. Vaccination is recommended for those 65 years of age or older and younger patients who are at high risk. A one-time repeat vaccination in 5 years is recommended for those who received their initial vaccination before the age of 65 years.

Prompt treatment with appropriate antibiotics almost always cures bacterial pneumonia, including *Mycoplasma* pneumonia. In uncomplicated cases, the patient responds to drug therapy within 48 to 72 hours.

A major problem today is pneumonia caused by multidrug-resistant (MDR) pathogens. Common culprits include methicillin-resistant *Staphylococcus aureus* and gram-negative bacilli. Risk factors for MDR pneumonia include advanced age, immunosuppression, history of antibiotic use, and prolonged mechanical ventilation. Antibiotic susceptibility tests can identify MDR organisms.

Currently, no definitive treatment exits for a majority of viral pneumonias. Care is generally supportive.

- Helpful measures include oxygen therapy, analgesics to relieve chest pain, and antipyretics, such as aspirin or acetaminophen. Individualize rest and activity to the patient's tolerance.
- Hydration is important. If the patient cannot maintain adequate oral intake, IV administration of fluids and electrolytes may be necessary. If the patient has heart failure, fluid intake is carefully monitored.
- Small, frequent meals are easier for patients with dyspnea to tolerate. Offer foods high in calories and nutrients.

Nursing Management

Goals

The patient with pneumonia will have clear breath sounds, normal breathing patterns, no signs of hypoxia, normal appearance on chest x-ray, normal WBC count, and no complications related to pneumonia.

Nursing Interventions

To reduce the risk of pneumonia, teach patients to practice good health habits such as frequent hand washing, proper nutrition, adequate rest, regular exercise, and coughing or sneezing into the elbow rather than hands. Avoiding cigarette smoke is 1 of the most important health-promoting behaviors. If possible, avoid exposure to people with upper respiratory infections (URIs). If a URI occurs, it should be treated promptly with supportive measures (e.g., rest, fluids). If symptoms persist for more than 7 days, the person should seek medical care. Encourage those at increased risk for pneumonia to obtain both influenza and pneumococcal vaccines.

The eNursing Care Plan 27-1 (on the website) for a patient with pneumonia applies to people both at home and in the hospital.

- Place the patient with altered consciousness in positions (e.g., side-lying, upright) that will prevent or minimize aspiration. Reposition the patient at least every 2 hours to promote lung expansion and mobilization of secretions.
- The patient who has a feeding tube requires attention to prevent aspiration.
- In the intensive care unit (ICU), strict adherence to "ventilator bundle" interventions reduces the incidence of VAP. These interventions are elevation of the head of the bed 30 to 45 degrees, daily "sedation holidays," assessment of readiness to extubate, prophylaxis for peptic ulcer disease and venous thromboembolism, and daily oral care with chlorhexidine.
- The patient who has difficulty swallowing (e.g., after a stroke) needs assistance in eating, drinking, and taking medication to prevent aspiration. After a patient has had local anesthesia to the throat, assess for a gag reflex before giving food or fluids.
- Patients with impaired mobility from any cause need assistance with turning and moving, as well as frequent encouragement to breathe deeply.
- Practice strict medical asepsis and adherence to infection control guidelines, including hand hygiene, to reduce the incidence of HAP.

▼ Patient and Caregiver Teaching

- Teach the patient about the importance of taking every dose of the prescribed antibiotic, any drug–drug and food–drug interactions for the prescribed antibiotic, and the need for adequate rest to promote recovery.
- Tell the patient to drink plenty of liquids (at least 6 to 10 glasses/day, unless contraindicated) and to avoid alcohol and smoking.
- A cool mist humidifier or warm bath may help the patient breathe easier.
- Provide information about influenza and pneumococcal vaccines.

PNEUMOTHORAX

Description

A *pneumothorax* is a complete or partial collapse of a lung as a result of an accumulation of air in the pleural space. Pneumothorax can be classified as *open* (air entering through an opening in the chest wall) or *closed* (no external wound).

Pathophysiology

Normally, negative (subatmospheric) pressure exists between the visceral pleura (surrounding the lung) and the parietal pleura (lining the chest cavity), allowing the lungs to be filled by chest wall expansion. The pleural space has only a few milliliters of lubricating fluid to reduce friction when the tissues move. When air enters the pleural space, the change in pressure (from negative to positive) causes a partial or complete lung collapse. As the volume of air in the pleural space increases, lung volume decreases.

Types of Pneumothorax

Spontaneous pneumothorax occurs as a result of the rupture of small blebs (air-filled sacs) located on the apex of the lung. These blebs occur in healthy, young people or from lung disease such as chronic obstructive pulmonary disease (COPD), asthma, cystic fibrosis, and pneumonia. Smoking increases the risk of bleb formation. Other risk factors include being tall and thin, male gender, family history, and previous spontaneous pneumothorax.

Traumatic pneumothorax can occur from either penetrating (open) or nonpenetrating (closed) chest trauma. A penetrating chest wound may be referred to as a "sucking chest wound," because air enters the pleural space through the chest wall during each inspiration (Fig. 18).

Iatrogenic pneumothorax can occur because of laceration or puncture of the lung during medical procedures. For example, transthoracic needle aspiration, subclavian catheter insertion, pleural biopsy, and transbronchial lung biopsy all have the potential to injure the lung. Barotrauma from excessive ventilatory pressure during manual or mechanical ventilation can rupture alveoli, creating a pneumothorax. Esophageal procedures may result in a pneumothorax from tearing of the esophageal wall.

Tension pneumothorax occurs when air enters the pleural space but cannot escape. The accumulation of air in the pleural space causes increasingly elevated intrapleural pressures. This results in compression of the lung on the affected side and pressure on the heart and great vessels, pushing them away from the affected side.

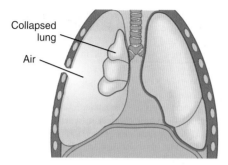

Fig. 18 Open pneumothorax resulting from collapse of lung following disruption of chest wall and outside air entering.

The mediastinum shifts toward the unaffected side, compressing the "good" lung, which further compromises oxygenation. As pressure increases, venous return is decreased and cardiac output falls. Tension pneumothorax may result from either an open or a closed pneumothorax.

Hemothorax is an accumulation of blood in the pleural space from injury to the chest wall, diaphragm, lung, blood vessels, or mediastinum. The patient with a traumatic hemothorax needs immediate insertion of a chest tube for evacuation of the blood, which can be recovered and reinfused for a short time after the injury.

Clinical Manifestations

If the pneumothorax is small, only mild tachycardia and dyspnea may be present. If it is a large pneumothorax, shallow, rapid respirations, dyspnea, air hunger, and oxygen desaturation may occur.

- Chest pain and a cough with or without hemoptysis may be present.
- No breath sounds are auscultated over the affected area.
- Chest x-ray shows air or fluid in the pleural space with reduced lung volume.

Interprofessional Management

Tension pneumothorax is a medical emergency, requiring urgent needle compression followed by chest tube insertion with water-seal drainage.

Emergency treatment of an open pneumothorax consists of covering the wound with an occlusive dressing secured on 3 sides (vent dressing). During inspiration, as negative pressure is created in the chest, the dressing pulls against the wound, preventing air from entering the pleural space. During expiration, as the pressure rises in the pleural space, the dressing is pushed out and air escapes through the wound and from under the dressing. If the object that caused the open chest wound is still in place, do not remove it. Stabilize the impaled object with a bulky dressing, and wait until a health care provider (HCP) is present, or, arrange transport to the nearest medical facility.

The most common treatment for a pneumothorax and hemothorax is to insert a chest tube and connect it to water-seal drainage (see Chest Tubes and Pleural Drainage, p. 679). If the patient with a small pneumothorax is stable, the condition may resolve spontaneously, or the pleural space can be aspirated with a large-bore needle (thoracentesis). Repeated spontaneous pneumothoraces be treated surgically by a partial pleurectomy, stapling, or pleurodesis to promote the adherence of pleurae to one another.

POLYCYSTIC KIDNEY DISEASE

Polycystic kidney disease (PKD) is 1 of the most common life-threatening genetic disease in the world. PKD is the fourth leading cause of end-stage renal disease (ESRD), affecting 5% of those with ESRD. A nongenetic PKD (acquired cystic kidney disease [ACKD]) is seen in those with severe kidney scarring and damage who typically require dialysis. After 5 years on dialysis, 90% of patients will have ACKD.

There are 2 forms of PKD. The *childhood form* is a rare autosomal recessive disorder that is often rapidly progressive. The *adult form* of PKD is an autosomal dominant disorder. Adult PKD is latent for many years and is usually manifested between 30 and 40 years of age. It involves both kidneys. The cortex and medulla are filled with large, thin-walled cysts that are several millimeters to several centimeters in diameter. The cysts enlarge and destroy surrounding tissue by compression.

Many people have no symptoms, which can delay diagnosis. Symptoms appear when the cysts begin to enlarge. Often the first manifestations are hypertension, hematuria (from rupture of cysts), or pain or a sensation of heaviness in the back, side, or abdomen. However, the first manifestation can be a urinary tract infection (UTI) or urinary stones. Bilateral, enlarged kidneys are often palpable on physical examination.

- Chronic pain can be constant and severe.
- The disease progresses to ESRD by age 60 years in 50% of patients.

- PKD can also affect the liver (liver cysts), heart (abnormal heart valves), blood vessels (aneurysms), and intestines (diverticulosis). The most serious complication is a ruptured cerebral aneurysm.

  Diagnosis is based on clinical manifestations, family history, ultrasound, or CT scan.

  There is no specific treatment for PKD. A major aim is to prevent or treat UTIs with appropriate antibiotics. Nephrectomy may be necessary for chronic pain, bleeding, or infection. When the patient begins to experience progressive renal failure, interventions are determined by the remaining renal function. Dialysis and kidney transplantation may be needed to treat ESRD.

  Nursing measures are those used for management of ESRD (see Kidney Disease, Chronic, pp. 358). They include diet modification, fluid restriction, drugs (e.g., antihypertensives), and assisting the patient and family in coping with the chronic disease process and financial concerns.

- The patient with the adult form of PKD often has children by the time the disease is diagnosed. Refer the patient and any adult children for genetic counseling.

POLYCYTHEMIA

P

Description

Polycythemia is the production and presence of increased number of red blood cells (RBCs). The increase in RBCs can be so great that blood circulation is impaired because of the increased blood viscosity (hyperviscosity) and volume (hypervolemia).

Pathophysiology

The 2 types of polycythemia are *primary polycythemia (polycythemia vera)* and *secondary polycythemia* (Fig. 19). Their etiologies and pathogeneses differ, although their complications and clinical manifestations are similar.

Polycythemia vera is a chronic myeloproliferative disorder. It involves not only RBCs but also white blood cells (WBCs) and platelets, leading to increased production of all these blood cells. This leads to enhanced blood viscosity and blood volume and congestion of organs and tissues with blood. Splenomegaly and hepatomegaly are common. Patients have hypercoagulopathies that predispose them to clotting. The disease develops insidiously and follows a chronic, vacillating course. The median age at diagnosis is 60 years, with a slight male predominance.

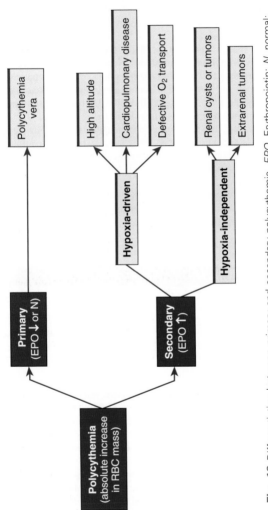

Fig. 19 Differentiating between primary and secondary polycythemia. *EPO,* Erythropoietin; *N,* normal; *RBC,* red blood cell.

- Polycythemia vera is associated with acquired gene mutations leading to increased production of blood cells.

Secondary polycythemia can be either hypoxia-driven or hypoxia-independent. In *hypoxia-driven polycythemia*, hypoxia stimulates erythropoietin (EPO) production in the kidney, which in turn stimulates RBC production. The need for O_2 may result from high altitude, lung or heart disease, defective O_2 transport, or tissue hypoxia. In *hypoxia-independent polycythemia*, cancer or benign tumor tissue makes extra EPO.

Clinical Manifestations

- Initial manifestations from hypertension caused by hypervolemia and hyperviscosity include headache, vertigo, dizziness, tinnitus, and visual changes.
- Blood vessel distention, circulatory stasis, thrombosis, and tissue hypoxia may cause angina, heart failure (HF), intermittent claudication, and thrombophlebitis.
- The most common serious acute complication is stroke from thrombosis.
- Hemorrhage caused by either vessel rupture from overdistention or inadequate platelet function may result in petechiae, ecchymoses, epistaxis, or gastrointestinal (GI) bleeding.

  Other clinical manifestations include:

- generalized pruritus related to histamine release from an increased number of basophils;
- hepatomegaly and splenomegaly may contribute to patient sensations of satiety and fullness;
- pain from peptic ulcer caused by increased gastric secretions;
- plethora (ruddy complexion);
- hyperuricemia from RBC destruction that follows excessive RBC production; gout.

Diagnostic Studies

Diagnostic study abnormalities include:

- high hemoglobin (Hgb) and RBC count with microcytosis;
- low to normal EPO level in polycythemia vera, high EPO level in secondary polycythemia;
- high WBC count with basophilia;
- high platelets (thrombocytosis) and platelet dysfunction;
- high leukocyte alkaline phosphatase, uric acid, and cobalamin levels;
- high histamine levels.

Bone marrow examination in polycythemia vera shows hypercellularity of RBCs, WBCs, and platelets.

Nursing and Interprofessional Management

Treatment of polycythemia vera is directed toward reducing blood volume and viscosity and bone marrow activity. Phlebotomy is the mainstay of treatment. The aim of phlebotomy is to reduce the hematocrit and keep it $< 45\%$. At the time of diagnosis 300 to 500 mL of blood may be removed every few days until the hematocrit is reduced to acceptable levels. Phlebotomy may be needed every 2 to 3 months, reducing the blood volume by about 500 mL each time. A person managed with repeated phlebotomies eventually becomes deficient in iron, although this effect is rarely symptomatic.

- Avoid iron supplementation.
- Hydration therapy can reduce the blood's viscosity. Assess fluid intake and output during hydration therapy to avoid fluid overload (which worsens circulatory congestion) or fluid deficit (which can make the blood even more viscous).
- Myelosuppressive agents, such as hydroxyurea, busulfan (Myleran), and chlorambucil (Leukeran), may be given. Ruxolitinib (Jakafi), which inhibits the expression of the JAK2 mutation, is given to patients who have not responded to hydroxyurea. α-Interferon (α-IFN) and pegylated interferon are given to women of childbearing age or those with intractable pruritus. Teach the patient about the side effects of the drugs.
- Begin activities and/or medications to decrease thrombus formation. Anagrelide (Agrylin), can reduce the platelet count and inhibit platelet aggregation. Low-dose aspirin is used to prevent clotting. Start active or passive leg exercises and ambulation when possible.
- Allopurinol (Zyloprim) may reduce the number of acute gouty attacks.
- Assess the patient's nutritional status, since inadequate food intake can result from GI symptoms of fullness, pain, and dyspepsia.

Because of its chronic nature, polycythemia vera requires ongoing evaluation. Assess the patient for complications.

PRESSURE INJURY

Description

A *pressure injury* is localized damage to the skin or underlying tissue. It usually occurs over a bony prominence or is related to a medical or other device. The injury occurs because of intense and/or prolonged pressure or pressure in combination with shear. The most common sites for pressure injuries are the sacrum and heels.

Factors influencing pressure injury development include amount of pressure (intensity), length of time pressure is exerted on skin (duration), and ability of patient's tissue to tolerate externally applied pressure. *Shear* (pressure exerted on skin when the surface layer adheres to bedding while deeper skin layers slide in the direction of body movement) and excessive moisture also contribute to pressure injury formation. The tolerance of soft tissue for pressure and shear are affected by microclimate, nutrition, perfusion, co-morbidities, and condition of the soft tissue.

- Patients at risk for the development of pressure injuries are those who are older, incontinent, unable to reposition or unaware of the need to reposition (e.g., spinal cord injury), and bed- or wheelchair-bound.
- Stage 3 or 4 (full-skin-thickness injury) pressure injury acquired after admission to a health care setting is considered a serious reportable event.

Clinical Manifestations

Pressure injuries are staged on the basis of the visible or palpable tissue in the injury bed. Table 68 shows the pressure injury stages. If the pressure injury becomes infected, the patient may display systemic signs of infection (e.g., leukocytosis, fever).

Nursing and Interprofessional Management

Pressure injury management requires local wound care as well as support measures such as adequate nutrition, pain management, and pressure relief. Both conservative and surgical strategies are used in the treatment of pressure injuries, depending on the wound's stage and condition.

Goals

The overall goals are that the patient with a pressure injury will have no deterioration of the wound, not develop an infection in the pressure injury, have healing of pressure injuries, and have no recurrence.

Nursing Interventions

Assess patients for pressure injury risk on admission and at periodic intervals, using a validated assessment tool, such as the Braden Scale (available at *www.bradenscale.com*). Reposition patients frequently to prevent pressure injuries. Although the past "standard" was every 2 hours, the frequency of turning and repositioning patients should be individualized on the basis of risk factors and

TABLE 68   Staging of Pressure Injuries

Definition and Description	Clinical Presentation
Stage 1 Pressure Injury: Nonblanchable Erythema of Intact Skin Intact skin with a localized area of nonblanchable erythema, which may appear differently in dark skin. Blanchable erythema or changes in sensation, temperature, or firmness may precede visual changes **Stage 2 Pressure Injury: Partial-Thickness Skin Loss With Exposed Dermis** Partial-thickness loss of skin with exposed dermis. The wound bed is viable, pink or red, and moist. May present as an intact or ruptured serum-filled blister. Adipose and deeper tissues are not visible. Often result from adverse microclimate and shear in the skin over the pelvis and shear in the heel. **Stage 3 Pressure Injury: Full-thickness Skin Loss** Full-thickness loss of skin, in which adipose is visible in the injury. Granulation tissue and epibole (rolled wound edges) are often present. Slough and/or eschar (types of dead tissue) may be visible. The depth of tissue damage varies by anatomic location; areas of significant adiposity can develop deep wounds. Undermining and tunneling may occur.	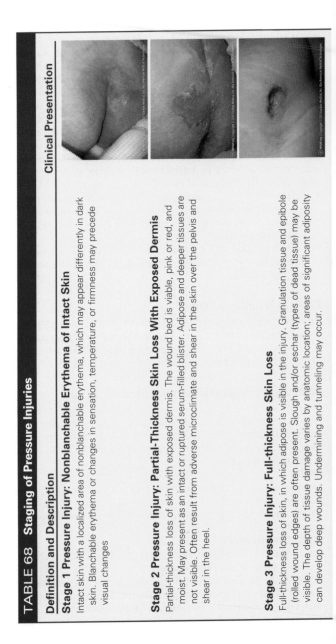

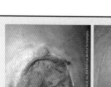
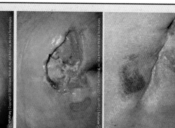

Stage 4 Pressure Injury: Full-thickness Skin and Tissue Loss

Full-thickness skin and tissue loss with exposed or directly palpable fascia, muscle, tendon, ligament, cartilage, or bone in the injury. Slough and/or eschar may be visible. Epibole, undermining and/or tunneling often occur. Depth varies by anatomic location.

Unstageable Pressure Injury: Obscured Full-Thickness Skin and Tissue Loss

Full-thickness skin and tissue loss in which the extent of tissue damage within the injury cannot be confirmed because it is obscured by slough or eschar. A Stage 3 or Stage 4 pressure injury is present after removing slough or eschar. Stable eschar (i.e. dry, adherent, intact without erythema or fluctuance) on the heel or ischemic limb should not be softened or removed.

Deep Tissue Pressure Injury (DTPI): Persistent Nonblanchable Deep Red, Maroon or Purple Discoloration

Intact or nonintact skin with localized area of persistent nonblanchable deep red, maroon, purple discoloration, or epidermal separation revealing a dark wound bed or blood-filled blister. Pain and temperature change often precede skin color changes. Discoloration may appear differently in dark skin. Results from intense and/or prolonged pressure and shear forces at the bone-muscle interface. May evolve rapidly to reveal the actual extent of tissue injury or may resolve without tissue loss. Visible necrotic tissue, subcutaneous tissue, granulation tissue, fascia, muscle, or other underlying structures indicates a full-thickness pressure injury (unstageable, Stage 3 or Stage 4). Do not use DTPI to describe vascular, traumatic, neuropathic, or dermatologic conditions.

Photos used with permission of the National Pressure Injury Advisory Panel.

P

TABLE 69 Patient and Caregiver Teaching

Pressure Injury

When teaching the patient or caregiver to prevent and care for pressure injuries, do the following:

1. Identify and explain risk factors and cause of pressure injuries to patient and caregiver.
2. Teach the caregiver techniques for incontinence. If incontinence occurs, cleanse skin at time of soiling and use absorbent pads or briefs.
3. Demonstrate correct positioning to decrease risk of skin breakdown. Teach caregiver to reposition a bed-bound patient at least every 2 hours, a chair-bound patient every hour. NEVER position the patient directly on the pressure injury if possible.
4. Review the available resources (i.e., caregiver's availability and skill, finances, equipment) of patients who need pressure injury care at home.
5. Teach patient and/or caregiver to place clean dressings over sterile dressings using "no touch" technique when changing dressings. Review the disposal of contaminated dressings.
6. Teach patient and caregiver to inspect skin daily. Tell them to report any significant changes to the HCP.
7. Teach patient and caregiver the importance of good nutrition to enhance injury healing.
8. Evaluate program effectiveness.

the type of support surface. For example, some high-risk patients may need to be turned and repositioned every hour.

- Implement prevention strategies for those identified as being at risk for a pressure injury. Table 69 lists guidelines for preventing pressure injuries.

If a pressure injury has developed, document its size, depth, and appearance. Initiate interventions based on the injury's characteristics (e.g., size, stage, location, presence of infection or pain) and the patient's general clinical status. Pressure injuries generally fall under the category of healing by secondary intention. Local injury care may involve debridement, wound cleaning, relief of pressure, and the application of a dressing.

- Necrotic tissue or eschar (except for dry, stable necrotic heels) must be removed by surgical, mechanical, enzymatic, or autolytic debridement methods. Once the pressure injury has been successfully debrided and has a clean granulating base, the goal is to provide an appropriate wound environment that supports moist wound healing and prevents disruption of newly formed granulation tissue.

- Reconstruction of the pressure injury site by operative repair, using skin grafts, skin flaps, musculocutaneous flaps, or free flaps, may be necessary.
- Pressure injuries should be cleaned with noncytotoxic solutions, such as normal saline, that do not kill or damage cells.
- After cleansing the pressure injury, cover it with an appropriate dressing. (Dressings are discussed in Table 11.9, Harding et al., Lewis' *Medical-Surgical Nursing,* ed 11.)
- Choose appropriate pressure-redistributing techniques (e.g., mattress replacement, mattress overlay, integrated bed system, seat cushion, seat cushion overlay) to move pressure off of areas of pressure injury. Whenever possible, do not turn the patient onto a body surface that has blanchable erythema. Massage is contraindicated in the presence of acute inflammation and where there is the possibility of damaged blood vessels or fragile skin.
- Sliding down in bed causes shear. Encourage patients to reposition themselves by lifting rather than sliding and to use a trapeze if needed. Lift sheets may be used to move patients up in bed or to transfer them.
- Maintaining adequate nutrition is an important nursing responsibility when caring for a patient with a pressure injury. Oral feedings must be adequate in calories, protein, fluids, vitamins, and minerals to meet the patient's nutritional requirements. Enteral feedings or parenteral nutrition can be used to supplement oral feedings.

▼ **Patient and Caregiver Teaching**

Because recurrence of pressure injuries is common, it is extremely important to teach the patient and caregiver about prevention techniques (see Table 69).

- Teach caregiver about the cause of pressure injuries, prevention techniques, early signs, nutritional support, and care techniques for pressure injuries.
- Because the patient with a pressure injury often requires extensive care for other health problems, the caregiver may need your psychosocial support.

PROSTATE CANCER

Description

Prostate cancer is a tumor of the prostate gland. It is the most common cancer among men, excluding skin cancer, and is the second leading cause of cancer death in men (exceeded only by lung cancer). A man has a 1 in 9 risk of developing prostate cancer in his lifetime. More than 2.9 million men in the United States are survivors of prostate cancer.

- Black men have a higher incidence of prostate cancer than any other population worldwide (except Jamaican men of African descent).

Pathophysiology

Prostate cancer is a slow growing androgen-dependent cancer. Tumor spread is by 3 routes: direct extension, through the lymph system, or through the bloodstream. Spread by direct extension involves the seminal vesicles, urethral mucosa, bladder wall, and external sphincter. Later spread occurs through the lymphatic system. The bloodstream is the route for spread to the pelvic bones, head of the femur, lower lumbar spine, liver, and lungs.

- The incidence of prostate cancer increases markedly after age 50 years, with a median age at diagnosis of 66 years.
- Dietary factors and obesity may be related to prostate cancer. A diet high in red and processed meats and high-fat dairy products along with a low intake of vegetables and fruits may increase the risk of prostate cancer.
- There is an increased prevalence of prostate cancer among farmers and commercial pesticide applicators, possibly caused by exposure to chemicals found in pesticides.
- It is not clear if smoking is a risk factor for prostate cancer.
- Persons with a family history of prostate cancer are at increased risk.

Clinical Manifestations

Prostate cancer usually has no early symptoms. Eventually the patient may have signs and symptoms similar to those of benign prostatic hyperplasia (BPH), including dysuria, hesitancy, dribbling, frequency, urgency, hematuria, nocturia, retention, interruption of urinary stream, and inability to urinate.

- Pain in the lumbosacral area that radiates down to the hips or legs, when coupled with urinary symptoms, may indicate metastasis. As the cancer spreads to the bones, spinal cord compression and bone destruction cause severe back and leg pain.

Diagnostic Studies

- Most men in the United States with prostate cancer are diagnosed by prostate-specific antigen (PSA) screening. Men should be told about the potential risks (e.g., evaluation and treatment that may be unnecessary) and benefits (early detection of prostate cancer) of PSA screening before being tested. The discussion about screening should take place at: (1) age

50 years for men who are at average risk of prostate cancer and are expected to live at least 10 more years; (2) age 45 years for men at high risk for development of prostate cancer, including blacks and men who have a first-degree relative (father, brother, or son) diagnosed with prostate cancer at an early age (younger than age 65 years); and (3) age 40 years for men at even higher risk (those with more than 1 first-degree relative who had prostate cancer at an early age). Mild elevations in PSA may occur with aging, BPH, recent ejaculation, constipation, or prostatitis, or after long bike rides. Decreases in the PSA level can occur with drugs such as finasteride (Proscar) and dutasteride (Avodart).

- When prostate cancer treatment is successful, PSA levels should fall to undetectable levels.
- On digital rectal examination (DRE), the prostate gland may feel hard, nodular, and asymmetric.
- Elevated prostatic acid phosphatase (PAP) levels are specific for prostate cancer.
- Biopsy using transrectal ultrasound can confirm the diagnosis.
- CT scan, bone scan, or MRI can assess cancer spread.
- Elevated serum alkaline phosphatase may indicate bone metastasis.

Interprofessional Management

Staging

The most common classification system for determining the extent of the prostate cancer is the tumor-node-metastasis (TNM) system (see p. 761).

The tumor is graded on the basis of tumor histology using 2 different grading systems: the Gleason scale, and the Grade Group. Gleason Grade 1 represents the most well-differentiated or lowest grade (most like original cells), and grade 5 represents the most poorly differentiated (unlike original cells) or highest grade. The 2 most commonly occurring patterns of cells are graded with the 2 scores, which are then added together to create a Gleason score. The Grade Group system grades the cells based on their differentiation. The Grade Group grades the tumor with 1 number on a scale from 1 to 5, with Grade Group 1 being lowest risk and Grade Group 5 being highest risk. Currently, the Gleason score and the Grade Group system are used together with the TNM system (Table 70) to determine the stage of the tumor.

- Most patients (93%) with prostate cancer are diagnosed when the cancer is in either a local or a regional stage. The 5-year survival rate with a diagnosis at these stages is 100%.

TABLE 70 **Staging of Prostate Cancer**

Stage	Tumor Size	Lymph Node Involvement	Metastasis	PSA Level	Gleason Score
I	Not felt on DRE Not seen by visual imaging	No	No	<10	≤6
II	Felt on DRE Seen by imaging Tumor confined to prostate	No	No	10–20	6–7
III	Cancer outside prostate Possible spread to seminal vesicles	No	No	Any level	Any score
IV	Any size	Any nodal involvement	Yes	Any level	Any score

DRE, Digital rectal examination; *PSA,* prostate-specific antigen.
Adapted from American Cancer Society: *How is prostate cancer staged?* Retrieved from *www.cancer.org/Cancer/ProstateCancer/DetailedGuide/prostate-cancer-staging.*

At all stages, there is more than 1 possible treatment option. The decision of which treatment course to pursue should be made jointly by patients, their partners, and the interprofessional team.

- A conservative approach to slow-growing tumors is active surveillance or "watchful waiting." This strategy is appropriate for: (1) a life expectancy of < 10 years (low risk of dying of the disease), (2) the presence of a low-grade, low-stage tumor, and (3) serious coexisting medical conditions. Patients are monitored with frequent PSA testing and DREs. Significant changes in PSA level, DRE findings, or symptoms warrant a reevaluation of treatment options.

Surgical Therapy

With radical prostatectomy, the entire prostate gland, seminal vesicles, and part of the bladder neck (ampulla) are removed. Retroperitoneal lymph node dissection is performed only on men with a high risk for metastatic disease. A pelvic lymph node dissection is typically done at the same time as prostatectomy to pathologically assess for nodal metastases in the local pelvic area. Typically, a higher number of lymph nodes are removed and dissected if the prostate cancer is higher grade/higher risk on biopsy. Surgery is not an option for advanced-stage disease, except to relieve symptoms associated with obstruction.

- Traditional approaches for radical prostatectomy are retropubic (low abdominal incision) and perineal (incision between the scrotum and anus).
- Robotic-assisted (e.g., da Vinci system) laparoscopic prostatectomy is associated with less bleeding, less pain, and a faster recovery.
- After surgery, the patient has a large indwelling catheter with a 20- or 30-mL balloon placed in the bladder via the urethra. A drain is left in the surgical site.

Two major adverse outcomes after a radical prostatectomy are erectile dysfunction (ED) and urinary incontinence. The incidence of ED depends on the patient's age, preoperative sexual functioning, whether nerve-sparing surgery was done, and the expertise of the surgeon. A nerve-sparing technique is sometimes used to reduce the risk of ED. Problems with urinary control may occur for the first few months because the bladder must be reattached to the urethra after the prostate is removed. Kegel exercises strengthen the pelvic floor muscles and the urinary sphincter and may help improve continence. Cryotherapy is a surgical technique that destroys cancer cells by freezing. The treatment takes about 2 hours, with the patient under general or spinal anesthesia.

A bilateral orchiectomy is the surgical removal of the testes that may be done alone or in combination with prostatectomy. For advanced stages of prostate cancer, an orchiectomy is 1 treatment option for cancer control.

Radiation Therapy

Radiation therapy is a common option for prostate cancer. Radiation therapy may be offered as the only treatment, or it may be offered in combination with surgery or hormonal therapy. Salvage radiation therapy given for cancer recurrence after a radical prostatectomy may improve survival.

- External beam radiation is the most widely used method. Brachytherapy using radioactive seed implants placed in the prostate gland is best suited for patients with early-stage disease.

Drug Therapy

The types of drug therapy available for the treatment of advanced or metastatic prostate cancer are androgen deprivation (hormone) therapy, chemotherapy, or a combination of both.

Prostate cancer growth is largely dependent on the presence of androgens. Androgen deprivation therapy (ADT) is focused on reducing the levels of circulating androgens to reduce the tumor growth. One of the biggest challenges with ADT is that almost all tumors treated will become resistant to this therapy *(hormone-refractory)* within a few years. Androgen deprivation can be produced by inhibiting androgen production or blocking androgen receptors.

- Luteinizing hormone–releasing hormone (LHRH) agonists (e.g., goserelin [Zoladex], leuprolide [Lupron, Eligard], triptorelin [Trelstar]) produce a chemical castration similar to the effects of an orchiectomy.
- Androgen receptor blockers (e.g., flutamide, nilutamide [Nilandron], enzalutamide (Xtandi), bicalutamide) compete with circulating androgens at the receptor sites.
- Combining an androgen receptor blocker with an LHRH agonist results in combined androgen blockade.

Chemotherapy is generally reserved for patients with hormone-refractory prostate cancer (HRPC) in late-stage disease. The goal of chemotherapy is mainly palliative.

- Men with advanced prostate cancer who have HRPC may receive a vaccine (sipuleucel-T [Provenge]). The vaccine stimulates the patient's system against the cancer and may prolong survival.

Nursing Management

Goals

The patient with prostate cancer will be an active participant in the treatment plan, have acceptable pain control, follow the therapeutic plan, understand the effect of the therapeutic plan on sexual function, and find an acceptable way to manage the impact on bladder or bowel function.

Nursing Interventions

One of your most important roles is to encourage patients (in consultation with their health care provider [HCP]) to have an annual prostate screening (PSA and DRE). See discussion of screening recommendations, pp. 500.

- Provide support for the patient and the family to help them cope with the cancer diagnosis.
- Care during the preoperative and postoperative phases of radical prostatectomy is similar to that with surgical procedures for BPH (see pp. 68).
- Refer to nursing interventions for the patient undergoing radiation therapy (p. 712) and chemotherapy (p. 674).
- Pain control is the primary nursing intervention for the terminally ill patient. It is managed through pain assessment, giving prescribed medications (both opioid and nonopioid agents), and nonpharmacologic methods of pain relief (e.g., relaxation breathing).
- In advanced prostate cancer, palliative and end-of-life care is often appropriate and beneficial.

▼ Patient and Caregiver Teaching

Teach appropriate catheter care for the patient discharged with an indwelling catheter in place.

- Teach the patient to clean the urethral meatus with soap and water once each day; maintain a high fluid intake; keep the collecting bag lower than the bladder at all times; keep the catheter securely anchored to the inner thigh or abdomen; and report any signs of bladder infection such as bladder spasms, fever, or hematuria.

If urinary incontinence is a problem, encourage the patient to practice pelvic floor muscle exercises (Kegel) with urination and throughout the day. Continuous practice during the 4- to 6-week healing process improves the success rate.

PSORIATIC ARTHRITIS

Psoriatic arthritis (PsA) is a progressive, inflammatory disease affecting about 30% of the people with psoriasis. *Psoriasis* is a common, benign, inflammatory skin disorder characterized by the presence of red, irritated, and scaly patches.

- Both PsA and psoriasis appear to have a genetic link with human leukocyte antigens (HLAs) in many patients. Although the exact cause of PsA is unknown, a combination of immune, genetic, and environmental factors is suspected.

PsA can occur in different forms. *Distal arthritis* primarily involves the ends of the fingers and toes, with pitting and color changes in the fingernails and toenails. *Asymmetric arthritis* involves different joints on each side of the body. *Symmetric* PsA resembles rheumatoid arthritis (RA) and affects joints on both sides of the body at the same time. It accounts for about 50% of cases. *Psoriatic spondylitis* is marked by pain and stiffness in the spine and neck. *Arthritis mutilans* is the most severe form of the disease, affecting only 5% of people with PsA but causing complete destruction of small joints.

- On x-ray, cartilage loss and erosion are similar to those seen in RA. Advanced cases of PsA often reveal widened joint spaces.
- A "pencil in cup" deformity is common in the distal interphalangeal (DIP) joints as a result of thin, weakened bone. In this deformity, the narrowed end of the affected metacarpals or phalanges inserts into the expanded end of the other (adjacent) bone sharing the joint.
- Elevated erythrocyte sedimentation rate (ESR), elevated serum uric acid, and mild anemia are seen in some patients. Therefore the diagnosis of gout must be excluded.

Treatment includes splinting, joint protection, and physical therapy. Nonsteroidal antiinflammatory drugs (NSAIDs) given early in the course of the disease may help with inflammation. Drug therapy also includes disease-modifying antirheumatic drugs (DMARDs) such as methotrexate, which is effective for both articular and cutaneous manifestations. Sulfasalazine, cyclosporine, and biologic response modifiers (e.g., etanercept, golimumab, adalimumab, infliximab) may also be used. Apremilast (Otezla), an inhibitor of the enzyme phosphodiesterase-4, may be given to treat adults with active PsA.

PULMONARY EMBOLISM

Description

Pulmonary embolism (PE) is the blockage of pulmonary arteries by a thrombus, fat, or air embolus or tumor tissue. Risk factors for PE include immobility or reduced mobility, surgery within the last 3 months (especially pelvic and lower extremity surgery), history of *deep vein thrombosis* (DVT), cancer, obesity, oral contraceptives, hormone therapy, cigarette smoking, prolonged air travel, heart failure, pregnancy, and clotting disorders.

Approximately 10% of patients with massive PE die within the first hour. Treatment with anticoagulants significantly reduces mortality.

Pathophysiology

Most PEs arise from DVT formed in the deep leg veins. Other sites of origin of PE include femoral or iliac veins, right side of the heart (atrial fibrillation), pelvic veins (especially after surgery or childbirth) or upper extremities.

An *embolus* is a mobile clot that travels with blood flow through ever-smaller blood vessels until it lodges and obstructs the pulmonary circulation. *Venous thromboembolism (VTE)* is the preferred term to describe the spectrum of pathologic conditions from DVT to PE.

Clinical Manifestations

Manifestations of PE are varied and nonspecific, making diagnosis hard.

- Dyspnea occurs in 85% of patients with PE.
- Other signs and symptoms are hypoxemia, tachypnea, cough, chest pain, hemoptysis, crackles, wheezing, fever, accentuation of the pulmonic heart sound, tachycardia, syncope, and sudden change in mental status from hypoxemia.
- Massive emboli may produce abrupt hypotension and shock.
- Small emboli may go undetected or cause vague, transient symptoms. However, in the patient with underlying cardiopulmonary disease, even small emboli may result in severe cardiopulmonary compromise.

Complications

Pulmonary infarction (death of lung tissue) is most likely when there is: (1) occlusion is of a large or medium-sized pulmonary vessel (more than 2 mm in diameter), (2) insufficient collateral blood flow from the bronchial circulation, or (3) preexisting lung disease. Infarction results in alveolar necrosis and hemorrhage with pleural effusion.

Pulmonary hypertension results from hypoxemia or involvement of more than 50% of the area of the normal pulmonary bed. A single embolus rarely causes pulmonary hypertension unless it is massive. Recurrent emboli may result in chronic pulmonary hypertension, leading to dilation and hypertrophy of the right ventricle. Depending on the degree of pulmonary hypertension and how quickly it develops, outcomes can vary. Some patients die within months and others live for decades (see Pulmonary Hypertension, p. 509).

Diagnostic Studies

- Spiral (or helical) CT scan is the most common test for diagnosis of PE. If the patient cannot have the contrast media used in a spiral CT, then a ventilation-perfusion (V/Q) scan is done.
- D-dimer testing assists in screening for an embolism.
- Arterial blood gases (ABGs) may show hypoxemia.

Interprofessional Management

Treatment is started as soon as PE is suspected. The goals are to: (1) provide adequate tissue perfusion and respiratory function, (2) prevent further growth or extension of thrombi in the lower extremities, (3) prevent embolization from the upper or lower extremities to the pulmonary vascular system, and (4) prevent further recurrence of PE. Supportive therapy for the patient's cardiopulmonary status varies according to the severity of the PE.

- O_2 needs are determined by ABG analysis. Mask, cannula, or endotracheal intubation and mechanical ventilation may be used to maintain adequate oxygenation.
- Respiratory measures such as turning, coughing, and deep breathing are important to help prevent or treat atelectasis.
- If shock is present, fluids and vasopressor agents may be necessary to support circulation. If heart failure is present, diuretics are used.

Immediate coagulation is required for patients with PE. Subcutaneous administration of low-molecular-weight heparin (LMWH) (e.g., enoxaparin [Lovenox], or fragmin [Dalteparin] or fondaparinux) is safer and more effective than unfractionated heparin. Warfarin (Coumadin) should be started at the time of diagnosis. Warfarin is usually administered for 3 months, then reevaluated. Alternatives to warfarin include apixaban (Eliquis), dabigitran (Pradaxa), and edoxaban (Savaysa).

- Fibrinolytic agents, such as the tissue plasminogen activator alteplase (Activase), dissolve the PE lesion as well as the clots at thrombus source.

Hemodynamically unstable patients with massive PE and contraindications to fibrinolytic therapy may be candidates for pulmonary embolectomy. This can be done via a diagnostic imaging (vascular catheter) or surgical approach.

Percutaneous catheter embolectomy or endovascular ultrasound delivered thrombolysis are newer, moderately invasive procedures for PE. In patients who are at high risk and patients for whom anticoagulation is contraindicated, an inferior vena cava (IVC) filter may be the treatment of choice.

Nursing Management

Nursing measures aimed at prevention of PE are similar to those for prophylaxis of VTE (see Venous Thrombosis, p. 651). These include the use of intermittent pneumatic compression devices, early ambulation, and anticoagulant medications.

The prognosis for a patient with PE is good if therapy is instituted promptly. Keep the patient in bed in a semi-Fowler's position to facilitate breathing. Maintain an IV line for drugs and fluid therapy. Administer O_2 therapy as ordered. Carefully monitor vital signs, ABGs, cardiac rhythm, pulse oximetry, and lung sounds to assess the patient's clinical status.

- The patient may be anxious because of pain, inability to breathe, and fear of death. Provide explanations, emotional support, and reassurance to help relieve the patient's anxiety.
- Monitor laboratory results to ensure therapeutic ranges of international normalized ratio (INR; for warfarin) and activated partial thromboplastin time (aPTT; for unfractionated IV heparin). Monitor platelet counts for thrombocytopenia and the possible development of heparin-induced thrombocytopenia (HIT). Observe the patient for complications of anticoagulant and fibrinolytic therapy (e.g., bleeding, hematomas, bruising).

▼ **Patient and Caregiver Teaching**
- Long-term management is similar to that for the patient with VTE (see p. 651).
- Patient teaching regarding long-term anticoagulant therapy is critical. Patients with recurrent emboli are treated with anticoagulants indefinitely. INR levels are obtained at intervals, and warfarin dosage is adjusted accordingly.
- Discharge planning is aimed at limiting the progression of the condition and preventing complications and recurrence. Reinforce the need for the patient to return to the health care provider (HCP) for regular follow-up examinations.

PULMONARY HYPERTENSION

Description

Pulmonary hypertension is elevated pulmonary pressure resulting from increased resistance to blood flow through the pulmonary circulation. Pulmonary hypertension can occur as a primary disease (idiopathic pulmonary arterial hypertension) or as a secondary complication of a respiratory, heart, autoimmune, hepatic, or connective tissue disorder (secondary pulmonary arterial hypertension).

Idiopathic pulmonary arterial hypertension (IPAH) is pulmonary hypertension that occurs without an apparent cause. It is associated with connective tissue diseases, cirrhosis, and human immunodeficiency virus (HIV) infection, but the relationship is unclear. If untreated, IPAH can rapidly progress, causing right-sided heart failure (HF) and death within a few years. Although new drug therapy has greatly improved survival, the disease is not curable.

Pathophysiology
The pathophysiology of IPAH is poorly understood. Some type of insult (e.g., hormonal, mechanical) to the pulmonary endothelium may cause a cascade of events leading to vascular scarring, endothelial dysfunction, and smooth muscle proliferation. IPAH affects females more often than males.

Clinical Manifestations
Classic manifestations are dyspnea on exertion and fatigue. Exertional chest pain, dizziness, and syncope are other symptoms. As the disease progresses, dyspnea occurs at rest. Pulmonary hypertension increases the workload of the right ventricle and causes right ventricular hypertrophy (a condition called *cor pulmonale*) (see Cor Pulmonale, p. 150) and eventually HF (see Heart Failure, p. 266).

- Right-sided cardiac catheterization is the definitive test to diagnose pulmonary hypertension. By the time patients become symptomatic, the pulmonary artery pressure is 2 to 3 times normal value.
- Confirmation of IPAH requires a thorough workup to exclude conditions that may cause secondary pulmonary arterial hypertension. Diagnostic evaluation includes electrocardiography (ECG), chest x-ray, pulmonary function testing, echocardiogram, and CT scan.

Nursing and Interprofessional Management
Treatment can relieve symptoms, improve quality of life, and prolong life. Drug therapy consists of agents that promote vasodilation of the pulmonary blood vessels, reduce right ventricular overload, and reverse remodeling. See Table 27.26, Harding et al., *Lewis' Medical-Surgical Nursing*, ed 11.

- Diuretics are used to manage peripheral edema.
- Anticoagulants are beneficial in pulmonary complications related to thrombus formation.
- Use of low-flow O_2 provides symptomatic relief by preventing the potent pulmonary vasoconstriction caused by hypoxia.
  Surgical interventions include pulmonary thromboendarterectomy (PTE), in which clots are removed from the pulmonary arteries.

Atrial septostomy is a palliative procedure that involves creating an intraatrial right-to-left shunt to decompress the right ventricle. It is used for a select group of patients awaiting lung transplantation. Lung transplantation is indicated for patients who do not respond to drug therapy and progress to severe right-sided HF.

Secondary Pulmonary Arterial Hypertension

Secondary pulmonary arterial hypertension (SPAH) occurs when another disease causes anatomic or vascular changes with a chronic increase in pulmonary artery pressures. SPAH can develop because of parenchymal lung disease, left ventricular dysfunction, intracardiac shunts, chronic PE, or systemic connective tissue disease.

Symptoms can reflect the underlying disease, but some are directly attributable to SPAH, including dyspnea, fatigue, lethargy, and chest pain. Diagnosis of SPAH is similar to that of IPAH.

- Treatment of SPAH consists mainly of treating the underlying primary disorder. When irreversible pulmonary vascular damage has occurred, therapies used for IPAH are started.

PYELONEPHRITIS

Description

Pyelonephritis is an inflammation of the renal parenchyma and collecting system (including the renal pelvis). *Urosepsis* is a systemic infection arising from a urologic source. If not treated promptly, it can lead to septic shock and death (see Shock, p. 549).

Pathophysiology

Pyelonephritis usually begins with colonization and infection of the lower urinary tract via the ascending urethral route. Bacteria normally found in the intestinal tract, including *Escherichia coli,* frequently cause pyelonephritis.

A preexisting factor is often present, such as *vesicoureteral reflux* (retrograde or backward movement of urine from lower to upper urinary tract) or dysfunction of lower urinary tract function, such as obstruction from benign prostatic hyperplasia or a urinary stone. Pregnancy-induced physiologic changes in the urinary system are one of the most important risk factors for acute pyelonephritis. For residents of long-term care facilities, catheter-associated urinary tract infections (CAUTIs) are common causes of pyelonephritis and urosepsis.

- *Acute pyelonephritis* often starts in the renal medulla and spreads to the adjacent cortex.

- In *chronic pyelonephritis* the kidneys become inflamed, develop fibrosis (scarring) leading to loss of renal function, and can atrophy (shrink). Chronic pyelonephritis is usually the result of significant anatomic abnormalities, such as vesicoureteral reflux or recurring infections involving the upper urinary tract. However, it may also occur in the absence of an existing infection, recent infection, or history of urinary tract infections (UTIs). It often progresses to end-stage renal disease (ESRD) when both kidneys are involved, even if the underlying infection or problem is successfully eradicated (see Kidney Disease, Chronic, p. 358).

Clinical Manifestations

The classic manifestations of acute pyelonephritis include: fever/chills, nausea/vomiting, malaise, and flank pain. They may include lower urinary tract symptoms such as dysuria, urgency, and frequency. Costovertebral angle (CVA) tenderness to percussion is typically present on the affected side.

Diagnostic Studies

- Urinalysis may show pyuria, bacteriuria, hematuria, and white blood cell (WBC) casts.
- Complete blood count (CBC) count with WBC differential identifies leukocytosis.
- Urine and blood cultures with sensitivities may be obtained.
- Ultrasound is used to identify anatomic abnormalities, hydronephrosis, renal abscesses, or stones.

Chronic pyelonephritis is diagnosed by radiologic imaging and biopsy rather than clinical features. Biopsy results indicate the loss of functioning nephrons, infiltration of the parenchyma with inflammatory cells, and fibrosis.

Nursing and Interprofessional Management

The patient with pyelonephritis will have normal renal function, normal body temperature, no complications, relief of pain, and no recurrence of symptoms.

Patients with severe infections or complicating factors, such as nausea and vomiting with dehydration, require hospital admission. Parenteral antibiotics are often given initially in the hospital to rapidly establish high serum and urinary drug levels.

The patient with mild symptoms may be treated as an outpatient with antibiotics for 7 to 14 days. Symptoms and signs typically improve or resolve within 48 to 72 hours after starting therapy. Relapses may be treated with a 6-week course of antibiotics. Antibiotic prophylaxis may also be used for recurrent infections.

- Teach the patient about the disease process with emphasis on continuing medications as prescribed, having a follow-up urine culture, and recognizing manifestations of recurrence or relapse. Stress the need for regular medical care.
- Encourage the patient to drink at least 8 glasses of fluid every day, even after the infection has been treated.

RAYNAUD'S PHENOMENON

Description

Raynaud's phenomenon is an episodic vasospastic disorder of the small cutaneous arteries, most often involving the fingers and toes. It occurs more often in women 15 to 40 years of age. Abnormalities in the vascular, intravascular, and neuronal mechanisms cause an imbalance between vasodilation and vasoconstriction.

Primary Raynaud's phenomenon occurs in isolation while secondary Raynaud's phenomenon occurs with an underlying disease (e.g., thyroid conditions, rheumatoid arthritis, scleroderma, systemic lupus erythematosus). Other contributing factors include use of vibrating machinery, work in cold environments or exposure to heavy metals (e.g., lead) and high homocysteine levels.

Clinical Manifestations

Exposure to cold, emotional upsets, tobacco use, and caffeine often trigger symptoms.

- The disorder is characterized by vasospasm-induced color changes (white, red, and blue) of fingers, toes, ears, and nose. Decreased perfusion results in pallor (white). The digits then become cyanotic (bluish purple). These changes are subsequently followed by rubor (red), caused by the hyperemic response when blood flow is restored.
- The patient usually describes cold and numbness in the vasoconstrictive phase, with throbbing and aching pain, tingling, and swelling in the hyperemic phase. An episode usually lasts only minutes but may persist for several hours.
- After frequent, prolonged attacks, the skin may become thickened and the nails brittle. Complications include punctate lesions (small holes) of the fingertips and superficial gangrenous ulcers in advanced stages.
- Diagnosis is based on persistent symptoms for at least 2 years.

Nursing and Interprofessional Management

Sustained-release calcium-channel blockers (e.g., nifedipine [Procardia]) are the first-line drug therapy. Calcium-channel blockers

R

relax smooth muscles of the arterioles by blocking the influx of calcium into the cells. This reduces the frequency and severity of vasospastic attacks.

- If calcium-channel blockers are not sufficient, other vasodilators (e.g., phosphodiesterase-5 inhibitors [sildenafil] or topical nitroglycerin 2% ointment may be used.

Prompt intervention is needed for patients with digital ulceration or critical ischemia. Treatment options include prostacyclin infusion therapy (e.g., iloprost), antibiotics, analgesics, and surgical debridement of necrotic tissue. Botulinum toxin A and statins may lessen the severity of Raynaud's phenomenon. Sympathectomy is considered in advanced cases.

▼ Patient and Caregiver Teaching

Teaching should be directed toward preventing recurrent episodes.

- Loose, warm clothing should be worn for protection from cold, including gloves for working in a refrigerator or freezer or handling cold objects.
- Temperature extremes should be avoided. Immersing hands in warm water often decreases the spasm.
- Patients should stop using all tobacco products and avoid caffeine and other drugs with vasoconstrictive effects (e.g., pseudoephedrine).
- Provide patients with information about stress management techniques.

REACTIVE ARTHRITIS

Reactive arthritis (Reiter's syndrome) is associated with a symptom complex that includes urethritis (in men) or cervicitis (in women), conjunctivitis, and mucocutaneous lesions. It occurs more often in young men than in young women.

- Although the exact cause is unknown, reactive arthritis appears to be a reaction triggered in the body after exposure to specific genitourinary or gastrointestinal (GI) tract infections. *Chlamydia trachomatis* is spread through sexual contact.
- Reactive arthritis is also associated with GI infections with *Shigella, Salmonella, Campylobacter,* or *Yersinia* species and other microorganisms.

Persons with inherited human leukocyte antigen (HLA)-B27 are at increased risk for developing reactive arthritis after sexual contact or exposure to certain enteric pathogens, supporting the suggestion of a genetic predisposition.

- Urethritis develops within 1 to 2 weeks after sexual contact or GI infection. Low-grade fever, conjunctivitis, and arthritis may occur over the next several weeks.
- This arthritis tends to be asymmetric, frequently involving the toes and the large joints of the lower extremities. Lower back pain may occur with severe disease.
- Mucocutaneous lesions commonly occur as small, painless, superficial ulcerations on the tongue, oral mucosa, and glans penis. Soft tissue manifestations include Achilles tendinitis or plantar fasciitis.
- The erythrocyte sedimentation rate (ESR) may be elevated.

Most patients recover within a few months of initial symptoms. Reactive arthritis is often associated with *C. trachomatis* infection, so treatment of patients and their sexual partners with doxycycline is widely recommended. Antibiotics have no effect on arthritis or other symptoms. Drug therapy may also include nonsteroidal antiinflammatory drugs (NSAIDs) and disease-modifying antirheumatic drugs (DMARDs). Physical therapy may be helpful during recovery.

REFRACTIVE ERRORS

Refractive errors are the most common visual problem. Irregularities in corneal curvature, lens-focusing power, or eye length prevent light rays from converging to a point on the retina. Types of refractive errors include:

- *Myopia* (nearsightedness), the most common refractive error, is an inability to accommodate for objects at a distance. It causes light rays to be focused in front of the retina. The person can see near objects but objects in the distance are blurred.
- *Hyperopia* (farsightedness) is an inability to accommodate for near objects. It causes the light rays to focus behind the retina. The person with hyperopia can see distant objects clearly.
- *Presbyopia* is an age-related loss of accommodation with an inability to focus on near objects. The lens becomes larger, firmer, and less elastic. The condition generally becomes noticeable in the early to mid-40s.
- *Astigmatism* is an uneven or irregular curvature of the cornea. Incoming light rays are bent unequally, causing visual distortion. Astigmatism can occur with any of the other refractive errors.

The major symptom of refractive errors is blurred vision. Additional complaints may include ocular discomfort, eye strain, or headaches. Vision correction may include eyeglasses, contact lenses, refractive surgery, or surgical implantation of an artificial lens.

R

RESPIRATORY FAILURE, ACUTE

Description

Acute respiratory failure (ARF) occurs when oxygenation, ventilation, or both are inadequate. Either not enough O_2 is transferred to the blood or inadequate CO_2 is removed from the lungs. ARF is not a disease. ARF occurs because of problems involving the lungs or other body systems (Table 71).

Problems that interfere with O_2 transfer result in *hypoxemia*. This is a decrease in arterial O_2 (PaO_2) and saturation (SaO_2) to less than the normal values. Insufficient CO_2 removal results in hypercapnia. This is an increase in arterial CO_2 ($PaCO_2$). Arterial blood gases (ABGs) are used to assess changes in pH, PaO_2, $PaCO_2$, bicarbonate, and SaO_2. We use pulse oximetry to assess arterial O_2 saturation (SpO_2).

ARF is classified as hypoxemic or hypercapnic.

- *Hypoxemic respiratory failure* is defined as a $PaO_2 < 60$ mm Hg when the patient is receiving an inspired O_2 concentration of 60% or more. In hypoxemic respiratory failure (also called *oxygenation failure*), the main problem is inadequate exchange of O_2 between the alveoli and pulmonary capillaries. The PaO_2 level shows low O_2 saturation in the patient receiving supplemental O_2.

- *Hypercapnic respiratory failure* (or *ventilatory failure*) is defined as a $PaCO_2 > 50$ mm Hg with acidemia (arterial pH < 7.35). The main problem is insufficient CO_2 removal. This causes the $PaCO_2$ to be higher than normal and acidemia occurs.

Major changes in PaO_2 and $PaCO_2$ occur with ARF. These may develop over minutes to hours. The patient may have hemodynamic instability (e.g., tachycardia, hypotension), increased respiratory effort, and decreased level of consciousness. Urgent intervention is required. *Chronic respiratory failure* develops more slowly, over several days to weeks. The patient is usually more stable as the body had time to compensate for the small, but subtle, changes that have occurred.

- Patients may have acute and chronic respiratory failure at the same time. This happens when a patient with a chronic respiratory problem develops a new acute problem. For example, a patient with chronic obstructive pulmonary disease (COPD) who has pneumonia could have "acute-on-chronic" respiratory failure.

Pathophysiology

Hypoxemic Respiratory Failure

Four physiologic mechanisms may cause respiratory failure: (1) mismatch between ventilation (V) and perfusion (Q), commonly

TABLE 71 Common Causes of Respiratory Failure

Hypoxemic Respiratory Failure	Hypercapnic Respiratory Failure
Respiratory System • Acute respiratory distress syndrome (ARDS) • Hepatopulmonary syndrome (e.g., low-resistance flow state, V/Q mismatch) • Massive pulmonary embolism (e.g., thrombus emboli, fat emboli) • Pneumonia • Pulmonary artery laceration and hemorrhage • Toxic inhalation (e.g., smoke inhalation) **Cardiac System** • Anatomic shunt (e.g., ventricular septal defect) • Cardiogenic pulmonary edema • Cardiogenic shock (decreasing blood flow through pulmonary vasculature) • High cardiac output states: diffusion limitation	**Respiratory System** • Asthma • Chronic obstructive pulmonary disease (COPD) • Cystic fibrosis **Central Nervous System** • Brainstem injury or infarction • Sedative and opioid overdose • Spinal cord injury • Severe head injury **Chest Wall** • Kyphoscoliosis • Pain • Severe obesity • Thoracic trauma (e.g., flail chest) **Neuromuscular System** • Amyotrophic lateral sclerosis • Critical illness polyneuropathy • Guillain-Barré syndrome • Muscular dystrophy • Multiple sclerosis • Myasthenia gravis • Phrenic nerve injury • Poliomyelitis • Toxin exposure or ingestion (e.g., botulinum, chemical nerve agents, tree tobacco, carbamate or organophosphate poisoning)

R

referred to as V/Q mismatch; (2) shunt; (3) diffusion limitation; and (4) hypoventilation. The most common causes are V/Q mismatch and shunt.

■ Many diseases and conditions cause *V/Q mismatch*. The most common ones involve increased secretions in the airways (e.g., COPD) or alveoli (e.g., pneumonia) or bronchospasms (e.g., asthma). V/Q mismatch may result from pain, alveolar collapse (atelectasis), or pulmonary emboli.

- *Shunt* occurs when blood exits the heart without having taken part in gas exchange. A shunt is an extreme V/Q mismatch. There are 2 types of shunt: anatomic and intrapulmonary. O_2 therapy alone is not effective in increasing the PaO_2 if hypoxemia is caused by shunt.

- *Diffusion limitation* occurs when gas exchange across the alveolar-capillary membrane is compromised by a process that damages or destroys the alveolar membrane or affects blood flow through the pulmonary capillaries. Conditions that cause the alveolar-capillary membrane to become thicker (fibrotic) slow gas transport. These include pulmonary fibrosis, interstitial lung disease, and acute respiratory distress syndrome (ARDS). An accumulation of fluid, white blood cells, or protein in the alveoli can decrease gas exchange between the alveolus and the capillary bed. A common example is pulmonary edema. The classic sign of diffusion limitation is hypoxemia that occurs with exercise.

- *Alveolar hypoventilation* is a decrease in ventilation that results in an increase in the $PaCO_2$. Alveolar hypoventilation may be caused by central nervous system (CNS) conditions, chest wall dysfunction, acute asthma, or restrictive lung diseases. Although alveolar hypoventilation is mainly a mechanism of hypercapnic respiratory failure, it contributes to hypoxemia.

Frequently, hypoxemic respiratory failure is caused by a combination of V/Q mismatch, shunt, diffusion limitation, and alveolar hypoventilation.

Hypercapnic Respiratory Failure

In acute hypercapnic respiratory failure (sometimes called *ventilatory failure*), the respiratory system cannot keep the CO_2 level within normal limits. This often occurs from increased CO_2 production or a decrease in alveolar ventilation. Hypercapnic respiratory failure can be acute or chronic. It often reflects significant problems with the respiratory system.

- Many conditions can cause impaired ventilation (see Table 71). They can be grouped into 4 categories: (1) CNS problems, (2) neuromuscular problems, (3) chest wall problems, and (4) conditions affecting the airways and/or alveoli.

Clinical Manifestations

Signs of respiratory failure are related to the extent of change in PaO_2 or $PaCO_2$, the speed of change (acute or chronic), and the patient's ability to compensate. A lack of O_2 affects all body systems.

One of the first signs of acute hypoxemic respiratory failure is a change in mental status because the brain is extremely sensitive to inadequate O_2 and acid-base balance. There may be restlessness, confusion, and agitation. Permanent brain damage can result if hypoxia is severe and prolonged. On the other hand, a morning headache and slow respiratory rate with decreased level of consciousness may indicate problems with CO_2 removal.

- Tachycardia, tachypnea, slight diaphoresis, and mild hypertension are early signs of ARF. These changes indicate attempts by the heart and lungs to compensate for decreased O_2 and rising CO_2 levels.
- Cyanosis is an unreliable indicator of hypoxemia. It is a late sign in ARF. It often does not occur until hypoxemia is severe (PaO_2 45 mm Hg or less).

Observing the patient's position helps assess the *work of breathing* (WOB), the effort needed by the respiratory muscles to move air into the lungs. In moderate distress, patients may be able to lie down but prefer to sit. With severe distress, they may be unable to breathe unless sitting upright.

- The tripod position helps decrease the WOB in patients with moderate to severe COPD and ARF. The patient sits with the arms propped on the overbed table or on the knees. Propping the arms increases the anteroposterior diameter of the chest and changes pressure in the thorax.

The patient in ARF may have a rapid, shallow breathing pattern (hypoxemia) or a slower respiratory rate (hypercapnia). Increased respiratory rates require a substantial amount of work and can lead to respiratory muscle fatigue. A change from a rapid rate to a slower rate in a patient in respiratory distress, such as that seen with acute asthma, suggests severe respiratory muscle fatigue and increased chance of respiratory arrest.

- The patient's ability to speak is related to the severity of dyspnea. The dyspneic patient may be able to speak only a few words at a time between breaths.
- Dyspneic patients may be using pursed-lip breathing. This technique increases PaO_2 by slowing respirations, increasing time for expiration, and preventing small bronchioles from collapsing.
- You may see *retraction* (inward movement) of the intercostal spaces or supraclavicular area and use of the accessory muscles (e.g., sternocleidomastoid) which often signifies a moderate degree of respiratory distress.
- *Paradoxical breathing* occurs with severe respiratory distress. With paradoxical breathing, the abdomen and chest move in the opposite manner—outward during exhalation and inward during inspiration.

R

Fine crackles may occur with pulmonary edema. Coarse crackles heard on expiration indicate fluid in the airways. This may be a sign of pneumonia or heart failure (HF). Absent or decreased breath sounds occur with atelectasis, pleural effusion, or hypoventilation. Bronchial breath sounds over the lung periphery occur with lung consolidation from pneumonia. You may hear a pleural friction rub if pneumonia involves the pleura.

Diagnostic Studies

- ABGs determine the levels of $PaCO_2$, PaO_2, bicarbonate, and pH.
- Chest x-ray helps identify possible causes of respiratory failure.
- A catheter may be inserted into a peripheral artery for monitoring BP and obtaining ABGs.
- Pulse oximetry monitors oxygenation status but reveals little about lung ventilation.
- Other studies may include complete blood count (CBC), serum electrolytes, urinalysis, and electrocardiography (ECG).
- Sputum and blood cultures determine sources of possible infection.
- If pulmonary embolus is suspected, a V/Q lung scan or CT scan may be done.

In severe respiratory failure, end-tidal CO_2 ($ETCO_2$) may be used to help confirm correct endotracheal tube placement immediately after intubation and to assess trends in lung ventilation.

Nursing and Interprofessional Management

Prevention of atelectasis, pneumonia, and complications of immobility, as well as optimizing hydration and nutrition, can potentially decrease the risk of respiratory failure in acutely ill patients. Consider age-related and acuity-related changes in physiology when assessing risk of acute respiratory failure.

Because many different problems cause ARF, initial management and specific care varies. Factors taken into consideration include patient age, severity of onset of respiratory failure, comorbidities, and most likely cause of the respiratory failure. We then tailor management strategies to what best meets the patient's unique needs. This section discusses general assessment and interventions most commonly used for patients with ARF. In acute care settings, collaboration between nursing and the interprofessional team (e.g., physicians, respiratory therapists, pharmacists), is essential. In severe ARF, the patient will be cared for in an intensive care unit (ICU).

- Additional information on care for the patient with acute respiratory failure is presented in eNursing Care Plan 67-1 (available on the website).

Respiratory Therapy

The goals of respiratory care include maintaining adequate oxygenation and ventilation and correcting acid-base imbalance. Interventions include O_2 therapy, mobilization of secretions, and positive pressure ventilation (PPV).

Oxygen Therapy. The primary goal of O_2 therapy is to correct hypoxemia (see Oxygen Therapy, p. 697). Always administer O_2 at the lowest possible FiO_2 (O_2 concentration) needed to keep SpO_2 and PaO_2 within patient-specific goals. Never withhold O_2 from a patient. It is essential to observe the patient's response to O_2 therapy. Closely monitor patients for changes in mental status, respiratory rate, and ABGs until their PaO_2 level has reached their baseline normal value. Ideally, the selected O_2 delivery device must maintain PaO_2 at 60 mm Hg or higher and SaO_2 at 90% or higher.

- Hypoxemia secondary to an intrapulmonary shunt is usually not responsive to high O_2 concentrations, and the patient usually requires PPV (see Mechanical Ventilation, p. 691).
- Chronic hypercapnia blunts the response of chemoreceptors to high CO_2 levels as a respiratory stimulant. Initial O_2 therapy may be provided to patients with chronic hypercapnia through a low-flow device, such as a nasal cannula at 1 to 2 L/minute or a Venturi mask at 24% to 28%. The patient with COPD who does not respond to O_2 therapy or other interventions may need mechanically ventilation with higher FiO_2.

Mobilization of Secretions. Retained pulmonary secretions may cause or worsen ARF. This occurs because the movement of O_2 into the alveoli and removal of CO_2 is severely limited or blocked. Secretions can be mobilized by proper positioning, effective coughing, chest physiotherapy, suctioning, humidification, hydration, and when possible, early ambulation.

Effective Coughing and Positioning. When secretions are present, encourage the patient to cough. Unfortunately, not all patients will have enough strength or force to produce a cough that will clear the airway of secretions.

- Augmented coughing (quad coughing) may help some patients. To aid with augmented coughing, place 1 or both hands at the anterolateral base of the patient's lungs. As you observe deep inspiration end and expiration begin, move your hands forcefully upward. This increases abdominal pressure and helps the patient cough. It increases expiratory flow and promotes secretion clearance.
- Position the patient upright. Either elevate the head of the bed at least 30 degrees or use a reclining chair or chair bed. This helps maximize respiratory expansion, decrease dyspnea, and mobilize secretions. Lateral or side-lying positioning may be used in

patients with disease involving only 1 lung, such as right-sided pneumonia. This position, termed *good lung down,* allows for improved V/Q matching in the affected lung.

Hydration and Humidification. Thick and viscous secretions are difficult to expel. Adequate fluid intake (2 to 3 L/day) keeps secretions thin and easier to remove. If the patient is unable to take sufficient fluids orally, IV hydration is used.

- Assess for signs of fluid overload by clinical evaluation (e.g., crackles, dyspnea) and invasive monitoring (e.g., increased central venous pressure) at regular intervals.
- Humidification helps with secretion management. We can thin secretions with aerosols of sterile normal saline or mucolytic drugs (e.g., acetylcysteine mixed with a bronchodilator) given by nebulizer.

Airway Suctioning. Suctioning may be needed if the patient cannot expectorate secretions. Suctioning through an artificial airway (e.g., endotracheal tube, tracheostomy) is only done as needed. (See Artificial Airways, p. 663). Perform suctioning beyond the posterior oropharynx with caution, while monitoring the patient for complications. These include hypoxia, increased intracranial pressure (ICP), dysrhythmias, hypotension (from sudden increase in intrathoracic pressure), hypertension and tachycardia (from noxious stimulation), and bradycardia (possible vasovagal response).

Positive Pressure Ventilation. If intensive measures fail to improve ventilation and oxygenation, and the patient continues to show signs of acute respiratory failure, ventilatory assistance may be initiated (see Mechanical Ventilation, p. 691). PPV may be provided invasively using orotracheal or nasotracheal intubation or noninvasively by a nasal or face mask.

Drug Therapy

Drug therapy depends on several factors. These include the cause of ARF, the patient's preexisting medical condition, and whether infection is present. Goals of drug therapy include: (1) reduce airway inflammation and bronchospasm; (2) relieve pulmonary congestion; (3) treat infection; and (4) reduce anxiety, pain, and restlessness.

Reduce Airway Inflammation and Bronchospasm. Corticosteroids (e.g., IV methylprednisolone) are often used in combination with other drugs, such as bronchodilators, to relieve inflammation and bronchospasm. It may take several hours to see their effects. Inhaled corticosteroids require 4 to 5 days for optimum therapeutic effects. So, they will not provide immediate relieve for ARF.

Relief of bronchospasm increases alveolar ventilation. In acute bronchospasm, short-acting bronchodilators (e.g., albuterol), may be given at 15- to 30-minute intervals until a response occurs. Give these drugs using a hand-held nebulizer or a metered-dose inhaler with a spacer. Side effects include tachycardia and hypertension. Prolonged use can increase the risk of dysrhythmias and cardiac ischemia. It is important to monitor the patient's vital signs and ECG for any changes.

Relieve Pulmonary Congestion. Interstitial fluid can accumulate in the lungs because of injury to the alveolar capillary membrane, HF, or fluid overload. Use of IV diuretics (e.g., furosemide [Lasix]), morphine, or nitroglycerin can decrease pulmonary congestion caused by HF. Use extreme caution when giving these drugs. Changes in heart rate and rhythm and significant decreases in BP are common.

Treat Infections. Lung infections (e.g., pneumonia, acute bronchitis) can result in excessive mucus production, fever, increased O_2 consumption, and inflamed, fluid-filled, and/or collapsed alveoli. Alveoli that are fluid filled or collapsed cannot take part in gas exchange. Infections can either cause or worsen ARF. IV antibiotics are often given to treat infection.

Reduce Anxiety, Pain, and Restlessness. Anxiety, pain, and restlessness may result from hypoxia. They increase O_2 consumption and CO_2 production (from an increased metabolic rate) and increase WOB. For the nonintubated patient, this may cause tachypnea and ineffective ventilation. For the intubated patient, this may cause ventilator dyssynchrony and increase the risk of unplanned extubation. Sedation and analgesia are used to decrease anxiety, agitation, and pain. Follow an evidence-based and goal-directed protocol using only the dosing needed to meet patient-specific goals.

Nutritional Therapy

Maintaining protein and energy stores is important in patients with ARF. The hypermetabolic state increases the caloric requirements needed to maintain body weight and muscle mass. Nutritional depletion causes a loss of muscle mass, including the respiratory muscles, which may delay recovery. Nutritional support should start early and focus on a diet that addresses the person's caloric, protein and nutrient requirements needs. Ideally, enteral nutrition (EN) should be started within 24 to 48 hours.

RESTLESS LEGS SYNDROME

Description and Pathophysiology

Restless legs syndrome (RLS), also known as *Willis-Ekbom disease* (WED), is a relatively common sleep and movement disorder with unpleasant sensory (paresthesia) and motor abnormalities of 1 or both legs. About 8% of the U.S. population has RLS. A small number have severe symptoms that affect their quality of life and require medication for treatment. RLS is more common in older adults. It is also more common in women than men.

There are 2 distinct types of RLS: primary (idiopathic) and secondary. Most people have primary RLS. Secondary RLS can occur with metabolic problems associated with iron deficiency, renal disease and hemodialysis, and neuropathy. Sleep deprivation, sleep apnea, pregnancy (especially third trimester) and use of certain medications (e.g., antiemetics, antidepressants that increase serotonin), can cause or worsen symptoms.

RLS is believed to be related to a dysfunction in the brain's basal ganglia circuits that use the neurotransmitter dopamine, which controls movements. In RLS, this dysfunction causes the urge to move the legs.

Clinical Manifestations

The severity of RLS sensory symptoms ranges from infrequent minor discomfort (numbness, tingling, "pins and needles" sensation) to severe pain. Sensory symptoms often appear first.

- Some persons compare the sensations to bugs crawling on the skin.
- The leg pain is localized within the calf muscles. Some patients have pain in the upper extremities and trunk.
- Pain at night can disrupt sleep. Physical activity, such as walking, stretching, rocking, or kicking, often relieves the pain.

Diagnostic Studies

- RLS is a clinical diagnosis based on the patient's history or the report of the bed partner related to nighttime activities. Diagnostic criteria include: (1) urge to move the legs, often accompanied by uncomfortable or unpleasant sensations in the legs; (2) urge to move the legs worsens during rest or inactivity; (3)) urge to move the legs is partially or totally relieved by movement, as long as the activity continues; (4) urge to move the legs becomes worse in the evening or night; and (5) these features are not caused by another medical or behavioral condition. Polysomnography studies during sleep distinguish RLS from other clinical conditions (e.g., sleep apnea) that disturb sleep.
- Blood tests, such as a complete blood count, serum ferritin, and renal function tests (e.g., serum creatinine), may help exclude secondary causes of RLS. A patient with diabetes may have paresthesia caused by peripheral neuropathy related to diabetes or RLS.

Nursing and Interprofessional Management

The goal of interprofessional management is to reduce discomfort and distress and improve sleep quality. When RLS is secondary to renal failure or iron deficiency, treatment of these conditions will decrease symptoms.

- Lifestyle changes may help persons with mild-to-moderate RLS. For example, decreasing the use of alcohol or tobacco, maintaining regular sleep habits, exercising, and massaging and stretching the legs may be helpful. The patient should avoid antihistamine containing medications (e.g., diphenhydramine).
- A vibratory counterstimulation device can compete with and diminish RLS sensations.

If nondrug measures fail to provide symptom relief, drug therapy is an option. The main drugs used to treat RLS aim to increase the amount of dopamine in the brain. They include dopamine precursors (e.g., carbidopa/levodopa) and dopamine agonists (e.g., ropinirole [Requip], pramipexole [Mirapex], rotigotine [Neupro]). The antiseizure drug gabapentin enacarbil (Horizant) may decrease the sensory sensations and nerve pain. The patient with iron deficiency anemia may need to start iron supplementation. Other drugs that may be used include antiseizure drugs and benzodiazepines. Clonidine (Catapres) and propranolol (Inderal) are effective in some patients. Low doses of opioids (e.g., oxycodone) are usually reserved for those patients with severe symptoms who fail to respond to other drug therapies.

RETINAL DETACHMENT

Description

Retinal detachment is a separation of the sensory retina and underlying pigment epithelium with fluid accumulation between the 2 layers. Almost all patients with an untreated, symptomatic retinal detachment become blind in the involved eye. Risk factors include increasing age, severe myopia, cataract surgery, eye trauma, and family or personal history of retinal detachment.

R

Pathophysiology

The most common cause is a retinal break, a full-thickness interruption in the retinal tissue. Retinal holes are spontaneous atrophic breaks. Retinal tears occur when the vitreous shrinks with aging and pulls on the retina.

Once there is a retinal break, liquid vitreous may leak between the layers, causing detachment.

Clinical Manifestations

Symptoms of a detaching retina include photopsia ("light flashes"), floaters, and a "cobweb" or ring in the vision field. Once the retina is detached, a painless loss of peripheral or central vision occurs "like a curtain" across the field of vision.

Diagnostic Studies

- Direct and indirect ophthalmoscopy or slit lamp microscopy
- Ultrasound to help identify a detachment

Interprofessional Management

For those retinal breaks less likely to progress to detachment, the ophthalmologist monitors the patient and instructs the patient to seek immediate evaluation for any signs or symptoms of impending detachment. The ophthalmologist usually refers the patient with a detachment to a retinal specialist.

Treatment objectives are to reattach the retina and seal any retinal breaks. Surgical treatment to seal breaks may include laser photocoagulation and cryopexy. Inward retinal traction can involve a scleral buckling procedure, pneumatic retinopexy, and vitrectomy.

- Visual prognosis depends on the extent, length, and area of detachment.

Nursing Management

In most cases, retinal detachment is an urgent situation requiring an unexpected surgery. Provide the patient with emotional support, especially during the immediate preoperative period.

- Give prescribed drugs for postoperative pain, and teach the patient to take these drugs as necessary when discharged.
- Begin discharge planning as early as possible because the patient may not be hospitalized for long.

▼ Patient and Caregiver Teaching

- Teach the patient with an increased risk of retinal detachment about the signs and symptoms of detachment and to seek immediate evaluation if any of these occur.
- Promote the use of protective eyewear to help avoid traumatic retinal detachment.
- Review the signs and symptoms of retinal detachment with the patient because the risk of detachment in the other eye is increased.

Patient and caregiver teaching after eye surgery is discussed in Table 22, p. 114.

RHEUMATIC FEVER AND HEART DISEASE

Description

Rheumatic fever (RF) is an acute inflammatory disease which can involve all the heart layers. RF occurs most frequently between the ages of 5 and 15 years. *Rheumatic heart disease* is a chronic scarring and deformity of the heart valves resulting from RF.

Pathophysiology

RF occurs as a complication 2 to 3 weeks after a group A streptococcal pharyngitis. Signs of RF appear to be from an abnormal immune response to bacterial antigens. RF affects the heart, skin, joints, and central nervous system (CNS).

Rheumatic heart disease, caused by RF, primarily affects young adults. RF has declined in developed countries because of the effective use of antibiotics to treat streptococcal infections.

About 50% of RF episodes are *rheumatic pancarditis*, involving all layers of the heart (endocardium, myocardium, pericardium).

- Rheumatic endocarditis is found mainly in the valves, with swelling and erosion of the valve leaflets. Vegetations form and initially create a fibrous thickening of the valve leaflets, fusion of commissures and chordae tendineae, and fibrosis of the papillary muscle. Stenosis and regurgitation may occur in valve leaflets. The mitral and aortic valves are most commonly affected.
- Nodules, called Aschoff's bodies, are formed by a reaction to inflammation, with swelling and fragmentation of collagen fibers. As the Aschoff's bodies age, they become more fibrous, and scar tissue forms in the myocardium.
- Rheumatic pericarditis affects both layers of the pericardium, which becomes thickened and covered with a fibrinous exudate.
- Systemic lesions of RF involve the skin, joints, and CNS. Painless subcutaneous nodules, arthralgias or arthritis, and chorea may develop.

Clinical Manifestations

The presence of 2 major criteria, or 1 major and 2 minor criteria, plus evidence of a preceding group A streptococcal infection indicates a high probability of acute RF.

Major Criteria

- *Carditis* is the most important manifestation of RF. It results in 3 signs: (1) an organic heart murmur or murmurs of mitral or aortic regurgitation, or mitral stenosis; (2) heart enlargement and heart failure (HF) occurring from myocarditis; and (3) pericarditis resulting in distant heart sounds, chest pain, a pericardial friction rub, or signs of effusion.

- *Monoarthritis or polyarthritis* is the most common finding in RF, occurring in up to 75% of patients. The larger joints (particularly the knees, ankles, elbows, and wrists) are most severely affected by swelling, warmth, redness, tenderness, and limitation of motion.
- *Sydenham's chorea* is the major CNS manifestation. It is characterized by involuntary movements (especially of the face and limbs), muscle weakness, and speech and gait problems.
- *Erythema marginatum* lesions are a less common feature. The bright pink, nonpruritic, maplike macular lesions occur mainly on the trunk and proximal extremities. The lesions intensify with heat (e.g., warm bath).
- *Subcutaneous nodules* are small, hard, painless swellings found over extensor surfaces of the joints, especially the knees, wrists, and elbows.

Minor Criteria

Minor clinical manifestations include fever, polyarthralgia, and certain laboratory tests (e.g., elevated C-reactive protein [CRP], elevated white blood cell [WBC] count).

Evidence of Infection

In addition to the major and minor criteria, there must also be evidence of a preceding group A streptococcal infection. Such evidence includes a positive result on a rapid antigen test for group A streptococci, an elevated antistreptolysin-O titer, or a positive throat culture.

Diagnostic Studies

- Chest x-ray may show an enlarged heart if HF is present.
- Echocardiogram may show valvular insufficiency and pericardial fluid or thickening.
- Electrocardiography (ECG) reveals a prolonged PR interval with delayed atrioventricular (AV) conduction.

Interprofessional Management

Treatment consists of drug therapy and supportive measures. Antibiotic therapy does not change the course of the acute disease or the development of carditis. It eliminates residual group A streptococci in the tonsils and pharynx and prevents the spread of organisms to close contacts. Salicylates, nonsteroidal antiinflammatory drugs (NSAIDs), and corticosteroids are the antiinflammatory agents most widely used to control the fever and joint manifestations.

Nursing Management

Goals

The goals for a patient with RF and rheumatic heart disease include: (1) normal or baseline heart function, (2) resumption of daily activities without joint pain, and (3) ability to manage the long-term antibiotic therapy.

Nursing Interventions

RF can be prevented by early detection and immediate treatment of group A streptococcal pharyngitis. Your role is to teach people in the community to seek medical attention for symptoms of streptococcal pharyngitis, and to emphasize the need for prompt and adequate treatment.

Administer antibiotics as ordered and teach the patient that oral antibiotics require adherence to the full course of therapy. Promote optimal rest to reduce cardiac workload and the body's metabolic needs. Position painful joints for proper alignment and apply heat for comfort. Give salicylates, NSAIDs, and corticosteroids as prescribed for joint pain.

- After acute symptoms have subsided, the patient without carditis can ambulate. If the patient has carditis with HF, strict bed rest restrictions apply.

▼ Patient and Caregiver Teaching

- Teach the patient that completing the full course of antibiotics is vital to successful treatment.
- Teach the patient with a history of previous RF about the disease process, possible sequelae, and the need for continuous prophylactic antibiotics.
- Patient and caregiver teaching should include good nutrition, hygiene practices, and adequate rest.
- Caution the patient about the possibility of developing valvular heart disease. Teach the patient to seek medical attention if excessive fatigue, dizziness, palpitations, or exertional dyspnea develops.

R

RHEUMATOID ARTHRITIS

Description

Rheumatoid arthritis (RA) is a chronic, systemic autoimmune disease characterized by inflammation of connective tissue in the diarthrodial (synovial) joints. RA is typically marked by periods of remission and exacerbation and frequently accompanied by extraarticular manifestations.

RA occurs globally, affecting all ethnic groups. However, incidence increases with age, peaking between the ages of 30 and 50 years. An estimated 1.5 million adult Americans are affected by RA. Almost 3 times as many women have the disease as men.

Pathophysiology

The exact cause of rheumatoid arthritis is unknown. However, it likely results from a combination of genetic and environmental triggers. An autoimmune theory suggests that changes associated with RA begin when a genetically susceptible person has an initial immune response to an antigen. The antigen, which is probably not the same in all patients, triggers formation of an abnormal immunoglobulin G (IgG). RA is marked by the presence of autoantibodies against this abnormal IgG. The autoantibodies, known as *rheumatoid factor* (RF), combine with IgG to form immune complexes that deposit on synovial membranes or superficial articular cartilage in the joints.

- Immune complex formation leads to complement activation and an inflammatory response. Neutrophils attracted to the site of inflammation release proteolytic enzymes that damage articular cartilage and cause the synovial lining to thicken.
- Other inflammatory cells include T helper (CD4$^+$) cells and proinflammatory cytokines, such as interleukin-1 (IL-1), interleukin-6 (IL-6), and tumor necrosis factor (TNF).
- Genetic predisposition is important in the development of RA.

RA has long been considered one of the most disabling forms of arthritis. Symptoms and outcomes can vary greatly. Without adequate treatment, patients may need mobility aids or joint reconstruction. They may also experience loss of independence and self-care ability. See Table 72 for the stages of disease progression. However, treatment advances have improved the prognosis for patients with newly diagnosed RA. The progression of joint damage can be slowed or stopped with aggressive, early treatment.

Clinical Manifestations

The onset of RA is typically subtle. Nonspecific manifestations, such as fatigue, anorexia, weight loss, and generalized stiffness, may precede the onset of joint symptoms. The stiffness becomes more localized after weeks to months.

Joint Manifestations

Articular involvement is marked by pain, stiffness, limitation of motion, and signs of inflammation (heat, swelling, tenderness). Joint symptoms occur symmetrically and frequently affect the small joints of the hands and feet, as well as the larger peripheral joints, including wrists, elbows, shoulders, knees, hips, ankles, and jaw.

TABLE 72 Stages of Rheumatoid Arthritis

Stage	Characteristics
I	• Synovitis marked by: • synovial membrane swelling with excess blood • membrane containing small areas of lymphocyte infiltration • high WBC counts in synovial fluid (5000 to 60,000/μL) • X-ray results: soft tissue swelling, possible osteoporosis; no evidence of joint destruction
II	• Increased joint inflammation, spreading across cartilage into joint cavity • Signs of gradual destruction in joint cartilage • Narrowing joint space from loss of cartilage
III	• Formation of synovial pannus • Joint cartilage becomes eroded, bone exposed • X-ray results: extensive cartilage loss, erosion at joint margins, possible deformity
IV	• End-stage: inflammatory process subsides • Loss of joint function • Formation of subcutaneous nodules

WBC, White blood cell.
Source: Rheumatoid Arthritis.net: a Health Union Community: Understanding RA stages and progressions. Retrieved from <http://rheumatoidarthritis.net/what-is-ra/stages-and-progression>.

- The patient typically has joint stiffness after periods of inactivity. (See Table 60, p. 434, for a comparison of the manifestations of RA and osteoarthritis [OA].)
- As RA progresses, inflammation and fibrosis of the joint capsule and supporting structures may cause deformity and disability. Muscle atrophy and tendon destruction around the joint can cause 1 articular surface to slip past the other *(subluxation).* Typical hand distortions include "ulnar drift," "swan neck," and boutonniere deformities.

Extraarticular Manifestations

RA can affect nearly every system in the body. Extraarticular manifestations are more likely to occur in the person with high levels of biomarkers, such as RF.

Rheumatoid nodules develop in about half of all patients with RA. They appear under the skim as firm, nontender, granuloma-type masses and are usually found over the extensor surfaces of joints, such as the fingers and elbows. Nodules at the base of the spine and back of the head are common in older adults.

R

Sjögren's syndrome can occur by itself or in conjunction with other arthritic disorders, such as RA and systemic lupus erythematosus (SLE). The inflammation of RA can also damage the tear-producing (lacrimal) glands, making the eyes feel dry and gritty. (See Sjögren's syndrome, p. 565.)

Felty syndrome is rare but can occur in patients with long-standing RA. It is characterized by an enlarged spleen and low white blood cell (WBC) count. Patients with Felty syndrome are at increased risk for infection and lymphoma.

Flexion contractures and hand deformities cause diminished grasp strength, affecting the patient's ability to perform self-care tasks. Cataract development and loss of vision can result from scleral nodules. Depression may also occur.

Diagnostic Studies

A diagnosis is often made based on history and physical findings. Some laboratory tests are useful to confirm the diagnosis and to monitor disease progression.

- Erythrocyte sedimentation rate (ESR) and C-reactive protein (CRP) are elevated as general indicators of active inflammation.
- Antinuclear antibody (ANA) titers may increase.
- High levels of antibodies to citrullinated peptide (anti-CCP) are more specific than RF for RA. Testing may allow an early, accurate diagnosis.
- Synovial fluid analysis in early disease often shows a straw-colored fluid with many fibrin flecks. The WBC count of synovial fluid is elevated (up to 25,000/μL).
- Tissue biopsy can confirm inflammatory changes in the synovium.
- X-rays alone are not diagnostic of RA. They may show only soft tissue swelling and possible bone demineralization in early disease. A narrowed joint space, articular cartilage destruction, erosion, subluxation, and deformity are seen in later disease. Poor alignment and fusion (ankyloses) may be noted in advanced disease.

Interprofessional Management

Care of the patient with RA begins with a thorough program of education and drug therapy. Teach the patient and caregivers about the disease process and home management strategies. Include information on correct drug administration, the need to report side effects, and importance of medical and laboratory follow-up visits. The physical therapist helps the patient maintain joint motion and muscle strength. An occupational therapist helps the patient maintain upper extremity function and encourages use of splints or other assistive devices for joint protection. A balance of rest and activity is also encouraged.

Drug Therapy

Drugs are the cornerstone of RA treatment. Because irreversible joint changes can occur as early as the first year of RA, health care providers (HCPs) aggressively prescribe disease-modifying antirheumatic drugs (DMARDs). These drugs may slow disease progression and lessen risk of joint erosion and deformity. The choice of drug is based on disease activity, the patient's functional level, and lifestyle considerations, such as the desire to become pregnant.

- Treatment of early RA often involves methotrexate (Rheumatrex) because it reduces clinical symptoms in days to weeks, is inexpensive, and has a lower toxicity compared with other drugs. Nausea and vomiting are the most frequent side effects. Methotrexate therapy requires frequent laboratory monitoring.
- Sulfasalazine (Azulfidine) and the antimalarial drug hydroxychloroquine (Plaquenil) may be effective DMARDs for mild to moderate disease.
- Leflunomide (Arava) is a synthetic DMARD that blocks immune cell overproduction and has efficacy similar to that of methotrexate and sulfasalazine.
- Tofacitinib (Xeljanz), a JAK (Janus kinase) inhibitor, is used to treat moderate to severe active RA. The drug interferes with JAK enzymes that contribute to joint inflammation in RA.

Biologic response modifiers (BRMs) (also called *biologics* or *immunotherapy agents*) are also used to slow disease progression in RA. They can be used alone or in combination therapy with a DMARD to treat patients with moderate to severe disease who have not responded to DMARDs.

- Tumor necrosis factor inhibitors include etanercept (Enbrel), infliximab (Remicade), adalimumab (Humira), certolizumab (Cimzia), and golimumab (Simponi). Other biologic and targeted inhibitors that may be used include anakinra (Kineret), tocilizumab (Actemra), sarilumab (Kevzara), abatacept (Orencia), and rituximab (Rituxan).

Additional drugs used infrequently for treating RA include antibiotics (minocycline [Minocin]), immunosuppressants (azathioprine [Imuran]), penicillamine (Cuprimine), and gold compounds (auranofin [Ridaura] or gold sodium thiomalate [Myochrysine]) may be used to manage symptoms during disease flare-ups. Corticosteroid therapy can be used to manage symptoms during disease flares. Intraarticular injections may temporarily reduce acute pain and inflammation.

Various nonsteroidal antiinflammatory drugs (NSAIDs) and salicylates, such as enteric-coated aspirin, are included in the drug regimen to treat arthritis pain and inflammation. Celecoxib (Cele-brex), the only available cyclooxygenase (COX)-2 inhibitor, is effective in RA as well as OA. All nonaspirin NSAIDs can increase the risk of blood clots, heart attack, and stroke.

Nursing Management

Goals

The patient with RA will have satisfactory pain relief and minimal loss of joint function, participate in planning and implementing the therapeutic regimen, maintain a positive self-image, and perform self-care to the maximum amount possible.

Nursing Interventions

Prevention of RA is not possible at this time. Community education should focus on symptom recognition to promote early diagnosis and treatment.

Interventions begin with a careful physical assessment (joint pain, swelling, range of motion, general health status), psychosocial assessment (family support, sexual satisfaction, emotional stress, financial constraints, vocation and career limitations), and environ-mental assessment (transportation, home, and work modifications).

- Inflammation may be effectively managed through the adminis-tration of NSAIDs, DMARDs, and biologic/targeted therapy agents. Discuss the action and side effects of each drug and the necessary laboratory monitoring. Make the drug regimen as understandable as possible.
- Nondrug management may include the use of therapeutic heat and cold, rest, relaxation techniques, joint protection, biofeed-back, transcutaneous electrical nerve stimulation (TENS), and hypnosis.
- Lightweight splints may be prescribed to rest an inflamed joint and prevent deformity from muscle spasms and contractures. Remove splints regularly to assess, give skin care, and perform range-of-motion (ROM) exercises. Reapply splints as prescribed.
- Plan care and procedures around the patient's morning stiffness. Sitting or standing in a warm shower, sitting in a tub with warm towels around the shoulders, or soaking the hands in a basin of warm water may relieve joint stiffness and allow the patient to perform activities of daily living comfortably.
- Alternating scheduled rest periods with activity helps relieve fatigue and pain. Help the patient identify activity modifications to avoid overexertion.
- Good body alignment while resting can be maintained with a firm mattress or bed board. Encourage positions of extension and teach the patient to avoid positions of flexion. Avoid pillows

under the knees. A small, flat pillow may be used under the head and shoulders.

- Assistive devices such as built-up utensils, button hooks, and raised toilet seats simplify tasks. A cane or a walker offers support and relief of pain when walking.
- Heat and cold therapy helps relieve stiffness, pain, and muscle spasm. Application of ice may help during periods of exacerbation. Moist heat appears to offer better relief of chronic stiffness.
- Reinforce participation in an exercise program and ensure correct performance of the exercises. Gentle ROM exercises are usually done daily to keep the joints functional.

▼ **Patient and Caregiver Teaching**
- Self-management requires that the patient understand the nature and course of RA, and the goals of therapy. Consider the patient's value system and perception of the disease.
- Help the patient recognize fears and concerns of living with a chronic illness.
- Evaluate the family support system. Financial planning may be needed. Community resources such as home care nurse visits, homemaker services, vocational rehabilitation, and self-help groups may provide support.

SCLERODERMA

Description

Scleroderma (systemic sclerosis) is a disorder of the connective tissue characterized by fibrotic, degenerative, and occasionally inflammatory changes in the skin, blood vessels, synovium, skeletal muscle, and internal organs. Two types of disease exist: *localized scleroderma,* which is the more common form, and *diffuse systemic scleroderma.*

Skin changes of localized disease are usually limited to a few places on the skin or muscle without involvement of the trunk or internal organs. The prognosis for patients with limited disease is generally better than for those with diffuse disease.

Scleroderma occurs in all ethnic groups. It is more common in blacks, Native Americans, and persons of Japanese descent. Most cases occur in women. The usual age at onset is between 30 and 50 years.

Pathophysiology

The exact cause of scleroderma is unknown. Immunologic dysfunction and vascular abnormalities are believed to play a role in the development of systemic disease. In scleroderma, collagen (protein that gives normal skin its strength and elasticity) is overproduced. This leads to progressive tissue fibrosis and occlusion of blood vessels. Collagen overproduction also disrupts normal function of internal organs such as the lungs, kidney, heart, and gastrointestinal (GI) tract.

- Vascular problems, which mainly involve the small arteries and arterioles, are almost always present. These changes are some of the earliest changes in scleroderma. Risk factors include environmental or occupational exposure to coal, plastics, and silica dust.

Clinical Manifestations

Manifestations of scleroderma range from benign limited skin disease to diffuse skin thickening with rapidly progressive and widespread organ involvement. Localized disease is often marked by the *CREST syndrome*:

*C*alcinosis: painful deposits of calcium in skin of fingers, forearms, pressure points

*R*aynaud's phenomenon: intermittent vasospasm of fingertips in response to cold or stress

*E*sophageal dysfunction: difficulty swallowing because of internal scarring

*S*clerodactyly: tightening of skin on fingers and toes

*T*elangiectasia: red spots on hands, forearms, palms, face, and lips from capillary dilation

Raynaud's phenomenon (sudden vasospasm of the digits) is the most common first symptom in localized scleroderma. Patients have decreased blood flow to the fingers and toes when exposed to cold (blanching or white phase). This is followed by cyanosis as hemoglobin releases O_2 to the tissues (blue phase), then erythema during rewarming (red phase). Numbness and tingling often occur (see Raynaud's Phenomenon, p. 513).

- About 20% of people with scleroderma develop secondary Sjögren's syndrome, a condition associated with dry eyes and dry mouth (see Sjögren's Syndrome, p. 565). Dysphagia, gum disease, and dental decay can result.
- Frequent reflux of gastric acid can occur because of esophageal fibrosis. If swallowing becomes difficult, the patient is likely to decrease food intake and lose weight. GI effects include constipation from colonic hypomotility and diarrhea caused by malabsorption from bacterial overgrowth.
- Lung involvement includes pleural thickening, pulmonary fibrosis, pulmonary artery hypertension, and abnormal pulmonary function.

- Primary heart disease consists of pericarditis, pericardial effusion, and dysrhythmias. Heart failure from myocardial fibrosis occurs most often in patients with systemic disease.
- Renal disease was previously a major cause of death in diffuse scleroderma. Recent improvements in dialysis, bilateral nephrectomy in patients with uncontrollable hypertension, and kidney transplantation have offered hope to patients with renal failure. The use of angiotensin-converting enzyme (ACE) inhibitors (e.g., lisinopril [Prinivil]) has had a marked impact on the treatment of renal disease.

Diagnostic Studies

- Blood studies may reveal mild hemolytic anemia.
- Anticentromere antibodies related to CREST syndrome are found in about 45% to 50% of people with localized scleroderma. Antibodies to topoisomerase-1 are present in about 30% of people with diffuse disease. Presence of either antibody is highly specific for diagnosis.
- If renal involvement is present, urinalysis may show proteinuria, microscopic hematuria, and casts.
- X-rays show evidence of subcutaneous calcification, distal esophageal hypomotility, and/or bilateral pulmonary fibrosis.
- Pulmonary function studies reveal decreased vital capacity and lung compliance.

Interprofessional Management

There is no specific treatment. Supportive care is directed to preventing or treating the complications of involved organs. Physical therapy helps maintain joint mobility and preserve muscle strength. Occupational therapy assists the patient in maintaining functional abilities.

Drug Therapy

Vasoactive agents are often prescribed in early disease. Calcium-channel blockers (nifedipine [Procardia], diltiazem [Cardizem]) and the angiotensin II blocker losartan are common treatments for Raynaud's phenomenon. Reserpine, an α-adrenergic blocking agent, increases blood flow to the fingers. Bosentan (Tracleer), an endothelin-receptor antagonist, and the vasodilator epoprostenol (Flolan) may improve blood flow to the lung.

Nonsteroidal antiinflammatory drugs (NSAIDs) and topical agents may give some relief from joint pain. Capsaicin cream may be useful not only as a local analgesic but also as a vasodilator. Other therapies prescribed to treat specific systemic problems include: (1) tetracycline for diarrhea caused by bacterial overgrowth, (2) histamine (H2) receptor blockers (e.g., cimetidine) and proton pump inhibitors (e.g., omeprazole) for esophageal symptoms, and (3) antihypertensive agent (e.g., captopril, propranolol, methyldopa) for hypertension with renal involvement.

- Immunosuppressive drugs (e.g., cyclophosphamide, mycophenolate mofetil) are used in severe cases.

Nursing Management

Because prevention is not possible, nursing interventions often begin during hospitalization for diagnostic purposes. Emotional stress and cold ambient temperatures may aggravate Raynaud's phenomenon.

Teach the patient to protect the hands and feet from cold exposure and possible burns or cuts that might heal slowly. Encourage the patient to avoid smoking because of its vasoconstricting effect. Alcohol-free lotions may help alleviate skin dryness and cracking but must be rubbed in for a long time because of skin thickness.

- A consultation with a dietitian is beneficial. Dysphagia may be reduced by eating small, frequent meals, chewing carefully and slowly, and drinking fluids. Decrease risk for heartburn by using antacids 45 to 60 minutes after each meal and sitting upright for at least 2 hours after eating. Using extra pillows or raising the head of the bed on blocks may reduce gastroesophageal reflux during the night.
- Job modifications are often needed because of problems with stair climbing, typing, writing, and cold exposure.
- Emphasize daily oral hygiene to avoid to tooth and gum disease.

Teach the patient to actively carry out therapeutic exercises. Encourage the use of moist heat applications or paraffin baths to promote skin flexibility in the hands and feet. Teach the patient to use assistive devices as needed and organize activities to preserve strength and reduce disability. Sexual dysfunction from body changes, pain, muscular weakness, limited mobility, decreased self-esteem, erectile dysfunction, and decreased vaginal secretions may require sensitive counseling.

SEIZURE DISORDER

Description

A *seizure* is a transient, uncontrolled electrical discharge of neurons in the brain that interrupts normal function. Seizures may accompany a variety of disorders, or they may occur without any apparent cause. *Seizure disorder*, also known as *epilepsy*, is a group of neurologic diseases marked by recurring seizures. It is the fourth most common neurologic disorder.

- Metabolic problems that cause seizures include acidosis, electrolyte imbalances, hypoglycemia, hypoxia, alcohol and barbiturate withdrawal, dehydration, and water intoxication.
- Extracranial disorders that cause seizures include systemic lupus erythematosus, diabetes, hypertension, sepsis, and heart, lung, liver, or kidney diseases.

Pathophysiology

The most common causes of seizure during the first 6 months of life are severe birth injury, congenital defects involving the central nervous system (CNS), infections, and inborn errors of metabolism.

In those 2 to 20 years of age, the main causes are birth injury, infection, head trauma, and genetic factors. In young adults 20 to 30 years of age, seizure disorder usually occurs from structural lesions such as trauma, brain tumors, or vascular disease. After 50 years of age, the main causes are stroke and metastatic brain tumors. However, one-third of all seizure cannot be attributed to a specific cause.

Seizure disorder is characterized by a group of abnormal neurons that seem to fire without a clear cause. Any stimulus that causes the neuron's cell membrane to depolarize can cause this firing. It spreads by physiologic pathways to involve near or distant areas of the brain. Localization of the seizure focus (the place where the seizure originates) is critical to the success of any possible surgical treatment.

Clinical Manifestations

Specific manifestations are determined by the site of the electrical disturbance. The preferred method of classifying epileptic seizures is based on the clinical and electroencephalographic (EEG) manifestations of seizures. This system divides seizures into 3 major classes: *generalized onset, focal onset*, and *unknown onset*. They are further described under each classification as *motor* or *nonmotor*.

Depending on the type, a seizure may progress through several phases: (1) *prodromal phase,* with sensations or behavior changes that precede a seizure by hours or days; (2) *aural phase,* with a sensory warning that is similar each time a seizure occurs; (3) *ictal phase,* from first symptoms to the end of seizure activity; and (4) *postictal phase,* the recovery period after the seizure.

Generalized-Onset Seizures

Generalized-onset seizures involve both sides of the brain and are characterized by bilateral synchronous epileptic discharge in the brain. In most cases the patient loses consciousness for a few seconds to several minutes.

- *Tonic-clonic* (formerly known as "grand mal") seizures are the most common generalized seizures. During a tonic-clonic seizure, the patient loses consciousness and falls to the ground, if upright. The body stiffens (tonic phase) for 10 to 20 seconds and the extremities jerk (clonic phase) for another 30 to 40 seconds. Cyanosis, excessive salivation, tongue or cheek biting, and incontinence may occur during the seizure. In the postictal phase, the patient usually has muscle soreness, feels tired, and may sleep for several hours. Some patients may not feel normal for several hours or days after a seizure. The patient has no memory of the seizure.
- Other types of generalized-onset motor seizures include tonic and clonic. A *tonic* seizure involves a sudden onset of increased tone in the extensor muscles, contributing to sudden stiff movements. Tonic seizures most often occur in sleep and affect both sides of the body. Patients will fall if they are standing when the seizure occurs. Tonic seizures usually last < 20 seconds. The patient usually remains aware. *Clonic* seizures begin with loss of awareness and sudden loss of muscle tone, followed by rhythmic limb jerking that may or may not be symmetric. Clonic seizures are rare.
- A generalized *atonic seizure* (or *drop attack*) involves either a tonic episode or a paroxysmal loss of muscle tone. It begins suddenly with the person falling to the ground. Seizures typically last < 15 seconds. The person usually remains conscious, and normal activity can be resumed immediately. Patients with this type of seizure are at great risk of head injury and often have to wear protective helmets.
- *Typical absence* ("petit mal") seizures usually occur only in children and rarely continue beyond adolescence. A simple absence seizure is a brief staring spell resembling "daydreaming" that lasts only a few seconds.
- In *atypical absence seizure*, the staring spell is accompanied by other signs and symptoms, such as eye blinking or jerking movements of the lips. A brief warning phase (aura) and confusion after the seizure are common.

Focal-Onset Seizures

Focal-onset seizures (formerly called *partial seizures*) begin in 1 hemisphere of the brain in a specific region of the cortex, as indicated by the EEG. They produce sensory, motor, cognitive, or emotional manifestations based on the function of the area of the brain involved. For example, if the discharging focus is located in the medial aspect of the postcentral gyrus, the patient may have paresthesias and tingling or numbness in the leg on the side opposite the focus.

Complications

Status epilepticus is a state of continuous seizure activity or a condition in which seizures recur in rapid succession without return to consciousness between seizures. It can occur with any type of seizure. Status epilepticus is the most serious complication of epilepsy and represents a neurologic emergency.

- During repeated seizures, the brain uses more energy than can be supplied. As neurons become exhausted and cease to function, permanent brain damage may result.
- *Convulsive status epilepticus* is the most dangerous because it can cause potentially fatal respiratory insufficiency, hypoxemia, dysrhythmias, hyperthermia, and systemic acidosis.
- Severe injury and death can result from physical trauma during a seizure. Patients who lose consciousness during a seizure are at greatest risk.

Perhaps the most common complication of seizure disorder is the effect it has on the patient's lifestyle. Antiseizure medications and the continued need to manage a chronic disease can contribute to depression. Patients may be victims of discrimination in employment and educational opportunities. Transportation may be difficult if state law does not allow the person to drive.

Diagnostic Studies

- Most important in diagnosis are accurate and comprehensive descriptions of the seizures and the patient's health history.
- EEG is useful only if it shows abnormalities. Some patients who do not have seizure disorder have abnormal EEG patterns, while many patients with seizure disorder have normal EEGs between seizures.
- Complete blood count (CBC), serum chemistry panel, studies of liver and kidney function, and urinalysis can rule out metabolic disorders.
- CT scan and MRI can rule out a structural lesion.
- Cerebral angiography, single-photon emission computed tomography (SPECT), magnetic resonance spectroscopy (MRS), magnetic resonance angiography (MRA), and positron emission tomography (PET) may be used.

Interprofessional Management

Most seizures are self-limiting and do not cause body injury. However, in cases of status epilepticus, significant body harm, or first-time seizure, medical care should be sought immediately. Table 58.7, Harding et al., *Lewis' Medical-Surgical Nursing*, ed 11, summarizes the emergency care of the patient with a generalized tonic-clonic seizure.

S

Drug Therapy

Seizure disorder is treated primarily with medications that stabilize the nerve cell membranes and preventing the spread of the epileptic discharge.

The principle of drug therapy is to begin with a single drug based on the patient's age and weight with consideration of the type, frequency, and cause of seizure. Then the dosage is increased until the seizures are controlled or toxic side effects occur. If seizure control is not achieved with a single drug, the drug dosage and timing or administration may be changed or a second drug may be added.

- The main drugs to treat tonic-clonic and focal onset seizures are phenytoin (Dilantin), carbamazepine (Tegretol), phenobarbital, and divalproex.
- The drugs used most often to treat generalized onset nonmotor and myoclonic seizures include ethosuximide (Zarontin), divalproex, and clonazepam (Klonopin). Some drugs are effective for multiple seizure types. Pregabalin (Lyrica) is used as an additional treatment for focal awareness or impaired awareness seizures not successfully controlled with 1 medication.
- Treatment of status epilepticus requires initiation of a rapid-acting antiseizure medication given IV. Drugs most commonly used are lorazepam (Ativan) and diazepam.
- Antiseizure drugs should not be discontinued abruptly after long-term use because this can precipitate seizures.

Surgical interventions are options for patients whose epilepsy cannot be controlled with drug therapy. Alternative therapies, such as vagal nerve stimulation and biofeedback, may also be used.

Nursing Management

Goals

The patient with seizures will be free from injury during a seizure, have optimal mental and physical functioning while taking antiseizure drugs, and have satisfactory psychosocial functioning.

Nursing Interventions

The patient with seizure disorder should practice good general health habits (e.g., maintaining a proper diet, getting adequate rest, exercising). Help the patient identify events or situations that cause seizures and provide suggestions for avoiding them or handling them better. Teach the patient to avoid excess alcohol intake, fatigue, and loss of sleep. Help the patient handle stress constructively.

Nursing care for a hospitalized patient or for a person who has had seizures as a result of metabolic factors should focus on observation and treatment of the seizure, teaching, and psychosocial intervention.

- Carefully observe and record details of the seizure event because the diagnosis and subsequent treatment often rest on the seizure description. What events preceded the seizure? When did the seizure occur? How long did each phase (aural [if any], ictal, postictal) last? What occurred during each phase?
- The description should include the exact onset of the seizure (which body part was affected first, and how); the course and nature of the seizure activity (loss of consciousness, tongue biting, automatisms, stiffening, jerking, total lack of muscle tone); the body parts involved and their sequence of involvement; and the presence of autonomic signs (dilated pupils, excessive salivation, altered breathing, cyanosis, flushing, diaphoresis, or incontinence).
- Assessment of the postictal period should include a detailed description of the level of consciousness (LOC), vital signs, memory loss, muscle soreness, speech disorders (aphasia, dysarthria), weakness or paralysis, sleep period, and the duration of each sign or symptom.
- During the seizure, you should do the following: maintain a patient airway for the patient, protect the patient's head, turn the patient to the side, loosen constrictive clothing, and ease the patient to the floor if seated. Do not restrain the patient or place any objects in the patient's mouth.
- After the seizure, the patient may require suctioning and oxygen.
- A seizure can be a frightening experience for the patient and others who witnessed it. Assess the level of their understanding and provide information about how and why the event occurred.

▼ Patient and Caregiver Teaching

Prevention of recurring seizures is the major goal in the treatment of epilepsy. Drugs must be taken regularly and continually, often for a lifetime. You have an important role in teaching the patient and caregivers. Guidelines for teaching are shown in Table 73.

TABLE 73 Patient and Caregiver Teaching

Seizure Disorder

Include the following information in the teaching plan for the patient with seizure disorder.

1. Take antiseizure medications as prescribed. Report all drug side effects to the HCP.
2. When needed, blood is drawn to ensure therapeutic drug levels. Schedule regular communication with the HCP to discuss treatment options.

S

Continued

TABLE 73 Patient and Caregiver Teaching

Seizure Disorder—cont'd

3. Use nondrug techniques, such as relaxation therapy, to try to reduce the number of seizures.
4. Be aware of community and online resources for education and help with tracking and explaining seizure activity.
5. Wear a medical alert bracelet or necklace and carry an identification card.
6. Avoid excess alcohol intake, fatigue, and loss of sleep.
7. Eat regular meals and snacks in between if feeling shaky, faint, or hungry.
8. Be knowledgeable as a woman of childbearing age about antiseizure medications and contraceptive use.

Caregivers should receive the following information.

Focal-Onset Seizures

1. Stay calm. Guide patient to safety to prevent injury but do not restrain.
2. Observe for asymmetry of activity and focus on specific actions, such as lip smacking and abnormal movements.
3. Assess patient's level of consciousness and ability to converse and respond appropriately.
4. Observe the time the event started and stopped. Take note of the time of return to baseline.
5. Provide respect and explanation of occurrence.

Generalized-Onset Tonic-Clonic Seizures

1. When seizure occurs outside the hospital setting, activate ERS if: (1) the duration is > 5 minutes; (2) events recur without the patient recovering to baseline; (3) the patient is unable to establish a normal breathing pattern, is injured or pregnant; or (4) you do not know if this is a first-time seizure event.
2. Maintain patient safety. Lower the patient to the floor or bed, remove glasses if worn, and loosen restrictive clothing.
3. Do not place anything in the patient's mouth. Patient's teeth/dentures may be damaged, and caregiver may be bitten.
4. Position patient on side (if possible) to improve the patient's ability to release oral secretions.
5. Observe the time event started and stopped. Take note of the time of return to baseline.
6. Assess for possible injury or any lingering motor weakness.

ERS, Emergency response services.

SEXUALLY TRANSMITTED INFECTIONS

Sexually transmitted infections (STIs) are diseases that spread through sexual contact with the penis, vagina, anus, mouth, or body fluids of an infected person. Mucosal tissues in the genitals (urethra in men, vagina in women), rectum, and mouth are especially susceptible to the bacteria and viruses that cause STIs. Common infections that are transmitted sexually are listed in Table 74.

Infections that are associated with sexual transmission can also be contracted by other routes, such as through blood or blood products or by *autoinoculation* (spread of infection by touching or scratching an infected area and transferring it to another part of the body). See Gonorrhea, p. 243; Syphilis, p. 595; Herpes, Genital, p. 296; Warts, Genital, p. 657; and Chlamydial Infection, p. 121.

TABLE 74 Causes of Sexually Transmitted Infections (STIs)

Sexually Transmitted Infection	Cause
Bacteria	
Chlamydia	*Chlamydia trachomatis*
Gonorrhea	*Neisseria gonorrhoeae*
Syphilis	*Treponema pallidum*
Viruses	
Genital herpes	Herpes simplex virus (HSV 1 or 2)
Genital warts (condylomata acuminata)	Human papillomavirus (HPV)
Human immunodeficiency virus (HIV) infection/acquired immunodeficiency syndrome (AIDS)	HIV
Hepatitis B and C	Hepatitis B and C viruses
Molluscum contagiosum	Poxvirus (molluscum contagiosum virus)
Parasites/Protozoa	
Trichomoniasis	*Trichomonas vaginalis*

S

An estimated 110 million people in the United States are infected with 1 or more STIs at any given time. In the United States, all cases of gonorrhea, chlamydia, and syphilis must be reported to the state or local public health authorities for surveillance and partner notification. Nurses and other health care providers (HCPs) are mandated to report these STIs to public health authorities.

Many factors contribute to the high rates of STIs (Table 75). Earlier reproductive maturity and increased longevity have resulted in a longer sexual life span.

- Other factors include greater sexual freedom, lack of barrier methods (e.g., condoms) during sexual activity, and an increased emphasis on sexuality in the media.
- Urbanization and easier travel are some of the global changes that contribute to increased opportunities for exposure to all infectious diseases, including STIs.
- Youth under age 25 years and those who are socially and economically disadvantaged are disproportionately affected by STIs.

TABLE 75   Risk Factors for Sexually Transmitted Infections (STIs)

High-Risk Behaviors

- Alcohol or drug use (inhibits judgment)
- Having new or multiple sexual partners
- Having more than 1 sexual partner
- Having sexual partners who have have/had multiple partners
- Inconsistent or incorrect use of condoms or other barrier methods
- Sharing needles used to inject drugs

High-Risk Medical History

High-Risk Populations

- Adolescents and young adults (age <25 yrs)
- Ethnicity (e.g., blacks, American Indian/Alaskan Native, Native Hawaiian/Other Pacific Islander, Hispanic)
- Men who have sex with men
- Persons in correctional facilities
- Transgender persons
- Victims of sexual assault
- Women

- Substance use can further contribute to unsafe sexual practices by impairing judgment.
- The male condom is considered to be the best form of protection (other than abstinence) against STIs. However, condoms are not often used in the general population.

Nursing and Interprofessional Management

The patient with an STI will demonstrate understanding of the mode of transmission and the risk posed by STIs, complete treatment and return for appropriate follow-up care, notify or assist in notification of sexual contacts about their need for testing and treatment, abstain from intercourse until infection is resolved, and demonstrate knowledge of safer sex practices.

The diagnosis of an STI may be met with a variety of emotions such as embarrassment, shame, guilt, anger, and even a desire for vengeance. Provide counseling and encourage the patient to voice feelings. A referral for professional counseling to explore the impact of an STI on a relationship may be indicated.

Single-dose treatment for gonorrhea, chlamydia, and syphilis helps prevent the problems associated with nonadherence with drug therapy. Give special instructions to the patient receiving multiple-dose therapy to complete the prescribed treatment. Patients should return to the treatment center for a repeat culture from infected sites or serologic testing at designated times to determine effectiveness of treatment.

- Advise the patient to inform sexual partners of the need for treatment, regardless of whether they are free of symptoms or experiencing symptoms.

Emphasize hygiene measures to the patient with an STI. An important measure is frequent hand washing and bathing.

- Bathing and cleaning of involved areas can provide local comfort and prevent secondary infection.
- Teach patients not to douche after sex. It can push bacteria higher into the reproductive tract.
- Sexual abstinence is needed during the communicable phase of the infection. After the patient has completed treatment, condoms or other barrier methods may prevent spread of infection and reinfection.

Be prepared to discuss decreasing exposure to STIs with all patients, young and old, regardless of sexual identity or preferences.

- "Safer" sex practices include abstinence, monogamy with an uninfected partner, avoiding certain high-risk sexual practices, harm reduction, and correct and consistent use of condoms and other barriers to limit contact with potentially infectious body fluids or lesions.

See Table 76 for a patient teaching guide regarding STIs.

TABLE 76 Patient Teaching

Sexually Transmitted Infections (STIs)

When teaching the patient with sexually transmitted infections:

1. Explain precautions to take, such as
   - Using condoms and other barrier methods with every sexual encounter
   - Being monogamous, defining what monogamy means with your partner
   - Asking potential partners about their sexual history
   - Asking potential partners if they have been tested for STIs
   - Avoiding sex with partners who have visible oral, inguinal, genital, perineal, or anal lesions, or those who use IV drugs
   - Voiding and washing genitalia and surrounding area after sex to flush out/wash-away organisms to reduce potential for transmitting infection
2. Explain the importance of taking all antibiotics or antiviral agents as prescribed. Symptoms will improve after 1–2 days of treatment, but organisms may still be present.
3. Teach patients diagnosed with gonorrhea, chlamydia, syphilis or trichomoniasis that all sexual partners need to be treated to prevent transmission and reinfection.
4. Teach patients to abstain from sexual contact during and for 7 days after treatment and to use condoms or other barrier methods when sexual activity is resumed to prevent spread of infection and reinfection.
5. Explain the importance of follow-up examination and retesting at least once after treatment (if appropriate) to confirm complete cure and prevent relapse.
6. Allow patients and partners to voice their concerns and clarify areas that need explanation.
7. Teach patients about the signs and symptoms of complications and need to report problems to their HCP to ensure proper follow-up and early treatment of reinfection.
8. Tell patients of the infectious nature of these infections to avoid a false sense of security, which may result in careless sexual practices or poor personal hygiene.
9. Tell patients about health department requirements for anonymously reporting certain STIs.

SHOCK

Description

Shock is a syndrome characterized by decreased tissue perfusion and impaired cellular metabolism. The 4 main categories of shock are cardiogenic, hypovolemic, distributive, and obstructive.

- Although the cause, initial presentation, and management strategies vary for each type, the physiologic responses of the cells to hypoperfusion are similar.

Cardiogenic Shock

Cardiogenic shock occurs when either systolic or diastolic dysfunction of the heart's pumping action results in reduced cardiac output (CO). The heart's inability to pump the blood forward is systolic dysfunction, most commonly caused by acute myocardial infarction (MI). The patient has impaired tissue perfusion and cellular metabolism because of cardiogenic shock.

- The patient presents with tachycardia, hypotension, and a narrowed pulse pressure. A low CO (< 4 L/min) and *cardiac index* (< 2.5 L/min/m^2) result from systolic dysfunction.
- Tachypnea and crackles are evidence of pulmonary congestion. The pulmonary artery wedge pressure (PAWP) and pulmonary vascular resistance are increased.
- Signs of peripheral hypoperfusion (e.g., cyanosis, pallor, diaphoresis, diminished pulses, delayed capillary refill) are apparent.
- Decreased renal blood flow results in sodium and water retention and decreased urine output.
- Anxiety, confusion, and agitation develop as cerebral perfusion is impaired.

Studies helpful in diagnosing cardiogenic shock include laboratory studies (e.g., cardiac biomarkers, b-type natriuretic peptide [BNP]), electrocardiogram (ECG), chest x-ray, and echocardiogram.

Hypovolemic Shock

Hypovolemic shock occurs when there is inadequate fluid volume in the intravascular space. The volume loss may be either absolute or relative.

- *Absolute hypovolemia* results when fluid is lost through hemorrhage, gastrointestinal (GI) loss (e.g., vomiting, diarrhea), fistula drainage, diabetes insipidus, or diuresis.
- In *relative hypovolemia,* fluid volume moves out of the vascular space into the extravascular space (e.g., intracavity space). This fluid shift is called *third spacing*. One example of relative volume loss is fluid leakage from the vascular space to the

S

interstitial space because of increased capillary permeability, as seen in burns.

A reduction in intravascular volume results in decreased venous return to the heart, decreased preload, decreased stroke volume, and decreased CO. A cascade of events results in decreased tissue perfusion and impaired cellular metabolism, the hallmarks of shock (Fig. 20). A total blood loss of 15% to 30% results in a sympathetic nervous system (SNS)–mediated response that increases heart rate, CO, and respiratory rate and depth. If hypovolemia is corrected at this time, tissue dysfunction is generally reversible.

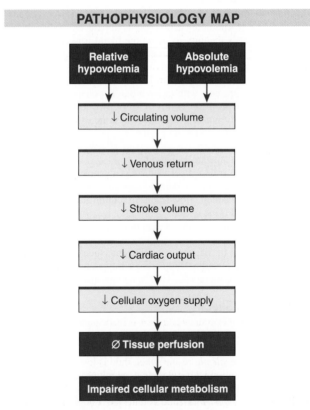

PATHOPHYSIOLOGY MAP

Fig. 20 The pathophysiology of hypovolemic shock. (Modified from Urden LD, Stacy KM, Lough ME: *Critical care nursing: diagnosis and management,* ed 6, St Louis, 2010, Mosby.).

- If volume loss is > 30%, it must be immediately replaced with blood products. A loss of more than 40% of the total blood volume results in irreversible tissue destruction.

Laboratory studies include serial measurements of hemoglobin and hematocrit levels, electrolytes, lactate, blood gases, and central venous oxygenation ($ScvO_2$), as well as hourly urine outputs.

Distributive Shock (Neurogenic, Anaphylactic, Septic)
Neurogenic Shock
Neurogenic shock is a hemodynamic phenomenon that can occur within 30 minutes of a spinal cord injury and last up to 6 weeks. The injury results in massive vasodilation without compensation because of the loss of SNS vasoconstrictor tone. This leads to a pooling of blood in the blood vessels, tissue hypoperfusion, and impaired cellular metabolism.

Spinal anesthesia can also temporarily block transmission of impulses from the SNS. Depression of the vasomotor center of the medulla from drugs (e.g., opioids, benzodiazepines) may result in decreased vasoconstrictor tone of the peripheral blood vessels and neurogenic shock.

- Manifestations are hypotension (from massive vasodilation) and bradycardia (from unopposed parasympathetic stimulation).

The patient in neurogenic shock may not be able to regulate body temperature. Initially, the patient's skin will be warm because of the massive vasodilation. As the heat disperses, the patient is at risk for hypothermia.

The pathophysiology of neurogenic shock is described in Fig. 66.4, Harding et al., *Lewis' Medical-Surgical Nursing*, ed 11.
Anaphylactic Shock
Anaphylactic shock is an acute and life-threatening hypersensitivity (allergic) reaction to a sensitizing substance such as a drug, chemical, vaccine, food, or insect venom. The reaction quickly causes massive vasodilation, release of vasoactive mediators, and an increase in capillary permeability.

- As capillary permeability increases, fluid leaks from the vascular space into the interstitial space. Anaphylactic shock can lead to respiratory distress as a result of laryngeal edema or severe bronchospasm, and to circulatory failure because of massive vasodilation.
- Patients present with a sudden onset of dizziness, chest pain, incontinence, swelling of the lips and tongue, wheezing, and stridor. Skin changes include flushing, pruritus, urticaria, and angioedema.
- A patient can develop a severe allergic reaction leading to anaphylactic shock after contact with, inhalation or ingestion of, or

S

injection with an antigen (allergen) to which the person has previously been sensitized.

Septic Shock

Septic shock is a subset of *sepsis* (systemic inflammatory response to infection). Septic shock is characterized by persistent hypotension, despite adequate fluid resuscitation, and inadequate tissue perfusion that results in tissue hypoxia. The main organisms that cause sepsis are gram-negative and gram-positive bacteria. Parasites, fungi, and viruses can also lead to the development of sepsis and septic shock. The pathophysiology of septic shock is described in Fig. 66.5, Harding et al., *Lewis' Medical-Surgical Nursing,* ed 11.

- When a microorganism enters the body, the normal immune/inflammatory cascade responses start. However, in severe sepsis and septic shock, the body's response is exaggerated. Inflammation and coagulation increase along with a decrease in fibrinolysis. Endotoxins from the microorganism cell wall stimulate the release of cytokines and other proinflammatory mediators. The combined effects of the mediators result in endothelial damage, vasodilation, increased capillary permeability, and neutrophil and platelet aggregation and adhesion to the endothelium.
- Manifestations include an initial decreased ejection fraction with the ventricles dilating to maintain stroke volume. The ejection fraction typically improves and the ventricular dilation resolves over 7 to 10 days. Persistence of a high CO and a low systemic vascular resistance (SVR) beyond 24 hours is an ominous finding often associated with development of severe hypotension and multiple organ dysfunction syndrome (MODS) (see Systemic Inflammatory Response Syndrome [SIRS] and MODS, p. 600).
- Respiratory failure is common. The patient initially hyperventilates, resulting in respiratory alkalosis. Once the patient can no longer compensate, respiratory acidosis develops.
- Other clinical signs include decreased urine output, alteration in neurologic status, and GI problems such as GI bleeding and paralytic ileus.

Obstructive Shock

Obstructive shock develops when a physical obstruction to blood flow occurs with a decreased CO. This can be caused from a restriction to diastolic filling of the right ventricle caused by compression (e.g., cardiac tamponade, tension pneumothorax, pulmonary embolism, superior vena cava syndrome). The pathophysiology of obstructive shock is described in Fig. 66.6, Harding et al., *Lewis' Medical-Surgical Nursing,* ed 11.

- Patients have decreased CO, increased afterload, and variable left ventricular filling pressures, depending on the obstruction. Other signs include jugular venous distention and pulsus paradoxus. Rapid assessment and immediate treatment are important to prevent further hemodynamic compromise and possible cardiac arrest.

Stages of Shock

Shock is categorized into 4 overlapping stages: (1) initial stage, (2) compensatory stage, (3) progressive stage, and (4) refractory stage.

Initial Stage

The *initial stage* of shock begins at the cellular level. This stage is usually not clinically apparent. Metabolism changes at the cellular level from aerobic to anaerobic, causing lactic acid buildup. Lactic acid is a waste product that is removed by the liver. However, this removal process requires oxygen, which is unavailable because of the decrease in tissue perfusion.

Compensatory Stage

In the *compensatory stage,* the body activates neural, hormonal, and biochemical mechanisms to try to overcome the increasing consequences of anaerobic metabolism and maintain homeostasis.

- One of the classic signs of shock is a drop in BP. The SNS stimulates vasoconstriction and the release of the potent vasoconstrictors epinephrine and norepinephrine. Blood flow to the heart and brain is maintained. Blood flow to the kidneys, GI tract, and lungs is diverted.
- The myocardium responds to SNS stimulation and the increase in oxygen demand by increasing heart rate and contractility. Increased contractility increases myocardial O_2 consumption.
- Shunting blood from the lungs has an important effect on the patient in shock. Areas of the lungs participating in ventilation are not perfused because of decreased blood flow to the lungs. The patient has a compensatory increase in the rate and depth of respirations.
- Decreased blood flow to the kidneys activates the renin-angiotensin-aldosterone system, resulting in vasoconstriction and sodium and water reabsorption.

If the cause of shock is corrected at this stage, the patient recovers with few or no residual effects. If the cause of shock is not corrected and the body is unable to compensate, the patient goes on to the progressive stage of shock.

Progressive Stage

The *progressive stage* of shock begins as compensatory mechanisms fail. Continued decreased cellular perfusion and altered

S

capillary permeability are distinguishing features of this stage. The patient may have profound edema *(anasarca)*. Aggressive interventions are needed to prevent the development of MODS.

- CO begins to fall, with a decrease in BP and peripheral perfusion, including a decrease in coronary artery, cerebral, and peripheral perfusion. Decreased perfusion results in dysrhythmias, myocardial ischemia, and possibly MI.
- The combined effects of pulmonary vasoconstriction and bronchoconstriction are impaired gas exchange, decreased compliance, and worsening ventilation-perfusion mismatch. The patient presents with tachypnea, crackles, and an overall increased work of breathing.
- As the blood supply to the GI tract is decreased, the normally protective mucosal barrier becomes ischemic, which predisposes the patient to ulcers and GI bleeding.
- The patient has a decreased urine output and an elevated blood urea nitrogen (BUN) and serum creatinine. Metabolic acidosis occurs from an inability to excrete acids and reabsorb bicarbonate.
- Loss of liver function leads to a failure to metabolize drugs and waste products such as ammonia and lactate. Jaundice results from accumulated bilirubin.
- Hematologic dysfunction places the patient at risk for the development of disseminated intravascular coagulation (DIC) (see Disseminated Intravascular Coagulation, p. 188).

Refractory Stage

In the last stage of shock, the *refractory stage,* decreased perfusion from peripheral vasoconstriction and decreased CO worsen anaerobic metabolism. The loss of intravascular volume worsens hypotension and tachycardia and decreases coronary blood flow. Cerebral blood flow cannot be maintained and cerebral ischemia results.

- The patient has profound hypotension and hypoxemia. In this stage, recovery is unlikely. The organs are failing, and the body's compensatory mechanisms are overwhelmed.

Diagnostic Studies

- Obtaining a thorough medical and surgical history and a history of recent events (e.g., surgery, chest pain, trauma) provides valuable data.
- Blood studies may include complete blood count (CBC), DIC screen, cardiac enzymes, BUN, glucose, electrolytes, arterial blood gases (ABGs), blood cultures, and liver enzymes.
- Decreased tissue perfusion in shock leads to an increased lactate level with a base deficit (the amount needed to bring the pH back

to normal). These laboratory changes reflect an increase in anaerobic metabolism.

- Twelve-lead ECG, continuous cardiac monitoring, and chest x-ray.
- Continuous pulse oximetry, invasive and non-invasive hemodynamic monitoring.

See Table 66.2, Harding et al., *Lewis' Medical-Surgical Nursing*, ed 11, for further information about laboratory findings seen in shock.

Interprofessional Management

Critical factors in management are early recognition and treatment. Prompt intervention in the early stages may prevent the decline to the progressive or irreversible stage. Successful management of the patient in shock includes: (1) identification of patients at risk for the development of shock; (2) integration of the patient's history, physical examination, and clinical findings to establish a diagnosis; (3) interventions to control or eliminate the cause of the decreased perfusion; (4) protecting target and distal organs from dysfunction; and (5) providing multisystem supportive care.

Emergency care of the patient in shock is presented in Table 77. General management strategies begin with ensuring that the patient is responsive and has a patent airway. Once the airway is established, with either a natural airway or an endotracheal tube, O_2 delivery must be optimized.

- Supplemental O_2 and mechanical ventilation may be needed to support oxygen delivery and maintain an arterial oxygen saturation of at least 90% (arterial partial pressure of O_2 [PaO_2] > 60 mm Hg) to avoid hypoxemia (see Artificial Airways: Endotracheal Tubes, p. 663, Oxygen Therapy, p. 697, and Mechanical Ventilation, p. 691). The mean arterial pressure and circulating blood volume are optimized with fluid replacement and drug therapy (see Tables 66.7 and 66.8 in Harding et al., *Lewis' Medical-Surgical Nursing*, ed 11).

In addition to general management of shock, there are specific interventions for different types of shock (Table 78).

Nursing Management
Goals

The overall goals for a patient in shock include: (1) evidence of adequate tissue perfusion, (2) restoration of normal or baseline BP, (3) recovery of organ function, (4) avoiding complications from prolonged states of hypoperfusion, and (5) preventing health care–associated complications of disease management and care.

S

TABLE 77 Emergency Management

Shock

Etiology[a]	Assessment Findings	Interventions
Surgical	• Anxiety	**Initial**
• Aortic dissection	• Chills	• If unresponsive, assess circulation, airway, and
• GI bleeding	• Confusion	breathing (CAB).
• Postoperative	• Cool, clammy skin (warm skin in	• If responsive, monitor airway, breathing, and
bleeding	early onset of septic and	circulation (ABC).
• Ruptured ectopic	neurogenic shock)	• Stabilize cervical spine as appropriate.
pregnancy or	• Cyanosis	• Control any external bleeding with direct pressure or
ovarian cyst	• Decreased level of	pressure dressing.
• Ruptured organ or	consciousness	• Give high-flow O_2 (100%) by nonrebreather mask or bag-
vessel	• Decreased O_2 saturation	valve-mask.
• Vaginal bleeding	• Dysrhythmias	• Anticipate need for intubation and mechanical
	• Extreme thirst	ventilation.
Medical	• Feeling of impending doom	• Establish IV access with 2 large-bore catheters (14- to 16-
• Addisonian crisis	• Hypotension	gauge) or an intraosseous access device; aid with central
• Dehydration	• Narrowed pulse pressure	line insertion.
• Diabetes	• Nausea and vomiting	• Begin fluid resuscitation with crystalloids (e.g., 30 mL/kg
• Diabetes insipidus	• Obvious hemorrhage or injury	repeated until hemodynamic improvement is noted).
• Myocardial infarction	• Pallor	• Draw blood for laboratory studies (e.g., blood cultures,
• Pulmonary embolus	• Rapid, weak, thready pulses	lactate, WBC).

- Sepsis

Trauma
- Fractures, spinal injury
- Multiorgan injury
- Ruptured or lacerated vessel or organ (e.g., spleen)

- Restlessness
- Tachypnea, dyspnea, or shallow, irregular respirations
- Temperature dysregulation
- Weakness

- Assess for life-threatening injuries (e.g., cardiac tamponade, liver laceration, tension pneumothorax).
- Consider vasopressor therapy if hypotension persists after fluid resuscitation.
- Insert an indwelling urinary catheter and nasogastric tube.
- Start antibiotic therapy after blood cultures if sepsis is suspected.
- Obtain 12-lead ECG and treat dysrhythmias.

Ongoing Monitoring
- ABCs
- Level of consciousness
- Vital signs, including pulse oximetry; peripheral pulses, capillary refill, skin color and temperature
- Respiratory status
- Heart rate and rhythm
- Urine output

[a]See Table 66.1 in Harding, et al., *Lewis' Medical-Surgical Nursing, ed 11,* for additional conditions associated with shock.
ECG, Electrocardiogram; *GI,* gastrointestinal; *WBC,* white blood cell.

S

TABLE 78 Interprofessional Care

Shock

Oxygenation	Circulation	Drug Therapies	Supportive Therapies
Cardiogenic shock			
• Provide supplemental O_2 (e.g., nasal cannula, nonrebreather mask) • Intubation and mechanical ventilation, if needed • Monitor $ScvO_2$ or SvO_2	• Restore blood flow with angioplasty with stenting, emergent coronary revascularization • Reduce workload of heart with circulatory assist devices: IABP, VAD	• Nitrates (e.g., nitroglycerin) • Inotropes (e.g., dobutamine) • Diuretics (e.g., furosemide) • β-Adrenergic blockers (contraindicated with ↓ ejection fraction)	• Treat dysrhythmias
Hypovolemic shock			

• Provide supplemental O_2
• Monitor $ScvO_2$ or SvO_2
	• Rapid fluid replacement using 2 large-bore (14-16 gauge) peripheral IV lines, an intraosseous access device, or central venous catheter
	• Restore fluid volume (e.g., blood or blood products, crystalloids)
	• End points of fluid resuscitation:
	  • CVP 15 mm Hg
	  • PAWP 10–12 mm Hg
		• No specific drug therapy	• Correct the cause (e.g., stop bleeding, GI losses)
			• Use warmed IV fluids, including blood products (if appropriate)

Septic shock

- Provide supplemental O_2
- Intubation and mechanical ventilation, if needed
- Monitor $ScvO_2$ or SvO_2

- Aggressive fluid resuscitation (e.g., 30 mL/kg of crystalloids repeated if hemodynamic improvement is noted)
- End points of fluid resuscitation are based on:
  1. Focused physical examination including vital signs, cardiopulmonary assessment, capillary refill, peripheral pulses, and skin or any 2 of the following:
     - $ScvO_2 > 70$ or $SvO_2 > 65$
     - CVP 8–12 mm Hg
     - Cardiovascular ultrasound
  2. Assessment of fluid responsiveness with passive leg raise or fluid challenge

- Antibiotics as ordered
- Vasopressors (e.g., norepinephrine)
- Inotropes (e.g., dobutamine)
- Anticoagulants (e.g., low-molecular-weight heparin)

- Obtain cultures (e.g., blood, wound) before beginning antibiotics
- Monitor temperature
- Control blood glucose
- Stress ulcer prophylaxis

Continued

S

TABLE 78 Interprofessional Care—cont'd

Shock

Oxygenation	Circulation	Drug Therapies	Supportive Therapies
Neurogenic shock			
• Maintain patent airway • Provide supplemental O_2 • Intubation and mechanical ventilation (if needed)	• Cautious administration of fluids	• Vasopressors (e.g., phenylephrine) • Atropine (for bradycardia)	• Minimize spinal cord trauma with stabilization • Monitor temperature
Anaphylactic shock			
• Maintain patent airway • Optimize oxygenation with supplemental O_2 • Intubation and mechanical ventilation, if needed	• Aggressive fluid resuscitation with colloids	• Epinephrine (IM or IV) • Antihistamines (e.g., diphenhydramine) • Histamine (H_2)-receptor blockers (e.g., ranitidine [Zantac]) • Bronchodilators: nebulized (e.g., albuterol) • Corticosteroids (if hypotension persists)	• Identify and remove offending cause • Prevent via avoidance of known allergens • Premedicate with history of prior sensitivity (e.g., contrast media)

Obstructive shock

- Maintain patent airway
- Provide supplemental O_2
- Intubation and mechanical ventilation, if needed

- Restore circulation by treating cause of obstruction
- Fluid resuscitation may provide temporary improvement in CO and BP

- No specific drug therapy

- Treat cause of obstruction (e.g., pericardiocentesis for cardiac tamponade, needle decompression or chest tube insertion for tension pneumothorax, embolectomy for pulmonary embolism)

CO, Cardiac output; *CVP,* central venous pressure; *GI,* gastrointestinal; *IABP,* intraaortic balloon pump; *MAP,* mean arterial pressure; *PAWP,* pulmonary artery wedge pressure; *ScvO2/SvO2,* central venous oxygenation/mixed venous oxygenation; *VAD,* ventricular assist device.

S

Nursing Interventions

You have an important role in the prevention of shock, beginning with the identification of patients at risk. In general, patients who are older or immunocompromised or have chronic illnesses are at an increased risk. Any person who has surgery or trauma is at risk for shock resulting from conditions such as hemorrhage, spinal cord injury, and sepsis.

Your role in shock involves: (1) monitoring the patient's ongoing physical and emotional status, (2) identifying trends to detect changes in the patient's condition, (3) planning and implementing nursing interventions and therapy, (4) evaluating the patient's response to therapy, (5) providing emotional support to the patient and caregiver, and (6) collaborating with other members of the inter-professional team to coordinate care.

Do not overlook or underestimate the effects of fear and anxiety on the patient and caregiver when faced with a critical, life-threatening situation. Fear, anxiety, and pain may aggravate respiratory distress and increase the release of catecholamines.

- Monitor the patient's mental state and level of pain using valid assessment tools. Provide drugs to decrease anxiety and pain as appropriate.
- Talk to the patient and encourage the caregiver to talk to the patient, even if the patient is intubated, sedated, or appears comatose. Patients who cannot respond may still be able to hear. If the intubated patient is capable of writing, provide a "magic slate" or a pencil and paper.
- Do not overlook the patient's spiritual needs. Offer to call a member of the clergy.

Caregivers can have a therapeutic effect on the patient. Encourage caregivers to perform simple comfort measures if desired. Provide privacy and assure the patient and caregivers that assistance is readily available.

Rehabilitation of the patient who has experienced critical illness requires correction of the precipitating cause, prevention or early treatment of complications, and education focused on disease management and/or prevention of recurrence.

- Continue to monitor the patient for complications throughout recovery, including decreased range of motion, decreased physical endurance, renal failure after acute tubular necrosis, and fibrotic lung disease because of acute respiratory distress syndrome (ARDS).
- Patients recovering from shock may require diverse services after discharge. These can include admission to transitional care units (e.g., for mechanical ventilation weaning) or rehabilitation

centers (inpatient or outpatient), or management by home health care agencies. Start planning a safe transition from the hospital to home as soon as the patient is admitted to the hospital.

- See also eNursing Care Plan 66-1: Patient in Shock, on the website.

SICKLE CELL DISEASE

Description

Sickle cell disease (SCD) is a group of inherited, autosomal recessive disorders characterized by an abnormal form of hemoglobin (Hgb) in the red blood cell (RBC). This abnormal Hgb, *hemoglobin S* (Hgb S), causes the erythrocyte to stiffen and elongate, taking on a sickle shape in response to low O_2 levels.

SCD is usually identified during routine neonatal screening. Although median survival can now exceed 45 to 65 years, the disease often results in irreversible damage of the lungs, kidneys, brain, retina or bones and significantly affects patients' quality of life.

Pathophysiology

Types of SCD include sickle cell anemia, sickle cell-thalassemia, sickle cell Hgb C disease, and sickle cell trait. *Sickle cell anemia* is the most severe of the SCD syndromes. It occurs when a person inherits Hgb S from both parents.

Sickle cell-thalassemia and *sickle cell Hgb C* occur when a person inherits Hgb S from 1 parent and another type of abnormal Hgb (e.g., thalassemia or Hgb C) from the other parent. These forms of SCD are less common and less severe than sickle cell anemia.

Sickle cell trait occurs when a person is heterozygous for Hgb S (Hgb AS). The person has inherited Hgb S from 1 parent and normal Hgb (Hgb A) from the other parent. Sickle cell trait is typically a mild condition.

The major pathophysiologic event of SCD is sickling of erythrocytes. Sickling episodes are most commonly triggered by low O_2 tension in the blood. Hypoxia or deoxygenation of the RBCs can be caused by viral or bacterial infection (most common factor), high altitude, emotional stress, surgery, and blood loss. Other triggering events include dehydration acidosis, decreased plasma volume, and low body temperature. A sickling episode can also occur without an obvious cause.

S

- Sickled RBCs become rigid and take on an elongated, crescent shape. Sickled cells cannot easily pass through capillaries or other small vessels and can cause vascular occlusion, leading to acute or chronic tissue injury. The resulting hemostasis promotes a self-perpetuating cycle of local hypoxia, deoxygenation of more erythrocytes, and more sickling.
- Circulating sickled cells are hemolyzed by the spleen, leading to anemia.
- Initially the sickling of cells is reversible with reoxygenation, but eventually the condition becomes irreversible because of cell membrane damage from recurrent sickling.

Sickle cell crisis is a severe, painful, acute exacerbation of erythrocyte sickling causing a vaso-occlusive crisis. As sickled cells impair blood flow, vasospasm occurs, further restricting blood flow. Tissue ischemia, infarction, and necrosis eventually occur from lack of oxygen. Shock is a possible life-threatening consequence because of severe tissue hypoxia and decreased circulating fluid volume. Sickle cell crisis can begin suddenly and persist for weeks.

- The frequency, extent, and severity of sickling episodes are unpredictable but largely depend on the percentage of Hgb S present. People with sickle cell anemia have the most severe form because erythrocytes contain a high percentage of Hgb S.

Clinical Manifestations

Many people with sickle cell anemia are in reasonably good health most of the time. However, they may have chronic health problems and pain because of organ hypoxia and damage (e.g., involving the kidneys or liver). The typical patient is anemic but asymptomatic except during sickling episodes.

- Because most persons with sickle cell anemia have dark skin, pallor is easier to detect by examining the mucous membranes. The skin may have a grayish cast. Because of the hemolysis, jaundice is common. Patients are prone to gallstones (cholelithiasis).
- During sickle cell crisis, the pain of tissue ischemia is quite severe. The back, chest, extremities, and abdomen are most often affected. Pain is accompanied by fever, swelling, tenderness, tachypnea, hypertension, and nausea and vomiting.

Complications

With repeated episodes of sickling, there is gradual involvement of all body systems, especially the spleen, lungs, kidneys, and brain.

- Infection is a major contributor to morbidity and mortality in patients with sickle cell disease. Pneumonia is the most common infection.
- The spleen becomes infarcted, dysfunctional, and small because of repeated scarring.
- *Acute chest syndrome* is a pulmonary complication that includes pneumonia, tissue infarction, and fat embolism, resulting in pulmonary hypertension, myocardial infarction (MI), and ultimately cor pulmonale.
- The kidneys may be injured from the lack of oxygen, resulting in renal failure.
- Stroke can result from thrombosis and infarction of cerebral blood vessels.
- The heart may become ischemic and enlarged, leading to heart failure.
- Retinal vessel obstruction may result in hemorrhage, scarring, retinal detachment, and blindness.
- Bone changes may include osteoporosis and osteosclerosis after infarction. Chronic leg ulcers can result from hypoxia.

Diagnostic Studies

- Peripheral blood smear may reveal sickled cells and abnormal reticulocytes.
- Hgb electrophoresis may be done to determine the amount of Hgb S and SCD from other variants.
- Findings of hemolysis (jaundice, elevated serum bilirubin levels) and abnormal laboratory test results (see Table 8, p. 33) may be present.
- Skeletal x-rays, MRI, and Doppler studies may be used to assess for bone and joint deformities, stroke, and deep vein thromboses, respectively.

Nursing and Interprofessional Management

Care is directed toward preventing and alleviating symptoms from complications of the disease, minimizing end-organ damage, and promptly treating serious sequelae such as acute chest syndrome. Teach patients with SCD to avoid high altitudes, maintain adequate fluid intake, and treat infections promptly. Teach about pain control. The pain during a crisis may be severe and require considerable analgesia.

- Immunizations for pneumococcus, *Haemophilus influenzae,* influenza, and hepatitis should be administered.
- Chronic leg ulcers may be treated with bed rest, antibiotics, warm saline soaks, mechanical or enzyme debridement, and grafting if necessary.

S

- Sickle cell crises may require hospitalization. O_2 may be administered to treat hypoxia and control sickling. Rest may reduce metabolic needs. Fluids and electrolytes are administered to reduce blood viscosity and maintain renal function.
- Priapism is managed with pain medication, fluids, and nifedipine (Procardia). If it does not resolve within a few hours, a urologist may be called.
- Transfusion therapy is indicated when an aplastic crisis occurs. These patients, like those with thalassemia major, may require chelation therapy to reduce transfusion-produced iron overload.
- During an acute crisis, optimal pain control usually includes large doses of continuous (rather than as needed [prn]) opioid analgesics along with breakthrough analgesia, often in the form of patient-controlled analgesia (PCA).
- Acute chest syndrome is treated with broad-spectrum antibiotics, O_2 therapy, and fluid therapy.
- Although many antisickling agents have been tried, hydroxyurea (Hydrea) is the only one to be beneficial. This drug increases the production of Hgb F (fetal Hgb), which is accompanied by reduced hemolysis, increased Hgb concentration, and decreased sickled cells and painful crises.
- Hematopoietic stem cell transplantation (HSCT) is the only available treatment that can cure some patients with SCD, but is not widely available.

SJÖGREN'S SYNDROME

Sjögren's syndrome is a relatively common autoimmune disease that targets the moisture-producing exocrine glands. This leads to xerostomia (dry mouth) and keratoconjunctivitis sicca (dry eyes). The nose, throat, airways, and skin can become dry. The disease may affect other glands, including those in the stomach, pancreas, and intestines (extraglandular involvement). The disease is usually diagnosed in people over age 40 years but can be found in all age groups. Women are 10 times more likely than men to have Sjögren's syndrome.

In primary Sjögren's syndrome, symptoms can be traced to problems with lacrimal and salivary glands. However, 20% to 40% of patients have extended disease affecting the lungs, liver, kidneys, and skin. This occurrence increases the risk for non-Hodgkin's lymphoma.

Sjögren's syndrome appears to be caused by genetic and environmental factors. One gene predisposes whites to the disease. Other genes are linked to the disease in people of Japanese, Chinese, and black ethnicity. The trigger may be a viral or bacterial infection that adversely stimulates the immune system.

In Sjögren's syndrome, lymphocytes attack and damage the lacrimal and salivary glands.

- Decreased tearing causes dry eyes, which leads to a gritty sensation in the eyes, burning, blurred vision, and photosensitivity.
- Dry mouth causes buccal membrane fissures, changes in taste, dysphagia, and increased mouth infection or dental decay.
- Dry skin and rashes, joint and muscle pain, and thyroid problems may be present. Other exocrine glands can be affected. For example, vaginal dryness may lead to painful intercourse (dyspareunia).

Autoimmune thyroid disorders, including Graves' disease and Hashimoto's thyroiditis, are common with Sjögren's syndrome. Histologic study shows lymphocyte infiltration of salivary and lacrimal glands. The disease may become more generalized and involve the lymph nodes, bone marrow, and visceral organs (pseudolymphoma).

Ophthalmologic examination (Schirmer's test for tear production), measures of salivary gland function, and lower lip biopsy of minor salivary glands aid in diagnosis. Treatment is symptomatic, including: (1) instillation of preservative-free artificial tears or ophthalmic antiinflammatory drops (e.g., cyclosporine [Restasis]) as needed for adequate hydration and lubrication, (2) surgical punctal occlusion, and (3) increased fluids with meals. Dental hygiene is important.

Pilocarpine (Salagen) and cevimeline (Evoxac) can be used to treat dry mouth. Increased humidity at home may reduce respiratory tract infections. Vaginal lubrication with a water-soluble product, such as K-Y jelly, may increase comfort during intercourse.

SPINAL CORD INJURY

Description
Spinal cord injury (SCI) can result in temporary or permanent alteration in spinal cord function. Some 282,000 persons in the United States are living with SCI.

- SCIs are usually caused by trauma, including motor vehicle collisions, falls, violence, and sports injuries. Young adult men ages 16 to 30 years have the greatest risk for SCI.

Pathophysiology
The extent of the neurologic damage caused by an SCI results from both *primary injury* (initial disruption of axons) and

secondary injury (processes such as ischemia, hypoxia, hemorrhage, and edema).

Primary SCI can be caused by cord compression by bone displacement, interruption of blood supply, or distraction from pulling on the cord. Penetrating trauma, such as gunshot and stab wounds, causes tearing and transection.

Secondary injury refers to ongoing, progressive damage after the primary injury. Possible causes include vascular changes resulting from hemorrhage, vasospasm, thrombosis, loss of autoregulation, breakdown of the blood-brain barrier, and infiltration of inflammatory cells that cause ischemia, edema, and cellular necrosis.

- *Apoptosis* (programmed cell death) may continue for weeks after injury and may contribute to postinjury demyelination. These processes lead to scar tissue formation, irreversible nerve damage, and permanent neurologic deficit. This ongoing destructive process makes it critical to initiate care and management of the patient with an SCI as soon as possible, to limit the damage.
- The extent of injury and prognosis for recovery are most accurately determined at 72 hours or more after injury. Fig. 21 shows the cascade of events causing secondary injury after traumatic SCI.

Spinal and Neurogenic Shock

Spinal shock may occur after acute SCI. It is characterized by loss of deep tendon and sphincter reflexes, loss of sensation, absent thermoregulation, and flaccid paralysis below the level of injury. This syndrome lasts days to weeks and may mask postinjury neurologic function.

Neurogenic shock results from the loss of vasomotor tone caused by injury and is characterized by hypotension and bradycardia. Loss of sympathetic innervation causes peripheral vasodilation, venous pooling, and decreased cardiac output. These effects are generally associated with a cervical or high thoracic injury.

Classification

SCIs are classified by the mechanism of injury, level of injury, and degree of injury. The major mechanisms of injury are flexion, flexion- rotation, hyperextension, vertical compression, extension-rotation, and lateral flexion. The level of injury may be cervical, thoracic, lumbar, or sacral. Cervical and lumbar injuries are the most common because these areas are associated with the greatest flexibility and movement. The degree of spinal cord involvement may be either complete or incomplete (partial).

- *Complete cord involvement* results in total loss of sensory and motor function below the level of the injury.

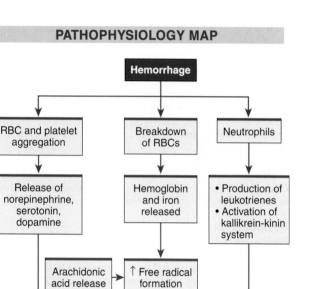

Fig. 21 Cascade of metabolic and cellular events that leads to spinal cord ischemia and hypoxia of secondary injury. *RBCs,* Red blood cells; *SCBF,* spinal cord blood flow.

- *Incomplete cord involvement* (partial transection) results in a mixed loss of voluntary motor activity and sensation and leaves some tracts intact. The degree of sensory and motor loss varies depending on the level of the injury and reflects the specific nerve tracts damaged.
- If the cervical cord is involved, paralysis of all 4 extremities results in *tetraplegia* (formerly termed *quadriplegia*). The lower the level of injury, the more function is retained in the arms.

S

- If the thoracic, lumbar, or sacral spinal cord is damaged, the result is *paraplegia* (paralysis and loss of sensation in the legs).

Clinical Manifestations

Manifestations of SCI are related to the level and degree of injury. The patient with an incomplete lesion may demonstrate a mixture of symptoms—the higher the injury, the more serious the effects because of the proximity of the cervical cord to the medulla and brainstem.

Movement and rehabilitation potential related to specific locations of the SCI are described in Table 60.2, Harding et al., *Lewis' Medical-Surgical Nursing,* ed 11. In general, sensory function closely parallels motor function at all levels.

Complications

Respiratory System

Cervical injuries above the level of C3 vertebra cause a total loss of respiratory muscle function. Injury or fracture at levels C3–C5 can result in diaphragmatic breathing with respiratory insufficiency and hypoventilation.

Cardiovascular System

Cord injury above the level of T6 leads to dysfunction of the sympathetic nervous system. The result is bradycardia, peripheral vasodilation, and hypotension (neurogenic shock).

Urinary System

Urinary retention is common in acute SCI and spinal shock. While the patient is in spinal shock, the bladder is atonic, and fails to empty (urinary retention). In the postacute phase, the bladder may become hyperirritable, with reflex emptying (urinary incontinence).

Gastrointestinal System

Decreased gastrointestinal (GI) motor activity contributes to gastric distention and development of paralytic ileus. Excessive release of hydrochloric acid (HCl) in the stomach may cause stress ulcers. Loss of voluntary control of the bowel after SCI results in neurogenic bowel.

- SCI above the level of the conus medullaris causes the anal sphincter to remain tight, and the ability to sense a full rectum is lost. Bowel movement occurs on a reflex basis when the rectum is full (incontinence).
- SCI at or below the conus medullaris causes the bowel to be areflexic. Peristalsis is impaired and stool propulsion is slow. The defecation reflex may be damaged and anal sphincter tone relaxed (retention). This leads to constipation, increased risk of incontinence, and possible impaction, ileus, or megacolon.

Integumentary System

Lack of movement and sensation increases the potential for skin breakdown over bony prominences. Pressure ulcers can occur quickly, leading to major infection or sepsis.

Thermoregulation

Poikilothermia is the inability to maintain a constant core temperature, with the patient assuming the temperature of the environment. It occurs because the interruption of the sympathetic nervous system prevents peripheral temperature sensations from reaching the hypothalamus. With SCI, there is decreased ability to sweat or shiver below the level of injury, which also affects body temperature regulation.

Peripheral Vascular Problems

Venous thromboembolism (VTE) is a common problem in the first 3 months. Pulmonary embolism is a leading cause of death in patients with SCI.

Pain

Pain after SCI can be nociceptive or neuropathic.

- *Nociceptive pain* in SCI can result from musculoskeletal, visceral, and/or other types of injury (e.g., skin ulceration, headache). Patients often describe musculoskeletal pain as dull or aching. It starts or worsens with movement. Visceral pain is located in the thorax, abdomen, and/or pelvis and may be dull, tender, or cramping.
- *Neuropathic pain* in SCI occurs from damage to the spinal cord or nerve roots. The pain can be located at or below the level of injury. Patients often identify neuropathic pain as hot, burning, tingling, "pins and needles," cold, and/or shooting. Even light touch can cause significant pain.

Autonomic Dysreflexia

Autonomic dysreflexia (also known as *hyperreflexia*) is a massive uncompensated cardiovascular reaction mediated by the sympathetic nervous system. It involves stimulation of sensory receptors below the level of the SCI. The intact sympathetic nervous system below the SCI responds to the stimulation by increasing BP, but the parasympathetic nervous system is unable to directly counteract these responses via the injured spinal cord. Baroreceptors in the carotid sinus and aorta sense the hypertension and stimulate the parasympathetic system. This results in a decreased heart rate, but visceral and peripheral vessels do not dilate because efferent impulses cannot pass through the injured spinal cord.

- *Autonomic hyperreflexia* is a life-threatening situation requiring immediate resolution to prevent status epilepticus, myocardial infarction, stroke, and even death.
- The most common precipitating cause is a distended bladder or rectum.

S

- Manifestations include hypertension, blurred vision, throbbing headache, marked diaphoresis above the level of the lesion, bradycardia (30 to 40 beats/minute), piloerection, nasal congestion, and nausea. Measure BP when the patient with an SCI reports a headache.
- Elevate the head of the bed 45 degrees or sit the patient upright, determine the cause, and notify the health care provider (HCP). If symptoms persist after the source has been relieved, a rapid-onset and short-duration agent, such as nitroglycerin, nitroprusside, or hydralazine, is administered. Continue careful monitoring until vital signs stabilize.
- Teach the patient and caregivers the causes and symptoms of autonomic hyperreflexia (see Table 60.7, Harding et al., *Lewis' Medical-Surgical Nursing,* ed 11). They must understand the life-threatening nature of this dysfunction, know how to relieve the cause, and be prepared to call for emergency care.

Diagnostic Studies

- CT scan is the preferred imaging study to diagnose the location and degree of injury and degree of spinal canal compromise. Cervical x-rays are obtained when CT scan is not readily available.
- MRI is used to assess soft tissue and neurologic changes and for neurologic deficits or worsening of neurologic status.
- Comprehensive neurologic examination is done along with assessment of the head, chest, and abdomen for additional injuries or trauma.
- Patients with cervical injuries who demonstrate altered mental status may need vertebral angiography to rule out vertebral artery damage.

Interprofessional Management

After stabilization at the injury scene, the person is transferred to a health care facility. A thorough assessment is done to evaluate the specific degree of deficit and establish the level and degree of injury. The patient may go directly to surgery after initial immobilization and assessment or to the intensive care unit (ICU) for monitoring and management.

Nonoperative Stabilization

Nonoperative treatments are focused on stabilization of the injured spinal segment and decompression, through either traction or realignment, to prevent secondary spinal cord damage caused by repeated contusion or compression.

Surgical Therapy

When cord compression is certain or the neurologic disorder progresses, immediate surgery may stabilize the spinal column. Early cord decompression is meant to reduce secondary injury.

- A fixation procedure involves attaching metal screws, plates, or other devices to the bones of the spine to help keep them aligned. This is usually done when 2 or more vertebrae have been injured. Small pieces of bone may be attached to the injured area to help the bones fuse into one solid piece.

Drug Therapy

Methylprednisolone is no longer approved by the U.S. Food and Drug Administration (FDA) for treatment in acute SCI.

- Low-molecular-weight heparin (LMWH) (e.g., enoxaparin [Lovenox]) is used to prevent VTE unless contraindicated.
- Vasopressor agents, such as phenylephrine or norepinephrine, are used in the acute phase to maintain mean arterial pressure and the perfusion to the spinal cord.

Nursing Management

Goals

The patient with an SCI will maintain an optimal level of neurologic functioning; have minimal or no complications of immobility; learn new skills, gain new knowledge, and acquire new behaviors to be able to care for self or direct others to do so; and return to home at an optimal level of functioning.

Nursing Interventions

High cervical injury resulting from flexion-rotation is the most complex SCI and is discussed in this section. Interventions for this type of injury can be modified for patients with less severe problems.

Immobilization.

- Proper immobilization of the neck involves maintenance of a neutral position. For cervical injuries, closed reduction with skeletal traction is used for early realignment (reduction) of the injury. Crutchfield or Gardner-Wells tongs or halo (halo ring) can provide this type of traction. A rope extends from the center of the device over a pulley to weights attached at the end. Traction must be maintained at all times. Possible displacement of the skull pins is a disadvantage of tongs. If pin displacement occurs, hold the patient's head in a neutral position and get help. Immobilize the head while the HCP reinserts the tongs.
- Infection at the sites of tong insertion is a potential problem. A common protocol involves cleansing the sites twice a day with chlorhexidine and applying an antibiotic ointment as a mechanical barrier to the entrance of bacteria.

After cervical fusion or other stabilization surgery, a hard cervical collar or sternal-occipital-mandibular immobilizer brace can be worn. A patient with a stable injury may have a halo fixation apparatus applied.

S

Respiratory Problems. The possibility of respiratory arrest requires careful monitoring and readiness for prompt action. If the patient is exhausted from labored breathing or if arterial blood gases indicate inadequate oxygenation or ventilation, endotracheal intubation or tracheostomy and mechanical ventilation are needed. (See Artificial Airways: Endotracheal Tubes, p. 663, Tracheostomy, p. 714, and Mechanical Ventilation, p. 691). Pneumonia and atelectasis may occur because of reduced vital capacity and the loss of intercostal and abdominal muscle function, resulting in diaphragmatic breathing, pooled secretions, and an ineffective cough.

- Regularly assess breath sounds, arterial blood gases (ABGs), tidal volume, vital capacity, skin color, breathing patterns (especially the use of accessory muscles), subjective comments about the effort to breathe, and the amount and color of sputum.
- Support gas exchange and ventilation by the administration of O_2, chest physiotherapy and assisted coughing, incentive spirometry, and tracheal suctioning.

Cardiovascular Instability. If bradycardia is symptomatic, an anticholinergic medication such as atropine is administered. A pacemaker may be inserted (see Pacemakers, p. 707). Hypotension is managed with fluid replacement and a vasopressor agent such as phenylephrine or norepinephrine. Monitor the patient for indications of hypovolemic shock secondary to hemorrhage, which may require blood transfusion.

- Use LMWH or low-dose heparin in combination with intermittent pneumatic compression devices (IPCs) or graduated compression stockings to promote venous return and reduce the risk of VTE.
- Perform range-of-motion (ROM) exercises and stretching regularly. Assess the thighs and calves of the legs for the signs of deep vein thrombosis (DVT) every shift (e.g., deep reddish color, edema).

Fluid and Nutritional Maintenance. If the GI tract stops functioning (paralytic ileus) during the first 48 to 72 hours after the injury, a nasogastric (NG) tube is inserted.

- Once bowel sounds are present or flatus is passed, and the patient is not receiving mechanical ventilation, a formal swallow evaluation should be done. If no risk of aspiration is identified, gradually introduce oral food and fluids.
- If the patient fails the swallow evaluation or is unable to eat because of an endotracheal tube or tracheostomy, a more secure feeding tube may be placed in the stomach or jejunum.

Bowel and Bladder Management. An indwelling catheter is inserted soon after the injury. Strict aseptic technique for catheter care is essential.

- *Catheter-acquired urinary tract infection* (CAUTI) is a common problem. After the patient is stabilized, assess the best means of managing long-term urinary function. Clean intermittent catheterization (CIC) is the preferred method for emptying the bladder.
- To combat constipation from neurogenic bowel, start a bowel program. This consists of a rectal stimulant (suppository or mini-enema) inserted daily, followed by gentle digital stimulation or manual evacuation.

Temperature Control. Monitor the environment and body temperature regularly. Because there is no vasoconstriction, piloerection, or heat loss through perspiration below the level of injury, temperature control is largely external to the patient.

Stress Ulcers. Stress ulcers can occur because of the physiologic response to severe trauma and psychologic stress. Peak incidence is 6 to 14 days after injury. Test stool and gastric contents daily for blood, and monitor hematocrit for a slow drop. Histamine (H_2)-receptor blockers (e.g., ranitidine) or proton pump inhibitors (e.g., pantoprazole, omeprazole) may be given prophylactically to decrease HCl secretion.

Pain Management. Musculoskeletal nociceptive pain can develop from injuries to bones, muscles, and ligaments. The pain is worse with movement or palpation. Antinflammatory drugs, such as ibuprofen (Motrin), may help with pain. Opioids may be used to manage nociceptive pain.

Visceral nociceptive pain is a dull, tender, or cramping pain in the thorax, abdomen, or pelvis. It may originate in the bladder or bowel. Assess the patient's bowel and bladder function to avoid bladder distention or constipation. Other causes of nociceptive pain include urinary tract infection (UTI) and renal stones. Notify the HCP if the patient has persistent pain despite treatment. Diagnostic imaging may be needed to determine the cause.

Neuropathic pain in the initial phase is usually at the level of SCI. It may occur on 1 or both sides of the body within the affected dermatome, and up to 3 levels below. The patient will describe hot, burning, tingling, shooting, electric pain. Pregabalin (Lyrica) is used to reduce pain.

Sensory Deprivation. To prevent sensory deprivation, compensate for the patient's absence of sensations by stimulating the patient above the level of injury. Conversation, music, and interesting foods can be a part of the nursing care plan. If the head of the bed must remain flat, provide prism glasses to help the patient read and watch television. Make every effort to prevent the patient from withdrawing from the environment.

S

Reflexes. Once spinal shock is resolved, reflexes often return with hyperactive and exaggerated responses. Penile erections can occur from a variety of stimuli, causing embarrassment and discomfort. Spasms ranging from mild twitches to convulsive movements below the level of the lesion may also occur. Reflex activity may be interpreted by the patient or caregiver as a return of function. Tactfully explain the reason for the activity. Spasms may be controlled with antispasmodic medications such as baclofen, dantrolene (Dantrium), or tizanidine (Zanaflex).

Rehabilitation. Physiologic and psychologic rehabilitation is complex. Many of the problems identified in the acute period may continue throughout life. Rehabilitation focuses on refined retraining of physiologic processes and extensive patient, caregiver, and family teaching about how to manage the changes resulting from injury.

Rehabilitation and long-term management of the SCI patient are further described in Chapter 60 of Harding et al., *Lewis' Medical-Surgical Nursing,* ed 11.

SPINAL CORD TUMORS

Description

Spinal cord tumors are classified as *primary* (arising from some component of cord, dura, nerves, or vessels) or *secondary* (from primary growths that have metastasized to the spinal cord).

Spinal cord tumors are further classified as *extradural* (outside the dura), *intradural-extramedullary* (between the spinal cord and dura), and *intramedullary* (within the substance of spinal cord itself) (see Fig. 60.12 and Table 60.13, Harding et al., *Lewis' Medical-Surgical Nursing,* ed 11).

Symptoms associated with spinal cord tumors are caused by the mechanical effects of slow compression and irritation of nerve roots, displacement of the spinal cord, or gradual obstruction of the vascular supply. The slow growth does not cause a secondary injury as in traumatic spinal cord injury (SCI), so complete function may be possible after the tumor is removed.

Clinical Manifestations

A common early symptom of a spinal cord tumor is back pain, with the location depending on the level of compression. The pain worsens with activity, coughing, straining, and lying down.

- Slowly increasing clumsiness, weakness, spasticity, and paralysis can develop.

- Sensory disruption occurs as coldness, numbness, and tingling in 1 or more extremities.
- Bladder problems are marked by urgency, with difficulty in starting the flow and progressing to retention with overflow incontinence.

Diagnostic Studies

Extradural tumors can be seen on routine spinal x-rays. Intradural and intramedullary tumors require MRI or CT scans or CT myelogram for detection. Cerebrospinal fluid (CSF) analysis may reveal tumor cells.

Nursing and Interprofessional Management

Spinal cord compression is an emergency. Relief of the ischemia related to the compression is the goal of therapy. Corticosteroids (e.g., dexamethasone) are given immediately to relieve tumor-related edema.

Indications for surgery vary depending on the type of tumor. Emergency surgery may be needed to decompress the spinal cord, obtain tissue for pathology, and determine appropriate adjunctive treatment. Primary spinal tumors may be removed with the goal of cure. In patients with metastatic tumors, treatment is primarily palliative, with the goal of restoring or preserving neurologic function, stabilizing the spine, and alleviating pain.

Radiation therapy and/or chemotherapy may be used to treat the tumor.

- Ensure that the patient receives pain medication as needed.
- Assess the patient's neurologic status before and after treatment. Depending on the neurologic dysfunction, the patient may require care similar to that of a patient recovering from an SCI. Rehabilitation of patients with spinal cord tumors is similar to SCI rehabilitation. (See Spinal Cord Injury, p. 567.)

SPLEEN DISORDERS

Many illnesses can affect the spleen. Most can cause some degree of *splenomegaly* (enlarged spleen). However, an enlarged spleen may be present in some people without any evidence of disease.

- The degree of splenic enlargement varies with the disease. Massive splenic enlargement occurs with chronic myelogenous leukemia and thalassemia major, whereas mild splenic enlargement occurs with heart failure and systemic lupus erythematosus. When the spleen enlarges, its normal blood cell filtering and

S

storage capacity increases, reducing the number of circulating blood cells.

A slight to moderate enlargement of the spleen is usually asymptomatic and found during routine examination of the abdomen. Massive splenomegaly may be tolerated. Patients report abdominal discomfort and early satiety. In addition to physical examination, other techniques to assess spleen size include radionuclide colloid liver-spleen scan, CT or positron emission tomography (PET) scan, MRI, and ultrasound scan.

Occasionally splenectomy is done for treatment of splenomegaly. Another indication for splenectomy is splenic rupture from trauma and diseases such as mononucleosis, malaria, and cancers. After a splenectomy, peripheral red blood cell (RBC), white blood cell (WBC), and platelet counts can increase dramatically.

Nursing responsibilities for patients with spleen disorders vary.

- Splenomegaly may be painful and require analgesics.
- Take care in moving, turning, and positioning; and evaluation of lung expansion, because spleen enlargement may impair diaphragmatic excursion.
- If anemia, thrombocytopenia, or leukopenia develops from splenic enlargement, institute nursing measures to support the patient and prevent life-threatening complications.
- If splenectomy was performed, observe the patient for hemorrhage and shock.
- After a splenectomy, patients may develop immunologic deficiencies and be at lifelong risk for infection from encapsulated organisms, such as pneumococcus. This risk is reduced by immunization with pneumococcal vaccine.

STOMACH CANCER

Description

Stomach (gastric) cancer is an adenocarcinoma of the stomach wall. The average age at diagnosis is 68 years. The overall 5-year survival rate of all people with stomach cancer is about 31%.

Pathophysiology

Many factors have been implicated in stomach cancer. Stomach cancer probably begins with a nonspecific mucosal injury as a result of infection (with *Helicobacter pylori*) or repeated exposure to irritants, such as bile, nonsteroidal antiinflammatory drugs (NSAIDs), or tobacco. Stomach cancer has also been associated with diets containing smoked foods, salted fish and meat, and pickled vegetables.

Other predisposing factors are obesity, family history, atrophic gastritis, pernicious anemia, adenomatous and hyperplastic polyps, and achlorhydria (absent or low production of gastric hydrochloric acid [HCl]). Consumption of whole grains and fresh fruits and vegetables is associated with reduced rates of stomach cancer.

Stomach cancer spreads by direct extension and typically infiltrates rapidly to the surrounding tissue and liver. Seeding of tumor cells into the peritoneal cavity occurs later in the disease.

Clinical Manifestations

Stomach cancers often spread to adjacent organs before any distressing symptoms occur. Clinical manifestations include unexplained weight loss, early satiety, indigestion, abdominal discomfort or pain, and signs and symptoms of anemia.

- Anemia occurs with chronic blood loss as the lesion erodes the stomach mucosa. The patient appears pale and weak with fatigue, dizziness, weakness, and positive occult stools.
- Supraclavicular lymph nodes that are hard and enlarged suggest metastasis via the thoracic duct. Ascites is a poor prognostic sign.

Diagnostic Studies

- Upper gastrointestinal (GI) endoscopy is the best diagnostic tool.
- Endoscopic ultrasound and CT and positron emission tomography (PET) scans can be used to stage the disease.
- Laparoscopy can be done to determine peritoneal spread.
- Blood studies detect anemia and also elevations in liver enzymes and serum amylase, which may indicate liver and pancreatic involvement.
- Stool examination provides evidence of occult or gross bleeding.

Interprofessional Management

Treatment of choice is surgical removal of the tumor. Surgical procedures used are similar to those used for peptic ulcer disease (see Peptic Ulcer Disease, p. 471).

Preoperative management focuses on correcting nutritional deficits and transfusing red blood cells (RBCs) to treat anemia. Gastric decompression may be needed if gastric outlet obstruction is present. Special preparation of the bowel is needed if the tumor has involved the colon.

- Therapy for localized stomach cancer is surgical resection followed by chemotherapy agents used in combination. These include fluorouracil, capecitabine (Xeloda), carboplatin, cisplatin, docetaxel (Taxotere), epirubicin (Ellence), irinotecan (Camptosar), oxaliplatin (Eloxatin), and paclitaxel. Intraperitoneal administration of

S

chemotherapy agents may also be used to treat metastatic disease (see Chemotherapy, p. 674).

- Trastuzumab (Herceptin) and ramucirumab (Cyramza) are targeted therapy agents used to treat stomach cancer. Ramucirumab binds to the receptor for vascular endothelial growth factor (VEGF) and prevents VEGF from binding to the receptor, thus preventing the growth and spread of cancer.

- The surgical aim is to remove the tumor and a margin of normal tissue. When the lesion is located in the fundus, a total gastrectomy with esophagojejunostomy is performed. Lesions located in the antrum or the pyloric region generally are treated by either a Billroth I or II procedure. When metastasis has occurred to adjacent organs, such as the spleen, ovaries, or bowel, the surgical procedure is modified and extended as necessary.

Radiation therapy may be used as a palliative measure to decrease tumor mass and provide temporary relief of obstruction (see Radiation Therapy, p. 712).

Nursing Management

Goals

The overall goals are that the patient with stomach cancer will experience minimal discomfort, achieve optimal nutritional status, and maintain a degree of spiritual and psychologic well-being appropriate to the disease stage.

Nursing Interventions

Your role in the early detection of stomach cancer focuses on identifying patients at risk, such as those with *H. pylori* infection, pernicious anemia, or achlorhydria. Encourage patients with a positive family history of stomach cancer to undergo diagnostic evaluation if manifestations of anemia, peptic ulcer disease, or vague epigastric distress are present.

When diagnostic tests confirm cancer, offer emotional and physical support, provide information, and clarify test results. Patient teaching is similar to that for peptic ulcer disease surgery (see p. 471 under Peptic Ulcer Disease).

Postoperative care is also similar to that after a Billroth I or II procedure for peptic ulcer disease. When a total gastrectomy is done, closely observe the patient for signs of fluid leakage at the site of anastomosis, as evidenced by an elevation in temperature and increasing dyspnea. Dumping syndrome may also occur with this procedure (see pp. 472 under Peptic Ulcer Disease).

- Postoperative wound healing may be impaired because of poor nutritional intake. IV or oral replacement of vitamins C, D, and K; the B complex vitamins; and cobalamin may be needed because they are normally absorbed in the duodenum.

▼ Patient and Caregiver Teaching
Before discharge, teach the patient and caregivers about comfort measures and the use of analgesics. Additional considerations include:

- Recurrence of cancer is common, and patients need regular follow-up examinations and imaging assessments.
- Teach wound care, if needed, to the primary caregiver in the home setting.
- Dressings, special equipment, or special services may be required for the patient's continued care at home.
- Provide a list of community resources and referral to Home Health services, if needed.

STROKE

Description
- *Stroke* occurs when there is ischemia to a part of the brain or hemorrhage into the brain that results in brain cell death. Movement, sensation, or emotions controlled by the affected brain area are lost or impaired. Severity of the stroke varies according to the location and extent of the damage. Stroke is the fifth most common cause of death in the United States. An estimated 800,000 people have a stroke annually, and 15% to 30% will live with permanent disability.
- The terms *brain attack* and *cerebrovascular accident* (CVA) are also used to describe stroke. The term *brain attack* communicates the urgency of recognizing the warning signs of a stroke and treating it as a medical emergency, as would be done with a heart attack (Table 79).

Risk factors associated with stroke can be divided into nonmodifiable and modifiable. Stroke risk increases with multiple risk factors.

Nonmodifiable risk factors include age, ethnicity or race, and family history or heredity. Two-thirds of all strokes occur in persons older than 65 years, but stroke can occur at any age. Strokes are more common in men, but more women die from stroke than men.

- Blacks have a higher incidence and a higher death rate from stroke than any other ethnic group. This may be related in part to an increased incidence of hypertension, obesity, and diabetes.
- People with a family history of stroke are at higher risk for stroke.

Modifiable risk factors include hypertension, heart disease, diabetes, smoking, obesity, sleep apnea, metabolic syndrome, lack of

S

TABLE 79 Patient and Caregiver Teaching

FAST for Warning Signs of Stroke

FAST is an easy way to remember the signs of stroke. Include the following information in the teaching plan for a patient at risk for stroke and the patient's caregiver.

F	Face drooping	Does one side of the face droop or is it numb? Ask the person to smile. Is the smile uneven?
A	Arm weakness	Is one arm weak or numb? Ask the person to raise both arms. Does one arm drift downward?
S	Speech difficulties	Is speech slurred? Is the person unable to speak or hard to understand? Ask the person to repeat a simple sentence like "The sky is blue." Is the sentence repeated correctly?
T	Time	Time is CRITICAL! If someone shows any of these signs (even if they go away), call 911 and get the person to the hospital. Note the time when the signs first appeared.

In addition, report the sudden onset of the following:
- confusion
- numbness or weakness, especially in one side of the body
- severe headache with no known cause
- trouble seeing in 1 or both eyes
- trouble walking, dizziness, loss of balance or coordination

Source: American Stroke Association: FAST. Retrieved from <www.strokeassociation.org/STROKEORG/WarningSigns/Stroke-Warning-Signs-and-Symptoms_UCM_308528_SubHomePage.jsp>.

physical exercise, poor diet, and drug or alcohol use. Hypertension is the most important modifiable risk factor. Proper treatment of hypertension reduces stroke risk by up to 50%.

Transient Ischemic Attack

A *transient ischemic attack* (TIA) is a transient episode of neurologic dysfunction caused by focal brain, spinal cord, or retinal ischemia, but without acute brain infarction. TIAs may be caused by microemboli that temporarily block the blood flow. Clinical symptoms typically last < 1 hour. TIAs are a warning sign of progressive CVA.

Most TIAs resolve. However, it is important to teach the patient to seek treatment for any stroke symptoms because there is no way to predict if a TIA will resolve. One-third of those who have a TIA will not have another one, one-third will have more TIAs, and one-third will progress to stroke.

TIA signs and symptoms depend on the blood vessel involved and the brain area that is ischemic.

- If the carotid system is involved, patients may have a temporary loss of vision in one eye, transient hemiparesis, numbness or loss of sensation, or a sudden inability to speak.
- Signs and symptoms of a TIA involving the vertebrobasilar system may include tinnitus, vertigo, darkened or blurred vision, ptosis, dysphagia, ataxia, and unilateral or bilateral numbness or weakness.

A TIA is a medical emergency. Teach people at risk for TIA to seek medical attention at once with any stroke-like symptom and to identify the time of symptom onset.

Pathophysiology

Strokes are classified as ischemic or hemorrhagic, based on the cause and underlying pathophysiology (Fig. 22 and Table 80).

Ischemic Stroke

An *ischemic stroke* results from inadequate blood flow to the brain from partial or complete occlusion of an artery. Ischemic strokes may be either thrombotic or embolic.

Thrombotic Stroke. A *thrombotic stroke* occurs from injury to a blood vessel wall and formation of a blood clot. The lumen of the blood vessel becomes narrowed, and if it becomes occluded, infarction occurs. It is the most common cause of stroke.

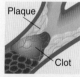

Thrombotic stroke. The process of clot formation (thrombosis) results in a narrowing of the lumen, which blocks the passage of the blood through the artery.

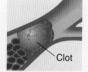

Embolic stroke. An embolus is a blood clot or other debris circulating in the blood. When it reaches an artery in the brain that is too narrow to pass through, it lodges there and blocks the flow of blood.

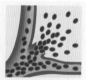

Hemorrhagic stroke. A burst blood vessel may allow blood to seep into and damage brain tissues until clotting shuts off the leak.

Fig. 22 Major causes of stroke.

TABLE 80 Types of Stroke

Gender and Age	Warning and Onset	Prognosis
Ischemic *Incidence:* accounts for 87% of strokes		
Embolic Men more than women	*Warning:* TIA (uncommon) *Onset:* sudden onset, most likely to occur during activity	Single event, signs and symptoms develop quickly, usually some improvement, recurrence common without aggressive treatment of underlying disease.
Thrombotic Men more than women Oldest median age	*Warning:* TIA (30%–50% of cases) *Onset:* often during or after sleep	Stepwise progression, signs and symptoms develop slowly, usually some improvement, recurrence in 20%–25% of survivors.
Hemorrhagic *Incidence:* Accounts for 13% of strokes		
Intracerebral Slightly higher in women	*Warning:* headache (25% of cases) *Onset:* activity (often)	Progression over 24 hr. Poor prognosis, fatality more likely with presence of coma.
Subarachnoid Slightly higher in women Youngest median age	*Warning:* headache (common) *Onset:* activity (often), sudden onset, most often related to head trauma	Usually single sudden event, fatality more likely with presence of coma.

- Thrombotic strokes are more common in older adults. Most thrombotic strokes are associated with hypertension or diabetes. The extent of the stroke depends on speed of onset, size of the lesion, and presence of collateral circulation. Many times, a TIA precedes a thrombotic stroke.
- Most patients do not have a decreased level of consciousness in the first 24 hours unless it is caused by a brainstem stroke or a condition such as seizures, increased intracranial pressure (ICP), or hemorrhage.
- Ischemic stroke symptoms may progress in the first 72 hours as infarction and cerebral edema increase.

Embolic Stroke. *Embolic stroke* occurs when an embolus lodges in and occludes a cerebral artery, resulting in infarction and edema of the area supplied by the involved vessel. Embolism is the second most common cause of stroke.

Most emboli originate in the heart. The embolus travels to the cerebral circulation and lodges where a vessel narrows. Heart conditions associated with emboli are atrial fibrillation, myocardial infarction (MI), and inflammatory and valvular heart conditions.

- The embolic stroke often occurs rapidly. The patient usually remains conscious, and may have a headache.
- Recurrence is common unless the underlying cause is aggressively treated.

Hemorrhagic Stroke

A *hemorrhagic stroke* results from bleeding into the brain tissue (intracerebral or intraparenchymal hemorrhage) or into the subarachnoid space or ventricles (subarachnoid hemorrhage [SAH]).

Intracerebral Hemorrhage. *Intracerebral hemorrhage* is bleeding within the brain caused by a rupture of a blood vessel. Hypertension is the most important cause of intracerebral hemorrhage. Other causes include vascular malformations, coagulation disorders, anticoagulant drugs, trauma, and ruptured aneurysm.

- Hemorrhage often occurs during periods of activity. Most often there is a sudden onset of symptoms, progressing over minutes to hours caused by ongoing bleeding.
- Manifestations include neurologic deficits, headache, nausea, vomiting, decreased level of consciousness, and hypertension. Extent of the symptoms varies depending on the amount, location, and duration of bleeding.
- Prognosis of patients with intracerebral hemorrhage is poor, with 40% to 80% of patients dying within 30 days, and 50% of the deaths occurring within the first 48 hours.

Subarachnoid Hemorrhage. *SAH* occurs when there is intracranial bleeding into the cerebrospinal fluid (CSF)–filled space between the arachnoid and pia mater membranes on the surface of the brain.

S

SAH is often caused by rupture of a cerebral aneurysm (a lesion of congenital or acquired weakness with ballooning of vessels). Other causes of SAH include arteriovenous malformations (AVMs), trauma, and cocaine use.

- The patient may have warning symptoms if the ballooning artery applies pressure to brain tissue. Minor warning symptoms may result from leaking of an aneurysm before major rupture. Sudden onset of a severe headache that is typically the "worst headache of one's life" is a characteristic symptom of a ruptured aneurysm.
- Loss of consciousness may occur, and the patient's level of consciousness may range from alert to comatose, depending on the severity of the bleeding.
- Other manifestations include focal neurologic deficits (including cranial nerve deficits), nausea, vomiting, seizures, and stiff neck.
- Despite improvements in surgical techniques and management, many patients with SAH die or are left with significant disability.

Clinical Manifestations

Neurologic manifestations do not significantly differ between ischemic and hemorrhagic stroke, because destruction of neural tissue is the basis of manifestations for both types of stroke. Manifestations are related to the location of the stroke. Manifestations seen with specific cerebral artery involvement are listed in Table 81. Fig. 23 illustrates manifestations of right- and left-sided stroke.

TABLE 81	Stroke Manifestations Related to Artery Involvement
Artery	**Manifestations**
Anterior cerebral	Motor and/or sensory deficit (contralateral), sucking or rooting reflex, rigidity, gait problems, loss of proprioception and fine touch
Middle cerebral	*Dominant side:* aphasia, motor and sensory deficit, hemianopsia *Nondominant side:* neglect, motor and sensory deficit, hemianopsia
Posterior cerebral	Hemianopsia, visual hallucination, spontaneous pain, motor deficit
Vertebral	Cranial nerve deficits, diplopia, dizziness, nausea, vomiting, dysarthria, dysphagia, and/or coma

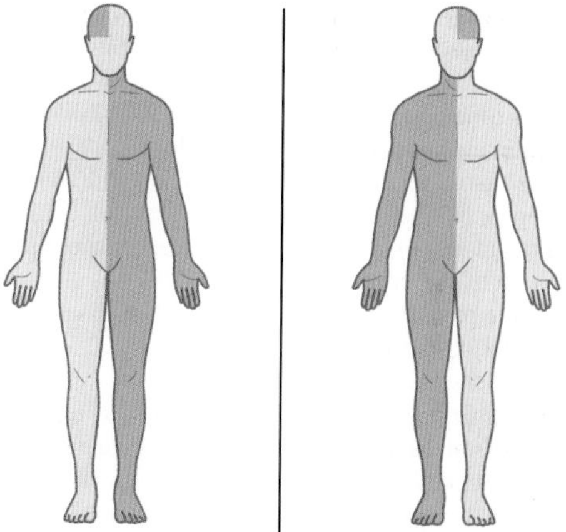

Right-brain damage
(stroke on right side of the brain)

- Paralyzed left side: hemiplegia
- Left-sided neglect
- Spatial-perceptual deficits
- Tends to deny or minimize problems
- Rapid performance, short attention span
- Impulsive, safety problems
- Impaired judgment
- Impaired time concepts

Left-brain damage
(stroke on left side of the brain)

- Paralyzed right side: hemiplegia
- Impaired speech/language aphasias
- Impaired right/left discrimination
- Slow performance, cautious
- Aware of deficits: depression, anxiety
- Impaired comprehension related to language, math

Fig. 23 Manifestations of right- and left-brain stroke.

Motor Function

Motor deficits are the most obvious effect of stroke. Motor deficits include impairment of: (1) mobility, (2) respiratory function, (3) swallowing and speech, (4) gag reflex, and (5) self-care abilities. Symptoms are caused by the destruction of motor neurons in the pyramidal pathway (nerve fibers from the brain that pass through the spinal cord to the motor cells). Because the pyramidal pathway crosses at the level of the medulla, a lesion on one side of the brain affects motor function on the opposite side of the brain (contralateral). Impaired spatial-perceptual orientation may further affect mobility.

S

- The initial *hyporeflexia* (depressed reflexes) progresses to *hyperreflexia* (hyperactive reflexes) for most patients.

Communication

The left hemisphere is dominant for language skills in all right-handed people and most left-handed people.

- Language disorders involve the expression and comprehension of written or spoken words. *Aphasia* (loss of comprehension and use of language) occurs when a stroke damages the dominant hemisphere of the brain.
- Many stroke patients have *dysarthria,* a disturbance in the muscular control of speech.

Affect

Patients who have had a stroke may have a hard time expressing emotions. Emotional responses may be exaggerated or unpredictable. Depression and feelings associated with changes in body image and loss of function can make this worse. Patients may be frustrated by mobility and communication problems.

Intellectual Function

Patients who have had a stroke may show impaired memory and judgment.

Diagnostic Studies

Diagnostic study results confirm manifestations of a stroke, identify likely causes, and guide decisions about therapy.

- MRI is more effective in identifying ischemic stroke than CT scans. However, CT scan is a rapid tool to rule out hemorrhage.
- CT angiography (CTA) provides visualization of cerebral blood vessels and an estimate of perfusion. CTA also detects filling defects in the cerebral arteries.
- Magnetic resonance angiography (MRA) can detect vascular lesions and blockages similar to CTA.
- Angiography can identify cervical and cerebrovascular occlusion, atherosclerotic plaques, and malformation of vessels.
- Intraarterial digital subtraction angiography (DSA) involves injection of a contrast agent to visualize vessels in the neck and circle of Willis.
- Transcranial Doppler (TCD) ultrasonography has been effective in detecting microemboli and vasospasm in the major cerebral arteries.
- If the suspected cause of the stroke includes emboli from the heart, diagnostic cardiac tests should be done.

Interprofessional Management

Prevention

The goals of stroke prevention include management of modifiable risk factors to prevent a stroke. Health promotion focuses on: (1) healthy diet, (2) weight control, (3) regular exercise, (4) not smoking, (5) limiting alcohol consumption, (6) BP management, and (7) routine health assessments. Patients with known risk factors such as DM, hypertension, obesity, high serum lipids, or cardiac problems require close management.

- Measures to prevent the development of a thrombus or embolus are used in patients with TIAs because they are at high risk for stroke. Antiplatelet drugs are usually the chosen treatment to prevent stroke in patients who have had a TIA. Aspirin at a dose of 81 mg/day is the most often used antiplatelet agent.
- Other drugs include ticlopidine, clopidogrel (Plavix), dipyridamole (Persantine), and combined dipyridamole and aspirin (Aggrenox).
- For patients who have atrial fibrillation, oral anticoagulation can include warfarin (Coumadin) and the direct factor Xa inhibitors: rivaroxaban (Xarelto), dabigatran (Pradaxa), and apixaban (Eliquis).
- Statins (simvastatin [Zocor], lovastatin) have been shown to be effective in the prevention of stroke for people who have had a TIA in the past.
- Surgical therapy for the patient with TIA from carotid disease includes carotid endarterectomy, transluminal angioplasty, and stenting.

Acute Care: Ischemic Stroke

The goals of acute care are preserving life, preventing further brain damage, and reducing disability. In the unresponsive person, acute care begins with managing the airway, breathing, and circulation. O_2 administration, artificial airway insertion, intubation, and mechanical ventilation may be required. Table 57.8, Harding et al., *Lewis' Medical-Surgical Nursing*, ed 11, outlines emergency management of the patient with a stroke.

- A key assessment is to determine the time of the onset of symptoms. This is important for all types of stroke, especially ischemic strokes since the time can affect treatment decisions.
- Once the person suspected of TIA or stroke arrives in the emergency department, it is important for the patient to rapidly undergo either a noncontrast head CT or MRI.
- After baseline neurologic assessment, patients are monitored closely for increasing neurologic deficits.
- Elevated BP is common right after a stroke and may be a protective response to maintain cerebral perfusion. After ischemic stroke in those patients who do not receive fibrinolytic therapy, the use of drugs to lower BP is recommended only if BP is markedly increased (systolic BP > 220 mm Hg or diastolic > 120 mm Hg).

S

■ Fluid and electrolyte balance must be controlled carefully. Adequate fluid intake is a priority but overhydration may increase cerebral edema. Managing increased ICP includes practices that improve venous drainage, such as elevating the head of the bed, maintaining head and neck in alignment, and avoiding hip flexion. For additional measures that reduce ICP, see Increased Intracranial Pressure, p. 331.

Drug Therapy. Recombinant tissue plasminogen activator (tPA) is given IV to reestablish blood flow and prevent cell death for patients with acute onset of ischemic stroke. This drug must be given within 3 to 4.5 hours of the onset of clinical signs. Patients are screened carefully before tPA is given, including a CT or MRI scan to rule out hemorrhagic stroke, blood tests for coagulation disorders, and screening for recent history of gastrointestinal (GI) bleeding, head trauma, or major surgery.

■ During tPA infusion, closely monitor the patient's vital signs to assess for improvement or deterioration related to intracerebral hemorrhage.

■ Control of BP is critical during and for 24 hours after treatment.

■ Aspirin may be started at a dose of 325 mg within 24 to 48 hours of an ischemic stroke.

■ For patients who have atrial fibrillation, oral anticoagulants include warfarin and the direct factor Xa inhibitors: rivaroxaban (Xarelto), dabigatran (Pradaxa), and apixaban (Eliquis). Platelet inhibitors include aspirin, ticlopidine, clopidogrel, and dipyridamole.

■ Statins are effective after an ischemic stroke.

Surgical Therapy. Stent retrievers (e.g., Solitaire FR, Trevo) are a way to open blocked arteries in the brain using a removable stent system. Stent retrievers are becoming the most effective way of managing ischemic stroke.

Acute Care: Hemorrhagic Stroke

Drug Therapy. Anticoagulants and platelet inhibitors are contraindicated in patients with hemorrhagic stroke. The main drug therapy for patients with hemorrhagic stroke is for managing hypertension. Oral and IV agents may be used to maintain BP within a normal to high-normal range (systolic BP < 160 mm Hg).

■ Seizure prophylaxis in the acute period after hemorrhagic stroke is situation-specific.

Surgical Therapy. Surgical interventions for hemorrhagic stroke include immediate evacuation of aneurysm-induced hematomas or cerebellar hematomas larger than 3 cm. Persons who have an AVM may have a hemorrhagic stroke if the AVM ruptures.

- Treatment of AVM is surgical resection and/or radiosurgery (i.e., gamma knife). Both may be preceded by interventional neuroradiology procedures to embolize the blood vessels that supply the AVM.

Subarachnoid hemorrhage is usually caused by a ruptured aneurysm. Patients may have multiple aneurysms. Treatment of an aneurysm involves clipping or coiling the aneurysm to prevent rebleeding.

- After aneurysmal occlusion via clipping or coiling, hyperdynamic therapy (hemodilution-induced hypertension achieved using vasoconstricting agents such as phenylephrine or dopamine and hypervolemia) may be instituted to increase the mean arterial pressure and cerebral perfusion. Volume expansion is achieved with crystalloid or colloid solution.
- Patients with SAH may receive the calcium-channel blocker, nimodipine, to treat cerebral vasospasms and minimize cerebral damage.
- SAH and intracerebral hemorrhage can involve bleeding into the ventricles of the brain. Insertion of a ventriculostomy can dramatically improve CSF drainage.

Rehabilitation Care

After the stroke has stabilized for 12 to 24 hours, care shifts from preserving life to lessening disability and reaching optimal function. Many of the interventions discussed in the acute phase are maintained during this phase.

Nursing Management
Goals

Establish the goals of nursing care together with the patient, caregiver, and family. Typical goals are that the patient will: (1) maintain a stable or improved level of consciousness, (2) achieve maximum physical functioning, (3) attain maximum self-care abilities and skills, (4) maintain stable body functions (e.g., bladder control), (5) maximize communication abilities, (6) maintain adequate nutrition, (7) avoid complications of stroke, and (8) maintain effective personal and family coping.

See eNursing Care Plan 57-1 for the patient with stroke on the website.

Nursing Interventions

Respiratory System. During the acute phase after a stroke, management of respiratory function is a nursing priority. An oropharyngeal airway may be used in comatose patients to prevent the tongue from falling back and obstructing the airway and to provide access for suctioning. Alternatively, a nasopharyngeal airway

S

may be used to provide airway protection and access. Interventions include frequently assessing airway patency and function, providing oxygenation, suctioning, promoting patient mobility, positioning the patient to prevent aspiration, and encouraging deep breathing.

Neurologic System. The primary clinical assessment tool to evaluate and document neurologic status in acute stroke patients is the National Institutes of Health (NIH) Stroke Scale (NIHSS), which measures stroke severity (see NIHSS in Table 57.11, Harding et al., *Lewis' Medical-Surgical Nursing,* ed 11). Other neurologic assessment includes mental status, pupillary responses, and extremity movement and strength. Closely monitor vital signs. A decreasing level of consciousness may indicate increasing ICP.

Cardiovascular System. Nursing goals for the cardiovascular system are aimed at maintaining homeostasis. Interventions include: (1) monitoring vital signs frequently; (2) monitoring cardiac rhythms; (3) calculating intake and output, noting imbalances; (4) regulating IV infusions; (5) adjusting fluid intake to the individual needs of the patient; (6) monitoring lung sounds for crackles and rhonchi indicating pulmonary congestion; and (7) monitoring heart sounds for murmurs or for S_3 or S_4 heart sounds.

- After a stroke, the patient is at risk for venous thromboembolism (VTE), especially in a weak or paralyzed lower extremity. The most effective prevention is to keep the patient moving. Teach active range-of-motion (ROM) exercises if the patient has voluntary movement in the affected extremity. For the patient with hemiplegia, perform passive ROM exercises several times each day.
- Other measures to prevent VTE include positioning to minimize the effects of dependent edema and the use of intermittent pneumatic compression devices.

Musculoskeletal System. The goal for the musculoskeletal system is to maintain optimal function, which is accomplished by prevention of joint contractures and muscle atrophy.

- In the acute phase, ROM exercises and positioning are important interventions. Passive ROM exercise is begun on the first day of hospitalization. Muscle atrophy from lack of innervation and inactivity can develop after a stroke, so exercise is important for rehabilitation and recovery.

Interventions to optimize musculoskeletal function include: (1) trochanter roll at the hip to prevent external rotation; (2) hand cones (not rolled washcloths) to prevent hand contractures; (3) arm supports with slings and lap boards to prevent shoulder displacement; (4) avoidance of pulling the patient by the arm to avoid shoulder displacement; (5) posterior leg splints, footboards, or high-top tennis shoes to prevent footdrop; and (6) hand splints to reduce spasticity.

Integumentary System. Interventions for preventing skin breakdown include: (1) pressure relief by position changes, special mattresses, or wheelchair cushions; (2) good skin hygiene; (3) emollients applied to dry skin; and (4) early mobility. An example of a position change schedule is side-back-side, with a maximum duration of 2 hours for any position.

- Position the patient on the weak or paralyzed side for no more than 30 minutes. Control of pressure is the single most important factor in both the prevention and treatment of skin breakdown (see Pressure Injury, p. 494.)

Gastrointestinal System. The most common bowel problem is constipation. Fluid and fiber intake goals are determined with the stroke team based on the patient's nutritional and fluid status. Physical activity also promotes bowel function. Laxatives, suppositories, or additional stool softeners may be ordered if the patient does not respond to increased fluid and fiber. Bowel retraining may be needed and continued into the rehabilitation phase.

Urinary System. In the acute stage of stroke, the primary urinary problem is poor bladder control, resulting in incontinence.

- Take steps to promote normal bladder function and avoid the use of an indwelling catheter.
- Long-term use of an indwelling catheter is associated with urinary tract infections and delayed bladder retraining. An intermittent catheterization program may be used for patients with urinary retention.

Nutrition. The patient may initially receive IV infusions to maintain fluid and electrolyte balance and to administer drugs. Patients should have their nutritional needs addressed in the first 72 hours of admission to the hospital, because nutrition is important for recovery and healing. Some patients may require enteral or parenteral nutrition support.

- Many patients have dysphagia after a stroke. Keep patients NPO until a speech therapist performs a swallowing evaluation within 24 hours after the stroke. Another member of the interprofessional team may perform the screen if a speech therapist is not available.
- To assess swallowing ability, elevate the head of the bed to an upright position (unless contraindicated) and give the patient a small amount of crushed ice or ice water to swallow. If the gag reflex is present and the patient is able to swallow safely, you may proceed with feeding.

S

- Place food on the unaffected side of the mouth. Follow feedings with scrupulous oral hygiene because food may collect on the affected side of the mouth.

Communication. During the acute stage, your role in meeting the psychologic needs of the patient is primarily supportive.

- An alert patient is usually anxious because of a lack of understanding of what has happened and the inability to communicate. Give the patient extra time to comprehend and respond to communication.

Sensory-Perceptual Alterations. *Homonymous hemianopsia* (blindness in the same half of each visual field) is common after a stroke.

- Initially help the patient by arranging the environment within the patient's perceptual field, such as arranging the food tray so that all food is on the right side or the left side to accommodate for field of vision.
- Later the patient learns to compensate for the visual defect by consciously attending to or scanning the neglected side. Weak or paralyzed extremities are carefully checked for adequacy of dressing, hygiene, and trauma.

Other visual problems may include diplopia, loss of the corneal reflex, and ptosis, especially if the stroke is in the vertebrobasilar arterial distribution. Diplopia is treated with an eye patch. If the corneal reflex is absent, prevent corneal abrasions with artificial tears or gel to keep the eyes moist and an eye shield (especially at night).

Coping. A stroke is usually a sudden, extremely stressful event for the patient, caregiver, and significant others.

- Reactions vary considerably but may involve fear, apprehension, denial of stroke severity, depression, anger, and sorrow.
- During the acute phase of caring for the patient and family, nursing interventions designed to facilitate coping involve providing information and emotional support.
- Explanations to the patient should be clear and understandable. Decision making and upholding the patient's wishes during this challenging time are of utmost importance.

Home Care and Rehabilitation. The patient is usually discharged from the acute care setting to home, an intermediate or long-term care facility, or a rehabilitation facility. You can prepare the patient and family through teaching and evaluating the transition plan for any barriers.

Follow-up care is carefully planned for continuing nursing, physical, occupational, and speech therapy, as well as medical care. Patient and caregiver can benefit from the combined expertise care of an interprofessional rehabilitation team. You can facilitate communication and coordination of care to achieve the patient's goals for successful rehabilitation.

The rehabilitation nurse assesses the patient, caregiver, and family with attention to: (1) rehabilitation potential of the patient, (2) physical status of all body systems, (3) presence of complications caused by the stroke or other chronic conditions, (4) cognitive status of the patient, (5) family resources and support, and (6) expectations of the patient and caregiver related to the rehabilitation program.

Rehabilitation and long-term management are further described in Chapter 57 of Harding et al., *Lewis' Medical-Surgical Nursing,* ed 11.

▼ **Patient and Caregiver Teaching**

■ Provide the caregiver with instruction and practice in home care while the patient is hospitalized. This allows for support and encouragement as well as opportunities for feedback. Adjustments in the home environment, such as the removal of a door to accommodate a wheelchair, can be made before discharge.

■ Your instruction related to home care should include exercise and ambulation techniques; dietary requirements; recognizing signs indicating the possibility of another stroke (e.g., headache, vertigo, numbness, visual changes); understanding emotional lability and the possibility of depression; medication routine; and time, place, and frequency of follow-up activities such as occupational therapy and physical therapy.

■ Assist the caregiver to stay healthy. Stress the importance of planning for respite or rest from caregiving activities on a regular basis.

SYPHILIS

Description

Syphilis is a sexually transmitted bacterial infection that can have serious long-term complications if not identified and treated effectively. The population most affected by syphilis is men who have sex with men (MSM), with the highest rates among black MSM between the ages of 25 and 29 years.

Pathophysiology

Syphilis is caused by *Treponema pallidum,* a bacterial spirochete. It is transmitted by direct contact with a syphilitic ulcer called a *chancre,* which can occur externally on the genitals, anus, or lips or internally in the vagina, rectum, mouth, tongue, or through the mucosal membranes of an infected person.

■ The incubation period can range from 10 to 90 days (average, 21 days).

- Having the infection does not provide protection from reinfection, even after successful treatment.
- An infected pregnant woman can transmit syphilis to her fetus during her pregnancy. There is a high risk for stillbirth or for having babies that develop complications after birth including seizures and death.

Clinical Manifestations

Signs and symptoms of syphilis mimic those of other infections. Consequently, it is hard to recognize syphilis. Without treatment, the infection progresses to the next stage.

- The *primary stage* is the development of a chancre at the site of transmission. This can appear days to months following infection. In most patients, it occurs by 3 weeks. Chancres can be found on the genitals but often go unnoticed when inside the mouth, vagina, or anus.
- In the *secondary stage,* syphilis is systemic. The classic maculopapular rash appears on the palms of the hands or soles of the feet, but often involves the trunk or extremities. Without treatment, the rash will resolve, but the patient still has syphilis and will remain infectious for some time. *Tertiary (late) syphilis*, is the final stage where patients will not have obvious symptoms. During this stage, the organism is silently causing organ damage over many years. The formation of gummas can lead to serious complications.

Complications

The *gummas* (destructive lesions) of late syphilis produce irreparable damage to bone, liver, or skin.

- In cardiovascular syphilis, the resulting aneurysm may press on structures, such as the intercostal nerves, causing pain. Scarring of the aortic valve results in aortic valve insufficiency and heart failure.
- Neurosyphilis causes mental deterioration. Visual impairment, tabes dorsalis (progressive locomotor ataxia), and dementia are rare, extreme manifestations.

Diagnostic Studies

- Detailed and accurate sexual history is important.
- Darkfield microscopy and direct fluorescent antibody tests of lesion exudate or tissue can confirm the diagnosis.
- To screen for syphilis, Venereal Disease Research Laboratory (VDRL) and rapid plasma reagin (RPR) testing can detect

nonspecific antitreponemal antibodies, which are usually positive 10 to 14 days after chancre appearance.
- To confirm a diagnosis of syphilis, the fluorescent treponemal
  antibody absorption (FTA-ABs) test, the *T. pallidum* particle
  agglutination (TP-PA) test, and the syphilis qualitative
  enzyme-linked immunoassay (EIA) can detect specific antitreponemal antibodies.

Interprofessional and Nursing Management

Management is aimed at starting treatment early. However, treatment cannot reverse damage that is already present in the late stage
of the disease.
- Penicillin G benzathine (Bicillin L-A) is the recommended treatment for all stages of syphilis. When penicillin is contraindicated, doxycycline or tetracycline may be used. Aqueous
  procaine penicillin G is the treatment of choice for neurosyphilis.
- It is important that all sexual contacts in the last 90 days be treated.
- Reexamination and follow-up testing are recommended every
  6 months for up to 2 years.
- Repeat human immunodeficiency virus (HIV) testing should be
  done on all HIV-negative patients diagnosed with primary or
  secondary syphilis given the higher risk of HIV transmission
  during these stages.

See Nursing Management: Sexually Transmitted Infections,
pp. 545.

SYSTEMIC EXERTION INTOLERANCE DISEASE

Description

Systemic exertion intolerance disease (SEID), formerly called
chronic fatigue syndrome, is a serious, complex, multisystem disease in which exertion of any sort (physical, emotional, cognitive)
is impaired and accompanied by profound fatigue. SEID is a poorly
understood condition that can have a devastating impact on the lives
of patients and their families.

SEID affects at least 1 million people in the United States. The
condition is 3 to 4 times more common in women than men. SEID
occurs in all ethnic and socioeconomic groups, but the illness is
more common in minorities and socioeconomically disadvantaged
groups. The true prevalence of SEID is unknown because many people with the disease have not been diagnosed.

S

Pathophysiology

The precise mechanisms of SEID remain unknown. Despite efforts to determine the cause and pathology of SEID, precise mechanisms are unknown. However, many theories exist about the cause of SEID.

- Neuroendocrine abnormalities have been implicated involving a hypofunction of the hypothalamic-pituitary-adrenal (HPA) axis and hypothalamic-pituitary-gonadal axis, which together regulate the stress response and reproductive hormone levels.
- Several microorganisms have been investigated as causative agents, including herpes viruses (e.g., Epstein-Barr virus [EBV], cytomegalovirus [CMV]), retroviruses, enteroviruses, *Candida albicans,* and *Mycoplasma.*
- Because many patients have cognitive deficits (e.g., decreased memory, attention, concentration), changes in the central nervous system (CNS) have been suggested as the cause of SEID.

Clinical Manifestations and Diagnostic Studies

Diagnosis of SEID requires that the patient have the following 3 symptoms: impaired function with profound fatigue lasting at least 6 months, postexertional malaise (total exhaustion after even minor physical or mental exertion that the patient sometimes describes as a "crash"), and unrefreshing sleep. The presence of either cognitive impairment or orthostatic intolerance (worsening of symptoms upon standing) is also required for diagnosis. Associated symptoms may vary in intensity over time.

- Severe fatigue is the most common symptom and the problem that causes the patient to seek health care.

SEID is often hard to distinguish from fibromyalgia because many clinical features are similar (Table 82). In about half the cases, SEID develops slowly, or the patient may have periodic episodes that gradually become chronic. SEID can arise suddenly in a previously active, healthy person. An unremarkable flu-like illness or other acute stress is often identified as a trigger.

- The patient may become angry and frustrated with health care providers (HCPs) who cannot diagnose a problem. The disorder may have a major impact on work and family responsibilities. Some people may need help with activities of daily living (ADLs).

Nursing and Interprofessional Management

Because no definitive treatment exists for SEID, supportive management is essential. Tell the patient what is known about the disease. Take complaints seriously.

TABLE 82   Common Features of Fibromyalgia and Systemic Exertion Intolerance Disease (SEID)
Occurrence
Previously healthy, young and middle-aged women
Etiology (theories)
Infectious trigger, dysfunction in HPA axis, CNS problem
Clinical Manifestations
Generalized musculoskeletal pain, malaise and fatigue, cognitive problems, headaches, sleep problems, depression, anxiety, fever
Disease Course
Variable intensity of symptoms, fluctuates over time
Diagnosis
No definitive laboratory tests or joint and muscle examinations
Mainly a diagnosis of exclusion
Management
Symptomatic treatment may include antidepressant drugs, such as amitriptyline and fluoxetine (Prozac).
Nondrug measures include heat, massage, regular stretching, biofeedback, stress management, and relaxation training.

CNS, Central nervous system; *HPA,* hypothalamic-pituitary-adrenal.

- Nonsteroidal antiinflammatory drugs (NSAIDs) can be used to treat headaches, muscle and joint aches, and fever. Antihistamines and decongestants can be used to treat allergic symptoms.
- Tricyclic antidepressants (e.g., doxepin, amitriptyline) and selective serotonin release inhibitors (SSRIs) (e.g., fluoxetine, paroxetine) can improve mood and sleep. Clonazepam (Klonopin) can be used to treat sleep problems and panic disorders.
- Use of low-dose hydrocortisone to decrease fatigue and disability is being studied.
- Teach the patient to avoid total rest because it can create a self-image of the patient as an invalid. On the other hand, strenuous exertion can worsen the exhaustion. Urge the patient to plan a carefully graduated exercise program.
- Behavioral therapy may be used to promote a positive outlook and improve overall disability and fatigue. One of the major problems facing many patients with SEID is economic security. When the illness strikes, they cannot work or must decrease work time. Loss of a job often leads to loss of medical insurance.

SEID does not appear to progress. Although most patients recover or at least gradually improve over time, some do not show substantial improvement. Recovery is more common in persons with a sudden onset of SEID.

S

SYSTEMIC INFLAMMATORY RESPONSE SYNDROME (SIRS) AND MULTIPLE ORGAN DYSFUNCTION SYNDROME (MODS)

Description

Systemic inflammatory response syndrome (SIRS) is a systemic inflammatory response to a variety of insults, including infection (referred to as "sepsis"), ischemia, infarction, and injury. Generalized inflammation in organs remote from the initial insult characterizes SIRS. Many different mechanisms can trigger SIRS, including:

- *mechanical tissue trauma*: burns, crush injuries, surgical procedures
- *abscess formation*: intraabdominal, extremities
- *ischemic* or *necrotic tissue*: pancreatitis, vascular disease, myocardial infarction
- *microbial invasion*: bacteria, viruses, fungi, parasites
- *endotoxin release*: gram-negative and gram-positive bacteria
- *global perfusion deficits*: postcardiac resuscitation, shock states
- *regional perfusion deficits*: distal perfusion deficits

Multiple organ dysfunction syndrome (MODS) is failure of 2 or more organ systems in an acutely ill patient such that homeostasis cannot be maintained without intervention. MODS results from SIRS.

- Prognosis for the patient with MODS is poor, with mortality rates at 40% to 60% when 3 or more organ systems fail.

Pathophysiology and Clinical Manifestations

When the inflammatory response is activated, consequences occur, including activation of inflammatory cells and release of mediators, direct damage to the endothelium, and hypermetabolism.

- An increase in vascular permeability allows mediators and protein to leak out of the endothelium and into the interstitial space.
- White blood cells (WBCs) begin to digest the foreign debris, and the coagulation cascade is activated.
- Hypotension, decreased perfusion, microemboli, and redistributed or shunted blood flow eventually compromise organ perfusion.

The respiratory system is often the first system to show signs of dysfunction in SIRS and MODS. Inflammatory mediators damage the pulmonary endothelium, causing increased capillary permeability. Fluid moves to the alveoli, causing alveolar edema. Alveoli collapse. This creates an increase in *shunt* (blood flow to the lungs that does not take part in gas exchange) and worsening ventilation-perfusion mismatch. The end result is acute respiratory distress syndrome (ARDS) (see p. 14).

Cardiovascular changes include myocardial depression and massive vasodilation in response to increasing tissue demands. To compensate for hypotension, heart rate and stroke volume increase, but increased capillary permeability decreases venous return and preload. Eventually, either perfusion of vital organs becomes insufficient or the cells are unable to use oxygen, and their function is further compromised.

Neurologic dysfunction manifests as mental status changes, an early sign of SIRS or MODS. Confusion, agitation, disorientation, lethargy, or coma may occur. These changes are caused by hypoxemia, the effect of inflammatory mediators, or impaired perfusion.

Acute kidney injury (AKI) is common in SIRS and MODS. Hypoperfusion and the effects of the mediators can cause AKI. Many antibiotics used to treat gram-negative bacteria (e.g., aminoglycosides) can be nephrotoxic, so careful monitoring of drug levels is needed.

In the early stages of SIRS and MODS, blood is shunted away from the gastrointestinal (GI) mucosa, making it highly vulnerable to ischemic injury. Decreased perfusion leads to a breakdown of the mucosal barrier and increases the risk for ulceration, GI bleeding, and bacterial movement from the GI tract into circulation.

Metabolic changes are pronounced in SIRS and MODS. Both syndromes trigger a hypermetabolic response, a catabolic state, and loss of lean body mass (muscle).

- The liver is unable to synthesize albumin needed to maintain plasma oncotic pressure. Intravascular fluid leaks to the interstitial space.
- The patient who is in a state of hypermetabolism is unable to convert lactate to glucose, and lactate accumulates (lactic acidosis). The liver is unable to maintain a glucose level, and the patient becomes hypoglycemic.

Disseminated intravascular coagulation (DIC) may result from dysfunction of the coagulation system. DIC causes microvascular clotting and bleeding at the same time because of the depletion of clotting factors and excessive fibrinolysis (see Disseminated Intravascular Coagulation, p. 188).

Electrolyte imbalances are common from hormonal and metabolic changes and fluid shifts. These changes exacerbate mental status changes, neuromuscular dysfunction, and dysrhythmias.

- Release of antidiuretic hormone and aldosterone cause sodium and water retention; aldosterone increases urinary potassium loss, and catecholamines cause potassium to move into the cells, resulting in hypokalemia.

- Metabolic acidosis results from hypoxia, impaired tissue perfusion, the shift to anaerobic metabolism, and progressive renal dysfunction.
- Hypocalcemia, hypomagnesemia, and hypophosphatemia are common.

The multisystem manifestations of SIRS and MODS are presented in Table 66.10, Harding et al., *Lewis' Medical-Surgical Nursing,* ed 11.

Nursing and Interprofessional Management

The most important goal in managing SIRS and MODS is to prevent SIRS from progressing to MODS. A critical component of the nursing role is vigilant assessment and ongoing monitoring to detect early signs of deterioration or organ dysfunction.

Interprofessional care of patients with MODS focuses on prevention and treatment of infection, maintenance of tissue oxygenation, nutritional and metabolic support, and appropriate support for individual failing organs.

- Aggressive infection control is essential to decrease the risk for health care–associated infections (HAIs). Early, aggressive surgery is recommended to remove necrotic tissue (e.g., early debridement of burn tissue) that provides a culture medium for microorganisms. Aggressive pulmonary management, including early ambulation, can reduce the risk of respiratory infection. Strict asepsis can decrease infections related to intraarterial lines, endotracheal tubes, urinary catheters, IV lines, and other invasive devices or procedures.
- Hypoxemia frequently occurs in patients with SIRS or MODS. Interventions to decrease oxygen demand and increase oxygen delivery are essential. Treating fever, chills, and pain decrease O_2 demand. Sedation, mechanical ventilation, analgesia, and rest may decrease oxygen demand O_2 delivery may be optimized by using individualized tidal volumes with positive end-expiratory pressure, increasing preload (e.g., fluids) or myocardial contractility to enhance cardiac output (CO), or reducing afterload to increase CO.
- Hypermetabolism in SIRS or MODS can result in profound weight loss, cachexia, and further organ failure. Providing early and adequate nutritional support decreases morbidity and mortality. The use of the enteral route is preferred to parenteral nutrition.

Support of any failing organ is a primary goal of therapy. For example, the patient with ARDS requires aggressive oxygen therapy and mechanical ventilation. Renal failure may require dialysis or continuous renal replacement therapy.

A final consideration may be that further interventions are futile. It is important to maintain communication between the health care team and the patient's family and caregivers about realistic goals and likely outcomes for the patient with MODS. Withdrawal of life support and providing end-of-life care may be the best option for the patient.

SYSTEMIC LUPUS ERYTHEMATOSUS

Description

Systemic lupus erythematosus (SLE) is a multisystem inflammatory autoimmune disease. It typically affects the skin, joints, and serous membranes (pleura, pericardium), and renal, hematologic, and neurologic systems. SLE is marked by a chronic unpredictable course, with alternating exacerbations and remissions.

About 1.5 million people in the United States have SLE. Blacks, Asian Americans, Hispanics, and Native Americans are more likely than whites to develop the disease. While SLE can affect anyone, 90% of those with SLE are women ages 15 to 45 years.

Pathophysiology

The cause of the abnormal immune response in SLE is unknown. It is a complex disorder of multifactorial origin resulting from interactions among genetic, hormonal, environmental, and immunologic factors.

- Hormones are known to play a role in the development of SLE. Onset or worsening of disease symptoms may occur after menarche, with the use of oral contraceptives, and during or after pregnancy. SLE symptoms worsen in the immediate postpartum period.
- Environmental factors believed to contribute to SLE include sun or ultraviolet light exposure, stress, and exposure to some chemicals and toxins. Infectious agents such as viruses also may stimulate immune hyperactivity. In addition, at least 45 medications currently in use may trigger SLE. Most cases have been associated with procainamide, hydralazine, and quinidine.

SLE is characterized by the production of various autoantibodies against nucleic acids (e.g., single- and double-stranded deoxyribonucleic acid [DNA]), erythrocytes, coagulation proteins, lymphocytes, and platelets. Autoimmune reactions are directed against the cell nucleus (antinuclear antibodies [ANA]), particularly DNA.

S

Circulating immune complexes containing antibody against DNA are deposited in the basement membranes of capillaries in the kidneys, heart, skin, brain, and joints. These complexes trigger inflammation that causes tissue destruction. An overaggressive autoimmune response is also related to activation of B and T cells. Specific disease effects depend on the involved cell types or organs.

Clinical Manifestations and Complications

No characteristic pattern occurs in the progression of SLE. General complaints, including fever, weight loss, joint pain *(arthralgia),* and excessive fatigue, may precede an exacerbation of disease activity.

Dermatology

Vascular skin lesions are most likely to develop in sun-exposed areas. Severe skin reactions can occur in people who are photosensitive. The classic butterfly rash over the cheeks and bridge of the nose occurs in about half of patients at some time during the disease.

- Oral or nasopharyngeal membrane ulcers can occur.
- Alopecia is common, and the scalp becomes dry, scaly, and atrophied.

Musculoskeletal

Polyarthralgia, pain in multiple joints, with morning stiffness is often the patient's first symptom. Arthritis occurs in 95% of patients with SLE. Diffuse swelling is accompanied by joint and muscle pain.

- Lupus-related arthritis is generally nonerosive, but it may cause deformities such as swan neck, ulnar deviation, and subluxation with hyperlaxity of the joints.

Cardiopulmonary

Tachypnea and cough in patients with SLE suggest restrictive lung disease. Cardiac involvement including dysrhythmias resulting from fibrosis of the sinoatrial (SA) and atrioventricular (AV) nodes indicates advanced disease.

- Hypertension and hypercholesterolemia from steroid use require aggressive treatment.

Renal

About 40% of persons with SLE have kidney damage. Renal involvement varies from mild proteinuria to rapid, progressive glomerulonephritis. Treatment typically includes corticosteroids, cytotoxic agents (cyclophosphamide), and immunosuppressive agents (azathioprine [Imuran], cyclosporine, and mycophenolate mofetil [CellCept]). Oral prednisone or pulsed IV methylprednisolone may also be used, especially in the initial treatment period when cytotoxic agents have not yet taken effect. Bilimumab (Benlysta) is a B-lymphocyte stimulator approved in 2011 to inhibit the inflammation of SLE.

Nervous System

Seizures are the most common neurologic manifestation. They are generally controlled by corticosteroids or antiseizure drugs.

- Cognitive problems may result from the deposition of immune complexes within the brain tissue. It is marked by disordered thinking, disorientation, and memory deficits.
- Various psychiatric disorders reported in SLE include depression, mood disorders, anxiety, and psychosis, although they may be related to the stress of having a major illness or to associated drug therapies.
- Occasionally a stroke or aseptic meningitis may be attributable to SLE. Headaches are common and can become severe during a flare (exacerbation).

Hematology

Abnormal blood conditions are common in SLE resulting from the formation of antibodies against blood cells. Anemia, leukopenia, thrombocytopenia, and coagulation disorders (excessive bleeding or clotting) are often present. Many patients with SLE benefit from high-intensity treatment with warfarin.

Infection

Patients with SLE appear to have increased susceptibility to infections, possibly related to defects in the ability to eliminate invading bacteria, deficiencies in the production of antibodies, and the immunosuppressive effect of many antiinflammatory drugs. Pneumonia is the most common infection.

Diagnostic Studies

- Diagnosis of SLE is based on distinct criteria. No specific test is diagnostic for SLE, but a variety of abnormalities may be present in the blood. SLE is marked by the presence of ANA in 97% of persons with the disease.
- Anti-DNA antibodies are found in one-half of the persons with SLE, but lupus can still be present if these antibodies are not identified.
- Anti-Smith (Sm) antibodies are found in 30% to 40% of persons with SLE and are almost always considered diagnostic.
- Nearly 30% of people with SLE have antiphospholipid antibodies. Antibodies to histone are most often seen in people with drug-induced SLE.
- Elevated erythrocyte sedimentation rate (ESR) and C-reactive protein (CRP) levels indicate inflammation and may be used to monitor disease activity.

Interprofessional Management

A major challenge in SLE treatment is to manage the active phase of the disease while preventing complications of treatment. The

S

prognosis of SLE can be improved with early diagnosis, prompt recognition of serious organ involvement, and effective therapeutic regimens.

Drug Therapy

Nonsteroidal antiinflammatory drugs (NSAIDs) are an important intervention, especially for patients with mild polyarthralgia or polyarthritis. Antimalarial agents such as hydroxychloroquine and chloroquine are often used to treat fatigue and moderate skin and joint problems, as well as to prevent flares.

Corticosteroid therapy should be limited to the lowest dose for the shortest possible time. For example, steroids can be used for a few weeks until a slower medication becomes effective. Taper the patient's dose of steroid slowly rather than stopping the medication abruptly

Immunosuppressive drugs such as azathioprine (Imuran) and cyclophosphamide may be prescribed to suppress the immune system and reduce end-organ damage.

- Topical immunomodulators are an alternative to corticosteroids for treating serious skin conditions. Tacrolimus (Protopic) and pimecrolimus (Elidel) suppress immune activity in the skin, including the butterfly rash and possibly discoid (round, coinshaped) lesions.

Nursing Management

Goals

The patient with SLE will have acceptable pain management, show awareness of and avoid activities that worsen the disease, and maintain optimal role function and positive self-image.

Nursing Interventions

During an SLE flare, the patient may quickly become very ill. Nursing interventions include accurately documenting the severity of symptoms and response to therapy. Specifically assess fever pattern, joint inflammation, limitation of motion, location and degree of discomfort, and fatigue.

- Monitor the patient's weight and fluid intake and output. This is especially important if corticosteroids are prescribed because of related fluid retention and possible renal failure. Collect 24-hour urine for protein and creatinine clearance as ordered.
- Observe for signs of bleeding that result from drug therapy, such as pallor, skin bruising, petechiae, or tarry stools.
- Carefully assess the patient's neurologic status. Assess for visual changes, headaches, personality changes, and forgetfulness. Psychosis may indicate central nervous system disease or may

be the effect of corticosteroid therapy. Nerve irritation of the extremities (peripheral neuropathy) may produce numbness, tingling, and weakness of the hands and feet.

- Explain the nature of the disease, treatments, and diagnostic procedures. Provide emotional support for the patient and caregiver, especially during a disease flare.

▼ **Patient and Caregiver Teaching**

Help the patient understand that even strong adherence to the treatment plan is not a guarantee against exacerbation, because the course of the disease is unpredictable. Several factors may increase disease activity, such as fatigue, sun exposure, emotional stress, infection, drugs, and surgery. Help the patient and caregiver eliminate or reduce exposure to such factors. Patient and caregiver teaching is outlined in Table 83.

- Many couples require pregnancy and sexual counseling. For the best outcome, pregnancy should be planned when the disease activity is minimal.
- Pain and fatigue may interfere with quality of life. Pacing techniques and relaxation therapy can help the patient remain involved in daily activities.

TABLE 83   Patient and Caregiver Teaching

Systemic Lupus Erythematosus

Include the following information in the teaching plan for a patient with systemic lupus erythematosus and the patient's caregiver.

- Disease process
- Names of drugs, actions, side effects, dosage, administration
- Pain management strategies
- Energy conservation and pacing techniques
- Therapeutic exercise, use of heat therapy (for arthralgia)
- Relaxation therapy
- Avoid physical and emotional stress
- Avoid exposure to those with infection
- Avoid drying soaps, powders, household chemicals
- Use of sunscreen protection (at least SPF 15) and protective clothing, with minimal sun exposure from 11:00 AM to 3:00 PM
- Regular medical and laboratory follow-up
- Marital and pregnancy counseling as needed
- Community resources and health care agencies

SPF, Sun protection factor.

S

TESTICULAR CANCER

Description
Testicular cancer is rare, but it is the most common type of cancer in men between 15 and 44 years of age. Testicular tumors are more common in men with undescended testicles (cryptorchidism) in infancy or with a family history of testicular cancer or anomalies. Most testicular cancers develop from 2 types of embryonic germ cells: seminomas and nonseminomas.

Clinical Manifestations
Testicular cancer may have a slow or rapid onset.

- The patient may notice a painless lump in his scrotum and scrotal swelling. The scrotal mass is usually nontender and very firm.
- Some patients report a dull ache or heavy sensation in the lower abdomen, perianal area, or scrotum.
- Manifestations associated with metastasis include lower back and/or chest pain, cough, and dyspnea.

Diagnostic Studies
- Palpation of scrotal contents is used to assess for masses and swelling.
- Ultrasound of the testes is indicated when testicular cancer is suspected.
- Blood serum levels of α-fetoprotein (AFP), lactate dehydrogenase (LDH), and human chorionic gonadotropin (hCG) are done if testicular cancer is suspected.
- Chest x-ray and CT scan of the abdomen and pelvis are used to detect metastasis.

Nursing and Interprofessional Management
Testicular cancer is one of the most curable types of cancer. Management generally involves a radical inguinal orchiectomy (surgical removal of the affected testis, spermatic cord, and regional lymph nodes). Retroperitoneal lymph node dissection and removal may also be done.

- Testicular germ cell tumors are more sensitive to systemic chemotherapy than any other adult solid tumor. Chemotherapy protocols use a combination of agents, including bleomycin, cisplatin. etoposide, and ifosfamide (Ifex).

The prognosis for patients with testicular cancer has improved, and 95% of patients obtain complete remission if the disease is detected early. All patients with testicular cancer, regardless of pathology or stage, require meticulous follow-up monitoring and regular physical examinations, chest x-ray, CT scan, and assessment of serum tumor markers (hCG, LDH, and AFP). The goal is to detect relapse when tumor burden is minimal.

- Because of the high risk for infertility after chemotherapy and/or pelvic radiation, the cryopreservation of sperm in a sperm bank before treatment begins should be sensitively discussed.

THALASSEMIA

Description

Thalassemia is a group of diseases involving inadequate production of normal hemoglobin (Hgb), which decreases red blood cell (RBC) production. Hemolysis also occurs in thalassemia.

- Thalassemia is commonly found in members of ethnic groups whose origins are near the Mediterranean Sea and equatorial or near-equatorial regions of southeastern Asia, the Middle East, India, Pakistan, China, Southern Russia, and Africa.

Pathophysiology

Thalassemia has an autosomal recessive genetic basis that results in an absent or reduced globulin protein. α-Globin chains are absent or reduced in α-thalassemia, and β-globin chains are absent or reduced in β-thalassemia. A person with thalassemia may have a heterozygous or homozygous form of the disease.

- In *thalassemia minor (thalassemic trait),* the person is heterozygous, with 1 thalassemic gene and 1 normal gene. Thalassemia minor is a mild form of the disease.
- In *thalassemia major,* the person is homozygous, with 2 thalassemic genes. Thalassemia major is a severe form of the disease.

Clinical Manifestations

- The patient with thalassemia minor may be asymptomatic, with mild to moderate anemia, microcytosis (small cells) and hypochromia (pale cells).
- The patient with thalassemia major has symptoms of anemia (see Anemia, p. 29). Marked splenomegaly, hepatomegaly, and jaundice result from hemolysis of RBCs. Chronic bone marrow hyperplasia leads to expansion of the marrow space. This may cause thickening of the cranium and the maxillary cavity walls.
- Cardiac complications from iron overload, lung disease, and hypertension contribute to early death.
- Endocrine problems (diabetes, growth retardation, hypogonadism), osteoporosis, pulmonary hypertension, and thrombosis may be present.

T

Nursing and Interprofessional Management

The laboratory findings in thalassemia major are summarized in Table 8, p. 30.

- Thalassemia minor requires no treatment because the body adapts to the reduction in normal Hgb.
- Thalassemia major is managed with blood transfusions or exchange transfusions. Chelating agents reduce the iron overloading that occurs with chronic transfusion therapy. Drugs used include oral deferasirox (Exjade, JadeNu) or deferiprone (Ferriprox), or IV or subcutaneous deferoxamine (Desferal).
- Ascorbic acid supplements may be used to increase urine excretion of iron. Ascorbic acid should only be taken with chelation therapy because it increases the absorption of dietary iron. It is given, along with folic acid, if there is evidence of hemolysis. Zinc supplements may be needed since zinc is reduced with chelation therapy. Iron supplements should not be given.
- Because RBCs are sequestered in the enlarged spleen, thalassemia may be treated by splenectomy.
- Although hematopoietic stem cell transplantation remains the only cure for patients with thalassemia, the risks associated with this procedure may outweigh its benefits.

THROMBOANGIITIS OBLITERANS

Thromboangiitis obliterans (Buerger's disease) is a nonatherosclerotic, segmental, recurrent inflammatory vaso-occlusive disorder of the small and medium-sized arteries and veins of the arms and legs. It occurs mostly in men under 45 years of age with a long history of tobacco or marijuana use, but without other cardiovascular disease (CVD) risk factors (e.g., hypertension, hyperlipidemia, diabetes).

In the acute phase of Buerger's disease, an inflammatory thrombus blocks the vessel. Over time, the thrombus becomes more organized, and the vessel wall inflammation subsides.

During the chronic phase, thrombosis and fibrosis in the vessel cause tissue ischemia. The symptoms of Buerger's disease are often confused with peripheral artery disease (PAD) and other autoimmune diseases (e.g., scleroderma).

- Patients may have intermittent claudication of the feet, hands, or arms. As the disease progresses, rest pain and ischemic ulcerations develop.

- Other signs and symptoms may include color and temperature changes of the limbs, paresthesia, superficial vein thrombosis, and cold sensitivity.

There are no laboratory or diagnostic tests specific to Buerger's disease. Diagnosis is based on the age at onset, history, symptoms, involvement of distal vessels, presence of ischemic ulcerations, and exclusion of other sources of emboli.

Treatment is the complete cessation of tobacco and marijuana use in any form. Conservative management includes avoiding limb exposure to cold temperatures, a supervised walking program, antibiotics to treat any infected ulcers, and analgesics to manage the ischemic pain. IV iloprost (Ventavis), a prostaglandin analog that promotes vasodilation, is used to manage rest pain, promote healing of ischemic ulcers, and decrease the need for amputation.

Teach patients to avoid trauma to the extremities. Painful ulcerations may require finger or toe amputations. The amputation rate in patients who continue tobacco use is much higher than in those who stop.

THROMBOCYTOPENIA

Description

Thrombocytopenia is a reduction of platelets below 150,000/µL (150×10^9/L). Acute, severe, or prolonged decreases from this normal range can result in prolonged bleeding from minor trauma or spontaneous bleeding without injury.

Platelet disorders can be inherited (e.g., Wiskott-Aldrich syndrome), but the vast majority are acquired. A common cause of acquired disorders is the ingestion of drugs such as quinine, aspirin, or myelosuppressive chemotherapy agents.

Some drugs can affect platelet aggregation. Aspirin doses as low as 81 mg can alter platelet aggregation. Normal function is restored when new platelets are made.

Immune Thrombocytopenia

Immune thrombocytopenia (ITP), the most common acquired thrombocytopenia, is an autoimmune destruction of circulating platelets. Antibody-coated platelets, mistakenly identified as foreign, are destroyed by macrophages in the spleen. ITP generally manifests as an acute condition in children and a chronic condition in adults.

Thrombotic Thrombocytopenic Purpura

Thrombotic thrombocytopenic purpura (TTP) is an uncommon syndrome characterized by hemolytic anemia, thrombocytopenia,

T

neurologic abnormalities, fever (in the absence of infection), and renal abnormalities. TTP is almost always associated with hemolytic-uremic syndrome (HUS).

- TTP is associated with enhanced agglutination of platelets, which form microthrombi in arterioles and capillaries.
- In most cases, the syndrome is caused by the deficiency of a plasma enzyme (ADAMTS13) that usually breaks down the von Willebrand (vWF) clotting factor into normal size.
- TTP is seen primarily in previously healthy adults.
- The syndrome may be idiopathic (autoimmune disorder with antibodies against ADAMTS13), caused by certain drug toxicities (e.g., chemotherapy, cyclosporine, quinine, oral contraceptives, valacyclovir, clopidogrel [Plavix]), pregnancy or preeclampsia, infection, or known autoimmune disorder such as systemic lupus erythematosus or scleroderma.
- TTP is a medical emergency because bleeding and clotting occur simultaneously

Heparin-Induced Thrombocytopenia

Heparin-induced thrombocytopenia (HIT), also called *heparin-induced thrombocytopenia* and *thrombosis syndrome* (HITTS), may develop 5 to 10 days after heparin therapy is initiated. In HIT, an immune-mediated response to heparin causes platelet destruction and vascular endothelial injury.

- Antibodies are created against a heparin-platelet complex, and platelets are removed prematurely from circulation, leading to thrombocytopenia and formation of platelet-fibrin thrombi.
- HIT leads to venous or arterial thrombosis. Deep vein thromboses and pulmonary emboli are common. Other complications may include arterial vascular infarcts resulting in skin necrosis, stroke, and end-organ damage (e.g., kidneys).
- As many as 3% of patients on heparin therapy develop HIT. Suspect HIT if the platelet count drops by more than 50% from baseline or if a thrombus forms while the patient is on heparin therapy.
- Symptoms of bleeding are unusual because the platelet count rarely drops below 20,000/μL.

Clinical Manifestations

Many patients with thrombocytopenia are asymptomatic. The major complication of thrombocytopenia is hemorrhage in any area of the body, including the joints, retina, and brain. Cerebral hemorrhage may be fatal.

- The most common symptom is bleeding, usually mucosal or cutaneous. Mucosal bleeding may manifest as epistaxis and gingival bleeding. Large bullous hemorrhages may appear on the buccal mucosa. Bleeding into the skin is seen as petechiae, purpura, or superficial ecchymoses.

- Prolonged bleeding after venipuncture or IM injection may indicate thrombocytopenia. Be aware of manifestations that reflect internal blood loss, including weakness, fainting, dizziness, tachycardia, abdominal pain, and hypotension.

Diagnostic Studies

- For comparison of laboratory results in various types of thrombocytopenia, see Table 30.12, Harding et al., *Lewis' Medical-Surgical Nursing*, ed 11.
- Platelet count is decreased below 150,000/μL (150 $\times$ 10^9/L). Spontaneous life-threatening hemorrhages (e.g., intracranial bleeding) may occur with counts below 20,000/μL (20 $\times$ 10^9/L).
- Specific assays for antigens help differentiate ITP from other types of thrombocytopenia.
- Bone marrow analysis may show normal or increased megakaryocytes (precursors of platelets). It is done to rule out leukemia, aplastic anemia, and other myeloproliferative disorders.
- Flow cytometry can be used to detect antiplatelet antibodies.

Interprofessional Management

Immune Thrombocytopenia

Multiple therapies are used to manage the patient with ITP. If the patient is asymptomatic, therapy may not be used unless the platelet count is below 10,000/μL. Corticosteroids (e.g., prednisone) are used initially to suppress the phagocytic response of splenic macrophages.

Splenectomy may be indicated if the patient is not responding to the conservative treatments. Approximately two-thirds of patients benefit from splenectomy, resulting in a sustained remission. High doses of IV immunoglobulin (IVIG) and a component of IVIG, anti-Rh$_o$(D) (anti-D, WinRho), may be used in the patient who is unresponsive to corticosteroids or splenectomy, or for whom splenectomy is not an option.

- Romiplostim (Nplate) and eltrombopag (Promacta) are used for patients with chronic ITP who have an insufficient response to the other treatments. These thrombopoietin receptor agonists drugs increase platelet production.

Platelet transfusions are not indicated until the count is < 10,000/μL (10 $\times$ 10^9/L) or for anticipated bleeding before a procedure.

Thrombotic Thrombocytopenic Purpura

TTP may be managed in a variety of ways. The first step is to treat the underlying disorder (e.g., infection) or remove an identified cause. Plasma exchange (plasmapheresis) may be needed to reverse

T

the process. Treatment should be continued daily until the patient's platelet counts normalize and hemolysis has ceased.

Corticosteroids may be added. Rituximab has been used for patients who are refractory to plasma exchange. Other immunosuppressants, such as cyclosporine or cyclophosphamide, may also be used. Splenectomy is considered. Administration of platelets is generally contraindicated because it may lead to new vWF-platelet complexes and increased clotting. If untreated, TTP usually results in irreversible renal failure and death.

Heparin-Induced Thrombocytopenia

All forms of heparin must be stopped when HIT is first recognized. This includes heparin flushes for vascular catheters.

To maintain anticoagulation, the patient should be started on a direct thrombin inhibitor, such as argatroban. Fondaparinux (Arixtra), a factor Xa inhibitor (indirect thrombin inhibitor), or bivalirudin (a synthetic thrombin inhibitor) may be used. Warfarin should be started only when the platelet count has reached at least 150,000/μL. If the clotting is severe, the most commonly used treatment modalities are plasmapheresis to clear the platelet-aggregating immunoglobulin (Ig) G from the blood, protamine sulfate to interrupt the circulating heparin, thrombolytic agents to treat the thromboembolic events, and surgery to remove clots. Platelet transfusions are not effective because they may enhance thromboembolic events.

Patients who have had HIT should never receive heparin or low-molecular-weight heparin (LMWH) again. This should be clearly marked in the patient's health record.

Nursing Management

The patient with thrombocytopenia will have no bleeding, maintain vascular integrity, and manage home care to prevent complications-related bleeding.

See eNursing Care Plan 30-2 for the patient with thrombocytopenia, available on the website for Harding et al, *Lewis' Medical-Surgical Nursing,* ed 11.

Discourage the use of over-the-counter (OTC) medications known to be causes of acquired thrombocytopenia and reduced platelet function. Some have aspirin as an ingredient. Aspirin reduces platelet adhesiveness, thus potentially contributing to bleeding.

The goal during acute episodes of thrombocytopenia is to prevent or control hemorrhage. In the patient with thrombocytopenia, bleeding is usually from superficial sites. Deep bleeding (into the muscles, joints, and abdomen) when clotting factors are diminished. Emphasize that a seemingly minor nosebleed or new petechiae may indicate potential hemorrhage and that the HCP should be notified.

- In a woman with thrombocytopenia, menstrual blood loss may exceed the usual amount and duration. Counting sanitary napkins used during menses is an important intervention to detect excess blood loss.
- Observe for early signs of thrombocytopenia in patients receiving cancer chemotherapy drugs.
- Proper administration of platelet transfusions is an important nursing responsibility.
- Monitor patients with ITP for response to therapy.

▼ **Patient and Caregiver Teaching**
- Teach the person with acquired thrombocytopenia to avoid causative agents when possible.
- Remind the patient to avoid injury or trauma during these periods and to observe for signs and symptoms of bleeding.
- Discuss the impact of the condition on the patient's quality of life.
- Patients with either ITP or acquired thrombocytopenia should plan periodic medical evaluations to assess their status and to treat situations in which exacerbations and bleeding are likely to occur.

For a more complete listing of precautions that patients should take when their platelet count is low, see Table 30.15, Harding et al., *Lewis' Medical-Surgical Nursing,* ed 11.

THYROID CANCER

Description
Thyroid cancer is the most common type of cancer of the endocrine system. The incidence of thyroid cancer has risen significantly in the past 25 years. Thyroid cancer affects more women than men, and the incidence is higher in whites and Asian Americans. Adults at increased risk include those who had head and neck radiation therapy during childhood, were exposed to radioactive fallout, or have a personal or family history of goiter.

Four main types of thyroid cancer are papillary, follicular, medullary, and anaplastic.

- *Papillary thyroid cancer* is the most common type, accounting for about 70% to 80% of all thyroid cancers. Papillary cancer tends to grow slowly and initially spreads to lymph nodes in the neck.
- *Follicular thyroid cancer* makes up about 10% to 15% of all thyroid cancers and tends to occur in older patients. Follicular

T

cancer first grows into the cervical lymph nodes and then spreads to the lungs and bones.

- *Medullary thyroid cancer* accounts for up to 10% of all thyroid cancers. It is more likely to occur in families and to be associated with other endocrine problems. It is diagnosed by genetic testing for a *protooncogene* called *RET*. Medullary thyroid cancer is a type of multiple endocrine neoplasia. This type of cancer is often poorly differentiated and associated with early metastasis.
- *Anaplastic thyroid cancer,* found in < 2% of patients with thyroid cancer, is the most advanced and aggressive thyroid cancer. It is the least likely to respond to treatment and has a poor prognosis.

Clinical Manifestations

The primary sign of thyroid cancer is a painless, palpable nodule or nodules in an enlarged thyroid gland. Patients or health care providers (HCPs) discover most of these nodules during palpation of the neck. Some patients may have difficulty swallowing or breathing because of tumor growth invading the trachea or esophagus.

Diagnostic Studies

Nodular thyroid gland enlargement or palpation of a mass requires further evaluation.

- Ultrasound is often the first diagnostic test used. CT, MRI, positron emission tomography (PET), and ultrasound-guided fine-needle aspiration (FNA) are other options.
- A thyroid scan may be done to evaluate for cancer. A nodule that does not take up radioactive iodine has a higher risk of being malignant.
- High serum calcitonin is associated with medullary thyroid cancer. In papillary and follicular cancers, serum thyroglobulin is high.

Nursing and Interprofessional Management

Surgical removal of the tumor is the main treatment for thyroid cancer. Surgical procedures may range from unilateral total lobectomy with removal of the isthmus to near-total thyroidectomy with bilateral lobectomy.

Radioactive iodine (RAI) may be given to some patients to destroy any remaining cancer cells after surgery. External beam radiation therapy may be given as palliative treatment for patients with metastatic thyroid cancer.

Many thyroid cancers are thyroid-stimulating hormone (TSH)-dependent, and thyroid hormone therapy in high doses is often prescribed to inhibit pituitary secretion of TSH. Chemotherapy, including doxorubicin, may be used for advanced disease. Vandetanib (Caprelsa), lenvatinib (Lenvima), sorafenib tosylate (Nexavar), and cabozantinib (Cometriq) are targeted therapy agents used for treatment of metastatic thyroid cancer. These drugs inhibit tyrosine kinases, which are enzymes that are involved in growth of cancer cells.

Nursing care for the patient with thyroid cancer is similar to that for the patient undergoing thyroidectomy (see Surgical Therapy section in Hyperthyroidism, p. 324). Because of the surgical site location and the potential for hypocalcemia, the patient requires frequent postoperative assessment.

- Assess the patient for airway obstruction, bleeding, and tetany, because a parathyroid gland may have been disturbed or removed during surgery.

TRIGEMINAL NEURALGIA

Description

Trigeminal neuralgia (TN) (tic douloureux) is characterized by sudden, usually unilateral, brief, recurrent episodes of severe stabbing pain in the distribution of the trigeminal nerve. It is seen more often in women than in men, and more often in people over age 40 years.

Pathophysiology

The trigeminal nerve is the fifth cranial nerve (CN V) and has both motor and sensory branches. The sensory branches, primarily the maxillary and mandibular branches, are involved in TN.

- Most TN cases result from vascular compression of the trigeminal nerve root by an abnormal loop of the superior cerebellar artery. Constant compression appears to lead to chronic injury, flattening and atrophy of the nerve and damage to the myelin sheath. TN may be related to underlying pathology, such as multiple sclerosis, shingles, or masses in the cerebellum or brainstem.

Clinical Manifestations

TN is classified as classic (TN 1) or atypical (TN 2). Patients may have both types.

TN 1 manifests with an abrupt onset of paroxysms of excruciating pain. It is described as burning or knifelike, or a lightning-like shock, in the lips, upper or lower gums, cheek, forehead, or side of the nose.

- Intense pain, twitching, grimacing, and frequent blinking and tearing of the eye occur during the acute attack (giving rise to the term *tic*). Some patients may have facial sensory loss.

T

- The attacks are usually brief, lasting seconds to 2 or 3 minutes, and are generally unilateral. Frequency ranges from 1 to over 50 times a day.
- After the refractory (pain-free) period, a phenomenon known as "clustering" is characterized by a cycle of pain and refractoriness that continues for hours.
- Pain episodes are usually triggered by light touch at a specific point (trigger zones) along the distribution of the nerve branches.
- Precipitating stimuli include chewing, toothbrushing, feeling a hot or cold blast of air on the face, washing the face, yawning, or even talking.
- As a result, the patient may neglect eating and hygiene practices, wear a cloth over the face, and withdraw from interaction. The patient may sleep excessively to cope with the pain.

The atypical form, TN 2, is distinguished by constant aching, burning, crushing, or stabbing pain. The pain has a lower intensity and does not subside completely. The distinct attacks associated with TN 1 do not occur in TN 2.

Diagnostic Studies

- The first episode of TN is sudden with a memorable onset. Diagnosis is based on history and examination.
- Neurologic assessment and CT scan or MRI of the brain are used to rule out any lesions, tumors, or vascular abnormalities.

Interprofessional Management

The goal of treatment is relief of pain. Antiseizure drug therapy may reduce pain by stabilizing the neuronal membrane and blocking nerve firing. These drugs are usually effective in treating TN 1 but less effective for TN 2. First-line drugs include carbamazepine (Tegretol) and oxcarbazepine (Trileptal). Topiramate (Topamax), clonazepam (Klonopin), phenytoin (Dilantin), lamotrigine (Lamictal), gabapentin, and valproic acid are other options. Tricyclic antidepressants, such as amitriptyline or nortriptyline, can be used to treat constant burning or aching pain. Analgesics or opioids are usually not effective in controlling pain in TN1 but may help with pain in TN2.

- Electrical stimulation of the nerves and nerve blocks with local anesthetics or botulinum toxin are treatment options.

If a conservative approach is ineffective or the patient is unable to tolerate adverse effects of prescribed drugs, surgical therapy is available. In percutaneous procedures, affected nerve fibers are damaged to eliminate pain. Although most patients are pain-free after such procedures, pain relief lasts longer with microvascular decompression.

Nursing Management

Monitor the patient's response to drug therapy and note any side effects. Discuss other pain management measures, such as acupuncture, biofeedback, and yoga.

Environmental management is essential during an acute period to decrease triggering stimuli. Keep the room at an even, moderate temperature and free of drafts.

Teach the patient about the importance of nutrition, hygiene, and oral care.

- Hygiene activities are best done when analgesia is at its peak. A small, soft-bristled toothbrush or a warm mouthwash assists in promoting oral care.
- Serve food high in protein and calories that is easily chewed and lukewarm. Offer food frequently. If the patient's nutritional status is compromised, a nasogastric (NG) tube can be inserted on the unaffected side for enteral feedings.

General postoperative nursing care for a craniotomy is appropriate if intracranial surgery has been performed. Compare the postoperative pain level with the preoperative level. Frequently evaluate the corneal reflex, extraocular muscle function, hearing, sensation, and facial nerve function.

- After a percutaneous radiofrequency procedure, apply an ice pack to the jaw on the operative side for 3 to 5 hours. To avoid injuring the mouth, the patient should not chew on the operative side until sensation has returned.

▼ **Patient and Caregiver Teaching**

Plan for regular follow-up care and teach the patient about the dosage and side effects of prescribed drugs. Encourage the patient to manage environmental stimuli and to use stress reduction methods.

Long-term management after surgical intervention depends on the residual effects of the procedure. If anesthesia is present or the corneal reflex is altered, teach the patient to: (1) chew on the unaffected side, (2) avoid hot foods or beverages that can burn the mucous membranes, (3) check the oral cavity after meals to remove food particles, (4) practice meticulous oral hygiene and continue with semiannual dental visits, (5) protect the face against extremes of temperature, (6) use an electric razor, (7) wear a protective eye shield and avoid rubbing the eyes, and (8) examine eye regularly for symptoms of infection or irritation.

TUBERCULOSIS

Description

Tuberculosis (TB) is an infectious disease caused by *Mycobacterium tuberculosis.* It usually involves the lungs, but can infect any organ, including brain, kidneys, and bones.

About one-third of the world's population are infected with TB. The incidence of TB worldwide declined until the mid-1980s. We are now seeing increasing rates of TB. This is attributed to human immunodeficiency (HIV) disease and the emergence of drug resistant strains of *M. tuberculosis.* TB is the leading cause of mortality in patients with HIV infection. Though the prevalence of TB in the United States has steadily declined, it has been suggested that it may be impossible to eradicate TB in the United States.

TB occurs disproportionately in the poor, underserved, and minorities. People most at risk include the homeless, residents of inner-city neighborhoods, foreign-born people, those living or working in institutions (long-term care facilities, prisons, shelters, hospitals), IV injecting drug users, overcrowded living conditions, less than optimal sanitation, and those with poor access to health care. Immunosuppression from any cause (e.g., HIV infection, cancer, long-term corticosteroid use) increases the risk of active TB infection.

- Once a strain of *M. tuberculosis* develops resistance to 2 of the most potent first-line antitubercular drugs (e.g., isoniazid [INH], rifampin [Rifadin]), it is defined as *multidrug-resistant tuberculosis* (MDR-TB). Extensively drug-resistant TB (XDR-TB) occurs when the organism is also resistant to any of the fluoroquinolones plus any injectable antibiotic agent. Resistance results from several problems, including incorrect prescribing, lack of public health case management, patient nonadherence to the prescribed regimen, and lack of funding for education and prevention.

Pathophysiology

M. tuberculosis is a gram-positive, aerobic acid-fast bacillus. It is usually spread from person to person by airborne droplets produced when speaking, breathing, sneezing, and coughing.

- TB is not highly infectious because transmission usually requires close contact and frequent or prolonged exposure. The disease cannot be spread by touching, sharing food utensils, kissing, or any other type of physical contact.
- Once inhaled by another person, *M. tuberculosis* particles lodge in bronchioles and alveoli. The organisms can grow in the lungs, kidneys, epiphyses of bone, cerebral cortex, and adrenal glands.

Classification

Several systems can be used to classify TB. The American Thoracic Society classifies TB based on development of the disease (Table 84). TB can also be classified according to: (1) its presentation—primary, latent, or reactivated—and (2) whether it is pulmonary or extrapulmonary.

Primary infection occurs when the bacteria are inhaled but there is an effective immune response and the bacteria become inactive.

TABLE 84 Classification of Tuberculosis (TB)

Class	Exposure or Infection	Description
0	No TB exposure	No TB exposure, not infected (no history of exposure, negative tuberculin skin test)
1	TB exposure, no infection	TB exposure, no evidence of infection (history of exposure, negative tuberculin skin test)
2	Latent TB infection, no disease	TB infection without disease (positive reaction to tuberculin skin test, negative bacteriologic studies, no x-ray findings compatible with TB, no clinical evidence of TB)
3	TB, clinically active	TB infection with clinically active disease (positive bacteriologic studies, or both a significant reaction to tuberculin skin test and clinical or x-ray evidence of current disease)
4	TB, but not clinically active	No current disease (history of previous episode of TB or abnormal, stable x-ray findings in a person with a positive reaction to tuberculin skin test. Negative bacteriologic studies if done. No clinical or x-ray evidence of current disease)
5	TB suspect	TB suspect (diagnosis pending). Person should not be in this classification for >3 mo.

Source: American Thoracic Society.

T

Most people have an effective immune response to encapsulate these organisms for the rest of their lives.

Latent TB infection (LTBI) occurs in a person who does not have active TB disease. People with LTBI have a positive skin test but are asymptomatic. They cannot transmit the TB bacteria to others but can develop active TB disease at some point. Immunosuppression, diabetes, poor nutrition, aging, pregnancy, stress, and chronic disease can reactivate the disease.

Active TB disease results if the initial immune response is not adequate, the body cannot contain the organisms, and the bacteria replicate. When active disease develops within the first 2 years of infection, it is termed *primary TB.* Postprimary TB, or *reactivation TB,* is defined as TB disease occurring 2 or more years after the initial infection.

Clinical Manifestations

- Active TB disease may initially present with fatigue, malaise, anorexia, unexplained weight loss, low-grade fevers, and night sweats.
- Sometimes TB has a more acute, sudden presentation. The patient may have a high fever, chills, generalized flu-like symptoms, pleuritic pain, a productive cough and acute respiratory failure.
- In patients with HIV infection, signs of TB, such as fever, cough, and weight loss, may be wrongly attributed to pneumonia caused by *Pneumocystis jiroveci* or other HIV-associated diseases.
- The manifestations of extrapulmonary TB depend on the organs infected. For example, renal TB can cause dysuria and hematuria. Bone and joint TB may cause severe pain. Headaches, vomiting, and lymphadenopathy may be present with TB meningitis.

Complications

Miliary TB results from widespread dissemination of the mycobacterium to distant organs. The infection may be fatal if left untreated.

- Manifestations may slowly progress over days, weeks, or months. Symptoms vary depending on which organs are infected.
- Hepatomegaly, splenomegaly, and generalized lymphadenopathy may be present.

Pleural TB is an infected fluid collection in the pleural space. *Empyema* may occur with large numbers of tubercular organisms in the pleural space.

Diagnostic Studies

- Tuberculin skin test (TST): induration (not redness) at the injection site means that the person has been exposed to TB and has

developed antibodies. See Chapter 25, Harding et al., *Lewis'
Medical-Surgical Nursing*, ed 11, for guidelines in performing
and interpreting TSTs.

- Interferon (INF)-gamma release assays (IGRAs)
- Blood test to detect response to mycobacterial antigens.
- Chest x-ray: diagnosis cannot be based solely on x-ray because
  other diseases may mimic TB.
- Bacteriologic studies: stained sputum smears for acid-fast bacilli
  (AFB test) can identify tubercle bacilli; cultures to grow tubercle
  bacilli confirm diagnosis.

Interprofessional Management

Most patients with TB are treated on an outpatient basis and continue to work and maintain their lifestyles with few changes. Hospitalization may be needed for severely ill or debilitated patients.
The mainstay of TB treatment is drug therapy.

Active Tuberculosis Disease

Because of the growing prevalence of MDR-TB, it is important to
manage the patient with active TB aggressively. Drug therapy is
divided into 2 phases: initial and continuation. The treatment for
patients with previously untreated TB is a 2-month initial phase with
4-drug therapy—isoniazid, rifampin, pyrazinamide, and
ethambutol.

- Nonadherence is a major factor in the emergence of multidrug
  resistance and treatment failures. Many people do not adhere
  to the treatment program.
- *Directly observed therapy* (DOT) involves providing the antitu-
  berculous drugs directly to patients and watching as they swallow the medications.

Latent Tuberculosis Infection

In people with LTBI, drug therapy helps prevent a TB infection from
developing into active TB disease. The standard treatment regimen
for LTBI is 9 months of daily INH.

Bacille Calmette-Guérin (BCG) vaccine is given to infants in
parts of the world with a high prevalence of TB. The BCG vaccine
should be considered for persons who meet specific criteria (e.g.,
health care workers who are continually exposed to MDR-TB and
when infection control precautions are not successful).

Nursing Management

Goals

The patient with tuberculosis will have normal pulmonary
function, adhere with the therapeutic regimen, take appropriate
measures to prevent the spread of the disease, and have no recurrence of disease.

T

Nursing Interventions

The ultimate goal is to eradicate TB worldwide.

- Screening programs in known high-risk groups are of value in detecting people with TB.
- Persons with a positive TST should have a chest x-ray to assess for active TB disease.
- Reducing prevalence of HIV infection, poverty, overcrowded living conditions, malnutrition, smoking, and drug and alcohol abuse can help minimize TB infection rates.

If hospitalization is needed for patients suspected of having TB, special measures should be taken.

- Airborne infection isolation is indicated for the patient with pulmonary or laryngeal TB until the patient is noninfectious (defined as effective drug therapy, clinical improvement, and 3 negative AFB smears).
- High-efficiency particulate air (HEPA) masks are worn by those entering the patient's room. Health care professionals should be "fit tested" each time a different brand or model of mask is used, to ensure proper mask size.

▼ **Patient and Caregiver Teaching**

- Teach hospitalized patients to cover the nose and mouth with paper tissues every time they cough, sneeze, or produce sputum.
- Teach the patient and caregivers about the prescribed regimen. Strategies to improve adherence include teaching and counseling, reminder systems, incentives or rewards, contracts, and DOT.
- Because about 5% of people have relapses, teach the patient to recognize and promptly report symptoms that indicate the recurrence of TB to the health care provider (HCP).
- Teach the patient about factors that could reactivate TB, such as immunosuppression or cancer.

ULCERATIVE COLITIS

Ulcerative colitis is an autoimmune disorder that, along with Crohn's disease, is referred to as *inflammatory bowel disease* (IBD). See Inflammatory Bowel Disease, p. 337, for a discussion of the disorder.

URETHRITIS

Description

Urethritis is inflammation of the urethra. Causes of urethritis include a bacterial or viral infection, *Trichomonas* or monilial infection (especially in women), chlamydial infection, and gonor-rhea (especially in men).

In *men,* purulent discharge can indicate gonococcal urethritis. A clear discharge typically signifies a nongonococcal urethritis. Ure-thritis produces bothersome lower urinary tract symptoms (LUTS), including dysuria, urgency, and frequent urination, similar to those seen with cystitis.

In *women,* urethritis is difficult to diagnose. It frequently pro-duces bothersome LUTS, but urethral discharge may not be present.

Nursing and Interprofessional Management

Treatment is based on identifying and treating the cause and provid-ing symptomatic relief.

- Drugs used to treat bacterial infections include trimethoprim/sulfamethoxazole, doxycycline (Vibramycin), ceftriaxone, and nitrofurantoin. Metronidazole (Flagyl) and clotrimazole) are options for treating *Trichomonas* infection. Nystatin, clotrima-zole, or fluconazole, may be used for monilial infections.
- In chlamydial infections, doxycycline or azithromycin may be used. For treatment of gonococcal urethritis, the preferred first-line treatment is azithromycin 1 g orally with 250 mg IM ceftriaxone.
- Warm sitz baths may temporarily relieve symptoms.

Teach female patients to avoid using vaginal deodorant sprays and to properly cleanse the perineal area after bowel movement or voiding. Teach all patients to avoid sexual intercourse for at least 7 days. Teach patients with sexually transmitted urethritis to refer their sex partners for evaluation and testing if they had sexual contact in the 60 days before onset of the symptoms or diagnosis.

URINARY INCONTINENCE

Description

Urinary incontinence (UI) is involuntary leakage of urine. Although it is more prevalent among older women and men, it is not a natural consequence of aging. Many cases of UI can be cured or signifi-cantly improved.

Pathophysiology

UI can result from anything that interferes with bladder or urethral sphincter control.

- Using the acronym *DRIP,* the causes of UI include *D: d*elirium, *d*ehydration, *d*epression; *R: r*estricted mobility, *r*ectal impaction;

I: *i*nfection, *i*nflammation, *i*mpaction; and *P:* *p*olyuria, *p*olypharmacy.

- UI disorders include stress, urge, overflow, and reflex incontinence. Patients may have more than one type of incontinence. The combination of stress and urge incontinence is referred to as mixed incontinence. (For a complete description of UI, see Table 45.16, Harding et al., *Lewis' Medical-Surgical Nursing,* ed 11.)

Diagnostic Studies

- A focused history, physical assessment, and a bladder log or voiding diary provide information about the onset of UI, factors that provoke urinary leakage, and associated conditions.
- Pelvic examination assesses for organ prolapse and evaluates pelvic floor muscle strength.
- Urinalysis can identify factors contributing to incontinence (e.g., urinary infection, diabetes).
- Measure postvoid residual (PVR) urine in the patient undergoing evaluation for UI. The PVR volume is obtained by asking the patient to void, followed by catheterization or use of bladder ultrasound within 10 to 20 minutes.
- Urodynamic testing may be indicated.
- Imaging studies of the upper urinary tract (e.g., ultrasound) are done when incontinence is associated with urinary tract infections or there is evidence of upper urinary tract involvement.

Interprofessional Management

Transient, reversible factors are corrected first, followed by management of the type of UI. In general, less invasive treatments are tried before more invasive methods are used.

Behavioral therapies may be used, including: (1) pelvic floor muscle training (Kegel exercises) to help patients manage stress, urge, or mixed UI; and (2) biofeedback to assist the patient identify, isolate, contract, and relax the pelvic muscles.

Drug Therapy

Drug therapy varies according to UI type.

- In stress UI, drugs have a limited role in the management. Bladder sphincter tone and urethral resistance may increase with αadrenergic agonists, but they have limited benefit.
- In *urge* and *reflex UI,* drugs play a key management role. Anticholinergic drugs (muscarinic receptor blockers) block the action of acetylcholine at muscarinic receptors. They relax the bladder muscle and inhibit overactive detrusor contractions. These preparations include immediate- and extended-release tolterodine (Detrol, Detrol LA); immediate- and extended-release

and transdermal oxybutynin (Ditropan XL, Oxytrol Transdermal System); twice-daily trospium chloride; extended-release solifenacin (VESIcare); and darifenacin (Enablex).

- Botox (onabotulinumtoxin A) can be used in the treatment of detrusor overactivity. Botox injected into the bladder results in relaxation of the bladder, an increase in its storage capacity, and a decrease in UI.

Surgical Therapy

Surgical techniques also vary according to the type of UI.

- Surgical correction of stress UI may reposition the urethra and/or create a backboard of support, or otherwise stabilize the urethra and bladder neck and make them better able to adapt to changes in intraabdominal pressure.
- Another technique for stress UI augments the urethral resistance of the intrinsic sphincter unit with a sling or periurethral injectable.
- Retropubic colposuspension and pubovaginal sling placement appear to be most effective. Typically, both procedures are done through low transverse incisions.
- Placement of a suburethral sling, using autologous fascia, cadaveric fascia, or a synthetic material, can correct stress UI in women.
- An artificial urethral sphincter can be inserted in men with intrinsic sphincter deficiency and severe stress UI.
- Bulking agents can be injected underneath the mucosa of the urethra to correct stress UI in women or men.

Nursing Management

Recognize both the physical and emotional problems associated with incontinence. Maintain and enhance the patient's dignity, privacy, and feelings of self-worth. Take a 2-step approach involving containment devices to manage existing urinary leakage and a definitive plan to reduce or resolve the factors leading to incontinence.

- Emphasize consuming an adequate volume of fluids and reducing or eliminating bladder irritants (particularly caffeine and alcohol) from the diet.
- Advise the patient to maintain a regular, flexible schedule of urination (usually every 2 to 3 hours while awake).
- Advise patients to quit smoking, because it increases the risk of stress UI.
- Teach patients to manage constipation, beginning with ensuring adequate fluid intake, increasing dietary fiber, lightly exercising, and judiciously using stool softeners.
- Behavioral treatments include bladder retraining and pelvic floor muscle training. (A patient teaching guide for pelvic floor muscle exercises is found in Table 45.18, Harding et al., *Lewis' Medical-Surgical Nursing*, ed 11.)

- Assess patient strategies and share information on products designed to contain urine.
- In inpatient or long-term care facilities, management of UI includes maximizing toilet access. Offer the urinal or bedpan, or assist the patient to the bathroom every 2 to 3 hours (or at scheduled times), and ensure privacy.

URINARY RETENTION

Description

Urinary retention is the inability to empty the bladder or the accumulation of urine in the bladder because of an inability to void. In some cases, it is associated with urinary leakage or postvoid dribbling, called overflow urinary incontinence (UI).

- *Acute urinary retention*, which is the total inability to pass urine via micturition, is a medical emergency.
- Chronic urinary retention is incomplete bladder emptying despite urination. The postvoid residual (PVR) volumes in patients with chronic urinary retention vary widely. Normal PVR is between 50 and 75 mL. Findings over 100 mL indicate the need to repeat the measurement. An abnormal PVR in the older patient of more than 200 mL obtained on 2 separate occasions needs further evaluation.

Pathophysiology

Urinary retention is caused by 2 different dysfunctions of the urinary system: bladder outlet obstruction and deficient detrusor (bladder wall muscle) contraction strength.

- *Bladder outlet obstruction* leads to urinary retention when the blockage is so severe that the bladder cannot evacuate its contents despite detrusor contraction. A common cause of obstruction in men is an enlarged prostate.
- Common causes of *deficient detrusor contraction strength* are neurologic diseases affecting the sacral vertebral segments 2, 3, and 4; long-standing diabetes; overdistention; long-term alcohol use; and drugs (e.g., anticholinergic drugs).

Diagnostic Studies

The diagnostic studies for urinary retention are the same as those for UI (see Urinary Incontinence, p. 625).

Interprofessional Management

Behavioral therapies for UI may also be used in the management of urinary retention. Scheduled toileting and double voiding may be effective in chronic urinary retention associated with moderate PVR volumes.

- Double voiding is an attempt to maximize bladder evacuation by having the patient urinate, sit on the toilet for 3 to 4 minutes, and urinate again before exiting the bathroom.
- If catheterization is required for urinary retention, intermittent catheterization is preferred, to decrease the risk of catheter-associated urinary tract infections (CAUTIs) and urethral irritation.

Drug Therapy

Several drugs may be given to promote bladder evacuation. For the patient with obstruction at the level of the bladder neck, an α-adrenergic blocker may be prescribed. These drugs relax the smooth muscle of the bladder neck and prostatic urethra, and may decrease urethral resistance.

Surgical Therapy

Surgical interventions are used to manage urinary retention caused by obstruction. Transurethral or open surgical techniques are used to treat benign or cancerous prostatic enlargement, bladder neck contracture, urethral strictures, or dyssynergia of the bladder neck.

- Pelvic reconstruction using an abdominal or transvaginal approach can correct bladder outlet obstruction in women with severe pelvic organ prolapse.
- Sacral neuromodulation involves a stimulator device and placement of a lead wire into the S3 foramen.
- An intraurethral valve pump can be placed to empty the patient's bladder as needed.

Nursing Management

Acute urinary retention is a medical emergency that requires prompt bladder drainage. Insert a catheter as prescribed. See Urinary Catheterization, p. 718.

- Teach the patient with or predisposed to acute urinary retention how to minimize risk, including avoiding rapid intake of large volumes of fluid.
- Advise the patient who is unable to urinate to drink a cup of coffee or brewed caffeinated tea to maximize urinary urgency, and then attempt to urinate while in a tub of warm water or a warm shower.
- If these measures do not lead to successful urination, have the patient seek immediate care.

Patients may manage chronic urinary retention with behavioral methods, an indwelling catheter, intermittent catheterization, surgery, or drugs. Scheduled toileting and double voiding are the primary behavioral interventions used for chronic retention.

URINARY TRACT CALCULI

Description

Calculi, or stones, can be found in various locations in the urinary tract. In their lifetime, 13% of men and 7% of women in the United States will have nephrolithiasis (kidney stone disease). The term *calculus* refers to the stone, and *lithiasis* refers to stone formation. Except for struvite (magnesium ammonium phosphate) stones associated with urinary tract infection (UTI), stone disorders are more common in men than in women. Most patients are middle-aged adults. Stone formation is more frequent in whites than in Blacks, Hispanics, and Asians.

- The incidence is higher in people with a family history of stone formation. Stones can recur in up to 50% of patients.
- Stone formation occurs more often in the summer months, supporting the possible contributing factors of a hot climate and dehydration.

Pathophysiology

Many factors are involved in the incidence and type of stone formation, including climatic, dietary, genetic, metabolic, and lifestyle influences. No single theory accounts for stone formation in all cases. We think kidney stones form when crystal-forming substances are not diluted by the kidney and/or there is reduced ability of the kidneys to keep the crystals from sticking together.

- Crystals in a supersaturated concentration can precipitate and unite to form a stone. Keeping urine dilute and free-flowing reduces the risk of recurrent stone formation.
- Urinary pH, solute load, and inhibitors in the urine affect the formation of stones. The higher the pH, the less soluble are calcium and phosphate. The lower the pH, the less soluble are uric acid and cystine.

Other important factors in stone development include obstruction with associated urinary stasis and UTI with urea-splitting bacteria (e.g., *Proteus, Klebsiella, Pseudomonas,* and some species of staphylococci). These bacteria cause the urine to become alkaline, contributing to the formation of struvite (calcium-magnesium-ammonium phosphate) stones.

- Infected stones, entrapped in the kidney, may assume a staghorn configuration as they enlarge. These stones can lead to hydronephrosis, renal infection, and loss of kidney function.

There are 5 major categories of stones: calcium oxalate, calcium phosphate, cystine, struvite, and uric acid. Stone composition may be mixed, although calcium stones are the most common.

Clinical Manifestations

The first symptom is usually sudden, severe pain in the flank area, back, or lower abdomen. People describe the pain as excruciating.

- *Renal colic* is the term used for the severe pain from the stretching, dilation, and spasm of the ureter in response to the obstructing stone. Nausea and vomiting may also occur.
- Urinary stones cause manifestations when they obstruct urinary flow. The type of pain is determined by the location of the stone. If the obstruction is in a calyx or the ureteropelvic junction (UPJ), the patient may have dull costovertebral flank pain or renal colic. Pain resulting from the passage of a stone calculus down the ureter is intense and colicky. The patient may be in mild shock, with cool, moist skin. As a stone nears the ureterovesical junction (UVJ), pain will be felt in the lateral flank and sometimes down into the groin and testicles or labia.
- Manifestations may include dysuria, fever, and chills.

Diagnostic Studies

- Noncontrast helical (spiral) CT scan, ultrasound, and intravenous pyelogram (IVP) may be used.
- Urinalysis is used to assess for hematuria, crystalluria, and urine pH. Measuring urine pH is useful in the diagnosis of struvite stones (tendency to alkaline or high pH) and uric acid or cystine stones (tendency to acidic or low pH).
- Retrieval and analysis of the stones are important in the diagnosis of the underlying problem contributing to stone formation.
- Serum calcium, phosphorus, sodium, potassium, bicarbonate, uric acid, and creatinine levels and blood urea nitrogen (BUN) are measured.

Interprofessional Management

Evaluation and management of the patient with renal stones involve 2 concurrent approaches. The *first approach* managing the acute attack by treating the pain, infection, or obstruction. Give opioids to relieve renal colic pain. Nonsteroidal antiinflammatory drugs (NSAIDs) can be considered if there is normal renal function. Many stones are 4 mm or less in size, so will pass spontaneously. However, such a stone may take weeks to pass. Tamsulosin (Flomax) or terazosin, α-adrenergic blockers that relax the smooth muscle in the ureter, can be given to facilitate stone passage.

The *second approach* is evaluating the cause of stone formation and preventing further stone development. Information obtained from the patient includes family history of stone formation, geographic location of residence, nutritional assessment (including fluid intake and intake of vitamins A, C, and D), activity pattern (active or sedentary), history of periods of prolonged illness with immobilization or dehydration, and history of disease or surgery involving the gastrointestinal (GI) or genitourinary (GU) tract. Include any prior episodes of stone formation, prescribed and over-the-counter (OTC) medications, and use of dietary supplements.

Adequate hydration, dietary sodium restrictions, dietary changes, and drugs minimize urinary stone formation.

- Various drugs are prescribed that prevent stone formation by altering urine pH, preventing excessive urinary excretion of a substance, or correcting a primary disease (e.g., hyperparathyroidism).

Treatment of struvite stones requires control of infection. Acetohydroxamic acid inhibits the chemical action caused by persistent bacteria and can slow struvite stone formation. The stone may have to be removed surgically if the infection cannot be controlled. Indications for open surgical, endourology, or lithotripsy stone removal include:

- stones too large for spontaneous passage (usually larger than 7 mm), associated with bacteriuria or symptomatic infection, or causing impaired renal function, persistent pain, nausea, or paralytic ileus;
- medical treatment not successful;
- patient with only 1 kidney.

Endourologic procedures include the use of endoscopes to reach stones in the urinary tract. *Cystoscopy* can remove small stones in the bladder. For large stones, a *cystolitholapaxy* is performed using a lithotrite to crush stones. A *cystoscopic lithotripsy* uses ultrasonic waves to break up stones. Complications with these procedures include hemorrhage, retained stone fragments, and infection. Flexible *ureteroscopes* can be used to remove stones from the renal pelvis and upper urinary tract with ultrasonic, laser, or electrohydraulic lithotripsy. The same types of lithotripsy can be used during a percutaneous nephrolithotomy when a nephroscope is inserted through the skin into the kidney pelvis.

Lithotripsy is a procedure for eliminating calculi from the urinary tract. Specific lithotripsy techniques include percutaneous ultrasonic lithotripsy, electrohydraulic lithotripsy, laser lithotripsy, and extracorporeal shock wave lithotripsy. Extracorporeal shock wave lithotripsy and laser lithotripsy are the most common.

Hematuria is common after lithotripsy procedures. A self-retaining ureteral stent is placed to prevent obstruction caused by sand buildup in the ureter, then removed 2 weeks later.

- If a stone is large or positioned in the mid or distal ureter, additional treatment may be needed.

Some patients need open surgical procedures because of pain, obstruction, or infection. The type of open surgery (e.g., *nephrolithotomy, pyelolithotomy, ureterolithotomy*) depends on location of the stone. For open surgery on the kidney or ureter, a flank incision directly below the diaphragm and across the side is usually preferred.

Nutritional Therapy

A high fluid intake (around 3 L/day) is recommended after an episode of urolithiasis to produce urine output of at least 2.5 L/day and prevent recurrent stones.

- Limit consumption of colas, coffee, and tea, because high intake of these beverages tends to increase the risk of recurring urinary stones.
- A low-sodium diet is recommended, because high sodium intake increases calcium excretion in the urine. Foods high in calcium, oxalate, and purines are listed in Table 45.12, Harding et al., *Lewis' Medical-Surgical Nursing*, ed 11.

Nursing Management

Goals

The overall goals are that the patient with urinary tract stones will have relief of pain, no urinary tract obstruction, and an understanding of measures to prevent recurrence of stones.

Nursing Interventions

Preventive measures related to the person who is on bed rest or is immobile for a prolonged period include maintaining an adequate fluid intake, turning the patient every 2 hours, and helping the patient sit or stand if possible to maximize urinary flow.

Pain management and patient comfort are primary nursing responsibilities in managing a person with an obstructing stone and renal colic.

- To retrieve any spontaneously passed stones, strain all urine voided by the patient, using gauze or a urine strainer.
- Encourage ambulation to promote movement of the stone to the lower urinary tract. To ensure safety, tell the patient who has acute renal colic to ask for help when ambulating, particularly if opioid analgesics are given.

▼ **Patient and Caregiver Teaching**

- Encourage adequate fluid intake to produce a urine output of approximately 2.5 L/day.
- Teach about dietary restriction of purines to lower risk for developing uric acid stones.
- Teach the patient the dosage, scheduling, and potential side effects of drugs used to reduce the risk of stone formation.
- Some patients may learn to self-monitor urinary pH or urinary output.

URINARY TRACT INFECTIONS

Description

Urinary tract infections (UTIs) are the second most common bacterial disease and the most common bacterial infection in women. *Escherichia coli (E. coli)* is the most common pathogen causing a UTI. *Candida albicans* is the second most common pathogen, causing UTIs associated with indwelling catheter use or asymptomatic colonization.

- Bacterial counts in the urine of 10^5 colony-forming units per milliliter (CFU/mL) or higher typically indicate a UTI. However, bacterial counts as low as 10^2 to 10^3 CFU/mL in a person with symptoms are also indicative of UTI.
- Fungal and parasitic UTIs are uncommon and seen in the patient who is immunosuppressed, has kidney disorders or diabetes or has taken multiple courses of antibiotics.

Classification

A UTI can be broadly classified as an upper or a lower UTI according to its location within the urinary system. Infection of the upper urinary tract (involving the renal parenchyma, pelvis, and ureters) typically causes fever, chills, and flank pain. A lower-urinary-tract infection does not usually have systemic manifestations.

Specific terms identify the UTI location. For example, *pyelonephritis* implies inflammation usually caused by infection of the renal parenchyma and collecting system. *Cystitis* indicates inflammation of the bladder wall, while *urethritis* is inflammation of the urethra. *Urosepsis* is a UTI that has spread systemically. It is a life-threatening condition requiring emergency treatment.

- *Uncomplicated UTIs* are those that occur in an otherwise normal urinary tract and usually involve only the bladder.
- *Complicated UTIs* are those associated with coexisting obstruction, stones, or catheters; abnormal genitourinary (GU) tract; DM or neurologic diseases; immunosuppression; pregnancy-induced changes; recurrent infection; or antibiotic resistance. The patient with a complicated infection is at risk for pyelonephritis, urosepsis, and renal damage.

Pathophysiology

The urinary tract above the urethra is normally sterile. Organisms that cause UTIs are usually introduced from the urethra. Gram-negative aerobic bacilli normally found in the gastrointestinal (GI) tract cause most UTIs. However, gram-positive organisms, such as streptococci, enterococci, and *Staphylococcus saprophyticus*, can also cause UTIs. Table 85 lists risk factors for UTIs.

TABLE 85 Risk Factors for Urinary Tract Infections

U

Anatomic Factors
- Congenital defects leading to obstruction or urinary stasis
- Fistula exposing urinary stream to skin, vagina, or fecal stream
- Obesity
- Shorter female urethra and colonization from normal vaginal flora

Foreign Bodies Factors Compromising Immune Response
- Aging
- Diabetes
- Human immunodeficiency virus infection

Factors Increasing Urinary Stasis
- Extrinsic obstruction (tumor, fibrosis compressing urinary tract)
- Intrinsic obstruction (stone, tumor of urinary tract, urethral stricture, benign prostatic hypertrophy)
- Renal impairment
- Urinary retention (e.g., neurogenic bladder)

Foreign Bodies
- Catheters (indwelling, external condom catheter, ureteral stent, nephrostomy tube, intermittent catheterization)
- Urinary tract instrumentation (cystoscopy)
- Urinary tract stones

Functional Disorders
- Constipation
- Voiding dysfunction with detrusor sphincter dyssynergia

Other Factors
- Habitual delay of urination ("nurse's bladder," "teacher's bladder")
- Pregnancy
- Menopause
- Multiple sex partners (women)
- Poor personal hygiene
- Use of spermicidal agents, contraceptive diaphragm (women), bubble baths, feminine sprays

- Urologic instrumentation (e.g., catheterization, cystoscopic examinations) allows bacteria normally present at the opening of the urethra to enter the urethra or bladder.

- Sexual intercourse promotes "milking" of bacteria from the vagina and perineum and may cause minor urethral trauma that predisposes women to UTIs.
- Blood-borne bacteria rarely invade the kidneys, ureters, or bladder unless there is a prior injury to the urinary tract,

UTIs are the most common health–care associated infection (HAI). They are primarily associated with use of an indwelling catheter. *Catheter-associated urinary tract infections (CAUTIs)* often are caused by *E. coli* and, less often, *Pseudomonas* organisms. CAUTIs are often underrecognized and undertreated, leading to extended hospital stays, increased health care costs, and patient morbidity and mortality.

Clinical Manifestations

Lower urinary tract symptoms (LUTS) are seen in patients with UTIs of both the upper and lower urinary tracts.

- Symptoms include dysuria, frequent urination (more often than every 2 hours), urgency, and suprapubic discomfort or pressure. Older adults tend to experience generalized abdominal discomfort, rather than dysuria and suprapubic pain.
- The urine may contain visible blood (hematuria) or sediment, giving it a cloudy appearance.
- Flank pain, chills, and fever indicate an infection involving the upper urinary tract (pyelonephritis).

Diagnostic Studies

- Dipstick urinalysis of a clean-catch specimen is done initially to identify presence of nitrites (indicating bacteriuria), white blood cells (WBCs), and leukocyte esterase (an enzyme present in WBCs indicating pyuria).
- After confirmation of bacteriuria and pyuria, a urine culture with sensitivity may be obtained.
- A CT urogram or ultrasound may be obtained when obstruction of the urinary system is suspected.

Interprofessional Management

Drug Therapy

Uncomplicated UTIs are treated with a short-term course of antibiotics, typically for 3 days. In contrast, complicated UTIs need a longer period of treatment, lasting 7 to 14 days or more.

- First-choice drugs to treat uncomplicated or initial UTIs are trimethoprim/sulfamethoxazole (TMP-SMX), nitrofurantoin, cephalexin, and fosfomycin. TMP-SMX has the advantages of being relatively inexpensive and taken twice daily. *E. coli* resistance to TMP-SMX, beta-lactams, and ciprofloxacin is an increasing problem in the United States.

- Other antibiotics used in the treatment of uncomplicated UTI include ampicillin, amoxicillin, and cephalosporins.
- Fluoroquinolones (e.g., levofloxacin, ciprofloxacin) are used to treat complicated UTIs.
- In patients with UTIs from fungi, fluconazole (Diflucan) is the preferred therapy.
- Prophylactic or suppressive antibiotics are sometimes given to patients who have repeated UTIs.
- A urinary analgesic, such as oral phenazopyridine, may relieve discomfort caused by severe dysuria.

Nursing Management

Goals

The goals for patient with a UTI are relief from bothersome LUTS, prevention of upper urinary tract involvement, and prevention of recurrence. See eNursing Care Plan 45-1 for the patient with a UTI on the website for Harding et al., *Lewis' Medical-Surgical Nursing,* ed 11.

Nursing Interventions

Health promotion activities, especially for persons who are at an increased risk for UTI, include teaching preventive measures, such as: (1) emptying the bladder regularly and completely, (2) evacuating the bowel regularly, (3) wiping the perineal area from front to back after urination and defecation, and (4) drinking an adequate amount of liquid each day.

- All patients undergoing instrumentation of the urinary tract are at risk for developing CAUTI. You have a major role in the prevention of these infections. Avoiding unnecessary catheterization and early removal of indwelling catheters are the most effective measures for reducing CAUTI. Always follow aseptic technique during these procedures.
- Wash your hands before and after contact with each patient. Wear gloves for care of urinary catheters. The American Nurses Association offers an evidence-based clinical tool for decreasing CAUTI.
- Acute intervention for the patient with a UTI includes adequate fluid intake. Fluid flushes out bacteria before they have a chance to colonize in the bladder. Caffeine, alcohol, citrus juice, chocolate, and highly spiced foods or beverages should be avoided because they may irritate the bladder.
- Application of local heat to the suprapubic area or lower back may relieve the discomfort associated with a UTI. A warm

shower or sitting in a tub of warm water filled to above the waist can provide temporary relief.

▼ **Patient and Caregiver Teaching**

Teach the patient about the prescribed drug therapy and side effects. Stress the importance of taking the full course of antibiotics.

- Teach patients to promptly report any of the following to their health care provider (HCP): (1) persistence of bothersome LUTS beyond the antibiotic treatment course, (2) onset of flank pain, or (3) fever. Recurrent symptoms associated with bacterial persistence or inadequate treatment typically occur within 1 to 2 weeks after completion of therapy.
- Teach the patient and caregiver about ongoing care, including taking antimicrobial drugs as ordered, maintaining adequate daily fluid intake, voiding regularly (approximately every 3 to 4 hours), urinating before and after intercourse, and temporarily discontinuing the use of a diaphragm.
- Teach patients prescribed phenazopyridine that the drug causes urine to turn orange or red.

VAGINAL, CERVICAL, AND VULVAR INFECTIONS

Definition

Infection and inflammation of the vagina, cervix, and vulva occur when the natural defenses of the acid vaginal secretions (maintained by a sufficient estrogen level) and the presence of *Lactobacillus* are disrupted. Aging, poor nutrition, and drugs (e.g., antibiotics, oral contraceptives, corticosteroids) can affect the microbiome of the vagina.

Pathophysiology

Organisms gain entrance to the lower genital tract through sexual intercourse, contact with contaminated hands or clothing, or douching. Table 86 presents the causes, manifestations and treatment of common infections of the female lower genital tract.

- Oral contraceptives, antibiotics, and corticosteroids may change the vaginal pH and trigger an overgrowth of the organisms present. For example, *Candida albicans* may be present in small numbers in the vagina. An overgrowth of this organism causes vulvovaginitis.
- Vulvar infections, such as herpes and genital warts, can be sexually transmitted when no visible lesions are present (see Herpes, Genital, p. 296, and Warts, Genital, p. 657).

TABLE 86 Infections of the Lower Genital Tract

Infection and Etiology	Manifestations	Treatment Considerations
Bacterial Vaginosis		
Corynebacterium vaginale *Gardnerella vaginalis*	Watery discharge with fish-like odor. May or may not have other symptoms.	Drug therapy based on cause: <ul><li>clindamycin (Clindesse)—vaginal</li><li>metronidazole (Flagyl)—oral or intravaginal</li><li>tinidazole (Tindamax)—oral</li></ul> *Lactobacillus acidophilus* taken orally by diet (e.g., yogurt, fermented soy products) or supplements can decrease unwanted vaginal bacteria
Cervicitis		
Chlamydia trachomatis *Neisseria gonorrhoeae* (most often)	Sexually transmitted. Mucopurulent discharge with postcoital spotting from cervical inflammation.	Drug therapy based on cause, common agents include azithromycin (Zithromax) and ceftriaxone Treat patient and partner. May be reportable according to state laws
Severe Recurrent Vaginitis (More Than 4 Episodes Per Year)		
Candida albicans (most often) or non-*albicans* strains	Depend on cause	Drug therapy based on cause All women who are unresponsive to first-line treatment should be offered HIV testing Common in women with uncontrolled diabetes or HIV infection

Continued

V

TABLE 86 Infections of the Lower Genital Tract—cont'd

Infection and Etiology	Manifestations	Treatment Considerations
Trichomonas Vaginitis		
Trichomonas vaginalis (protozoa)	Sexually transmitted. Itching, frothy greenish or gray discharge. Hemorrhagic spots on cervix or vaginal walls.	Antifungal agents • metronidazole (Flagyl) • tinidazole (Tindamax) Treat patient and partner
Vulvovaginal Candidiasis		
C. albicans (fungus)	Itching, thick white curd-like discharge.	Antifungal agents • clotrimazole (Gyne-Lotrimin, Mycelex) • fluconazole (Diflucan) • miconazole (Monistat) • terconazole (Terazol)

HIV, Human immunodeficiency virus; *KOH,* potassium hydroxide.

Clinical Manifestations

Abnormal vaginal discharge and a reddened vulva are common signs of infection. See Table 86 for additional manifestations of lower genital tract infections.

Diagnostic Studies

Evaluation of genital problems includes a history, physical examination, and appropriate laboratory and diagnostic studies. Because many problems relate to sexual activity, a sexual history is essential.

- Ulcerative lesions are cultured for herpesvirus.
- Vulvar dystrophies are examined by colposcope, with biopsy specimens taken.
- Vaginal discharge is evaluated by examining the discharge under a microscope and obtaining specimens for culture.
- With cervicitis, endocervical cultures are obtained for chlamydia and gonorrhea.
- Sexually transmitted infections (STIs) are discussed on p. 545.

Interprofessional and Nursing Management

Antibiotics taken as directed will cure bacterial infections. Women with vaginal conditions or cervical infection should abstain from intercourse for at least 1 week. Sexual partners must be evaluated and treated if the patient is diagnosed with trichomoniasis, chlamydial infection, gonorrhea, syphilis, or human immunodeficiency virus (HIV) infection.

Treatment of vulvar skin conditions is symptomatic, controlling the itching and hence the scratching. High-potency topical corticosteroid ointment, such as clobetasol, helps relieve itching. Interrupting the "itch-scratch cycle" prevents further secondary damage to the skin.

Teach women about common genital conditions and how to reduce their risks. Recognize symptoms that indicate a problem and help women seek care in a timely manner.

- Teach patients how to properly take prescribed drugs and to get follow-up care. Partners should be treated so that reinfection does not occur.
- When a woman is using a vaginal medication such as an antifungal cream for the first time, show her the applicator and how to fill it. Also teach where and how the applicator should be inserted by using visual aids or models.
- Vaginal creams should be inserted before going to bed so that the medication will remain in the vagina for a long period of time. Women using vaginal creams or suppositories may wish to use panty liners during the day, when the residual medication drains out.

VALVULAR HEART DISEASE

Description

Valvular heart disease is defined according to the affected valve or valves (mitral, aortic, tricuspid, pulmonary) and the type of dysfunction: *stenosis* or *regurgitation.*

- The pressures on either side of an open valve normally are equal. However, in *stenosis,* the valve opening is smaller, impeding the forward flow of blood and creating a pressure difference on the 2 sides of the open valve. The degree of stenosis (constriction or narrowing) is reflected in the pressure differences (i.e., the higher the gradient, the greater the stenosis).
- In *regurgitation* (also called *incompetence* or *insufficiency*), incomplete closure of valve leaflets results in backward flow of blood.

Congenital heart conditions are the most common cause of valve disorders in children and adolescents. Aortic stenosis and mitral regurgitation are in older adults with heart disease. Other causes of valve disease in adults are related to acquired immunodeficiency syndrome (AIDS) and the use of some antiparkinsonian drugs.

Clinical manifestations of valvular heart disease are presented in Table 87.

Mitral Valve Stenosis

Pathophysiology

Worldwide, the most common cause of mitral valve stenosis is rheumatic heart disease. Less common causes include congenital mitral stenosis, rheumatoid arthritis, radiation exposure, and systemic lupus erythematosus (SLE).

- Rheumatic endocarditis causes scarring of valve leaflets and chordae tendineae. Contractures and adhesions develop between the commissures (the junctional areas).
- The stenotic mitral valve takes on a "fish mouth" shape because of the thickening and shortening of mitral valve structures. Flow obstruction increases left atrial pressure and volume, resulting in higher pulmonary vasculature pressure and eventually involving the right ventricle.

Clinical Manifestations

The main symptom is exertional dyspnea caused by reduced lung compliance. Fatigue and palpitations from atrial fibrillation may also occur. Heart sounds include a loud first heart sound and a low-pitched, rumbling diastolic murmur (best heard at the apex with the stethoscope bell).

Other clinical manifestations are identified in Table 87.

TABLE 87 Manifestations of Valvular Heart Disease

Type	Manifestations
Mitral valve prolapse	Palpitations, dyspnea, chest pain, activity intolerance, syncope, holosystolic murmur
Mitral valve regurgitation	*Acute:* generally poorly tolerated. New systolic murmur with pulmonary edema. Cardiogenic shock develops rapidly. *Chronic:* weakness, fatigue, exertional dyspnea, palpitations, S_3 gallop, holosystolic murmur
Mitral valve stenosis	Dyspnea on exertion, hemoptysis, fatigue. Atrial fibrillation on ECG. Palpitations. Loud, accentuated S_1. Low-pitched, diastolic murmur
Aortic valve regurgitation	*Acute:* abrupt onset of profound dyspnea, chest pain, left ventricular failure and cardiogenic shock. *Chronic:* fatigue, exertional dyspnea, orthopnea, PND. Water-hammer pulse, heaving precordial impulse, decreased or absent S_1, S_3, or S_4. Soft high-pitched diastolic murmur, Austin Flint murmur
Aortic valve stenosis	Angina, syncope, dyspnea on exertion, heart failure, normal or soft S_1, decreased or absent S_2, systolic murmur, prominent S_4
Tricuspid and pulmonic stenosis	*Tricuspid:* peripheral edema, ascites, hepatomegaly. Diastolic low-pitched murmur with increased intensity during inspiration. *Pulmonic:* fatigue, loud midsystolic murmur

ECG, Electrocardiogram; *PND,* paroxysmal nocturnal dyspnea.

Mitral Valve Regurgitation

Pathophysiology

Mitral valve function depends on the integrity of mitral leaflets, chordae tendineae, papillary muscles, left atrium (LA), and left ventricle (LV). A defect in any of these structures can cause regurgitation. Myocardial infarction with left ventricular failure increases the risk for rupture of the chordae tendineae and acute mitral regurgitation (MR).

- Most cases of MR are caused by myocardial infarction, chronic rheumatic heart disease, mitral valve prolapse, ischemic papillary muscle dysfunction, and infective endocarditis (IE).
- MR allows blood to flow backward from the LV to the LA because of incomplete valve closure during systole. Both chambers of the left side of the heart must work harder to preserve an adequate cardiac output (CO).
- In acute MR, the sudden increase in pressure and volume is transmitted to the pulmonary bed. This results in pulmonary edema and, if not treated, cardiogenic shock.
- In chronic MR, the added volume load results in left atrial enlargement and left ventricular dilation and hypertrophy, and, finally, a decrease in CO.

Clinical Manifestations

Patients with acute MR have thready peripheral pulses and cool, clammy extremities. A low CO may mask a new systolic murmur. Rapid assessment (e.g., cardiac catheterization) and intervention (e.g., valve repair or replacement) are critical for a positive outcome.

Patients with chronic MR may remain asymptomatic for years until the development of some degree of left ventricular failure. Manifestations are identified in Table 87.

Mitral Valve Prolapse

Pathophysiology

Mitral valve prolapse (MVP) is an abnormality of the mitral valve leaflets and papillary muscles or chordae that allows the leaflets to prolapse, or "buckle," back into the left atrium during systole. It is the most common form of valvular heart disease in the United States.

- MVP is usually benign, but serious complications can occur, including MR, IE, sudden cardiac death, and cerebral ischemia.
- There is an increased familial incidence in some patients resulting from a connective tissue defect affecting only the valve, or as part of Marfan's syndrome or other hereditary conditions that influence the structure of collagen in the body.

Clinical Manifestations

MVP covers a broad spectrum of severity. Most patients are asymptomatic for their entire lives. Clinical manifestations may include those identified in Table 87.

- Patients may or may not have chest pain. If chest pain occurs, episodes tend to occur in clusters, especially during periods of emotional stress. Chest pain may occasionally be accompanied by dyspnea, palpitations, and syncope and does not respond to antianginal treatment (e.g., nitrates).

TABLE 88   **Patient and Caregiver Teaching**

Mitral Valve Prolapse

Include the following information in the teaching plan for a patient with mitral valve prolapse (MVP) and the patient's caregiver.

- Take drugs as prescribed (e.g., β-adrenergic blockers to control palpitations, chest pain).
- Adopt healthy eating habits.
- Avoid caffeine because it is a stimulant and may worsen symptoms.
- If you use diet pills or other over-the-counter drugs, check for common ingredients that are stimulants (e.g., caffeine, ephedrine) because these can worsen symptoms.
- Begin or maintain an exercise program to achieve optimal health.
- Contact the health care provider (HCP) or emergency medical services if symptoms develop or worsen (e.g., palpitations, fatigue, shortness of breath, anxiety).

Patients with MVP generally have a benign course unless problems related to MR develop. Table 88 provides a teaching plan for patients with MVP.

Aortic Valve Stenosis

Pathophysiology

Congenital aortic stenosis is found in childhood, adolescence, or young adulthood. In older patients, *aortic stenosis* is a result of rheumatic fever or degeneration similar to that in coronary artery disease.

- In rheumatic valve disease, fusion and calcification cause the valve leaflets to stiffen and retract, resulting in stenosis.
- Aortic stenosis causes obstruction of flow from the LV to the aorta during systole. The result is left ventricular hypertrophy and increased myocardial oxygen consumption because of the increased myocardial mass.
- As the disease progresses and compensation fails, reduced CO leads to pulmonary hypertension and heart failure.

Clinical Manifestations

Symptoms of aortic stenosis (AS) develop when the valve orifice becomes about one-third of its normal size. Symptoms include the classic triad of angina, syncope, and exertional dyspnea, reflecting left ventricular failure. Auscultation of AS often reveals a normal or soft S1, a decreased diminished or absent S2, a crescendo-decrescendo systolic murmur, with radiation to the carotids. Common manifestations are presented in Table 87.

Aortic Valve Regurgitation
Pathophysiology
Aortic regurgitation may be the result of primary disease of the aortic valve leaflets, the aortic root, or both.

- Acute aortic regurgitation is caused by IE, trauma, or aortic dissection and constitutes a life-threatening emergency.
- Chronic aortic regurgitation is generally the result of rheumatic heart disease, a congenital bicuspid aortic valve, syphilis, a connective tissue problem, or a postsurgical cause.
- Aortic regurgitation causes retrograde blood flow from the ascending aorta into the LV, resulting in volume overload.
- Myocardial contractility eventually declines, and blood volume increases in the LA and pulmonary bed. This leads to pulmonary hypertension and right ventricular failure.

Clinical Manifestations
Clinical manifestations of acute and chronic aortic valve regurgitation are presented in Table 87.

Tricuspid and Pulmonic Valve Disease
Diseases of the tricuspid and pulmonic valves are uncommon, with stenosis occurring more frequently than regurgitation. Tricuspid stenosis results in right atrial enlargement and elevated systemic venous pressures. Pulmonic stenosis results in right ventricular hypertension and hypertrophy. Table 87 presents clinical manifestations of these valve diseases.

Diagnostic Studies: Valvular Heart Disease
- Electrocardiogram (ECG) shows variations in heart rate (HR), rhythm, and possible ischemia or chamber enlargement.
- Echocardiogram reveals valve structure, function, and heart chamber size.
- Transesophageal echocardiography and Doppler color-flow imaging help diagnose and monitor valvular heart disease progression.
- Real-time 3-dimensional echocardiography helps assess mitral valve and congenital heart disease.
- Chest x-ray reveals heart size, altered pulmonary circulation, and valve calcification.
- Cardiac catheterization detects chamber pressure changes and pressure gradients (differences) across the valves.

Interprofessional Management: Valvular Heart Disease
Overall treatment focuses on preventing exacerbations of heart failure, acute pulmonary edema, thromboembolism, and recurrent

endocarditis. Heart failure is treated with vasodilators, positive inotropes, β-adrenergic blockers, diuretics, and a low-sodium diet.

- Anticoagulant therapy is used in patients with atrial fibrillation to prevent systemic or pulmonary emboli.
- Atrial dysrhythmias are common and treated with calcium-channel blockers, β- blockers, antidysrhythmic drugs, or electrical cardioversion.
- An alternative treatment for some patients with valvular stenosis is the *percutaneous transluminal balloon valvuloplasty* (PTBV) procedure in a heart catheterization laboratory. A balloon-tipped catheter is threaded from the femoral artery to the stenotic valve so that the balloon may be inflated to separate valve leaflets.
- The Sapien Transcatheter Heart Valve (THV) is used for some patients with AS. The insertion process is similar to the PTBV.

Surgical Therapy

The type of valve repair or replacement depends on the valves involved, disease pathology severity, and the patient's symptoms.

- Valve repair is preferred over replacement when appropriate. Repair has a lower operative mortality rate than valve replacement, but may not restore total valve function.
- Open surgical *valvuloplasty* involves repairing the valve by suturing the torn leaflets, chordae tendineae, and papillary muscles. It is primarily used to treat mitral regurgitation or tricuspid regurgitation.
- For patients with mitral or tricuspid regurgitation, further valve repair or reconstruction using annuloplasty is an option. *Annuloplasty* involves reconstruction of the annulus, with or without the aid of prosthetic rings.

Valve Replacement. Valve replacement may be required for mitral, aortic, tricuspid, or pulmonic valve disease.

- *Mechanical valves* are made of combinations of metal alloys, pyrolite carbon, and Dacron. Biologic valves are constructed from bovine, porcine, and human (cadaver) cardiac tissue.
- Mechanical prosthetic valves are more durable than biologic tissue valves, but they carry an increased risk of thromboembolism and patients need long-term anticoagulant therapy. Anticoagulation therapy is not needed with biologic valves. However, they are less durable and tend to develop early calcification, tissue degeneration, and stiffening of leaflets. Both valve types are subject to leaking and endocarditis.
- Long-term anticoagulation is needed for those patients with biologic valves who have atrial fibrillation. Some patients with biologic valves or annuloplasty with prosthetic rings may need anticoagulation the first few months after surgery, until the suture lines are covered by endothelial cells (endothelialized).

- The choice of valves depends on many factors. A mechanical valve may be best for a younger patient because it is more durable. If a patient cannot take an anticoagulant (e.g., women of childbearing age), a biologic valve is considered. Frail patients with co-morbidities should be referred to a qualified heart team for a full evaluation before considering surgery.

Nursing Management: Valvular Heart Disease
Goals
The overall goals for the patient with valve disease include: (1) normal heart function, (2) improved activity tolerance, and (3) an understanding of the disease process and health maintenance measures.
Nursing Interventions
Encouraging early treatment of streptococcal infection and providing prophylactic antibiotics for patients with a history of rheumatic fever are critical to prevent acquired rheumatic valve disease. Patients at risk for endocarditis and any patients with certain high-risk heart conditions must receive prophylactic antibiotics.

- Teach the person with a history of rheumatic fever, endocarditis, or congenital heart disease the symptoms of valvular heart disease to report.
- Design activities considering the patient's limitations. An appropriate exercise plan can increase cardiac tolerance. Activities that cause fatigue and dyspnea should be limited.
- Develop your patient's care plan to emphasize conserving energy, setting priorities, and taking planned rest periods.
- Consider referral to a vocational counselor if the patient has a physically or emotionally demanding job.
- Perform ongoing cardiac assessments to monitor the effectiveness of medications. Teach the actions and side effects of drugs to increase adherence. Reinforce the importance of prophylactic antibiotic therapy to prevent IE.
- The patient on anticoagulants (e.g., warfarin) after surgery for valve replacement must have the international normalized ratio (INR) checked regularly to determine adequacy of therapy. INR values of 2.5 to 3.5 are therapeutic for patients with mechanical valves.

▼ **Patient and Caregiver Teaching**
- Teach the patient to notify the health care provider (HCP) about any signs or symptoms of infection, heart failure, or bleeding.
- Encourage patients to wear a medical identification (Medic Alert) device.

VARICOSE VEINS

Description

Varicose veins (varicosities) are dilated (to 3 mm or larger in diameter), tortuous superficial veins, often found in the saphenous vein system. They may be small and innocuous or large and bulging.

- *Primary* varicose veins (idiopathic), caused by weakness of the vein walls, are more common in women.
- *Secondary* varicosities typically result from result from direct injury, a previous venous thromboembolism (VTE), or excessive vein distention. Secondary varicose veins may also occur in the esophagus (esophageal varices), vulva, spermatic cords (varicoceles), and anorectal area (hemorrhoids), and as abnormal arteriovenous (AV) connections.

Pathophysiology

Risk factors include family history of chronic venous disease, weakness of the vein structure, female gender, Hispanic ethnicity, tobacco use, increasing age, obesity, multiparity, history of VTE, venous obstruction resulting from extrinsic pressure by tumors, phlebitis, previous leg injury, and occupations that require prolonged standing or sitting.

- In primary varicose veins, weak vein walls allow the vein valve ring to enlarge so that the leaflets no longer fit together properly (incompetent). Incompetent vein valves allow backward blood flow, particularly when the patient is standing. This results in increased venous pressure and further venous distention.

Clinical Manifestations

Discomfort from varicose veins varies dramatically and tends to be worse after episodes of superficial thrombophlebitis. The most common varicose vein symptoms include a heavy, achy pain after prolonged standing or sitting, which is relieved by walking or limb elevation. Some patients feel pressure or a cramplike, burning sensation. Swelling and/or nocturnal leg cramps may also occur.

Superficial venous thrombosis is the most frequent complication of varicose veins and may occur spontaneously or after trauma, surgical procedures, or pregnancy.

Diagnostic Studies

- Superficial varicose veins can be diagnosed by appearance.
- Duplex ultrasound detects obstruction and reflux in the venous system.

Interprofessional Management

Conservative treatment involves rest with limb elevation, graduated compression stockings, leg-strengthening exercise such as walking, and weight loss if indicated.

Venoactive drugs have been used to treat varicose veins and advanced chronic venous disease. These include micronized purified flavonoid fraction, rutosides (e.g., horse chestnut seed extract [*Aesculus hippocastanum*]), proanthocyanidins (from grapes and apples), and Ruscus (butcher's broom). Therapeutic benefits of venoactive drugs include pain relief, edema reduction, and decreased leg cramping and restless legs symptoms. These drugs have been widely used in Europe. They are not approved by the U.S. Food and Drug Administration (FDA); however, many are available over the counter as dietary or herbal supplements.

Sclerotherapy involves the injection of a substance that obliterates venous telangiectasias (i.e., spider veins) and small superficial varicose veins. Direct IV injection of a sclerosing agent, such as hypertonic saline, induces inflammation and causes thrombosis of the vein. After injection, a graduated compression stocking or compression bandage is recommended. Patients should not travel long distances during the first week after sclerotherapy to minimize the risk of a VTE.

- Other noninvasive options include transcutaneous laser therapy for telangiectasias and high-intensity pulsed-light therapy for reticular veins.

Surgical intervention is needed for recurrent superficial vein thrombosis or when chronic venous insufficiency cannot be controlled. Traditional surgical intervention involves ligating the entire vein (usually the greater saphenous) and removing its incompetent branches. An alternative but time-consuming technique is ambulatory phlebectomy, which involves pulling the varicosity through a "stab" incision, followed by excision of the vein.

Nursing Management

Prevention is a key factor related to varicose veins. Teach the patient to avoid sitting or standing for long periods, maintain ideal body weight, avoid injury to the extremities, avoid wearing constrictive clothing, and walk daily.

After vein ligation surgery, check extremities regularly for color, movement, sensation, temperature, presence of edema, and pedal pulses. Some bruising and discoloration are considered normal.

- Elevate the patient's legs 15 degrees to decrease edema.
- Apply graduated compression stockings or bandages. Remove them every 8 hours for a short period and then reapply them.

Long-term management of varicose veins is directed toward improving circulation, relieving discomfort, improving cosmetic appearance, and avoiding complications such as superficial thrombophlebitis and ulceration. Varicose veins can recur in other veins after surgery.

▼ **Patient and Caregiver Teaching**

- Teach the patient to apply custom-fitted graduated compression stockings in bed, before rising in the morning.
- Stress the importance of periodically positioning the legs above heart level.
- The overweight patient may need assistance with weight loss.
- Patients with a job that requires long periods of standing or sitting need to frequently flex and extend their hips, legs, and ankles and change positions.

VENOUS THROMBOSIS

Description

Venous thrombosis involves the formation of a thrombus (blood clot) with vein inflammation. It is the most common disorder of the veins.

Superficial vein thrombosis is the formation of a thrombus in a superficial vein, usually the greater or lesser saphenous vein.

Deep vein thrombosis (DVT) is a disorder involving a thrombus in a deep vein, often the iliac or femoral vein. *Venous thromboembolism* (VTE) is the preferred term to represent the spectrum from DVT to pulmonary embolism (PE). Table 89 compares superficial vein thrombosis and VTE.

Pathophysiology

Three key factors *(Virchow's triad)* that cause venous thrombosis are venous stasis, damage of the endothelium (inner lining of the vein), and hypercoagulability of the blood. The patient at risk for the development of VTE usually has a predisposing condition to these 3 disorders.

Venous stasis occurs when the venous valves are dysfunctional or the muscles of the extremities are inactive. Venous stasis occurs more often in people who are obese, have chronic heart failure or atrial fibrillation, have been on long trips without regular exercise, undergo a prolonged surgical procedure, or are immobile for long periods (e.g., with spinal cord injury or hip fracture).

Damage to the endothelium of the vein may be caused by direct (e.g., surgery, intravascular catheterization, trauma, fracture, burns,

TABLE 89 Comparison of Superficial Vein Thrombosis (SVT) and Venous Thromboembolism (VTE)

	SVT	VTE
Usual Location	Typically, superficial leg veins (e.g., varicosities) Sometimes, superficial arm veins	Deep veins of arms (e.g., axillary, subclavian), legs (e.g., femoral), pelvis (e.g., iliac, inferior or superior vena cava), and pulmonary system
Clinical Findings	Tenderness, itchiness, redness, warmth, pain, inflammation, and induration along the course of the superficial vein Vein appears as a palpable cord. Edema rarely occurs.	Tenderness to pressure over involved vein, induration of overlying muscle, venous distention Edema of affected extremity May have mild to moderate pain, deep reddish color to area caused by venous congestion *Note:* Some patients may have no obvious physical changes in the affected extremity.
Sequelae	If untreated, clot may extend to deeper veins, and VTE may occur.	Embolization to lungs (pulmonary embolism) may occur and may result in death[a] Pulmonary hypertension and postthrombotic syndrome with or without venous leg ulceration may develop.

[a]See Pulmonary Embolism, p. 506.

prior VTE) or indirect (chemotherapy, vasculitis, sepsis, diabetes) injury. Damaged endothelium has decreased fibrinolytic properties, which predispose the patient to thrombus development.

Hypercoagulability of the blood occurs in many disorders, including severe anemias, polycythemia, malignancies (e.g., cancers of the breast, brain, pancreas, and gastrointestinal tract), nephrotic syndrome, hyperhomocysteinemia, and protein C, protein S, and antithrombin deficiency.

- Women who use tobacco, are of childbearing age and take estrogen-based oral contraceptives, are postmenopausal on oral hormone therapy, are over 35 years old, and have a family history of VTE, are at a very high risk for VTE.

Localized platelet aggregation and fibrin entrap red blood cells (RBCs), white blood cells (WBCs), and more platelets to form a thrombus. A frequent site of thrombus formation is the valve cusps of veins.

- As the thrombus enlarges, blood cells and fibrin collect behind it, making a larger clot with a "tail" that eventually occludes the lumen of the vein.
- If a thrombus only partially blocks the vein, the thrombus becomes covered by endothelial cells and the thrombotic process stops.
- If the thrombus does not detach, it undergoes lysis or becomes firmly organized and adherent within 5 to 7 days.
- The organized thrombus may detach and result in an embolus that flows through the venous circulation to the heart and lodges in the pulmonary circulation, resulting in PE.

Superficial Vein Thrombosis
Clinical Manifestations and Diagnosis
The patient may have a palpable, firm, subcutaneous cordlike vein. The surrounding area may be itchy, tender to the touch, reddened, and warm. A mild temperature elevation and leukocytosis may be present. Edema of the extremity may occur.

Duplex ultrasound is used to confirm the diagnosis (5 cm or larger clot) and to rule out clot extension to a deep vein.
Interprofessional and Nursing Management
For patients with a lower leg superficial vein thrombosis, subcutaneous fondaparinux (Arixtra) reduces symptomatic VTE, and superficial vein thrombosis extension and recurrence without causing major bleeding problems.

If the superficial vein thrombosis affects a very short vein segment (< 5 cm) and is not near the saphenofemoral junction, anticoagulants may not be needed, and oral nonsteroidal antiinflammatory drugs (NSAIDs) can ease symptoms.

- Other interventions to relieve SVT symptoms include telling the patient to wear graduated compression stockings or bandages, elevate the affected limb above level of heart, apply topical NSAIDs, apply warm compresses, and perform mild exercise such as walking.

Venous Thromboembolism
Clinical Manifestations and Diagnosis
The patient with lower extremity VTE may have unilateral leg edema, pain, tenderness with palpation, dilated superficial veins, a sense of fullness in the thigh or the calf, paresthesias, warm skin, erythema, or a systemic temperature $> 100.4°$ F ($38°$ C).

- If the inferior vena cava is involved, both legs may be edematous and cyanotic. If the superior vena cava is involved, similar symptoms may occur in the arms, neck, back, and face.

Diagnosis of an initial VTE is based on clinical assessment combined with D-dimer testing and ultrasound.

Complications
The most serious complications of VTE are PE, chronic thromboembolic pulmonary hypertension, and postthrombotic syndrome (PTS).

- *PTS* can result from chronic venous hypertension caused by valvular destruction (from inflammation and scarring), stiff noncompliant vein walls, and persistent venous obstruction. Symptoms include pain, aching, sensation of heaviness, cramps, itching, and tingling. Signs include persistent edema, increased pigmentation, eczema, secondary varicosities, and lipodermatosclerosis.

Diagnostic Studies
- Platelet count, hemoglobin (Hgb), hematocrit (Hct), D-dimer testing, and coagulation tests (bleeding time, prothrombin time [PT], and partial thromboplastin time [PTT]) may be altered if underlying blood dyscrasias are present.
- Venous compression ultrasound evaluates deep femoral, popliteal, and posterior tibial veins.
- Duplex ultrasound and color-flow Doppler determine the location and extent of venous thrombi.

Interprofessional Management
In patients at risk for VTE, a variety of interventions are used. Patients on bed rest should change position every 2 hours. Unless contraindicated, teach patients to flex and extend their feet, knees, and hips at least every 2 to 4 hours while awake. Patients who can get out of bed should be in a chair for meals and ambulate at least 4 to 6 times per day as able. Tell the patient and the caregiver about the importance of these measures.

- Graduated compression stockings (e.g., thromboembolic deterrent [TED] hose) are a part of VTE prevention in hospitalized patients. VTE prevention is enhanced if the stockings are used along with anticoagulation.
- *Intermittent pneumatic compression devices* (IPCs) use inflatable sleeves or boots to compress the calf and thigh and/or foot and ankle to improve venous return. IPCs may be used with

elastic compression stockings. IPCs are not worn when a patient
has an active VTE because of the risk of PE.

Anticoagulants are used routinely for VTE prevention and treatment. The goal of anticoagulant therapy for VTE prophylaxis is to
prevent clot formation. The goals for treatment of a confirmed VTE
are to prevent further clot development and embolization.

Three major classes of anticoagulants are available: (1) vitamin K
antagonists, (2) thrombin inhibitors (both indirect and direct), and
(3) factor Xa inhibitors. Anticoagulant therapy does not dissolve
the clot. Clot lysis begins naturally through the body's intrinsic fibrinolytic system (see Table 37.10 on anticoagulant therapy, Harding
et al., *Lewis' Medical-Surgical Nursing*, ed 11).

Another treatment option for patients with a thrombus is catheter-
directed administration of a thrombolytic drug (e.g., urokinase, tissue plasminogen activator [tPA]). It dissolves the clot(s), reduces the
acute symptoms, improves deep venous flow, reduces valvular
reflux, and may help decrease the incidence of PTS. Catheter-
directed thrombolysis is an option for select patients who are at a
low bleeding risk and present with an acute, extensive, symptomatic, proximal VTE. Systemic anticoagulation is needed before, during, and after catheter-directed thrombolysis.

- Vena cava interruption devices (e.g., Greenfield, Vena Tech,
  TrapEase filters) can be inserted percutaneously through the
  right femoral or right internal jugular vein. The filters act as a
  sieve, permitting filtration of clots without interruption of
  blood flow.

The interventional radiology procedures for an occluded vein are
similar to those used in the treatment of lower extremity peripheral
arterial disease (PAD). Such procedures include mechanical throm-
bectomy, placement of a pharmacomechanical device, and post-
thrombus extraction, angioplasty, and/or stenting.

Some patients with extensive, acute, proximal VTE who are not
candidates for catheter-directed thrombolysis and/or interventional
radiology therapies (because of high bleeding risk) may undergo
surgery.

Nursing Management

Goals. The patient with VTE will have pain relief, decreased edema,
no skin ulceration, no bleeding complications, and no evidence
of PE.

Nursing Interventions

Focus your nursing care for the patient with VTE on the prevention
of thrombi and reduction of inflammation. Review with the patient
any drugs, vitamins, minerals, and dietary and herbal supplements
that may interfere with anticoagulant therapy.

- Check the results of pertinent tests before initiating, administering, or adjusting anticoagulant therapy.
- Monitor for and reduce the risk of bleeding with anticoagulant therapy.
- Early ambulation after VTE results in a more rapid decrease in edema and limb pain. Teach the patient and the caregiver the importance of exercise, and assist the patient in ambulating several times a day.

▼ Patient and Caregiver Teaching

- Focus discharge teaching on modification of VTE risk factors, use of elastic compression stockings, importance of monitoring laboratory values, dietary and medication instructions, and guidelines for follow-up care. Once the edema is resolved, measure the patient for custom-fitted elastic compression stockings. Use of such stockings (or sleeves in the case of upper extremity VTE) is recommended for at least 2 years after VTE.
- Advise the patient to avoid all nicotine products.
- Teach the patient to avoid constrictive clothing.
- When traveling long distances, tell patients to frequently exercise the calf muscles, take short walks, and drink beverages without alcohol or caffeine. For those at high risk for VTE who are planning a long trip, recommend properly fitted, knee-high graduated compression stockings during travel to decrease edema and VTE risk.
- Teach the patient and caregiver about signs and symptoms of PE, such as sudden onset of dyspnea, tachypnea, and pleuritic chest pain.
- Instruct the patient and caregiver about drug dosage, actions, and side effects; the need for routine blood tests; and what symptoms need immediate medical attention.
- Teach patients taking low-molecular-weight heparin (LMWH) or fondaparinux and their caregivers how to give the drug subcutaneously.
- Teach patients taking warfarin (Coumadin) to follow a consistent diet of foods containing vitamin K (e.g., dark green leafy vegetables) and to avoid any supplements containing vitamin K. Encourage proper hydration to prevent additional hypercoagulability of the blood, which may occur with dehydration.
- Active patients need to avoid contact sports and high-risk (for trauma) activities (e.g., skiing). Teach older patients about safety precautions to prevent falls (e.g., avoid use of throw rugs).
- Help the patient develop an exercise program with an emphasis on leg strength training and aerobic activity.

WARTS, GENITAL

Description

Genital warts (condylomata acuminata) are caused by the human papillomavirus (HPV). There are around 100 types of papillomavirus types. More than 40 types can be sexually transmitted. About 355,000 people are diagnosed each year. Most sexually active men and women will be infected with some type of HPV at some point in their lives. In most states, HPV is not a reportable infection.

Pathophysiology

"Low-risk" strains of the virus can cause warts on the skin. "High-risk" strains can lead to cancers of the genital tract, anus, or oropharynx in some patients. HPV types 6 and 11 cause about 90% of genital and anal wart cases. HPV is transmitted by skin-to-skin contact, most often during vaginal, anal, or oral sex, but it can be transmitted during nonpenetrative sexual activity. The basal epithelial cells infected with HPV undergo transformation and proliferation to form a warty growth. The incubation period can range from weeks to years. Infection with one type of HPV does not prevent infection with another type.

Clinical Manifestations

Most people who have HPV do not know they are infected, because they are asymptomatic. Genital warts are discrete, single, or multiple papillary growths that are white to gray and flesh–colored or hyperpigmented, depending on the skin type. They may grow and coalesce to form large, cauliflower-like masses.

- In men, the warts may occur on the penis and scrotum, around the anus, or in the urethra.
- In women, the warts may be located on the vulva, vagina, and cervix and in the perianal area.
- Itching or bleeding on defecation may occur with anal warts.

Diagnostic Studies

- A diagnosis can be made based on the appearance of the lesions.
- Biopsy provides a definitive diagnosis.

Interprofessional and Nursing Management

Genital warts are difficult to treat and often require multiple office visits. The primary goal is the removal of symptomatic warts.

- In-office treatment consists of chemical or ablative (removal with laser or electrocautery) methods. A common treatment is the use of trichloroacetic acid (TCA) or bichloroacetic acid (BCA) applied directly to the wart surface.

- Options include patient-applied treatments, such as Podofilox (Condylox) liquid or gel or Imiquimod cream (Aldara, Zyclara).

Treatment of warts may or may not decrease infectivity as the HPV causing these may still be present. Anogenital warts are hard to treat and often need more than one treatment or modality. Therapy should be modified if a patient has not improved or cannot tolerate the side effects of certain treatments.

- If the warts do not resolve with topical therapies, treatments such as cryotherapy with liquid nitrogen, electrocautery, laser therapy, local α-interferon injections, or surgical excision may be needed. Teach patients that because treatment does not destroy the virus (merely the infected tissue), recurrence and reinfection are possible, and long-term follow-up is advised.

HPV vaccines offer protection against strains causing 90% of genital warts and 70% (Gardasil) to 90% (Gardasil-9) of cervical cancers. They may offer protection from anal and certain types of throat cancer. Ideally, a person should receive a vaccine before the start of sexual activity, but even those who are infected with HPV can still get protection against HPV types not already acquired.

See Nursing Management: Sexually Transmitted Infections, pp. 547.

PART TWO

Treatments and Procedures

AMPUTATION

Description

An *amputation* is the removal of a body extremity by trauma or surgery. An estimated 2 million people in the United States are living with limb loss. Most amputations are done because of peripheral vascular disease (PVD), especially in older patients with diabetes. These patients often have peripheral neuropathy that progresses to deep ulcers and gangrene. Amputation in young people is usually because of trauma (e.g., motor vehicle crashes, farming-related accidents). Battle injuries have affected over 1700 U.S. veterans since 2003, with several losing more than 1 limb.

- The goal of amputation surgery is to preserve extremity length and function while removing all infected, pathologic, or ischemic tissue. (For the levels of amputation of the upper and lower extremities, see Fig. 62.23 in Harding et al., *Lewis' Medical-Surgical Nursing,* ed 11.)

Nursing Management

Control of illnesses, such as PVD, diabetes, chronic osteomyelitis, and pressure injuries, can prevent or delay the need for amputation.

- Teach patients with these conditions to carefully examine the lower extremities daily for signs of skin infection or breakdown. Teach the patient to report problems to the HCP. These include decreased or absent sensation, tingling, burning pain, cuts, abrasions, and changes in skin color or temperature.
- Review safety precautions for people taking part in recreational activities and potentially hazardous work. This responsibility is especially important for the occupational health nurse.
- Be aware of the tremendous psychologic and social implications of an amputation. The disruption in body image often results in the patient going through the grieving process. Use therapeutic communication to assist the patient and caregiver to develop a realistic attitude about the future.

Preoperative Care

Before surgery, reinforce information that the patient and caregiver have received about the reasons for the amputation, proposed prosthesis, and mobility-training program.

- Teach the patient upper extremity exercises, such as push-ups in bed or the wheelchair, to promote arm strength for crutch walking and gait training.

- If a compression bandage will be used after surgery, instruct the patient about its purpose and application. If an immediate prosthesis is planned, discuss general ambulation expectations.

Tell the patient that it may feel as if the amputated limb is still present after surgery. This phenomenon, termed *phantom limb sensation,* occurs in many amputees.

Postoperative Care

Monitor the patient's vital signs and the operative site dressing for hemorrhage. Careful attention to sterile technique during dressing changes reduces the potential for wound infection.

- If an immediate postoperative prosthesis has been applied, careful surveillance of the surgical site is needed. Keep a surgical tourniquet available for emergency use. If excess bleeding occurs, notify the surgeon at once.
- Not all patients are candidates for prostheses. The seriously ill or debilitated patient may not have the upper body strength or energy required to use a prosthesis. Mobility with a wheelchair may be the most realistic goal in this situation.

Flexion contractures may delay the rehabilitation process. The most common and debilitating contracture is hip flexion. Patients should avoid sitting in a chair for more than 1 hour with hips flexed or with pillows under the surgical extremity. Unless specifically contraindicated, patients should lie on their abdomen for 30 minutes 3 to 4 times each day and position the hip in extension while prone.

- As recovery and ambulation progress, phantom limb sensation and pain usually subside, although the pain can become chronic. The patient may report shooting, burning, or crushing pain and feelings of coldness, heaviness, and cramping.

▼ Patient and Caregiver Teaching

As the patient's overall condition improves, the health care provider (HCP) and physical therapist start and supervise an exercise program.

- Active range-of-motion exercises of all joints should be started as soon as possible after surgery.
- Crutch walking starts as soon as the patient is physically able. Follow prescribed weight-bearing guidelines to avoid disrupting the skin flap and delaying the healing process.
- Instruct the patient and the caregiver about residual limb care, ambulation, prevention of contractures, recognition of complications, exercise, and follow-up care. Table 90 outlines patient and caregiver teaching after an amputation.

TABLE 90 Patient and Caregiver Teaching After an Amputation

After an amputation, include the following instructions when teaching the patient and the caregiver.

- Inspect the residual limb daily for signs of skin irritation, especially redness, excoriation, and odor. Especially evaluate areas prone to pressure.
- Stop using the prosthesis if irritation develops. Have the area checked before resuming use of the prosthesis.
- Wash the residual limb thoroughly each night with warm water and a bacteriostatic soap. Rinse thoroughly and dry gently. Expose the residual limb to air for 20 minutes.
- Do not use any substance, such as lotions, alcohol, powders, or oil, on residual limb unless prescribed by the HCP.
- Wear only a residual limb sock that is in good condition and supplied by the prosthetist.
- Change residual limb sock daily. Launder in a mild soap, squeeze, and lay flat to dry.
- Use prescribed pain management techniques.
- Perform range of motion (ROM) to all joints daily. Perform general strengthening exercises, including the upper extremities, daily.
- Do not elevate the residual limb on a pillow.
- Lie prone with hip in extension for 30 minutes 3–4 times daily.

ARTIFICIAL AIRWAYS: ENDOTRACHEAL TUBES

Description

An artificial airway is created by inserting a tube into the trachea, bypassing upper airway and laryngeal structures. The tube is placed into the trachea through the mouth or nose past the larynx *(endotracheal [ET] intubation)* or through a stoma in the neck *(tracheostomy)*. ET intubation is common in intensive care unit (ICU) patients requiring mechanical ventilation for <2 weeks. Fig. 24 shows the parts of an ET tube.

- Indications for ET intubation include upper airway obstruction, apnea, high risk of aspiration, ineffective clearance of secretions, and respiratory distress. It is done quickly and safely at the bedside by a health care provider (HCP) or respiratory therapist.

In *oral ET intubation,* the ET tube is passed through the mouth and between the vocal cords and into the trachea with the aid of a laryngoscope or bronchoscope. Oral ET intubation is preferred for

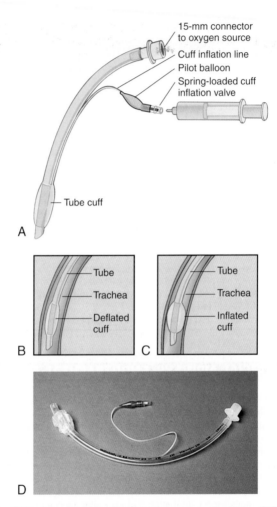

Fig. 24 Endotracheal tube. (A) Parts of an endotracheal tube. (B) Tube in place with cuff deflated. (C) Tube in place with the cuff inflated. (D) Photo of tube before placement.

most emergencies because the airway can be secured rapidly and a larger-diameter tube is used. A larger-bore tube provides less airway resistance and allows easier performance of suctioning and bronchoscopy, if needed.

- There are risks associated with oral ET intubation. It is hard to place the tube in patients with limited head and neck mobility (e.g., suspected spinal cord injury). Teeth can be chipped or accidentally removed during the procedure. Salivation increases and swallowing is difficult. The patient can obstruct the ET tube by biting down on the tube. Sedation, along with a bite block or oropharyngeal airway, can be used to avoid tube obstruction. The ET tube and bite block (if used) should be secured (separately) to the face. Mouth care is a challenge.

In *nasal ET intubation,* the ET is placed blindly (i.e., without seeing the larynx) through the nose and nasopharynx and past the vocal cords. We use nasal ET intubation when oral intubation is not possible (e.g., unstable cervical spine injury, dental abscess, epiglottitis).

- Nasal intubation is contraindicated in patients with facial fractures or suspected fractures at the base of the skull and postoperatively after cranial surgery.

Nursing and Interprofessional Management

Unless ET intubation is emergent, consent is obtained. Tell the patient and caregiver the reason for ET intubation and the steps in the procedure. Explain that while intubated, the patient will not be able to speak, but that you will provide other means of communication. Also explain that the patient may have removable mitts or soft wrist restraints placed as a reminder not to move the tube.

- Have a self-inflating bag-valve-mask (BVM) device (e.g., Ambu bag) available and attached to O_2; have suctioning equipment ready at the bedside; and establish IV access. ET intubation is described in Chapter 65 of Harding et al., Lewis' *Medical-Surgical Nursing,* ed 11.

Managing a patient with an artificial airway is often shared between the registered nurse (RN) and Respiratory Therapist (RT). Agency policy dictates specific management tasks. Nursing responsibilities for the patient with an artificial airway may include: (1) maintaining correct tube placement, (2) maintaining proper cuff inflation, (3) monitoring oxygenation and ventilation, (4) maintaining tube patency, (5) assessing for complications, (6) providing oral care and maintaining skin integrity, and (7) fostering comfort and communication.

Continuously monitor the patient with an ET tube for proper tube placement. Observe for symmetric chest wall movement, and auscultate to confirm bilateral breath sounds.

- It is an emergency if the ET tube is not positioned properly. If malpositioning occurs, stay with the patient, try to maintain the airway, support ventilation with a BVM and 100% O_2, and call for help to immediately assess or reposition the tube. It may be necessary to ventilate the patient with a BVM device (Ambu bag) and 100% O_2. If a dislodged tube is not repositioned, no oxygen will be delivered to the lungs, or the entire volume will be delivered to 1 lung. This places the patient at risk for pneumothorax.

The cuff is an inflatable, pliable sleeve encircling the lower, outer wall of the ET tube. The cuff stabilizes and seals the ET tube within the trachea and prevents the escape of ventilating gases.

Excess volume in the ET tube cuff can cause tracheal damage. To avoid this, inflate the cuff with air, then measure and maintain the cuff pressure at 20 to 25 cm H_2O. Record cuff pressure after intubation and on a routine basis (e.g., every 8 hours) using the *minimal occluding volume* (MOV) *technique* or the *minimal leak technique* (MLT).

- The steps in the MOV technique for cuff inflation are as follows: (1) for the mechanically ventilated patient, place a stethoscope over the trachea and inflate the cuff to MOV by adding air until no air leak is heard at peak inspiratory pressure (end of ventilator inspiration); (2) for the spontaneously breathing patient, inflate until no sound is heard after a deep breath or after inhalation with a BVM; (3) use a manometer to verify that cuff pressure is between 20 and 25 mm Hg; and (4) record cuff pressure in the chart.
- If adequate cuff pressure cannot be maintained or larger volumes of air are needed to keep the cuff inflated, the cuff could be leaking or there could be tracheal dilation at the cuff site. In such situations, notify the HCP.

The procedure for MLT is similar with 1 exception. Remove a small amount of air from the cuff until a slight air leak is auscultated at peak inflation.

- Closely monitor the patient with an ET tube for adequate oxygenation and ventilation by assessing clinical findings, arterial blood gases (ABGs), arterial oxygen saturation by pulse oximetry (SpO_2), and other indicators of oxygenation status.
- Do not routinely suction a patient. Regularly assess the patient to determine the need for suctioning. Indications for suctioning include: (1) visible secretions in the ET tube, (2) sudden onset of respiratory distress, (3) suspected aspiration of secretions, (4) increase in respiratory rate or frequent coughing, and (5) sudden decrease in SpO_2. Other signs that may indicate the patient needs suctioning include an increase in peak airway pressure and auscultation of adventitious breath sounds over the trachea or bronchi. See Table 91 for open and closed suctioning techniques.

A

TABLE 91 Suctioning Procedures for Patient on Mechanical Ventilator

General Measures for Open- and Closed-Suction Techniques

1. Gather all supplies and equipment.
2. Wash hands and don personal protective equipment and gloves.
3. Explain procedure and patient's role in assisting with secretion removal by coughing.
4. Monitor patient's cardiopulmonary status (e.g., vital signs, SpO_2, SvO_2 or $ScvO_2$, ECG, level of consciousness) before, during, and after suctioning.
5. Turn on suction and set vacuum to 100–120 mm Hg.
6. Pause ventilator alarms.

Open-Suction Technique

7. Open sterile catheter package using the inside of the package as a sterile field. NOTE: Suction catheter should be no wider than one-half the diameter of the ET tube (e.g., for a 7-mm ET tube, select a 10-F suction catheter).
8. Fill the sterile solution container with sterile normal saline or water.
9. Don sterile gloves.
10. Pick up sterile suction catheter with dominant hand. Using nondominant hand, secure the connecting tube (to suction) to the suction catheter.
11. Check equipment for proper functioning by suctioning a small volume of sterile saline solution from the container. *(Go to step 13.)*

Closed-Suction Technique

12. Connect the suction tubing to the closed suction port.
13. Hyperoxygenate the patient for 30 seconds using one of the following methods:
    - Activate the suction hyperoxygenation setting on the ventilator using nondominant hand. This is the safest method to hyperoxygenate the patient and should be used when available.
    - Increase FIO_2 to 100%. *Note:* remember to return FIO_2 to baseline level when done suctioning, if not done automatically after preset time by ventilator.
    - Disconnect the ventilator tubing from the ET tube and manually ventilate the patient with 100% O_2 using a BVM device. Attach a PEEP valve to the BVM for patients on >5 cm

Continued

TABLE 91 Suctioning Procedures for Patient on Mechanical Ventilator—cont'd

H_2O PEEP. Give 5 or 6 breaths over 30 seconds. Having a second person to deliver the manual breaths significantly increases the V_T delivered.

14. With suction off, gently and quickly insert the catheter using the dominant hand. When you meet resistance, pull back 1/2 inch.

15. Apply continuous or intermittent suction using the nondominant thumb. Withdraw the catheter over 10 seconds or less.

16. Hyperoxygenate once more for another 30 seconds as described in step 13.

17. If secretions remain and the patient has tolerated suctioning, perform two or three suction passes as described in steps 14 and 15. Rinse the suction catheter with sterile saline solution between suctioning passes as needed. Maintaining a closed circuit at all times is best to reduce the risk of infection.

18. Reconnect patient to ventilator (open-suction technique).

19. Rinse the catheter and connecting tubing with the sterile saline solution.

20. Suction oral pharynx. NOTE: Use a separate catheter for this step when using the closed-suction technique.

21. Discard the suction catheter and rinse the connecting tubing with the sterile saline solution (open-suction technique).

22. Reset FIO_2 (if needed) and ventilator alarms.

23. Reassess patient for signs of effective suctioning.

BVM, Bag-valve-mask; *ECG*, electrocardiogram; *ET*, endotracheal; *FIO₂*, fraction of inspired oxygen; *PEEP*, positive end-expiratory pressure; *SpO₂*, arterial oxygen saturation by pulse oximetry; *SvO₂*, mixed venous oxygen saturation; *ScvO₂*, central venous oxygen saturation; *V_T*, tidal volume.
Adapted from Wiegand DL: *AACN procedure manual for high acuity, progressive, and critical care*, ed 7, St Louis, 2017, Elsevier.

- With an oral ET tube in place, the patient's mouth is always open. Moisten the lips, tongue, and gums with saline or water swabs to prevent mucosal drying. Proper oral care provides comfort and prevents injury to the gums and dental plaque formation.
- Meticulous care is needed to prevent skin breakdown on the face, lips, tongue, and/or nares because of pressure from the ET tube or from the method used to secure the ET tube to the patient's face. Reposition and resecure or retape the ET tube every 24 hours and as needed.

For the nasally intubated patient, remove the old tape and clean the skin around the ET tube with saline-soaked gauze. For the orally intubated patient, remove the bite block (if present) and the old tape. Provide oral hygiene then reposition the ET tube to the opposite side of the mouth. Replace the bite block (if appropriate) and reconfirm proper cuff inflation and tube placement. Secure the ET tube again per agency policy.

- Two staff members should always perform the repositioning procedure to prevent accidental ET tube dislodgment. Monitor the patient for respiratory distress throughout the procedure. Monitor the patient for signs of respiratory distress throughout the procedure.

B

BASIC LIFE SUPPORT FOR HEALTH CARE PROVIDERS

Description

Basic life support (BLS) consists of a series of actions and skills performed by the rescuer(s) based on assessment findings.

- The first action the rescuer performs on finding an adult victim is to assess for responsiveness. This is done by tapping or shaking the victim's shoulder and asking, "Are you all right?" If the victim does not respond, simultaneously scan the victim's chest for signs of breathing and perform a pulse check (described later).
- If the rescuer is alone, the rescuer shouts for help. If someone responds, the rescuer asks him or her to activate the emergency response system (ERS) (e.g., through the use of a mobile phone) and get an automatic external defibrillator (AED) (if available). If no one responds and the rescuer does not have a mobile phone, the rescuer should leave to activate the ERS, get an AED (if available), and return to the victim before beginning cardiopulmonary resuscitation (CPR) and defibrillation if necessary.

Cardiopulmonary Resuscitation

Cardiac arrest is characterized by the absence of a pulse and breathing in an unconscious victim. The current approach for cardiopulmonary resuscitation (CPR) is the chest *compressions–airway–breathing* (CAB) sequence.

- The first step in CPR is to perform a pulse check by palpating the carotid pulse for at least 5 but no more than 10 seconds. While maintaining a head-tilt position with 1 hand on the victim's forehead, locate the victim's trachea using 2 or 3 fingers of your other hand. Slide these fingers into the groove between the trachea and neck muscles where the carotid pulse can be felt. The technique is more easily performed on the side nearest you.
- If a pulse is felt, give 1 rescue breath every 5 to 6 seconds (10 to 12 breaths/minute) and recheck the pulse every 2 minutes. If no pulse is felt, start CAB.

- Chest compression technique consists of fast and deep applications of pressure on the lower half of the sternum. The victim must be in the supine position when the compressions are performed. The victim must be lying on a flat, hard surface, such as a CPR board (specially designed for use in CPR), a headboard from a unit bed, or, if necessary, the floor. Position yourself close to the side of the victim's chest. More frequently, mechanical chest compression devices are being used to provide chest compressions both prehospital and in the emergency department.
- Chest compressions are combined with rescue breathing for an effective resuscitation effort of the adult victim of cardiac arrest. The compression-ventilation ratio for 1- or 2-rescuer CPR is 30 compressions to 2 breaths (Table 92). However, if the patient has an advanced airway (e.g., endotracheal tube, laryngeal mask

---

TABLE 92   Adult 1- and 2-Rescuer Basic Life Support With Automatic External Defibrillator (AED)

Assess
- Determine unresponsiveness: tap or shake victim's shoulder; shout, "Are you all right?"
- Check for no breathing or abnormal breathing (e.g., gasping) while simultaneously performing a pulse check (5–10 sec).

Activate Emergency Response System (ERS)
- Activate ERS (e.g., call 911) and get the AED (if available) (outside of hospital).
- Call a code and ask for the AED or crash cart (in hospital).

Begin High-Quality CPR
- (See Figs. A.1 and A.2 in Appendix A of Harding et al., *Lewis' Medical-Surgical Nursing,* ed 11).
- If victim has a pulse but is not breathing or not breathing adequately, begin rescue breathing at a rate of 1 breath every 3–5 sec, or about 12–20 per minute. Recheck the pulse every 2 minutes.
- If there is no pulse, expose the victim's chest and immediately begin chest compressions
- Deliver compressions at a rate of 100–120 per minute.
- Compress the chest at least 2 inches but not > 2.4 inches.
- Allow for complete chest recoil after each compression.
- Deliver a compression-ventilation ratio of 30 compressions to 2 breaths.[a]

TABLE 92   Adult 1- and 2-Rescuer Basic Life Support With Automatic External Defibrillator (AED)—cont'd

- Minimize interruptions in compressions by delivering the 2 breaths in <10 sec.

Deliver Effective Breaths
- Open airway adequately.
- Deliver breath to produce a visible chest rise.
- Avoid excessive ventilation.

Integrate Prompt Use of the AED
- Use AED as soon as possible.
- If rhythm is shockable, deliver 1 shock and then resume chest compressions immediately after delivery of shock.
- If the rhythm is not shockable, resume CPR and recheck rhythm every 5 cycles.

Continue CPR
- Continue CPR between rhythm checks and shocks, and until ACLS providers arrive or the victim shows signs of movement.

[a]For patients with ongoing CPR and an advanced airway in place, a ventilation rate of 1 breath every 6 seconds (10 breaths per minute) is recommended.
CPR, Cardiopulmonary resuscitation.
Sources: American Heart Association: *BLS for healthcare providers—student manual,* Dallas, 2015, The Association; and American Heart Association: *Highlights of the 2015 American Heart Association guidelines update for CPR and ECC,* Dallas, 2015, The Association.

airway), do not pause between compressions for breaths and deliver 1 breath every 6 seconds (10 breaths/minute).
- If a mechanical chest compression device is not used, then it is preferable to have two persons performing CPR. One rescuer, positioned at the victim's side, performs chest compressions while the second rescuer, positioned at the victim's head, maintains an open airway and performs ventilations. To maintain the quality and rate of compressions, rescuers should change roles every 2 minutes. Interruptions in CPR should be limited.
- When the AED or advanced cardiovascular life support (ACLS) team arrives, assess the victim's rhythm. If the victim has a shockable rhythm (e.g., ventricular tachycardia, ventricular fibrillation), deliver 1 shock followed by 5 cycles of CPR before

checking the rhythm. If the rhythm is not a shockable rhythm, resume CPR and recheck the rhythm every 5 cycles.

- If the victim has a pulse but is gasping (e.g., agonal breathing) or not breathing, establish an open airway and begin rescue breathing. Open an adult's airway by hyperextending the head. Use the *head tilt–chin lift maneuver.* This involves tilting the head back with 1 hand and lifting the chin forward with the fingers of the other hand. Use the *jaw-thrust maneuver* if you suspect a cervical spine injury. Try to ventilate the victim using a mouth-to-barrier (recommended) device (e.g., face mask, bag-valve-mask) or by mouth-to-mouth resuscitation. Give ventilations with the victim's nostrils pinched. Take a regular (not deep) breath and tightly seal your lips around the victim's mouth. Give 1 breath and watch for a rise in the victim's chest. Continue rescue breaths at a rate of 10 to 12 per minute.
- If the victim cannot be ventilated, proceed with CPR. When providing the next rescue breaths, look for and remove any visible objects from the victim's mouth (Table 93 and Fig. 25).

TABLE 93 Management of the Adult Choking Victim

Conscious Adult Choking Victim

Assess Victim for Severe Airway Obstruction

Look for any of the following signs:
- Poor or no air exchange
- Clutching the neck with the hands, making the universal choking sign
- Weak, ineffective cough or no cough at all
- High-pitched noise while inhaling or no noise at all
- Increased respiratory difficulty
- Possible cyanosis

Ask the victim if he or she is choking. If the victim nods yes and cannot talk or has any of the symptoms noted earlier, severe airway obstruction is present and you must take immediate action.

Abdominal Thrusts (Heimlich Maneuver) With Standing or Sitting Victim

1. Stand or kneel behind victim and wrap arms around the victim's waist.
2. Make fist with 1 hand.
3. Place thumb side of fist against victim's abdomen. Position fist midline, slightly above navel and well below breastbone.
4. Grasp fist with other hand and press fist into victim's abdomen with a quick, forceful upward thrust.

TABLE 93   Management of the Adult Choking Victim—cont'd

5. Give each new thrust with a separate, distinct movement to relieve the obstruction. CAUTION: If victim is pregnant or obese, give chest thrusts instead of abdominal thrusts. Position hands (as described) over lower portion of the breastbone and apply quick backward thrusts.
6. Repeat thrusts until object is expelled or victim becomes unresponsive.

Unconscious Adult Choking Victim

If you see a choking victim collapse and become unresponsive:
1. Activate the emergency response system (ERS).
2. Lower the victim to the ground and begin CPR, starting with compressions (do not check for a pulse).
3. Open the victim's mouth wide each time you prepare to give breaths. Look for the object. If you see the object and can easily remove it, do so with your fingers. If you do not see the object, continue with CPR using the chest compression–airway–breathing sequence.
4. If efforts to ventilate are unsuccessful, continue with CPR.

CPR, Cardiopulmonary resuscitation.
Source: American Heart Association: *BLS for healthcare providers—student manual,* Dallas, 2015, The Association.
Note: guidelines are updated on an ongoing basis and are available at <https://eccguidelines.heart.org/index.php/circulation/cpr-ecc-guidelines-2>.

B

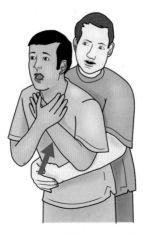

Fig. 25 Abdominal thrusts *(Heimlich maneuver)* administered to a conscious (standing) choking victim.

Hands-Only Cardiopulmonary Resuscitation

Hands-only CPR can be used to help adult victims who suddenly collapse from cardiac arrest outside of a health care setting. If you witness this event (as a bystander), you can choose to provide conventional CPR (described previously) or chest compressions only (push fast and deep in the center of the chest). Both methods are effective in the first few minutes of an out-of-hospital cardiac arrest.

CHEMOTHERAPY

Description

Chemotherapy (antineoplastic therapy) is the use of chemicals as a systemic therapy for cancer. It is a primary cancer treatment for most solid tumors and hematologic cancers (e.g., leukemias, lymphomas). The goal of chemotherapy is to eliminate or reduce the number of cancer cells present in the primary and metastatic tumor site(s).

- The two major categories of chemotherapeutic drugs are *cell cycle phase–nonspecific* and *cell cycle phase–specific*. These agents are often given together to maximize effectiveness by using drugs that function in different ways and throughout the cell cycle.

Classification of Chemotherapeutic Drugs

Chemotherapy drugs are generally classified according to their molecular structure and mechanisms of action (Table 94).

TABLE 94 **Drug Therapy Chemotherapy**	
Mechanisms of Action	**Examples**
Alkylating Agents	
Cell Cycle Phase–Nonspecific Agents	
Damage DNA by causing breaks in the double-stranded helix. If repair does not occur, cells will die immediately (cytocidal) or when they try to divide (cytostatic).	bendamustine (Treanda), busulfan (Myleran), chlorambucil (Leukeran), cyclophosphamide, dacarbazine, ifosfamide (Ifex), mechlorethamine (Mustargen), melphalan, temozolomide (Temodar), thiotepa

TABLE 94 Drug Therapy Chemotherapy—cont'd

Mechanisms of Action	Examples

Antimetabolites

Cell Cycle Phase–Specific Agents

Mimic naturally occurring substances, thus interfering with enzyme function or DNA synthesis. Primarily act during S phase. Purine and pyrimidine are building blocks of nucleic acids needed for DNA and RNA synthesis

Mechanisms of Action	Examples
• Interfere with purine metabolism	cladribine, clofarabine (Clolar), fludarabine, mercaptopurine (Purixan), nelarabine (Arranon), pentostatin (Nipent), thioguanine
• Interfere with pyrimidine metabolism	capecitabine (Xeloda); cytarabine, floxuridine, fluorouracil, gemcitabine (Gemzar)
• Interfere with folic acid metabolism	methotrexate (Trexall), pemetrexed (Alimta)
• Interfere with DNA synthesis	hydroxyurea (Hydrea, Droxia)

Antitumor Antibiotics

Cell Cycle Phase–Nonspecific Agents

Mechanisms of Action	Examples
Bind directly to DNA, thus inhibiting the synthesis of DNA and interfering with transcription of RNA.	bleomycin, dactinomycin (Cosmegen), daunorubicin, doxorubicin (Doxil), epirubicin (Ellence), idarubicin, mitomycin, mitoxantrone, valrubicin (Valstar)

Mitotic Inhibitors

Cell Cycle Phase–Specific Agents

Taxanes

Mechanisms of Action	Examples
Antimicrotubule agents that interfere with mitosis. Act during the late G_2 phase and mitosis to stabilize microtubules, thus inhibiting cell division.	albumin-bound paclitaxel (Abraxane), docetaxel (Taxotere), paclitaxel (Taxol)

Vinca Alkaloids

Mechanisms of Action	Examples
Act in M phase to inhibit mitosis.	vinblastine, vincristine, vinorelbine (Navelbine)

Others

Mechanisms of Action	Examples
Microtubular inhibitors.	estramustine (Emcyt), ixabepilone (Ixempra), eribulin (Halaven)

C

Continued

TABLE 94 Drug Therapy Chemotherapy—cont'd	
Mechanisms of Action	**Examples**
Nitrosoureas	
Cell Cycle Phase–Nonspecific Agents	
Like alkylating agents, break DNA helix, interfering with DNA replication. Cross blood-brain barrier.	carmustine (BiCNU, Gliadel), lomustine (Gleostine), streptozocin (Zanosar)
Platinum Drugs	
Cell Cycle Phase–Nonspecific Agents	
Bind to DNA and RNA, miscoding information and/or inhibiting DNA replication, and cells die.	carboplatin, cisplatin, oxaliplatin
Topoisomerase Inhibitors	
Cell Cycle Phase–Specific Agents	
Inhibit topoisomerases (normal enzymes) that function to make reversible breaks and repairs in DNA that allow for flexibility of DNA in replication.	etoposide, irinotecan (Camptosar), topotecan (Hycamtin)

Note: Many of these drugs are irritants or vesicants that require special attention during administration to avoid extravasation. It is important to know this information about a drug before administering it.

Methods of Administration
The IV route is the most common route for giving chemotherapy. Major concerns associated with IV chemotherapy include venous access problems, device- or catheter-related infection, and *extravasation* (infiltration of drugs into tissues surrounding the infusion site). Many chemotherapy drugs are either irritants or vesicants.

- *Irritants* will damage the intima of the vein, causing phlebitis and sclerosis and limiting future peripheral venous access.
- *Vesicants* may cause severe local tissue breakdown and necrosis if inadvertently infiltrated into the skin. It is extremely important to monitor for and promptly take action if extravasation of a vesicant occurs.

To minimize discomfort, emotional distress, and risks of infection and infiltration, systemic IV chemotherapy can be given through a central vascular access device placed in a large blood vessel.

Regional chemotherapy delivers the drug directly to the tumor site. Examples of this type of administration include intraarterial, intraperitoneal, intrathecal (intraventricular), and intravesical bladder chemotherapy.

Effects of Chemotherapy

Chemotherapy agents cannot selectively distinguish between normal cells and cancer cells. Chemotherapy-induced side effects are caused by the destruction of normal cells that are rapidly proliferating. These cells include the bone marrow, lining of the gastrointestinal system, and integumentary system (skin, hair, and nails).

The adverse effects of these drugs can be classified as acute, delayed, or chronic.

- *Acute toxicity* includes anaphylactic and hypersensitivity reactions, extravasation or a flare reaction, anticipatory nausea and vomiting, and dysrhythmias.
- *Delayed effects* are numerous and include delayed nausea and vomiting, mucositis, alopecia, skin rashes, bone marrow depression, altered bowel function, and a variety of neurotoxicities.
- *Chronic toxicities* involve damage to organs, such as the heart, liver, kidneys, and lungs.

Nursing management of side effects and problems caused by chemotherapy and radiation therapy is provided in Table 15.11, Harding et al., *Lewis' Medical-Surgical Nursing,* ed 11.

Nursing Management: Chemotherapy and Radiation Therapy

You have an important role in helping patients deal with the side effects of chemotherapy and radiation therapy.

- Myelosuppression is one of the most common effects of chemotherapy. To a lesser extent, it can occur with radiation therapy. Treatment-induced myelosuppression can result in life-threatening and distressing effects. These include infection, hemorrhage, and overwhelming fatigue. Monitor the complete blood count (CBC), particularly the neutrophil, platelet, and red blood cell (RBC) counts.
- Fatigue is a persistent subjective sense of tiredness that interferes with usual day-to-day functioning. Help patients recognize that fatigue is a common effect of therapy. Ignoring fatigue may lead to an increase in symptoms. However, maintaining exercise and

activity within tolerable limits is often helpful in managing fatigue.

The intestinal mucosa is sensitive to chemotherapy and radiation therapy, resulting in nausea and vomiting, diarrhea, mucositis, and anorexia. These problems can affect the patient's hydration and nutritional status and sense of well-being.

- Nausea and vomiting can be successfully managed with antiemetic regimens, dietary modification, and other nondrug interventions. Assess patients for signs and symptoms of dehydration and metabolic alkalosis.
- Both radiation therapy– and chemotherapy-induced diarrhea are best managed with diet modification, antidiarrheals, antimotility agents, and antispasmodics (see Table 42.2, Harding et al., *Lewis' Medical-Surgical Nursing,* ed 11).
- Mucositis can be alleviated with systemic and/or topical analgesics and antibiotics if infection is present. Monitor and get prompt treatment for oral candidiasis (which often occurs with mucositis). Meticulous oral care during and for a long time after treatment reduces the risk of cavities, which may occur because of decreased saliva. Saliva substitutes may be offered to patients with xerostomia. Many patients find that drinking small amounts of water frequently has a similar effect.
- Monitor the patient with anorexia to ensure that weight loss does not become excessive. Also observe for dehydration. Small, frequent meals of high-protein, high-calorie bland foods are better tolerated than large meals.

Skin changes with chemotherapy range from mild redness and hyperpigmentation to more distressing effects, such as acral erythema or desquamation. Alopecia caused by chemotherapy is usually reversible. Hair generally begins to grow back 3 to 4 weeks after the drugs are discontinued.

- With radiation therapy, skin effects occur only locally, in the treatment field. Basic skin care instructions are presented in Table 15.12, Harding et al., *Lewis' Medical-Surgical Nursing,* ed 11. Verify these guidelines with your agency's radiation oncology department.

▼ **Patient and Caregiver Teaching**

Teaching is an important part of your role related to chemotherapy.

- Explore the patient's attitude about treatment. You can promote the development of a hopeful attitude about cancer and support the patient and family during the various stages of the process of cancer.
- To decrease the fear and anxiety often associated with chemotherapy and radiation therapy, tell the patient what to expect

during a course of treatment. Good nursing judgment is essential to determine the amount of information that the patient and caregiver can assimilate.
- Assess the psychosocial concerns and emotional responses of patients and their families so that you can connect patients with appropriate supportive care resources.

CHEST TUBES AND PLEURAL DRAINAGE

C

Description
When fluid or air accumulates in the pleural space, the pressure becomes positive and the lung collapses. Chest tubes are inserted to drain the pleural space, reestablishing negative pressure to allow for lung reexpansion. Tubes may also be inserted in the mediastinal space postoperatively to remove air and fluid.

Chest Tube Insertion
Chest tube insertion can be performed in the emergency department (ED), in the operating room, or at the patient's bedside. Time permitting, a chest x-ray is used to confirm the affected side. The patient is positioned with the arm raised above the head on the affected side to expose the midaxillary area, the standard site for insertion.
- The area is cleansed with antiseptic solution, and the chest wall is infiltrated with a local anesthetic. A small incision is made over a rib. The chest tube is then advanced up and over the top of the rib, to avoid the intercostal nerves and blood vessels (Fig. 26).
- Once inserted, the tube is connected to a pleural drainage system. Two tubes may be connected to the same drainage unit with a Y-connector.
- The incision is closed with sutures and the chest tube is secured. The wound is covered with an occlusive dressing.
- Insertion of a chest tube and its presence in the pleural space are painful. Monitor the patient's comfort and use appropriate pain-relieving interventions.

Pleural Drainage
There are 2 types of pleural drainage systems used to remove air from the pleural space (Fig. 27). The first type is a *flutter valve* (Heimlich valve). This device consists of a 1-way rubber valve within a rigid plastic tube. It is attached to the external end of the chest tube. It has two nozzles. The inlet nozzle allows the air to pass in the valve through the chest drainage tube attached to it. The outlet

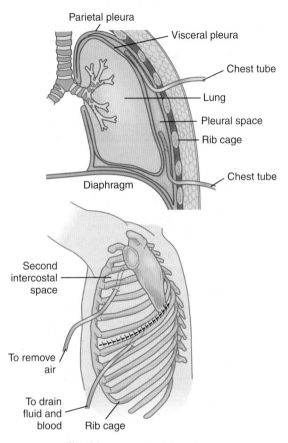

Fig. 26 Placement of chest tubes.

nozzle allows the air to pass to the environment or a collecting device during expiration. During inspiration, when pressure in the chest is decreased, the valve closes. During expiration, when intrathoracic pressure increases, the valve opens. The flutter valve can be used during emergency transport and to manage a small to moderate-sized pneumothorax.

The second type of pleural drainage system is larger and has 3 basic compartments. A variety of commercial chest drainage systems are available.

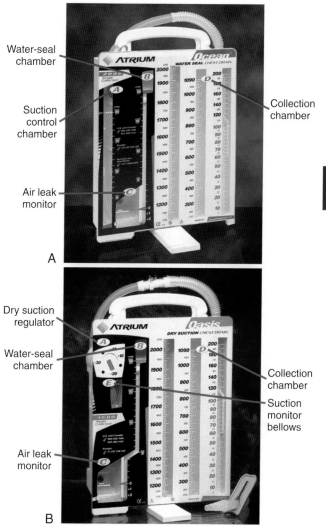

Fig. 27 Chest drainage units. Both units have 3 chambers: (1) collection chamber, (2) water-seal chamber, and (3) suction control chamber. Suction control chamber requires a connection to a wall suction source that is dialed up higher than the prescribed level. (A) Water suction. This unit uses water in the suction control chamber to control the wall suction pressure. (B) Dry suction. This unit controls wall suction by using a regulator control dial. (Courtesy Atrium Medical Corporation, Hudson, New Hampshire.)

- The first compartment, or collection chamber, receives fluid and air from the pleural space. The drained fluid stays in this chamber.
- The second chamber, called the *water-seal chamber*, contains 2 cm of water and acts as a one-way valve. Air enters from the collection chamber and bubbles up through the water. The water prevents backflow of air into the patient from the system. Initially, brisk bubbling of air occurs in the suction chamber when a pneumothorax is evacuated. During normal use, there will be intermittent bubbling because of an increase in intrathoracic pressure during exhalation, coughing, or sneezing. Eventually, the air leak seals and the lung fully expands.
- A third compartment, the suction control chamber, applies suction to the chest drainage. The amount of suction applied to the chest drainage unit is regulated by the amount of water in this chamber and not by the amount of suction applied to the system from the wall regulator.

Dry suction chest drainage systems do not contain water. They often have a visual alert that shows if the suction is working.

Nursing Management: Chest Drainage

General guidelines for nursing care of the patient with chest tubes and water-seal drainage systems are presented in Table 27.21, Harding et al., *Lewis' Medical-Surgical Nursing,* ed 11.

- Assess vital signs, lung sounds, and pain level. Assess for and notify health care provider (HCP) about signs of reaccumulating air and fluid in the chest (decreased or absent breath sounds), significant bleeding (>100 mL/hr), chest drainage site infection (drainage, redness, fever, increased white blood cell [WBC] count), or poor wound healing. Evaluate for subcutaneous emphysema at the chest tube site.
- Encourage the patient to periodically cough and breathe deeply to facilitate lung expansion, and encourage range-of-motion exercises to the shoulder on the affected side. Encourage incentive spirometry hourly while the patient is awake, to prevent atelectasis or pneumonia.
- Use meticulous sterile technique during dressing changes to reduce the incidence of infection.

Drainage System

- Keep tubing coiled loosely below chest level without kinking or compression.
- Keep all connections among the chest tubes, drainage tubing, and drainage collector tight, and tape at connections.

- Mark the time of measurement and fluid level on the chamber. Report changes in the quantity or characteristics of drainage to the HCP.
- Observe for air fluctuations and bubbling in the water-seal chamber. If tidaling is not observed, the drainage system is blocked, the lungs are reexpanded, or the system is attached to suction. If bubbling increases, there may be an air leak.
- Suspect a leak when bubbling is continuous. Retape tubing connections and ensure that the dressing is air occlusive. If a leak persists, briefly clamp the chest tube at the patient's chest. If the leak stops, then the air leak is coming from the patient.
- High fluid levels in the water seal indicate residual negative pressure. The chest system may need to be vented by using the high-negativity release valve available on the drainage system to release residual pressure from the system.
- Never elevate the drainage system to the level of the patient's chest because this will cause fluid to drain back into the lungs.
- Clamping chest tubes during transport is no longer advocated. The danger of rapid accumulation of air in the pleural space, causing tension pneumothorax, is far greater than that of a small amount of atmospheric air that enters the pleural space.
- If a chest tube becomes disconnected, the immediate priority is to reestablish the water-seal system. If the drainage system unit is overturned and the water seal is disrupted, return it to an upright position and encourage the patient to take a few deep breaths, followed by forced exhalations and cough maneuvers.
- Milking or stripping chest tubes is not recommended because these practices can dangerously increase intrapleural pressures and damage lung tissue. Position tubing so that drainage flows freely to negate the need for milking or stripping.

Chest Tube Removal

Chest tubes are removed when the lungs are reexpanded and fluid drainage has ceased or is minimal. Suction is usually discontinued and gravity drainage is used for 24 hours before tube removal. In most settings, the tube is removed by the HCP or an advanced practice nurse.

- To remove the tube: (1) cut the suture; (2) have the patient take a deep breath, exhale, and bear down (Valsalva maneuver); and (3) remove the tube.
- The site is immediately covered with an airtight dressing, and the pleura will seal off. The wound heals in several days.
- A chest x-ray is done to evaluate for pneumothorax or fluid reaccumulation.

DIALYSIS

Dialysis is a technique in which substances move from the blood through a semipermeable membrane and into a dialysis solution (dialysate). It corrects fluid and electrolyte imbalances and removes waste products in renal failure. It also can be used to treat drug overdose.

The two methods of dialysis are *peritoneal dialysis* (PD) and *hemodialysis* (HD) (Table 95).

TABLE 95 Comparison of Peritoneal Dialysis and Hemodialysis

Advantages	Disadvantages
Peritoneal Dialysis	
• Immediate initiation in almost any hospital	• Bacterial or chemical peritonitis
• Less complicated than hemodialysis	• Protein loss into dialysate
• Portable system with CAPD	• Exit site and tunnel infections
• Fewer dietary restrictions	• Self-image problems with catheter placement
• Rather short training time	• Hyperglycemia
• Usable in patient with vascular access problems	• Surgery for catheter placement
• Less cardiovascular stress	• Contraindicated in patients with multiple abdominal surgeries, traumatic injury, unrepaired hernia
• Home dialysis possible	• Requires completion of education program
• Preferable for diabetic patient	• Catheter can migrate
	• Best instituted with willing partner
Hemodialysis	
• Rapid fluid removal	• Vascular access problems
• Rapid removal of urea and creatinine	• Dietary and fluid restrictions
• Effective potassium removal	• Heparinization may be necessary
• Less protein loss	• Extensive equipment necessary
• Lowering of serum triglycerides	• Hypotension during dialysis
• Home dialysis possible	• Added blood loss that contributes to anemia
	• Specially trained personnel necessary

TABLE 95 Comparison of Peritoneal Dialysis and Hemodialysis—cont'd	
Advantages	**Disadvantages**
• Temporary access can be placed at bedside	• Surgery for permanent access placement • Self-image problems with permanent access

CAPD, Continuous ambulatory peritoneal dialysis.

- In PD, the peritoneal membrane acts as the semipermeable membrane.
- In HD, an artificial membrane (usually made of cellulose-based or synthetic materials) is used as the semipermeable membrane and is in contact with the patient's blood.

Dialysis is begun when the patient's uremia can no longer be adequately treated with conservative medical management. In general, this is when the glomerular filtration rate (GFR) (or creatinine clearance) is <15 mL/min/1.73 m^2. The nephrologist determines when to start dialysis on the basis of the patient's clinical status. Certain uremic complications, including encephalopathy, neuropathies, uncontrollable hyperkalemia, pericarditis, and accelerated hypertension, indicate the need for immediate dialysis.

Most patients with end-stage renal disease (ESRD) are treated with dialysis because: (1) there is a lack of donated organs, (2) some patients are physically or mentally unsuitable for transplantation, or (3) some patients do not want transplants.

- An increasing number of individuals, including older adults and those with complex medical problems, receive maintenance dialysis. Age is not a factor in determining candidacy. Factors that are important are the patient's ability to cope and the existing support system.

Dialysis is discussed in detail in Chapter 46 of Harding et al., *Lewis' Medical-Surgical Nursing,* ed 11.

ENTERAL NUTRITION

Enteral nutrition (EN, also known as *tube feeding*) is nutrition (e.g., liquefied food or formula) delivered directly into the gastrointestinal (GI) tract, bypassing the oral cavity. EN is used for the patient who has a functioning GI tract but is unable to take any or enough oral nourishment, or when it is unsafe to do so.

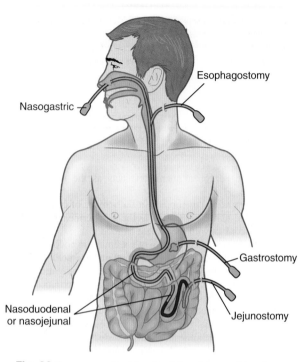

Fig. 28 Common enteral feeding tube placement locations.

EN is easily administered, safer, more physiologically efficient, and typically less expensive than parenteral nutrition. Fig. 28 shows the location of commonly used enteral feeding tubes.

- EN is given via a tube, catheter, or stoma. The type of enteral access depends on the anticipated length of time enteral feeding will be required, degree of risk for aspiration, patient's clinical status, adequacy of digestion and absorption, and patient's anatomy (e.g., extreme obesity).
- Nasally and orally placed tubes (orogastric, nasogastric [NG], nasoduodenal, or nasojejunal) are most commonly used for short-term feeding (<4 weeks).
- Nasoduodenal and nasojejunal tubes are transpyloric tubes. These tubes are used when pathophysiologic conditions, such as risk of aspiration, warrant delivering the feeding below the patient's pyloric sphincter. Placement into the small intestine decreases the chance of regurgitating gastric contents into the esophagus and subsequent aspiration. However, the patient

can still aspirate gastric secretions if the stomach is not emptying properly.

If the feedings are necessary for an extended time, other tubes are placed in the stomach or small bowel by surgical, endoscopic, or fluoroscopic procedures.

Common delivery options are continuous infusion or intermittent (bolus) feedings by infusion pump, bolus feedings by gravity, and bolus feedings by syringe. Continuous infusion is most often used for critically ill patients. Bolus feeding may be preferred as the patient improves or at home.

Tube Feedings and Safety

Aspiration and dislodged tubes are important safety concerns. You have a critical role to ensure that tube feedings are safely administered. Obtain x-ray confirmation of newly inserted nasal or orogastric tubes before feeding or administering medications. Maintain proper placement of the tube after feedings are started.

To determine if a feeding tube has maintained the proper position, mark the exit site of the feeding tube at the time of the initial x-ray, and observe for a change in the external tube length during feedings. Recheck the tube insertion length at regular intervals.

- Elevate the patient's head of bed to a minimum of 30 degrees, but preferably 45 degrees, to prevent aspiration. Check institution policy for suspending feeding while the patient is supine. If intermittent delivery is used, the head of the bed should remain elevated for 30 to 60 minutes after feeding.
- Follow your agency policy for checking gastric residual volumes (GRV). Common protocols call for checking GRV every 6 to 8 hours in noncritically ill patients and before each bolus feeding.

The types of problems encountered for patients receiving tube feedings and corrective measures are presented in Table 39.12, Harding et al., *Lewis' Medical-Surgical Nursing,* ed, 11.

Patient teaching includes skin care, tube care, feeding administration, and potential complications.

IMMUNOTHERAPY AND TARGETED THERAPY

Description

Immunotherapy and targeted therapy are cancer treatment modalities that can be effective alone or in combination with surgery, chemotherapy, and radiation therapy.

- *Immunotherapy* uses the immune system, the body's main defense against infection and disease, to fight cancer. Some types of immunotherapy are called *biologic therapy*. Immunotherapy can boost or manipulate the immune system and create an environment that is not conducive for cancer cells to grow or attack cancer cells directly. Various types of immunotherapy include cytokines, vaccines, and monoclonal antibodies. Immunotherapy consists of agents that modify the relationship between host and tumor by altering the biologic response of the host to the tumor cell (Table 96).

TABLE 96 Select Immunotherapies and Targeted Therapies

Mechanism of Action	Examples
Angiogenesis Inhibitors	
Bind vascular endothelial growth factor (VEGF), thereby inhibiting angiogenesis	bevacizumab (Avastin) pazopanib (Votrient) ramucirumab (Cyramza)
CD20 Monoclonal Antibodies	
Bind CD20 antigen, causing cytotoxicity and radiation injury	ibritumomab tiuxetan/ yttrium-90 (Zevalin)
Bind CD20 antigen, causing cytotoxicity	ofatumumab (Arzerra) rituximab (Rituxan)
CD52 Monoclonal Antibody	
Bind CD52 antigen (found on T and B cells, monocytes, NK cells, neutrophils)	alemtuzumab (Campath)
Cytokines	
Inhibit DNA and protein synthesis. Suppress cell proliferation. Increase cytotoxic effects of natural killer (NK) cells	α-interferon (Intron A)
Stimulate proliferation of T and B cells Activate NK cells	interleukin-2 (aldesleukin [Proleukin])
Human Epidermal Growth Factor Receptor-2	
Monoclonal antibody to HER-2 that attaches to the antigen. It is taken into the cells and eventually kills them	pertuzumab (Perjeta) trastuzumab (Herceptin)
Trastuzumab connected to a chemotherapy drug called DM1	ado-trastuzumab emtansine (Kadcyla)

TABLE 96 Select Immunotherapies and Targeted Therapies—cont'd

Mechanism of Action	Examples
Immunomodulatory Drugs (IMIDS)	
Inhibit production of TNF, IL-6, and VEGF (which leads to its antiangiogenic effects). Stimulate T and NK cells and increase γ-interferon and IL-2 production	apremilast (Otezla) lenalidomide (Revlimid) pomalidomide (Pomalyst) thalidomide (Thalomid)
Kinase Inhibitors	
Anaplastic Lymphoma Kinase (ALK) Inhibitors	
Inhibit anaplastic lymphoma kinase (ALK)	ceritinib (Zykadia) crizotinib (Xalkori)
BCR-ABL Tyrosine Kinase Inhibitors	
Inhibit BCR-ABL TK. Primarily used in chronic myeloid leukemia	bosutinib (Bosulif) dasatinib (Sprycel) imatinib (Gleevec) nilotinib (Tasigna)
BRAF and MEK Kinase Inhibitors	
Inhibit BRAF and MEK enzymes	dabrafenib (Tafinlar) trametinib (Mekinist) vemurafenib (Zelboraf) cobimetinib (Cotellic)
EGFR Tyrosine Kinase (TK) Inhibitors	
Inhibit epidermal growth factor receptor (EGFR) TK	cetuximab (Erbitux) erlotinib (Tarceva) gefitinib (Iressa) panitumumab (Vectibix)
Inhibit EGFR-TK and binds HER-2	lapatinib (Tykerb)
Multi-Tyrosine Kinase Inhibitors	
Inhibit multiple TKs	axitinib (Inlyta) cabozantinib (Cometriq) pazopanib (Votrient) regorafenib (Stivarga) sorafenib (Nexavar) sunitinib (Sutent) vandetanib (Caprelsa)

Continued

TABLE 96 Select Immunotherapies and Targeted Therapies—cont'd	
Mechanism of Action	**Examples**
mTOR Kinase Inhibitors	
Inhibit a specific protein known as the mechanistic target of rapamycin (mTOR)	everolimus (Afinitor) temsirolimus (Torisel)
Programmed Death Receptor (PD)-1 Blockers	
Block PD-1, a protein on T cells that normally helps keep these cells from attacking other cells. Thus boosts immune response against cancer cells	nivolumab (Opdivo) pembrolizumab (Keytruda)
Proteasome Inhibitors	
Inhibit proteasome activity, which functions to regulate cell growth	bortezomib (Velcade) carfilzomib (Kyprolis)
Vaccines	
Live attenuated strain of *Mycobacterium bovis* induces immune response. Used intravesically to treat bladder cancer	BCG vaccine
Vaccine against prostate cancer that stimulates the immune system against the cancer	sipuleucel-T (Provenge)

BRAF, B-Raf; *HER-2*, human epidermal growth factor receptor 2; *IL*, interleukin; *TNF*, tumor necrosis factor.

- *Targeted therapy* interferes with cancer growth by targeting specific cellular receptors and pathways that are important in tumor growth (see Table 96). Targeted therapy agents are selective for specific molecular targets. They can kill cancer cells with less damage to normal cells compared with chemotherapy agents.

  Types of targeted therapy agents include various tyrosine kinase inhibitors, monoclonal antibodies, angiogenesis inhibitors, and proteasome inhibitors.

- *Tyrosine kinase inhibitors* block an important enzyme that activates the signaling pathways that regulate cell proliferation and survival.

- *Monoclonal antibodies* bind to specific target cells. They may also stimulate an immunologic response in the patient.
- *Angiogenesis inhibitors* prevent the vascularization of tumors.
- *Proteasome inhibitors* promote protein accumulation and cause altered cell function.

Nursing Management

The effects of immunotherapy and targeted therapy are acute and dose-limited. Capillary leak syndrome and pulmonary edema are problems that require critical care nursing. Bone marrow depression that occurs with immunotherapy is usually more transient and less severe than that seen with chemotherapy.

- Fatigue associated with immunotherapy can be so severe that it is a dose-limiting toxicity. As agents are combined, therapy-related effects increase.
- Acetaminophen given before treatment and every 4 hours after treatment can help relieve the flulike syndrome. IV meperidine (Demerol) has been used to control the severe chills associated with some immunotherapy.

Other nursing measures include monitoring vital signs and temperature, planning for periods of rest for the patient, assisting with activities of daily living (ADLs), and monitoring for adequate oral intake.

MECHANICAL VENTILATION

Description

Mechanical ventilation is the process by which room air or oxygen-enriched air is moved into and out of the lungs by a mechanical ventilator. Mechanical ventilation is not curative. It is a means of supporting patients until they recover the ability to breathe independently or until a decision is made to stop ventilatory support. Indications for mechanical ventilation include apnea, inability to breathe or protect the airway, acute respiratory failure, severe hypoxia, and respiratory muscle fatigue.

Types of Mechanical Ventilation

The two major types of mechanical ventilation are negative pressure ventilation and positive pressure ventilation (PPV).

- *Negative pressure ventilation* involves the use of chambers that encase the chest or body and surround it with intermittent subatmospheric or negative pressure. Intermittent negative pressure around the chest wall pulls chest outward. This reduces intrathoracic pressure. Air rushes in through the upper airway, which is outside the sealed chamber. Expiration is passive; the machine cycles off, allowing chest retraction. This type of ventilation is like normal ventilation in that decreased intrathoracic pressures produce inspiration and expiration is passive. Negative pressure ventilation is noninvasive and does not require an artificial airway.

- Several portable negative pressure ventilators are available for home use for patients with neuromuscular diseases, central nervous system disorders, diseases and injuries of the spinal cord, or severe chronic obstructive pulmonary disease (COPD). They are not used routinely for acutely ill patients.
- *Positive pressure ventilation* (PPV) is the main method used with acutely ill patients. During inspiration, the ventilator pushes air into the lungs under positive pressure. Intrathoracic pressure is raised during lung inflation rather than lowered as occurs in spontaneous ventilation. Expiration occurs passively, as in normal expiration. PPV units are categorized as either volume or pressure ventilators. With volume ventilation, a predetermined tidal volume (VT) is delivered with each inspiration. With pressure ventilation, the peak inspiratory pressure is predetermined.

Nursing Management

For nursing management of the patient receiving mechanical ventilation, see eNursing Care Plan 65-1, available on the website for Harding et al., *Lewis' Medical-Surgical Nursing,* ed 11.

OSTOMIES

Description

An *ostomy* is a surgically created opening on the abdomen that allows for the discharge of body waste. The outermost portion that is visible is a *stoma.* The stoma is the result of the large or small bowel being brought to the outside of the abdomen and sutured in place. When a stoma is created as a fecal diversion, feces will drain through the stoma instead of the anus.

An ostomy is necessary when the normal elimination route is no longer possible. For example, if the person has stage III transverse colon cancer, the diseased portion of the colon is surgically removed with a margin of healthy tissue. Sometimes the tumor can be resected, leaving enough healthy tissue to immediately *anastomose* (reconnect) the two remaining ends of healthy bowel, and no ostomy is necessary. If the tumor involves the rectum and is large enough to necessitate the removal of the anal sphincters, the anus is sutured shut and a permanent ostomy is created.

Types of Ostomies

Ostomies are named according to location and type (Fig. 29). An ostomy in the ileum is an *ileostomy*. An ostomy in the colon is a *colostomy*. The ostomy is further characterized by its site (e.g., sigmoid or transverse). The more distal the ostomy, the more the intestinal contents resemble feces. A comparison of colostomies and ileostomies is shown in Table 97.

The major types of ostomies are end stoma, loop, and double-barrel ostomies.

- An *end stoma* is created by dividing the bowel and bringing the proximal end as a single stoma. The distal portion of the gastrointestinal (GI) tract is surgically removed or it is oversewn and left in the abdominal cavity. If the distal bowel is removed, then the stoma is permanent.
- A *loop stoma* is constructed by bringing a loop of bowel to the abdominal surface and then opening the anterior part of the bowel to provide fecal diversion. This results in 1 stoma with a proximal and distal opening and an intact posterior bowel wall that separates the 2 openings. A loop stoma is usually temporary.
- In a *double-barrel stoma,* the bowel is divided, and both the proximal and distal ends are brought through the abdominal wall as 2 separate stomas. The proximal one is the functioning stoma; the distal, nonfunctioning stoma is referred to as the mucus fistula. The double-barreled stoma is usually temporary.

The procedures used to perform ostomy surgeries are further discussed in Chapter 42 in Harding et al., *Lewis' Medical-Surgical Nursing,* ed 11.

Nursing Management

Preoperative Care

Psychologic preparation and emotional support are important as the person copes with the change in body image and a loss of control over elimination and its odors.

- A wound, ostomy, and continence nurse (WOCN) should choose the site where the ostomy will be and mark the abdomen before surgery. The site should be within the rectus muscle, on a flat surface, and in a place that the patient is able to see.

Postoperative Care

Postoperative nursing care includes assessment of the stoma and provision of an appropriate pouching system that protects the skin and contains drainage and odor. The stoma should be dark pink to red. A dusky blue stoma indicates ischemia, and a brown-black

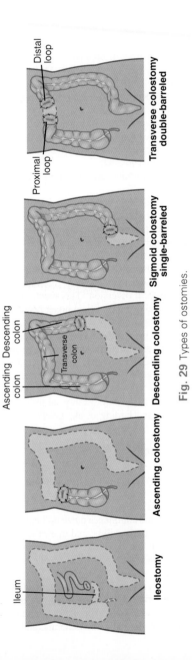

Fig. 29 Types of ostomies.

TABLE 97	Comparison of Ileostomy and Colostomy			
		COLOSTOMY		
Characteristic	**Ileostomy**	**Ascending**	**Transverse**	**Sigmoid**
Stool consistency	Liquid to semiliquid	Semiliquid	Semiliquid to semiformed	Formed
Fluid requirement	Increased	Increased	Possibly increased	No change
Bowel regulation	No	No	No	Yes (if there is a history of a regular bowel pattern)
Pouch and skin barriers	Yes	Yes	Yes	Dependent on regulation
Indications for surgery	Ulcerative colitis, Crohn's disease, diseased or injured colon, familial polyposis, trauma, cancer	Perforating diverticulum in lower colon, trauma, rectovaginal fistula, inoperable tumors of colon, rectum, or pelvis	Same as for ascending	Cancer of the rectum or rectosigmoidal area, perforating diverticulum, trauma

0

stoma indicates necrosis. Assess and document stoma color every 4 hours. Teach the patient that the stoma will be mildly to moderately swollen the first 2 to 3 weeks after surgery.

Nursing care for the patient with an ostomy is presented in eNursing Care Plan 42-3 on the website.

Colostomy Care

A colostomy in the ascending and transverse colon produces semiliquid stools. Instruct the patient to use a drainable pouch. A colostomy in the sigmoid or descending colon produces semiformed or formed stools and sometimes can be regulated by the irrigation method. The patient may or may not wear a drainage pouch. A well-balanced diet and adequate fluid intake are important.

Colostomy irrigations may be used to stimulate emptying of the colon. Regularity is possible only when the stoma is in the distal colon or rectum. With bowel control achieved, there should be little or no spillage between irrigations and the patient may need to wear only a pad or cover over the stoma. Irrigation requires manual dexterity and adequate vision. People who irrigate regularly should have ostomy bags available in case they develop diarrhea.

▼ Patient and Caregiver Teaching

Colostomy

- Pouching systems consist of an adhesive skin barrier and a bag or pouch to collect the feces. The skin barrier is a piece of pectin-based or karaya wafer that has a measurable thickness and hydrocolloid adhesive properties. Teach the patient to perform a pouch change, provide appropriate skin care, control odor, care for the stoma, and identify signs and symptoms of complications.
- Instruct the patient about the importance of adequate fluids and a healthy diet and when to seek health care.
- Recommend home care and outpatient follow-up by a WOCN. Give patients written information about the particular ostomy, instructions for pouch changes, supplies and where to purchase them, and outpatient follow-up appointments.
- Emotional support, interventions from skillful WOCNs, and visits from people who have successfully learned to manage their ostomies will help patients learn to cope with and manage the new stoma. Resources such as the United Ostomy Associations of America (*www.ostomy.org*) may also be helpful.
- For ostomy teaching guidelines, see Table 42.28, Harding et al., *Lewis' Medical-Surgical Nursing,* ed 11.

Ileostomy Care

- Because the stool from an ileostomy is caustic to the skin, a secure pouching system is important. An open-ended, drainable pouch is preferable for easy emptying. The drainable pouch is usually worn for 4 to 7 days before being changed unless leakage occurs.

- In the first 24 to 48 hours after surgery, the amount of drainage from the stoma may be negligible. Once peristalsis returns, the patient may experience a period of high-volume output of 1500 to 1800 mL/day. Later, the average amount can be 500 mL/day.

▼ **Patient and Caregiver Teaching**
Ileostomy

- Instruct the patient to drink at least 2 to 3 L/day when there are excessive fluid losses from heat and sweating. Patients must learn signs and symptoms of fluid and electrolyte imbalance so they can take appropriate action.
- A low-fiber diet is ordered initially. Reintroduce fiber-containing foods gradually.
- A stoma bleeds easily because it has a high vascular supply. Tell the patient that minimal oozing of blood is normal.
- Encourage the patient to share concerns and ask questions. Provide accurate information in a clear manner. Recommend support services and assist patients to develop confidence in managing the stoma.
- Help the patient understand if specific aspects of surgery and treatment may affect sexual function or sexual activity. Encourage the patient to discuss concerns.

OXYGEN THERAPY

Description

O_2 therapy is often used in the treatment of chronic obstructive pulmonary disease (COPD) and other problems associated with hypoxemia. Long-term continuous O_2 therapy (LTOT) increases survival and improves exercise capacity and mental status in hypoxemic patients. Improved survival occurs in patients with COPD who receive LTOT (more than 15 hr/day) to treat hypoxemia.

Goals for O_2 therapy are to keep the arterial oxygen saturation (SaO_2) above 90% during rest, sleep, and exertion, or partial pressure of oxygen in arterial blood (PaO_2) >60 mm Hg. O_2 is given to treat hypoxemia and many other problems, such as shock, pneumonia, and pulmonary emboli. O_2 therapy must be tailored to meet each patient's unique circumstances and physiological needs.

Methods of Administration

Various methods of O_2 administration are used (Table 98). The device used depends on factors the patient's underlying condition, fraction of inspired O_2 (FIO_2) needed by the patient and delivered by the device, humidification requirements, patient cooperation, comfort, cost, and financial resources.

O_2 delivery systems are classified as low- or high-flow systems. Most methods of O_2 delivery are low-flow devices that provide O_2 in concentrations that vary with the person's respiratory pattern. Low-flow devices pull in a proportion of room air. This makes the range of FIO_2 known but the exact FIO_2 hard to determine. Nasal prongs and nonrebreather masks are examples of low-flow O_2 systems. High-flow O_2 delivery devices deliver fixed concentrations of O_2 (e.g., 28%, 35%) independent of the patient's respiratory pattern. The Venturi mask and mechanical ventilators are examples of a high-flow O_2 delivery systems.

- O_2 obtained from oxygen cylinders or wall systems is dry. Dry O_2 has an irritating effect on mucous membranes and dries secretions. Humidification involves the addition of sterile distilled water, attached to the O_2 delivery device, to prevent breathing dry air.

Complications

O_2 supports combustion and increases the rate of burning, so it is important to prohibit smoking or open flames in the area where O_2 is in use. A "No Smoking" sign should be prominently displayed on the patient's door. Caution the patient against smoking cigarettes with an O_2 cannula in place because it can easily ignite and cause significant burns and life-threatening airway issues.

Chemoreceptors in the respiratory center that control the drive to breathe respond to CO_2 and O_2. Normally, an increase in CO_2 in the blood is the major stimulant of the respiratory center. Over time, some patients with COPD who have hypercapnia develop a tolerance for high CO_2 levels (the respiratory center loses its sensitivity to the elevated CO_2 levels). For these people, a major "drive" to breathe is hypoxemia. As a result, there is concern about the dangers of giving O_2 to COPD patients and reducing their drive to breathe. It is better to give oxygen to a patient who needs it because the danger of not giving oxygen to a patient far outweighs the risk.

- Pulse oximetry and/or arterial blood gases (ABGs) are used to determine what FIO_2 level is needed. Safe administration of O_2 can be achieved by gradually increasing the concentration of oxygen, with close monitoring of both PaO_2 and partial pressure of carbon dioxide in arterial blood ($PaCO_2$). The goal is a pulse O_2 saturation (SpO_2) of at least 90% or a PaO_2 of at least

(Text Continues on page 48)

TABLE 98 Methods of Oxygen Administration

Description	Nursing Interventions
Low-Flow Delivery Devices	
Nasal Cannula	
• Most commonly used device	• Stabilize nasal cannula when caring for a restless patient.
• O_2 delivered via plastic nasal prongs	• Amount of O_2 inhaled depends on room air and patient's breathing pattern.
• Safe and simple method that allows some freedom of movement. Patient can eat, talk, or cough while wearing device.	• Most patients with COPD can tolerate 2 L/min via cannula.
• Used for a patient requiring low O_2 concentrations	• Assess patient's nares and ears for skin breakdown. May need to pad cannula where it sits on ears
• Obtains O_2 concentrations of 24% (at 1 L/min) to 44% (at 6 L/min)	• If flow rates are >5 L/min, nasal membranes may dry and place patient at risk for nose bleeding

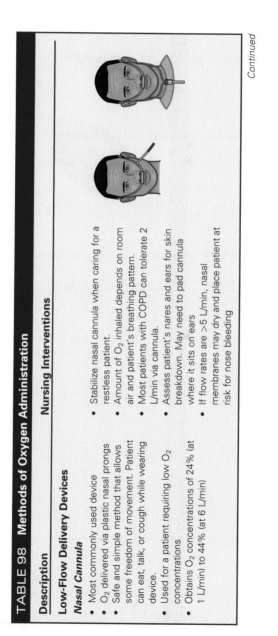

Continued

TABLE 98 Methods of Oxygen Administration—cont'd

Description	Nursing Interventions
Simple Face Mask	
• Covers patient's nose and mouth	• Wash and dry under mask q4h and PRN.
• Used only for short periods, especially when transporting patients	• Mask must fit snugly.
• Longer use is typically not tolerated because of tight seal and heat generated around nose and mouth from mask.	• Nasal cannula may be provided while patient is eating.
• Achieves O_2 concentrations of 35%–50% with flow rates of 6–12 L/min	• Watch for pressure necrosis at top of ears from elastic straps if patient wears for a longer time. Gauze or other padding may alleviate this problem.
• Mask provides adequate humidification of inspired air.	

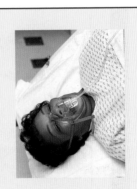

Partial and Nonrebreather Masks

- Used for short-term (24 hour) therapy for patients needing higher O_2 concentrations (60%–90% at 10–15 L/min)
- O_2 flows into reservoir bag and mask during inhalation.
- Bag allows patient to rebreathe about first third of exhaled air (rich in O_2) in conjunction with flowing O_2.
- Vents stay open on partial mask only.
- Some agencies prefer this over nonrebreather as a safety issue.

- O_2 flow rate must be sufficient to keep bag from deflating during inspiration to avoid CO_2 buildup and rebreathing of CO_2.
- If deflation occurs, increase flowrate on flowmeter on wall to keep bag inflated.
- Mask should fit snugly.
- With nonrebreather masks, make sure valves are open during expiration and closed during inhalation to prevent decrease in FIO_2 or build-up in CO_2
- Monitor patient closely, since more advanced interventions may be needed, such as CPAP, BiPAP, or intubation with mechanical ventilation.

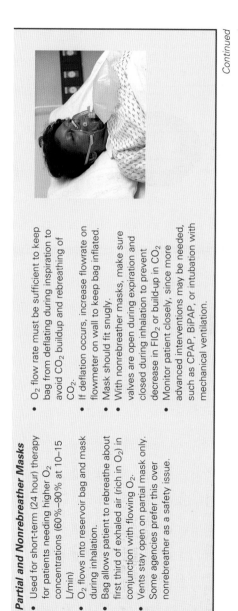

Continued

TABLE 98 Methods of Oxygen Administration—cont'd

Description	Nursing Interventions
Oxygen-Conserving Cannula • Generally indicated for long-term O_2 therapy at home vs. during hospitalization (e.g., pulmonary fibrosis, pulmonary hypertension) • Looks like a "moustache" (Oxymizer) or "pendant" type • Cannula has a built-in reservoir that ↑ O_2 concentration and allows patient to use lower flow, usually 30%–50%, which increases comfort, lowers cost, and can be increased with activities. • Can deliver O_2 up to 8L/min.	• May cause necrosis over tops of ears. Tubing can be padded. • Cannula cannot be cleaned. Manufacturer recommends changing cannula every week. • More expensive than standard cannulas and may need evaluation with ABGs and oximetry to determine correct flow for patient. • Cannula is highly visible.

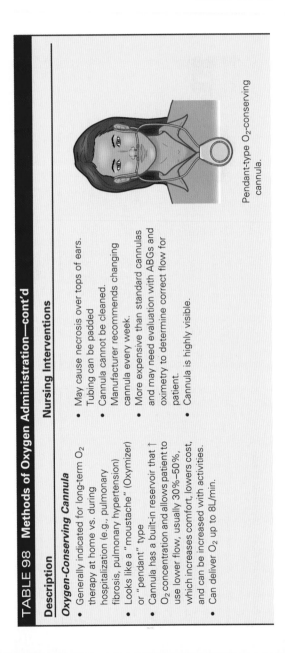

Pendant-type O_2-conserving cannula.

Continued

High-Flow Delivery Devices

Tracheostomy Collar

- Collar attaches to neck with elastic strap and can deliver humidity and O_2 via tracheostomy.
- Some O_2 concentration is lost into atmosphere because collar does not fit tightly.
- Venturi device can be attached to flowmeter and thus can deliver exact amounts of O_2 via collar.

- Secretions collect inside collar and around tracheostomy. Remove collar and clean at least q4hr and PRN to prevent aspiration of fluid and infection.
- Because condensation occurs in tubing, periodically drain tubing distal to tracheostomy.

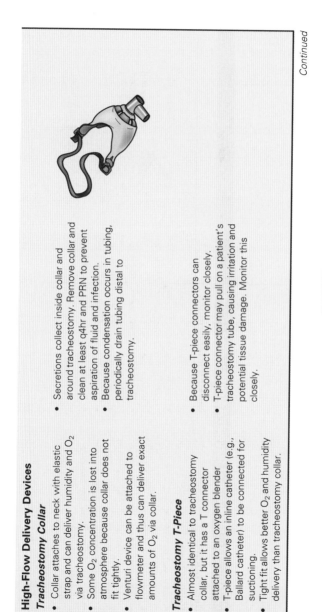

Tracheostomy T-Piece

- Almost identical to tracheostomy collar, but it has a T connector attached to an oxygen blender.
- T-piece allows an inline catheter (e.g., Ballard catheter) to be connected for suctioning.
- Tight fit allows better O_2 and humidity delivery than tracheostomy collar.

- Because T-piece connectors can disconnect easily, monitor closely.
- T-piece connector may pull on a patient's tracheostomy tube, causing irritation and potential tissue damage. Monitor this closely.

O

TABLE 98 Methods of Oxygen Administration—cont'd

Description	Nursing Interventions
Venturi Mask • Mask can deliver precise, high-flow rates of O_2. • Lightweight plastic, cone-shaped mask Masks are available for delivery of 24%, 28%, 31%, 35%, 40%, and 50% O_2. • Method is especially helpful for giving low, constant O_2 concentrations to patients with COPD. • Adaptors can be applied to increase humidification.	• Entrainment device on mask must be changed to deliver higher concentrations of O_2. • Air entrainment ports must not be occluded. • Uncomfortable. • Must be removed when patient eats. • Patient can talk but voice may be muffled.

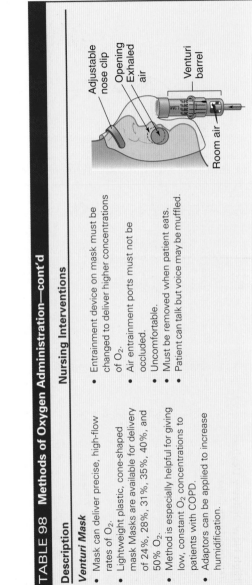

Adjustable nose clip

Opening
Exhaled air

Venturi barrel

Room air

High-Flow Nasal Cannula

- Blends O_2 with compressed air to generate FIO_2 up to 1.0 at flow rate of up to 60 L/min.
- Active heated humidifier capable of providing 100% body humidity
- Soft and flexible nasal prongs.
- More comfortable than mask

- Nasal cannula must be smaller than 50% of nares to allow flow during exhalation and flush out end-expiratory CO_2.
- Patients can eat and drink with device in place.
- Well tolerated
- Patient may describe feeling of always having to blow nose ("rainout") because of humidification

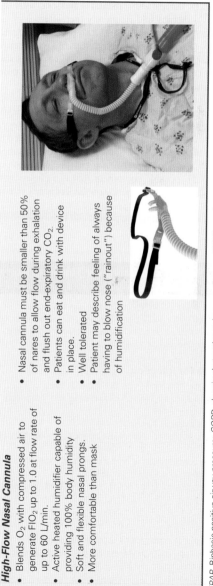

BiPAP, Biphasic positive airway pressure; COPD, chronic obstructive pulmonary disease; CPAP, continuous positive airway pressure; FIO_2, fraction of inspired O_2.

60 mmHg. Assess the patient's mental status and vital signs before starting O_2 therapy and frequently thereafter.

Pulmonary oxygen toxicity may result from prolonged exposure to a high level of O_2 (PaO_2). High concentrations of O_2 can result in a severe inflammatory response because of oxygen free radicals damage to alveolar-capillary membranes, resulting in severe pulmonary edema, shunting of blood, and hypoxemia.

- To prevent toxicity, the amount of O_2 administered should be just enough to maintain the PaO_2 within a normal or acceptable range for the patient.

Infection can be a complication of O_2 administration. Heated nebulizers present the highest risk. Constant use of humidity supports bacterial growth. *Pseudomonas aeruginosa* is the most common infecting organism. Disposable equipment that is a closed system should be used. Each agency has a policy on the frequency of equipment changes.

A home care guide for teaching the patient and family about home O_2 use is given in Table 99.

TABLE 99 Patient and Caregiver Teaching Home Oxygen Use

The company that provides the prescribed O_2 therapy equipment will teach the patient about equipment care. The following are some general instructions that you may include when teaching the patient and caregiver about the use of home O_2.

Decreasing Risk for Infection

- Brush teeth or use mouthwash several times a day.
- Wash nasal cannula (prongs) with a liquid soap and thoroughly rinse once or twice a week.
- Replace cannula every 2–4 weeks.
- If you have a cold, replace the cannula after your symptoms pass.
- Always remove secretions that are coughed out.
- If you use an O_2 concentrator, unplug the unit and wipe down the cabinet with a damp cloth and dry it daily.
- Ask the company providing the equipment how often to change the filter.

Safety Issues

- Post "No Smoking" warning signs outside the home.
- O_2 will not "blow up," but it will increase the rate of burning because it is combustible.

TABLE 99   Patient and Caregiver Teaching Home Oxygen Use—cont'd
• Do not allow smoking in the home, and do not smoke while wearing an O_2 cannula or other device. Nasal cannulas and masks can catch fire, causing serious burns to face and airways.
• Do not use flammable liquids, such as paint thinners, cleaning fluids, gasoline, kerosene, oil-based paints, or aerosol sprays while receiving O_2.
• Do not use blankets or fabrics that carry a static charge, such as wool or synthetics.
• Inform your electric company if you are using a concentrator. In case of a power failure, the company will know the medical urgency of restoring your power.

Adapted from <www.YourLungHealth.org>.

PACEMAKERS

Description

The artificial cardiac pacemaker is an electronic device used to pace the heart when the normal conduction pathway is damaged. The basic pacing circuit consists of a power source (battery-powered pulse generator), 1 or more conducting leads (pacing leads), and the myocardium. The electrical signal (stimulus) travels from the pacemaker, through the leads, to the wall of the myocardium. The heart muscle is stimulated to contract.

Demand pacemakers, which are the most common, sense the heart's electrical activity and fire only when the heart rate (HR) drops below a preset rate. Demand pacemakers have two distinct features: (1) a sensing device that inhibits the pacemaker when the HR is adequate, and (2) a pacing device that triggers the pacemaker when no QRS complexes occur within a preset time.

Permanent pacemakers are implanted entirely within the patient's body. The power source is implanted subcutaneously, usually over the pectoral muscle on the patient's nondominant side. It is attached to pacer leads, which are threaded transvenously (through a vein) to the right atrium and 1 or both ventricles. Indications for insertion of a permanent pacemaker are listed in Table 100.

New technology and research are focused on miniaturized, leadless permanent pacemakers. Single component devices have the battery, sensors, electronics, and stimulating electrodes in a small capsule that is placed in the ventricle using a deflatable sheath. A multicomponent device has a small "seed" that is placed in a cardiac chamber. It acts as an energy transducer while an outside piece

P

TABLE 100 Indications for Permanent Pacemakers

- Acquired AV block
- Second-degree AV block
- Third-degree AV block
- Atrial fibrillation with a slow ventricular response
- Bundle branch block
- Cardiomyopathy (dilated or hypertrophic)
- Heart failure
- SA node dysfunction
- Symptomatic bradycardia with unknown cause
- Tachydysrhythmias (e.g., ventricular tachycardia)

AV, Atrioventricular; *SA,* sinoatrial.

beams ultrasound (or radio waves) to the "seed." The seed converts the energy to a pacing pulse. The lack of a transvenous lead and subcutaneous pulse generator is a major shift in cardiac pacing.

Cardiac resynchronization therapy (CRT) is a pacing technique that resynchronizes the heart cycle by pacing both ventricles (biventricular pacing). This is used for patients with heart failure to improve ventricular function.

A *temporary pacemaker* is one that has the power source outside the body. Temporary pacemakers are used until short-term cardiac conduction problem resolve or until more definitive therapy is available. There are 3 types of temporary pacemakers: transvenous, epicardial, and transcutaneous. Table 101 lists common reasons for temporary pacing.

TABLE 101 Common Indications for Temporary Pacemakers

- Maintenance of adequate HR and rhythm during special circumstances, such as surgery and postoperative recovery, during cardiac catheterization or coronary angioplasty, with drug therapy that may cause bradycardia, and before implantation of a permanent pacemaker
- Prophylaxis after open heart surgery
- Acute anterior MI with second- or third-degree AV block or bundle branch block
- Acute inferior MI with symptomatic bradycardia and AV block
- Electrophysiologic studies to evaluate patient with bradydysrhythmias and tachydysrhythmias

AV, Atrioventricular; *HR,* heart rate; *MI,* myocardial infarction.

- A *transvenous pacemaker* consists of a lead or leads that are threaded transvenously to the right atrium and/or right ventricle and attached to the external power source.
- In *epicardial pacemakers,* atrial and ventricular pacing leads are attached to the epicardium during heart surgery in case pacing is required during the surgical recovery period. The leads are passed through the chest wall and attached to the external power source.
- A *transcutaneous pacemaker* can provide adequate HR and rhythm to the patient in an emergency. This type of pacemaker involves the use of external electrode pads that are connected to the external power source.

Nursing Management

Patients with temporary or permanent pacemakers are monitored by electrocardiogram (ECG) to evaluate the status of the pacemaker. Pacemaker malfunction primarily involves a failure to sense or a failure to capture.

- *Failure to sense* occurs when the pacemaker fails to recognize spontaneous atrial or ventricular activity and fires inappropriately. Failure to sense is caused by fibrosis around the tip of the pacing lead, battery failure, sensing set too high, or electrode displacement.
- *Failure to capture* occurs when the electrical charge to the myocardium is insufficient to produce atrial or ventricular contraction. This can result in serious bradycardia or asystole. Failure to capture may be caused by pacer lead fracture, battery failure, electrode displacement, electrical charge set too low, or fibrosis at the electrode tip.
- *Failure to pace* occurs if the pacemaker does not initiate an electrical stimulus when it should fire. This can be caused by a wire fracture, lead displacement, oversensing, or electrical interference.
  After the pacemaker insertion, the patient can be out of bed once stable. Have the patient limit arm and shoulder activity on the operative side to prevent dislodging the newly implanted pacing leads.
- Observe the insertion site for signs of bleeding, and check that the incision is intact. Note any temperature elevation or pain at the insertion site. Stable patients are discharged by the next day.
- After discharge, patients need to check pacemaker function on a regular basis. This can include outpatient visits to a pacemaker clinic or home monitoring using telephone transmitter devices.
- The goals of pacemaker therapy include enhancing physiologic functioning and quality of life. Emphasize these goals to the patient and the caregiver, and provide specific advice on activity restrictions. Table 102 outlines patient and caregiver teaching about pacemakers.

P

TABLE 102   Patient and Caregiver Teaching Pacemaker

Include the following information in the teaching plan for a patient with a pacemaker and the patient's caregiver.

1. Maintain follow-up care with your health care provider (HCP) to begin regular pacemaker function checks. This is often done by interrogating the device using a telephone.
2. Report any signs of infection at incision site (e.g., redness, swelling, drainage) or fever to your HCP immediately.
3. Keep incision dry for 4 days after implantation, or as ordered.
4. Avoid lifting arm on pacemaker side above shoulder until approved by your cardiologist.
5. Avoid direct blows to pacemaker site.
6. Avoid close proximity to high-output electric generators, since these can interfere with the function of the pacemaker.
7. You should not have an MRI scan unless the pacemaker is approved as MRI-safe or there is a protocol in place for patient safety during the procedure.
8. Microwave ovens are safe to use and do not interfere with pacemaker function.
9. Avoid standing near antitheft devices in doorways of department stores and public libraries. Walk through them at a normal pace.
10. Travel is not restricted. Tell security (e.g., airport, train station, public buildings) of presence of pacemaker because it may set off the metal detector. If handheld screening wand is used, it should not be placed directly over the pacemaker. Manufacturer information may vary about the effect of metal detectors on the function of the pacemaker.
11. Monitor pulse and tell your HCP if heart rate drops below predetermined rate.
12. Always carry pacemaker information card and a current list of your medications.
13. Obtain and wear a Medic Alert ID at all times.
14. Consider joining a pacemaker support group (e.g., <https://www.pacemakerclub.com>).

PARENTERAL NUTRITION

Description

Parenteral nutrition (PN) is a nutrient solution delivered directly into the bloodstream. PN is used when the gastrointestinal (GI) tract cannot be used for the ingestion, digestion, and absorption of essential nutrients (Table 103).

TABLE 103 Common Indications for Parenteral Nutrition

- Chronic severe diarrhea and vomiting
- Complicated surgery or trauma
- GI obstruction
- GI tract anomalies and fistulas
- Intractable diarrhea
- Severe anorexia nervosa
- Severe malabsorption
- Short bowel syndrome

GI, Gastrointestinal.

Administration of Parenteral Nutrition

PN may be administered by central or peripheral techniques. Both central and peripheral forms of PN are used in the patient who is not a candidate for enteral nutrition (EN). The patient receiving PN must be able to tolerate a large volume of fluid.

- *Central PN* is indicated when long-term nutritional support is needed or when the patient has high protein and caloric requirements. Central PN may be administered using a central venous catheter that originates at the subclavian or jugular vein and whose tip lies in the superior vena cava. Central PN may also be administered using peripherally inserted central catheters (PICCs) that are placed into the basilic or cephalic vein and then advanced into the distal end of the superior vena cava.

- *Peripheral PN* (PPN) is administered using a large-bore catheter in a large peripheral vein. PPN is used when nutritional support is needed for only a short time, protein and caloric requirements are not high, the risk of a central catheter is too great, or to supplement inadequate enteral intake.

Commercially prepared PN base solutions that contain dextrose and protein in the form of amino acids are available. The pharmacy adds the prescribed electrolytes (e.g., sodium, chloride, calcium, magnesium, phosphate), vitamins, and trace elements (e.g., zinc, copper, chromium, selenium, manganese) to meet the patient's needs. A 3-in-1 or total nutrient admixture containing an IV fat emulsion, dextrose, and amino acids is widely used.

Refeeding syndrome can occur any time a malnourished patient starts aggressive nutritional support. It is characterized by fluid retention and electrolyte imbalances (low phosphate, potassium, magnesium). It is associated with dysrhythmias, respiratory arrest, and neurologic problems (e.g., paresthesias).

P

TABLE 104   Complications of Parenteral Nutrition

Metabolic Problems

- Altered renal function
- Essential fatty acid deficiency
- Hyperglycemia, hypoglycemia
- Hyperlipidemia
- Liver dysfunction
- Refeeding syndrome

Catheter-Related Problems

- Air embolus
- Catheter-related sepsis
- Dislodgment
- Hemorrhage
- Occlusion
- Phlebitis
- Pneumothorax, hemothorax, and hydrothorax
- Thrombosis of vein

- Conditions that predispose patients to refeeding syndrome include long-standing malnutrition states, such as chronic alcohol use, vomiting and diarrhea, chemotherapy, and major surgery. Other complications of PN are listed in Table 104.

Home Nutritional Support

Home PN nutrition is an accepted mode of therapy for the person who needs continued nutritional support. Nutritional therapies are expensive. Specific criteria must be met for expenses to be reimbursed. The discharge planning team needs to be involved early on to help address such issues.

- Teach the patient and caregiver about catheter or tube care, proper technique in handling the solutions and tubing, and side effects and complications.
- Tell the family about support groups such as the Oley Foundation (<www.oley.org>) that provide peer support and advocacy.

RADIATION THERAPY

Description

Radiation therapy is one of the oldest methods of cancer treatment. Delivery of high-energy beams, when absorbed into tissue, produces ionization of atomic particles. The energy in ionizing radiation acts to break the chemical bonds in DNA and cause cell death.

Different types of ionizing radiation are used to treat cancer, including electromagnetic radiation (i.e., x-rays, gamma rays) and particulate radiation (alpha particles, electrons, neutrons, protons).

- Historically, the radiation dose was expressed in *rad* (radiation absorbed dose) units. Now we use, *gray* (Gy) or *centigray* (cGy) units are used. One cGy is equal to 1 rad, and 100 cGy equal 1 Gy.
- Once the total dose to be delivered is determined, that dose is divided into daily fractions. Doses between 180 and 200 cGy/ day are considered standard. They are typically delivered once a day Monday through Friday for a period of 2 to 8 weeks, depending on the desired total dose.
- Radiation only affects tissues in the treatment field, so it is not used as the main treatment for systemic disease. However, radiation therapy may be used by itself or in combination with chemotherapy or surgery to treat primary tumors or for palliation of metastatic lesions.
- Radiation can be delivered externally *(external beam radiation therapy)* or internally *(brachytherapy)*.

Rapidly dividing cells in the gastrointestinal (GI) tract, oral mucosa, and bone marrow exhibit early acute responses to radiation. Tissues with slowly proliferating cells, such as cartilage, bone, and kidneys, show later responses to radiation. Some cancers are more susceptible to radiation than others (Table 105).

Nursing Management: Radiation Therapy and Patient and Caregiver Teaching

See Chemotherapy, p. 674.

TABLE 105 Tumor Radiosensitivity

High Radiosensitivity
- Hodgkin's lymphoma
- Neuroblastoma
- Non-Hodgkin's lymphoma
- Ovarian dysgerminoma
- Testicular seminoma
- Wilms' tumor

Moderate Radiosensitivity
- Bladder carcinoma
- Breast adenocarcinoma
- Esophageal carcinoma
- Oropharyngeal carcinoma
- Prostate carcinoma
- Uterine and cervical carcinoma

Mild Radiosensitivity
- Colon adenocarcinoma
- Gastric adenocarcinoma
- Renal adenocarcinoma
- Soft tissue sarcomas (e.g., chondrosarcoma)

Poor Radiosensitivity
- Malignant glioma
- Malignant melanoma
- Osteosarcoma
- Testicular nonseminoma

R

TRACHEOSTOMY

Description

A *tracheostomy* is a surgically created stoma (opening) in the trachea to establish an airway, or the procedure for creating this opening. It is used to: (1) establish a patent airway, (2) bypass an upper airway obstruction, (3) facilitate removal of secretions, (4) permit long-term mechanical ventilation, and (5) facilitate weaning from mechanical ventilation.

Most surgical tracheostomy procedures are done in the operating room using general anesthesia. These are typically done electively for patients already intubated who require prolonged mechanical ventilation. When swelling, trauma, or upper airway obstruction prevents endotracheal intubation, an emergent cricothyroidotomy (also known as a "cricothyrotomy") is needed. This procedure, which can be completed in minutes, involves making an incision through the skin and cricothyroid membrane on the anterior surface of the neck.

A *percutaneous tracheostomy* can also be performed using local anesthesia and sedation and analgesia. A needle is placed into the trachea, followed by a guide wire. The opening is progressively dilated until it is large enough for insertion of a tracheostomy tube.

- A tracheostomy tube provides a more secure airway and allows more freedom of movement than an endotracheal tube. There is less risk of long-term damage to the vocal cords. Airway resistance and work of breathing are decreased. Patients may be more comfortable without a tube in the mouth.

- The patient can eat with a tracheostomy because the tube enters lower in the airway (Fig. 30). Speaking is also possible once the tracheostomy cuff can be deflated.

After the tracheostomy tube is removed, care involves applying a sterile occlusive dressing and monitoring the site for bleeding. The dressing must be changed if it gets soiled or wet. If necessary, close the stoma with tape strips. Instruct the patient to splint the stoma with the fingers when coughing, swallowing, or speaking.

- Epithelial tissue begins to form in 24 to 48 hours, and the opening closes in several days.

Nursing Management

Before the tracheostomy, explain the purpose of the procedure and inform the patient and family that the patient will not be able to speak if an inflated cuff is used. A variety of tubes are available to meet patient needs (see Fig. 30). Characteristics and nursing

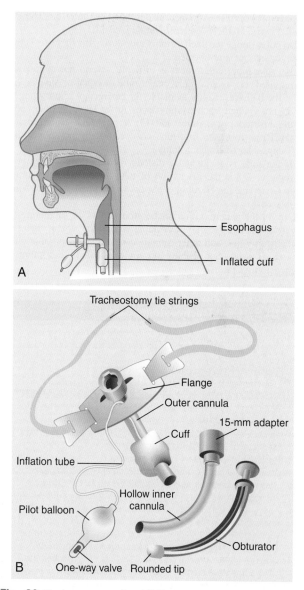

Fig. 30 Tracheostomy tube. (A) Tracheostomy tube inserted in airway with inflated cuff. (B) Parts of a tracheostomy tube.

management of tracheostomies are described in Table 26.6, Harding et al., Lewis' *Medical-Surgical Nursing,* ed 11.

Do not dislodge the tracheostomy tube during the first 5 to 7 days, when the stoma is not healed.

- Because tube replacement is difficult, several precautions are required: (1) keep a replacement tube of equal or smaller size at the bedside, readily available for emergency reinsertion; (2) do not change tracheostomy tapes for at least 24 hours after the insertion procedure; and (3) let a health care provider (HCP) perform the first tube change, usually no sooner than 7 days after the tracheostomy.
- If the tube is accidentally dislodged, immediately attempt to replace it. See the discussion of tube replacement techniques in Chapter 26 in Harding et al., *Lewis' Medical-Surgical Nursing,* ed 11.

Care of the patient with a tracheostomy involves suctioning the airway to remove secretions, cleaning around the stoma, changing tracheostomy ties, and inner cannula care if a nondisposable inner cannula is used. See Table 106 for a detailed description of tracheostomy care.

TABLE 106 Tracheostomy Care

The following are general guidelines for basic tracheostomy care. Become familiar with the specific policies and/or procedures in your institution.

1. Explain procedure to patient.
2. Use tracheostomy care kit or collect necessary sterile equipment (e.g., suction catheter, 1 pair sterile gloves, 1 pair nonsterile gloves, water basin, tracheostomy ties, tube brush or pipe cleaners, 4 × 4 gauze pads, sterile water or normal saline, and tracheostomy dressing [optional]). Note: clean rather than sterile technique is used at home.
3. Position patient in semi-Fowler's position.
4. Assemble needed materials on bedside table next to patient.
5. Wash hands. Put on personal protective equipment (goggles and clean gloves).
6. Auscultate chest sounds. If wheezes or coarse crackles are present, suction the airway if the patient is unable to cough up secretions (Table 26.8, Harding et al., *Lewis' Medical-Surgical Nursing,* ed 11). Remove soiled dressing and clean gloves.
7. Open sterile equipment, pour sterile H_2O or normal saline into 2 compartments of sterile container or 2 basins, and put on sterile gloves. Note: hydrogen peroxide (3%) is no longer recommended unless an infection is present. If it is used, rinse

TABLE 106 Tracheostomy Care—cont'd

the inner cannula and skin with sterile H_2O or normal saline afterward, to prevent trauma to tissue.

8. If present, unlock and remove inner cannula. Many tracheostomy tubes do not have inner cannulas. Care for these tubes includes all steps except for inner cannula care.

9. If disposable inner cannula is used, replace with new cannula. If a nondisposable cannula is used:
   • Immerse inner cannula in sterile solution and clean inside and outside of cannula using tube brush or pipe cleaners.
   • Rinse cannula in sterile solution. Remove from solution and shake to dry.
   • Insert inner cannula into outer cannula with the curved part downward, and lock in place.

10. Remove dried secretions from stoma using 4 × 4 gauze pad soaked in sterile water or saline. Gently pat area around the stoma until dry. Be sure to clean under the tracheostomy flange (faceplate), using cotton swabs to reach this area.

11. Place dressing around tube. Use a precut tracheostomy dressing or unlined gauze. Do not cut the gauze because threads may be inhaled or wrap around the tracheostomy tube. Change the dressing as required. Wet dressings promote infection and stoma irritation.

12. Change tracheostomy tapes using 2-persons change technique. Tie tracheostomy tapes securely with room for 2 fingers between tapes and skin. To prevent accidental tube removal, secure the tracheostomy tube by gently applying pressure to the flange of the tube during the tape changes. Do not change tracheostomy tapes for 24 hours after the tracheostomy procedure.

13. Some patients prefer tracheostomy tapes made of self-gripping fabric (Velcro), which are easier to adjust.

14. Repeat care three times/day and as needed.

▼ **Patient and Caregiver Teaching**
- Assess ability of the patient and caregiver to provide care at home.
- Include instructions for tracheostomy tube care, stoma care, suctioning, airway care, and responding to emergencies.
- Make a referral to a home health care nurse to provide ongoing assistance and support.
- Teach patient and caregiver the signs and symptoms to report to health care professionals, such as changes in secretions (color and consistency) and elevated temperature.

T

URINARY CATHETERIZATION

Indications for short-term urinary catheterization are listed in Table 107. Two unacceptable reasons are routine acquisition of a urine specimen for laboratory analysis and convenience of the nursing staff or the patient's family.

- Complications seen with long-term use (more than 30 days) of indwelling catheters include catheter-associated urinary tract infection (CAUTI), bladder spasms, periurethral abscess, chronic pyelonephritis, urosepsis, urethral trauma or erosion, fistula or stricture formation, and stones.

Catheterization for sterile urine specimens may be needed when a patient has a history of complicated urinary tract infection (UTI). A catheter should be the last resort to provide the patient with a dry

---

TABLE 107 Indications for Urinary Catheterization

Indwelling Catheter

- Relieve urinary retention caused by lower urinary tract obstruction, paralysis, or inability to void
- Bladder decompression preoperatively and operatively for lower abdominal or pelvic surgery
- Facilitate surgical repair of urethra and surrounding structures
- Splinting of ureters or urethra to facilitate healing after surgery or other trauma in area
- Accurate measurement of urine output in critically ill patient
- Contamination of stage III or IV pressure ulcers with urine that has impeded healing, despite appropriate personal care for the incontinence
- Terminal illness or severe impairment, which makes positioning or clothing changes uncomfortable, or which is associated with intractable pain

Intermittent (Straight, in-and-out) Catheter

- Relieve urinary retention caused by lower urinary tract obstruction, paralysis, or inability to void
- Study of anatomic structures of urinary system
- Urodynamic testing
- Collect sterile urine sample in certain situations
- Instill medications into bladder
- Measure residual urine after voiding (postvoid residual [PVR]) if portable ultrasound not available

environment to prevent skin breakdown and protect dressings or skin lesions.

Strict aseptic technique is mandatory when a urinary catheter is inserted. See Table 108 for urinary catheter management. Address patient concerns, which may include embarrassment related to

TABLE 108 Management of Patient With Urethral Catheter

The following measures can be used to manage the patient with a urethral catheter and prevent catheter-associated urinary tract infection (CAUTI).

1. Teach catheter care to the patient, particularly one who is ambulatory.
2. Use a sterile, closed drainage system in short-term catheterization. Do not disconnect the distal urinary catheter and proximal drainage tube except for catheter irrigation (if ordered and indicated).
3. Maintain unobstructed downhill flow of urine. Empty the collecting bag regularly, and keep it below the level of the bladder.
4. Provide perineal care (once or twice a day and when necessary), including cleansing the meatus-catheter junction with soap and water. Do not use lotion or powder near the catheter.
5. Anchor catheter using some type of securement device. Anchor catheter to upper thigh in women and lower abdomen in men, to prevent catheter movement and urethral tension.
6. Use sterile technique whenever the collecting system is open. If frequent irrigations are necessary in short-term catheterization to maintain catheter patency, a triple-lumen catheter may be preferable, permitting continuous irrigations within a closed system.
7. If ordered, aspirate small volumes of urine for culture from the catheter sampling port by means of a sterile syringe and needle. First prepare the puncture site with an antiseptic solution.
8. When the patient is catheterized for <2 weeks, routine catheter change is not necessary. For long-term use of an indwelling catheter, replace the catheter as indicated by patient assessment and not on a routine schedule.
9. With long-term use of a catheter, a leg bag may be used. If the collection bag is reused, wash it in soap and water and rinse thoroughly. When it is not reused immediately, fill it with ½ cup of vinegar and drain. The vinegar is effective against *Pseudomonas* and other organisms and eliminates odors.

Continued

TABLE 108   Management of Patient With Urethral Catheter—cont'd
10. Remove the catheter as early as possible. Intermittent catheterization and external catheters are alternatives that may be associated with fewer cases of bacteriuria and urinary tract infection (UTI) than with chronic indwelling urethral catheters.

exposure of the body, an altered body image, and fear that care of the catheter will result in increased dependency.

- Catheters vary in construction materials, tip shape, and lumen size.
- Catheters are sized according to the French scale. Each French unit (F) equals 0.33 mm of diameter. The diameter listed is the internal diameter of the catheter. The size used varies with the patient's size and the purpose of catheterization. In women, urethral catheter sizes 14F to 16F are the most common. In men, sizes 14F to 18F are used. Balloon sizes are either 5 or 30 mL.

The most common route of catheterization is *urethral catheterization*, insertion of the catheter through the external meatus into the urethra, past the internal sphincter, and into the bladder.

Suprapubic catheterization is the simplest and oldest method of urinary diversion. The 2 methods of insertion of a suprapubic catheter into the bladder are: (1) through a small incision in the abdominal wall, and (2) using a trocar. A suprapubic catheter is placed while the patient is under general anesthesia for another surgical procedure or at the bedside with a local anesthetic. The catheter may be sutured in place.

- The suprapubic catheter is used in temporary situations, such as during bladder, prostate, and urethral surgery. It is used long term in some patients.
- The care of the catheter is similar to that of the urethral catheter. Tape the catheter to prevent dislodgement. A pectin-base skin barrier (e.g., Stomahesive) is effective in protecting the skin around the insertion site from breakdown.
- A suprapubic catheter is prone to poor drainage because of mechanical obstruction of the catheter tip by the bladder wall, sediment, and clots. To ensure patency of the tube: (1) prevent tube kinking by coiling the excess tubing and maintaining gravity drainage, (2) have the patient turn from side to side, and (3) milk the tube. If these measures are not effective, obtain a health care provider (HCP)'s order to irrigate the catheter with sterile technique.

- If the patient has bladder spasms that are hard to control, urinary leakage may result. Oxybutynin (Ditropan XL) or other oral antispasmodics or belladonna and opium (B&O) suppositories may be prescribed to decrease bladder spasms.

An alternative approach to a long-term indwelling catheter is *intermittent catheterization* of the urethra, also referred to as "straight" or "in-and-out" catheterization. It is used in conditions, such as neurogenic bladder (e.g., spinal cord injuries, chronic neurologic diseases) or bladder outlet obstruction in men. This type of catheterization may be used in the oliguric and anuric phases of acute kidney injury to reduce the chance of infection from an indwelling catheter. Intermittent catheterization is used postoperatively, often after a surgical procedure to treat urinary incontinence.

- The technique consists of inserting a urethral catheter into the bladder every 3 to 5 hours. Some patients perform intermittent catheterization only once or twice each day to measure residual urine and ensure an empty bladder.
- Instruct patients to wash and rinse the catheter and their hands with soap and water before and after catheterization. Lubricant is necessary for men and may make catheterization more comfortable for women.
- The patient, caregiver, or HCP may insert the catheter.
- In the hospital or long-term care facility, sterile technique is used for catheterizations. For home care, a clean technique that includes good hand washing with soap and water is used.
- Teach the patient to observe for signs of UTI so that treatment can be instituted early.

PART THREE

Reference Appendix

ABBREVIATIONS

ABG	arterial blood gas
ACE	angiotensin-converting enzyme
ACLS	advanced cardiac life support
ACS	acute coronary syndrome
ACTH	adrenocorticotropic hormone
ADH	antidiuretic hormone
AED	automated external defibrillator
AIDS	acquired immunodeficiency syndrome
AKA	above-knee amputation
AKI	acute kidney injury
ALL	acute lymphocytic leukemia
ALS	amyotrophic lateral sclerosis
AMI	acute myocardial infarction
ANA	antinuclear antibody
ANS	autonomic nervous system
AORN	Association of periOperative Registered Nurses
APD	automated peritoneal dialysis
aPTT	activated partial thromboplastin time
ARDS	acute respiratory distress syndrome
ATN	acute tubular necrosis
BCLS	basic cardiac life support
BKA	below-knee amputation
BMI	body mass index
BMR	basal metabolic rate
BMT	bone marrow transplantation
BPH	benign prostatic hyperplasia
BSE	breast self-examination
BUN	blood urea nitrogen
CABG	coronary artery bypass graft
CAD	coronary artery disease; circulatory assist device
CAPD	continuous ambulatory peritoneal dialysis
CAVH	continuous arteriovenous hemofiltration
CBC	complete blood count
CCU	coronary care unit; critical care unit
CDC	Centers for Disease Control and Prevention
CIS	carcinoma in situ
CKD	chronic kidney disease
CLL	chronic lymphocytic leukemia
CML	chronic myelocytic leukemia
CMP	cardiomyopathy
CN	cranial nerve
CNS	central nervous system

Continued

ABBREVIATIONS—cont'd

CO	cardiac output
COPD	chronic obstructive pulmonary disease
CPAP	continuous positive airway pressure
CPR	cardiopulmonary resuscitation
CRRT	continuous renal replacement therapy
CRNA	certified registered nurse anesthetist
CSF	cerebrospinal fluid
CT	computed tomography
CVA	cerebrovascular accident; costovertebral angle
CVAD	central venous access device
CVI	chronic venous insufficiency
CVP	central venous pressure
D&C	dilation and curettage
DDD	degenerative disc disease
DI	diabetes insipidus
DIC	disseminated intravascular coagulation
DJD	degenerative joint disease
DKA	diabetic ketoacidosis
DM	diabetes mellitus; diastolic murmur
DRE	digital rectal examination
DVT	deep vein thrombosis
ECF	extracellular fluid
ECG	electrocardiogram
ED	emergency department; erectile dysfunction
EEG	electroencephalogram
EMG	electromyogram
ENT	ear, nose, and throat
ERCP	endoscopic retrograde cholangiopancreatography
ERS	emergency response system
ESR	erythrocyte sedimentation rate
ESRD	end-stage renal disease
ET	endotracheal
FEV	forced expiratory volume
FRC	functional residual capacity
FUO	fever of unknown origin
GCS	Glasgow Coma Scale
GERD	gastroesophageal reflux disease
GFR	glomerular filtration rate
GH	growth hormone
GTT	glucose tolerance test
GU	genitourinary
GYN, Gyn	gynecologic
H&P	history and physical examination

ABBREVIATIONS—cont'd

HAV	hepatitis A virus
HBV	hepatitis B virus
HCP	health care provider
Hct	hematocrit
HCV	hepatitis C virus
HD	hemodialysis; Huntington's disease
HDL	high-density lipoprotein
HF	heart failure
Hgb	hemoglobin
HIV	human immunodeficiency virus
HPV	human papillomavirus
HSCT	hematopoietic stem cell transplantation
I&D	incision and drainage
IABP	intraaortic balloon pump
IBS	irritable bowel syndrome
ICP	intracranial pressure
IE	infective endocarditis
IFG	impaired fasting glucose
IGT	impaired glucose tolerance
INR	international normalized ratio
IOP	intraocular pressure
IPPB	intermittent positive pressure breathing
ITP	idiopathic thrombocytopenic purpura
IUD	intrauterine device
IV	intravenous
IVP	intravenous push
JVD	jugular venous distention
KUB	kidney, ureters, and bladder (x-ray)
KS	Kaposi sarcoma
KVO	keep vein open
LAD	left anterior descending
LDL	low-density lipoprotein
LLQ	left lower quadrant
LMN	lower motor neuron
LMP	last menstrual period
LOC	level of consciousness
LP	lumbar puncture
LUQ	left upper quadrant
LVH	left ventricular hypertrophy
MAP	mean arterial pressure
MD	muscular dystrophy
MDS	myelodysplastic syndrome

Continued

ABBREVIATIONS—cont'd

MG	myasthenia gravis
MI	myocardial infarction
MICU	medical intensive care unit
MODS	multiple organ dysfunction syndrome
MRB	manual resuscitation bag
MS	multiple sclerosis
MVP	mitral valve prolapse
NAFLD	nonalcoholic fatty liver disease
NASH	nonalcoholic steatohepatitis
NG	nasogastric
NHL	non-Hodgkin's lymphoma
NPO	nothing by mouth
NS	normal saline
NSR	normal sinus rhythm
OA	osteoarthritis
OD	right eye; optical density; overdose
OOB	out of bed
OR	operating room
ORIF	open reduction and internal fixation
OS	left eye
OSA	obstructive sleep apnea
OTC	over-the-counter
PA	posteroanterior; physician's assistant
PAC	premature atrial contraction
$PaCO_2$	partial pressure of carbon dioxide in arterial blood
PaO_2	partial pressure of oxygen in arterial blood
PACU	postanesthesia care unit
PAD	peripheral artery disease
PAP	pulmonary artery pressure
PAWP	pulmonary artery wedge pressure
PCA	patient-controlled analgesia
PCI	percutaneous coronary intervention
PCO_2	partial pressure of carbon dioxide
PCWP	pulmonary capillary wedge pressure
PD	Parkinson's disease; peritoneal dialysis
PE	pulmonary embolism; physical examination
PEEP	positive end-expiratory pressure
PEFR	peak expiratory flow rate
PERRLA	pupils equal, round, and reactive to light and accommodation
PET	positron emission tomography
PICC	peripherally inserted central catheter
PID	pelvic inflammatory disease

ABBREVIATIONS—cont'd

PKD	polycystic kidney disease
PMH	past medical history
PMI	point of maximal impulse
PMS	premenstrual syndrome
PN	parenteral nutrition
PND	paroxysmal nocturnal dyspnea
PNS	peripheral nervous system
PO, po	orally
PO_2	partial pressure of oxygen
POC	point-of-care
PPD	purified protein derivative
PSA	prostate-specific antigen
PT	prothrombin time
PTT	partial thromboplastin time
PVC	premature ventricular contraction
PUD	peptic ulcer disease
R/O	rule out
RA	rheumatoid arthritis
REM	rapid eye movement
RF	rheumatic fever
RHD	rheumatic heart disease
RLQ	right lower quadrant
RLS	restless legs syndrome
ROM	range of motion
ROS	review of systems
RUQ	right upper quadrant
SA	sinoatrial
SCD	sickle cell disease; sudden cardiac death
SCI	spinal cord injury
SDB	sleep-disordered breathing
SICU	surgical intensive care unit
SIRS	systemic inflammatory response syndrome
SLE	systemic lupus erythematosus
SNS	sympathetic nervous system
SOB	shortness of breath
STI	sexually transmitted infection
SVR	systemic vascular resistance
SVT	superficial vein thrombosis
TAH	total abdominal hysterectomy
TB	tuberculosis
TBSA	total body surface area

Continued

ABBREVIATIONS—cont'd

TCDB	turn, cough, and deep breathe
TENS	transcutaneous electrical nerve stimulation
THR	total hip replacement
TIA	transient ischemic attack
TJC	The Joint Commission
TKO	to keep open
TNM	tumor, node, metastasis
TPR	temperature, pulse, and respirations
TURP	transurethral resection of the prostate
UA	unstable angina
UAP	unlicensed assistive personnel
UGI	upper gastrointestinal
UI	urinary incontinence
UMN	upper motor neuron
URI	upper respiratory infection
UTI	urinary tract infection
VAD	venous access device; ventricular assist device
VDH	valvular disease of the heart
VF	ventricular fibrillation
VS	vital signs
VT	ventricular tachycardia
VTE	venous thromboembolism
WHR	waist-to-hip ratio
WNL	within normal limits

THE JOINT COMMISSION OFFICIAL "DO NOT USE" LIST[a]

A

Do Not Use	Potential Problem	Use Instead
U (unit)	Mistaken for "0" (zero), the number "4" (four) or "cc"	Write "unit"
IU (International Unit)	Mistaken for IV (intravenous) or the number 10 (ten)	Write "International Unit"
D., QD, q.d., qd (daily)	Mistaken for each other	Write "daily"
Q.O.D., QOD, q.o.d., qod (every other day)	Period after the Q mistaken for "I" and the "O" mistaken for "I"	Write "every other day"
Trailing zero (X.0 mg)[b]	Decimal point is missed	Write X mg
Lack of leading zero (.X mg)		Write 0.X mg
MS	Can mean morphine sulfate or magnesium sulfate	Write "morphine sulfate"
MSO₄ and MgSO₄	Confused for one another	Write "magnesium sulfate"

[a]Applies to all orders and all medication-related documentation that is handwritten (including free-text computer entry) or on preprinted forms.
[b]Exception: a "trailing zero" may be used only where required to demonstrate the level of precision of the value being reported, such as for laboratory results, imaging studies that report size of lesions, or catheter/tube sizes. It may not be used in medication orders or other medication-related documentation.

Additional Abbreviations, Acronyms, and Symbols

Do Not Use	Potential Problem	Use Instead
> (greater than) < (less than)	Misinterpreted as the number "7" (seven) or the letter "L" confused for one another	Write "greater than" Write "less than"
Abbreviations for drug names	Misinterpreted because of similar abbreviations for multiple drugs	Write drug names in full
Apothecary units	Unfamiliar to many practitioners Confused with metric units	Use metric units
@	Mistaken for the number "2" (two)	Write "at"
cc	Mistaken for U (units) when poorly written	Write "mL" or "ml" or "milliliters" ("mL" is preferred)
μg	Mistaken for mg (milligrams), resulting in 1000-fold overdose	Write "mcg" or "micrograms"

BLOOD GASES

Normal Values

	Arterial (Sea Level)
pH	7.35–7.45
PaO_2[a]	80–100 mm Hg (10.6–13.33 kPa)
$PaCO_2$	35–45 mm Hg (4.66–5.98 kPa)
HCO_3	21–28 mEq/L (21–28 mmol/L)
O_2 saturation	>95%

[a]In a patient >60 years of age, normal PaO_2 is equal to 80 mm Hg minus 1 mm Hg for every year over 60. When supplemental oxygen is provided, expected $PaO_2 = FIO_2 \times 5$.

B

Interpreting Arterial Blood Gases (ABGs)

1. Check pH
   $\uparrow$ = Alkalosis; $\downarrow$ = acidosis
2. Check $PaCO_2$
   $\uparrow$ = CO_2 retention (hypoventilation); respiratory acidosis or compensating for metabolic alkalosis
   $\downarrow$ = CO_2 blown off (hyperventilation); respiratory alkalosis or compensating for metabolic acidosis
3. Check HCO_3
   $\uparrow$ = Nonvolatile acid is lost; HCO_3 is gained (metabolic alkalosis or compensating for respiratory acidosis)
   $\downarrow$ = Nonvolatile acid is added; HCO_3 is lost (metabolic acidosis or compensating for respiratory alkalosis)
4. Determine imbalance
5. Determine if compensation exists

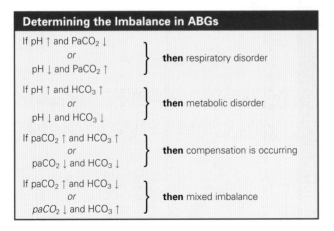

Determining the Imbalance in ABGs

If pH $\uparrow$ and $PaCO_2$ $\downarrow$
or
pH $\downarrow$ and $PaCO_2$ $\uparrow$ } **then** respiratory disorder

If pH $\uparrow$ and HCO_3 $\uparrow$
or
pH $\downarrow$ and HCO_3 $\downarrow$ } **then** metabolic disorder

If $paCO_2$ $\uparrow$ and HCO_3 $\uparrow$
or
$paCO_2$ $\downarrow$ and HCO_3 $\downarrow$ } **then** compensation is occurring

If $paCO_2$ $\uparrow$ and HCO_3 $\downarrow$
or
$paCO_2$ $\downarrow$ and HCO_3 $\uparrow$ } **then** mixed imbalance

BLOOD PRODUCTS[a]

Description	Special Considerations	Indications for Use
Albumin		
Prepared from plasma Can be stored for 5 yr Available in 5% or 25% solution Heat treated and does not transmit viruses	Albumin 25% expands the blood volume by about 3.5 times Hyperosmolar solution acts by moving water from extravascular to intravascular space	Hypovolemic shock, hypoalbuminemia, after large-volume paracentesis, replacement in plasmapheresis
Cryoprecipitates and Commercial Concentrates		
Prepared from fresh frozen plasma 10–15 mL/bag Can be stored for 1 yr Once thawed, must be used within 5 days		Replacement for fibrinogen deficiency, usually because of DIC, severe liver disease, or massive transfusion Has other clotting factors, especially factor VIII, factor XIII, and von Willebrand factor
Fresh Frozen Plasma		
Liquid portion of whole blood is separated from cells and frozen	Use in treating hemorrhagic shock is being replaced by pure preparations, such as albumin and plasma expanders	Bleeding caused by deficiency in clotting factors (e.g., DIC, hemorrhage, massive transfusion, liver disease, vitamin K deficiency, excess warfarin)

One unit contains about 250 mL

Rich in clotting factors but contains no platelets

Can be stored for up to 1 yr, depending on storage

Must be used within 24 hr after thawing

Frozen RBCs

Prepared from RBCs using glycerol for protection and frozen

Can be stored for 10 yr

Must be used within 24 hr of thawing. Successive washings with saline solution remove most WBCs and plasma proteins

Autotransfusion. Stockpiling or rare donors for patients with alloantibodies

Packed RBCs

Prepared from whole blood by sedimentation or centrifugation

One unit contains 250–350 mL

Use of RBCs for treatment allows remaining components of blood (e.g., platelets, albumin, plasma) to be used for other purposes

Less danger of fluid overload

Severe or symptomatic anemia, acute blood loss

One unit of RBCs can be expected to increase Hgb by 1 g/dL or Hct by 3% in a typical adult

Continued

B

BLOOD PRODUCTS—cont'd

Description	Special Considerations	Indications for Use
Can be stored up to 42 days depending on processing (anticoagulants and preservatives)	Preferred RBC source because they are more component specific Leukocyte depletion (leukoreduction) by filtration, washing, or freezing is frequently used Decreases nonhemolytic febrile or mild allergic reactions in patients who receive frequent transfusions Reduces transmission of Cytomegalovirus	One unit can replace a blood loss of 500 mL
Platelets		
Prepared from fresh whole blood	Can obtain multiple units from one donor by plateletpheresis	Bleeding caused by thrombocytopenia
An apheresed single donation is usually 200–400 mL in volume	Can be kept at room temperature in the Blood Bank under gentle agitation for 1–5 days depending on type of collection and storage bag used	May be contraindicated in thrombotic thrombocytopenic purpura and HITTS except in life-threatening hemorrhage Average corrected count increment is $10 \times 10^9/L$
May be pooled from multiple donors	For patients who receive frequent transfusions and become refractory, may give leukocyte reduced, HLA, or type specific to prevent alloimmunization to HLA antigens	Failure to have an increase may be caused by fever, sepsis, splenomegaly, or DIC or development of antibodies (refractory)

[a]Component therapy has replaced the use of whole blood, which is rarely used. Granulocyte transfusions are not included here because they are rarely used. DIC, Disseminated intravascular coagulation; Hct, hematocrit; Hgb, hemoglobin; HITT, heparin-induced thrombocytopenia and thrombotic syndrome; HLA,

BREATH SOUNDS

Auscultation Finding	Description	Common Etiology and Significance
Absent breath sounds	No sound heard over entire lung or area of lung	Pneumothorax, pleural effusion, mainstem bronchi obstruction, large atelectasis, pneumonectomy, lobectomy
Bronchophony, whispered pectoriloquy	Spoken or whispered syllable more distinct than normal on auscultation	Pneumonia
Coarse crackles	Louder, discontinuous, low-pitched sounds caused by air passing through airway intermittently occluded by mucus, unstable bronchial wall. May be heard on inspiration, expiration, or both. Similar sound to blowing through straw under water	Excess fluid within the lungs, heart failure, pulmonary edema, pneumonia with severe congestion, COPD
Egophony	Spoken "E" similar to "A" on auscultation because of altered transmission of voice sounds	Pneumonia, pleural effusion
Fine crackles	Short, discontinuous, high-pitched sounds heard just before the end of inspiration. Result of rapid equalization of gas pressure when collapsed alveoli or terminal bronchioles suddenly snap open. Similar sound to that made by rolling hair between fingers	Interstitial edema (early pulmonary edema), alveolar filling (pneumonia), loss of lung volume (atelectasis), early phase of heart failure, idiopathic pulmonary fibrosis

Continued

B

BREATH SOUNDS—cont'd

Auscultation Finding	Description	Common Etiology and Significance
Pleural friction rub	Creaking or grating sound from roughened, inflamed pleural surfaces rubbing together. Evident during inspiration, expiration, or both. No change with coughing. Often uncomfortable, especially on deep inspiration	Pleurisy, pneumonia, pulmonary infarct
Stridor	Continuous musical or crowing sound of constant pitch. Result of partial obstruction of larynx or trachea	Croup, epiglottitis, vocal cord edema after extubation, foreign body
Wheezes	Continuous high-pitched squeaking or musical sound caused by rapid vibration of bronchial walls. First evident on expiration but possibly evident on inspiration as obstruction of airway increases. May be audible without stethoscope	Bronchospasm (caused by asthma), airway obstruction (caused by foreign body, tumor), COPD

COPD, Chronic obstructive pulmonary disease.

COMMONLY USED FORMULAS

Parameter	Formula	Normal Range
Anion gap	$Na - (HCO_3^- + Cl)$	8–16 mEq/L
Body mass index (BMI)	$\dfrac{\text{Weight in pounds}}{\text{Height in inches}^2} \times 703$	18.5–24.9 kg/m²
Cardiac index (CI)	$\dfrac{CO}{\text{Body surface area(BSA)}}$	2.2–4.0 L/min/m²
Cardiac output (CO)	$HR \times SV$	4–8 L/min
Cerebral perfusion pressure (CPP)	$MAP - ICP$	80–100 mm Hg
Ejection fraction (EF)	$\dfrac{SV}{\text{End-diastolic volume}} \times 100$	55% or greater
Mean arterial pressure (MAP)	$\dfrac{2(DBP) + SBP}{3}$	70–105 mm Hg
Stroke volume (SV)	$\dfrac{CO}{HR}$	60–150 mL/beat

DBP, Diastolic blood pressure; *HR,* heart rate; *ICP,* intracranial pressure; *SBP,* systolic blood pressure.

CHARACTERISTICS OF COMMON DYSRHYTHMIAS

Normal Rhythm/ Dysrhythmia	Rate and Rhythm	PATTERN		
		P Wave	PR Interval	QRS Complex
Normal sinus rhythm (NSR)	60–100 beats/min and regular	Normal	Normal	Normal
Sinus bradycardia	<60 beats/min and regular	Normal	Normal	Normal
Sinus tachycardia	101–200 beats/min and regular	Normal	Normal	Normal
Premature atrial contraction (PAC)	Usually 60–100 beats/min and irregular	Abnormal shape	Normal	Normal (usually)
Paroxysmal supraventricular tachycardia (PSVT)	150–220 beats/min and regular	Abnormal shape, may be hidden in the preceding T wave	Normal or shortened	Normal (usually)
Atrial flutter	*Atrial:* 200–350 beats/min and regular *Ventricular:* > or <100 beats/min and may be regular or irregular	Flutter (F) waves (sawtoothed pattern); more flutter waves than QRS complexes; may occur in a 2:1, 3:1, 4:1 (etc.) pattern	Not measurable	Normal (usually)
Atrial fibrillation	*Atrial:* 350–600 beats/min and irregular *Ventricular:* > or <100 beats/min and irregular	Fibrillatory (f) waves	Not measurable	Normal (usually)

Junctional dysrhythmias	40–180 beats/min and regular	Inverted; may be hidden in QRS complex	Shortened, if present	Normal (usually)
First-degree AV block	Normal and regular	Normal	>0.20 sec	Normal
Second-degree AV block				
• Type I (Mobitz I, Wenckebach heart block)	Atrial: Normal and regular Ventricular: Slower and irregular	Normal	Progressive lengthening	Normal QRS width, with pattern of 1 nonconducted (blocked) QRS complex
• Type II (Mobitz II heart block)	Atrial: Usually normal and regular Ventricular: Slower and regular or irregular	More P waves than QRS complexes (e.g., 2:1, 3:1)	Normal or prolonged but consistent for every QRS	Widened QRS, preceded by ≥ 2 P waves, with nonconducted (blocked) QRS complex

Continued

C

CHARACTERISTICS OF COMMON DYSRHYTHMIAS—cont'd

Normal Rhythm/ Dysrhythmia	Rate and Rhythm	PATTERN		
		P Wave	PR Interval	QRS Complex
Third-degree AV block (complete heart block)	Atrial: Regular but may appear irregular because of P waves hidden in QRS complexes Ventricular: 20–60 beats/min and regular	Normal, but no connection with QRS complex	Inconsistent	Normal or widened, no relationship with P waves
Premature ventricular contraction (PVC)	PVCs occur at variable rates Underlying rhythm can be regular or irregular	Not usually visible, hidden in the PVC	Not measurable	Wide and distorted
Ventricular tachycardia (VT)	150–250 beats/min and regular or irregular	Not usually visible	Not measurable	Wide and distorted
Accelerated idioventricular rhythm	40–100 beats/min and regular	Not usually visible	Not measurable	Wide and distorted
Ventricular fibrillation (VF)	Not measurable and irregular	Absent	Not measurable	Not measurable

AV, Atrioventricular.

ELECTROCARDIOGRAM (ECG) MONITORING

ECG Waveforms and Normal Sinus Rhythm

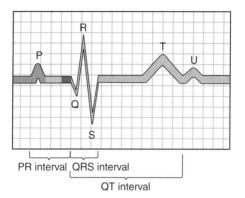

ECG Waveforms and Intervals and Sources of Potential Variations[a]

Description	Normal Duration (sec)	Source of Possible Variation
P wave		
Represents time for the passage of the electrical impulse through the atrium causing atrial depolarization (contraction). Should be upright.	0.06–0.12	Disturbance in conduction within atria
PR interval		
Measured from beginning of P wave to beginning of QRS complex. Represents time taken for impulse to spread through the atria, AV node and bundle of His, bundle branches, and Purkinje fibers, to a point immediately before ventricular contraction.	0.12–0.20	Disturbance in conduction usually in AV node, bundle of His, or bundle branches but can be in atria as well
QRS complex		
Q wave: first negative (downward) deflection after the P wave, short and narrow, not present in several leads.	<0.03	MI may result in development of a pathologic Q wave that is wide (≥0.03 sec) and deep (≥25% of the height of the R wave)
R wave: first positive (upward) deflection in the QRS complex.	Not usually measured	
S wave: First negative (downward) deflection after the R wave.	Not usually measured	

QRS interval

Measured from beginning to end of QRS complex. Represents time taken for depolarization (contraction) of both ventricles (systole).

<0.12

Disturbance in conduction in bundle branches or in ventricles

ST segment

Measured from the S wave of the QRS complex to the beginning of the T wave. Represents the time between ventricular depolarization and repolarization (diastole). Should be isoelectric (flat).

0.12

Disturbances (e.g., elevation, depression) usually caused by ischemia, injury, or infarction

T wave

Represents time for ventricular repolarization. Should be upright.

0.16

Disturbances (e.g., tall, peaked; inverted) usually caused by electrolyte imbalances, ischemia, or infarction

QT interval[b]

Measured from beginning of QRS complex to end of T wave. Represents time taken for entire electrical depolarization and repolarization of the ventricles. Normal adult women have slightly longer QT intervals than men.

0.34–0.43

Disturbances usually affecting repolarization more than depolarization and caused by drugs, electrolyte imbalances, and changes in heart rate

[a] Heart rate influences the duration of these intervals, especially the PR and QT intervals (e.g., QT interval shortens in duration as heart rate increases).
[b] A corrected QT interval (QTc) is calculated to account for the influence of heart rate.
AV, Atrioventricular; MI, myocardial infarction.

E

GLASGOW COMA SCALE

Appropriate Stimulus	Response	Score
Eyes Open		
Approach to bedside	Spontaneous response	4
Verbal command	Opening of eyes to name or command	3
Pain	Lack of opening of eyes to previous stimuli but opening to pain	2
	Lack of opening of eyes to any stimulus	1
	Untestable[a]	U
Best Verbal Response		
Verbal questioning with maximum arousal	Appropriate orientation, conversant—correct identification of self, place, year, and month	5
	Confusion—conversant, but disorientation in 1 or more spheres	4
	Inappropriate or disorganized use of words (e.g., cursing), lack of sustained conversation	3
	Incomprehensible words, sounds (e.g., moaning)	2
	Lack of sound, even with painful stimuli	1
	Untestable[a]	U

GLASGOW COMA SCALE—cont'd

Appropriate Stimulus	Response	Score
Best Motor Response		
Verbal command (e.g., "raise your arm," "hold up 2 fingers")	Obedience of command	6
Pain (pressure on proximal nail bed)	Localization of pain, lack of obedience but presence of attempts to remove offending stimulus	5
	Flexion withdrawal,[a] flexion of arm in response to pain without abnormal flexion posture	4
	Abnormal flexion, flexing of arm at elbow and pronation, making a fist	3
	Abnormal extension, extension of arm at elbow usually with adduction and internal rotation of arm at shoulder	2
	Lack of response	1
	Untestable[a]	U

[a]Added to the original scale by some centers.

HEART SOUNDS

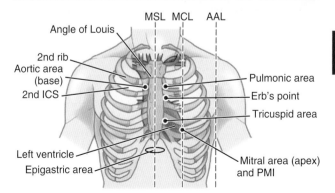

HEART SOUNDS—cont'd

Sound	Auscultation Site	Clinical Occurrence
S_1 (M_1 T_1)	Apex	Closing of mitral and tricuspid valves; signals the beginning of systole
S_2 (A_2 P_2)	A_2 at second ICS, RSB; P_2 at second ICS, LSB	Closing of aortic and pulmonic valves; signals the beginning of diastole
S_2 physiologic split	Second ICS, LSB (pulmonic area)	Can be normal and is a split sound that corresponds with the respiratory cycle caused by a normal delay of pulmonic valve during inspiration; can be abnormal if heard during expiration or if it is constant during the respiratory cycle; accentuated during exercise or in individuals with thin chest walls; heard most often in children and young adults
S_3 (ventricular gallop)	Apex	Low-intensity vibration of the ventricular wall usually associated with decreased compliance of the ventricles during filling; heard closely after S_2; common in children and young adults and during last trimester of pregnancy
S_4 (atrial gallop)	Apex	Low-frequency vibration caused by atrial filling and contraction against increased resistance in ventricle; precedes S_1 of next cycle; may be normal in infants, children, and athletes; pathologic in patients with heart disease

Murmurs	Apex Second ICS, LSB, or RSB	Produced by turbulent blood flow across diseased heart valves. They are graded on a 6-point Roman numeral scale of loudness and recorded as a ratio. The numerator is the intensity of the murmur, and the denominator is always VI, which indicates that the 6-point scale is being used. Grade I/VI indicates a murmur that is barely audible, heard only in a quiet room and then not easily; grade VI/VI indicates a murmur that can be heard with stethoscope lifted off chest wall.
Pericardial friction rubs	Usually heard best at the apex, with patient upright and leaning forward, and after expiration	Caused by friction that occurs when inflamed surfaces of pericardium (pericarditis) move against each other. They are high-pitched, scratchy sounds that may be transient or intermittent and may last several hours to days.

ICS, Intercostal space; *LSB,* left sternal border; *RSB,* right sternal border.

H

INTRACRANIAL PRESSURE MONITORING

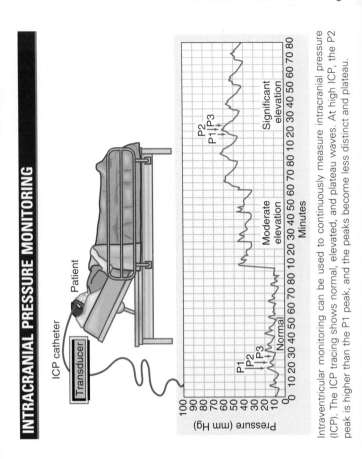

Intraventricular monitoring can be used to continuously measure intracranial pressure (ICP). The ICP tracing shows normal, elevated, and plateau waves. At high ICP, the P2 peak is higher than the P1 peak, and the peaks become less distinct and plateau.

LABORATORY VALUES

Test	Conventional Units	SI Units[a]
Complete Blood Count		
Red blood cells (RBCs)	*Male:* 4.7–6.1 × 10^6/μL *Female:* 4.2–5.4 × 10^6/μL	*Male:* 4.7–6.1 × 10^{12}/L *Female:* 4.2–5.4 × 10^{12}/L
White blood cells (WBCs)	5000–10,000/mm^3	5.0–10.0 × 10^9/L
Hemoglobin (Hgb)	*Male:* 14–18 g/dL *Female:* 12–16 g/dL	*Male:* 140–180 g/L *Female:* 120–160 g/L
Hematocrit (Hct)	*Male:* 42%–52% *Female:* 37%–47%	*Male:* 0.42–0.52 *Female:* 0.37–0.47
Chemistry		
Alanine aminotransferase (ALT)	4–36 U/L	
Albumin	3.5–5 g/dL	35–50 g/L
Aspartate aminotransferase (AST)	0–35 U/L	0–0.58 μkat/L
Ammonia	10–80 mcg/dL	6–47 μmol/L
Amylase	60–120 Somogyi U/dL	30–220 U/L
Bicarbonate	21–28 mEq/L	21–28 mmol/L
Bilirubin		
• Total	0.3–1.0 mg/dL	5.1–17 μmol/L
• Direct	0.2–0.8 mg/dL	3.4–12.0 μmol/L
• Indirect	0.1–0.3 mg/dL	1.7–5.1 μmol/L
b-Type natriuretic peptide (BNP)	<100 pg/mL	<100 pmol/L
Calcium (total)	9.0–10.5 mg/dL	2.25–2.62 mmol/L
Calcium (ionized)	4.5–5.6 mg/dL	1.05–1.3 mmol/L
Cholesterol	<200 mg/dL	<5.2 mmol/L
• High-density lipoprotein (HDL)	*Male:* >45 mg/dL *Female:* >55 mg/dL	*Male:* >0.75 mmol/L *Female:* >0.91 mmol/L
• Low-density lipoprotein (LDL)	*Recommended:* <130 mg/dL	
• Very low-density lipoproteins (VLDLs)	7–32 mg/dL	

Continued

LABORATORY VALUES—cont'd

Test	Conventional Units	SI Units
Chloride	98–106 mEq/L	98–106 mmol/L
Creatinine	*Male*: 0.6–1.2 mg/dL	*Male*: 53–106 μmol/L
	Female: 0.5–1.1 mg/dL	*Female*: 44–97 μmol
Glucose (fasting)	74–106 mg/dL	4.1–5.9 mmol/L
Hemoglobin, glycosylated (A1C)	4.0%–5.6%	4.0%–5.6%
Iron, total	*Male:* 80–180 mcg/dL	*Male:* 14–32 μmol/L
	Female: 60–160 mcg/dL	*Female:* 11–29 μmol/L
Lactic dehydrogenase (LDH)	100–190 U/L	100–190 U/L
Lipase	0–160 U/L	
Magnesium	1.3–2.1 mEq/L	0.65–1.05 mmol/L
Osmolality	285–295 mOsm/kg	285–295 mmol/kg
Phosphorus (phosphate)	3.0–4.5 mg/dL	0.97–1.45 mmol/L
Phosphatase, alkaline	30–120 U/L	0.5–2.0 μkat/L
Potassium	3.5–5.0 mEq/L	3.5–5.0 mmol/L
Protein (total)	6.4–8.3 g/dL	64–83 g/L
Sodium	136–145 mEq/L	136–145 mmol/L
Triglyceride	*Male*: 40–160 mg/dL	*Male*: 0.45–1.81 g/L
	Female: 35–135 mg/dL	*Female*: 0.40–1.52 g/L
Urea nitrogen (BUN)	10–20 mg/dL	3.6–7.1 mmol/L
Coagulation		
Activated partial thromboplastin time (aPTT)	30–40 sec	30–40 sec
Fibrin split (degradation) products, FSP	<10 mcg/mL	<10 mg/L
Platelets (thrombocytes)	150–400 × 10^3/μL	150–400 × 10^9/L
Prothrombin time (Protime, PT)	11–12.5 sec	11–12.5 sec

[a]*SI,* Système International (i.e., International System of Units).

LUNG VOLUMES AND CAPACITIES

Parameter	Definition	Normal Value[a]
Volumes		
Tidal volume (VT)	Volume of air inhaled and exhaled with each breath. Only a small proportion of total capacity of lungs	0.5 L
Expiratory reserve volume (ERV)	Additional air that can be forcefully exhaled after normal exhalation is complete	1.0 L
Residual volume (RV)	Amount of air remaining in lungs after forced expiration. Air available in lungs for gas exchange between breaths	1.5 L
Inspiratory reserve volume (IRV)	Maximum volume of air that can be inhaled forcefully after normal inhalation	3.0 L
Capacities		
Total lung capacity (TLC)	Maximum volume of air that lungs can contain (TLC = IRV + VT + ERV + RV)	6.0 L
Functional residual capacity (FRC)	Volume of air remaining in lungs at end of normal exhalation (FRC = ERV + RV). Increase or decrease possible with lung disease	2.5 L
Vital capacity (VC)	Maximum volume of air that can be exhaled after maximum inspiration (VC = IRV + VT + ERV). Higher VC for men (generally)	4.5 L
Inspiratory capacity (IC)	Maximum volume of air that can be inhaled after normal expiration (IC = VT + IRV)	3.5 L

[a]Normal values vary with patient's height, weight, age, race, and gender.

L

MEDICATION ADMINISTRATIONS

Equivalent Weights and Measures

Metric	Apothecary	Household
Weight		
1 kg	2.2 pounds	
1000 mg = 1 g	gr xv	
60 or 65 mg	gr i	
30 mg	gr ss (one-half)	
0.4 mg	1/150 gr	
1 mcg = 0.0001 mg		
Volume		
1000 mL = 1 L	Approx. 1 quart	Approx. 1 quart
1 L distilled water weighs	1 kg	
500 mL	Approx. 1 pint	16 ounces
240 or 250 mL	viii (8 ounces)	1 cup
30 mL	i (1 fluid ounce)	2 tablespoons
15 mL	iv (4 fluid drams)	1 tablespoon
4 to 5 mL	i (1 fluid dram)	1 teaspoon
1 mL	Minims xv or xvi	

Drug Calculations

Ratio and Proportion

1. To set up a ratio and proportion, put on the right-hand side what you already have, or what you already know (e.g., 1000 mg : 1 mL).
2. On the left-hand side put X, or what you want to know (e.g., 750 mg : X).
3. The equation should look like this:

$$750 \text{ mg} : X = 1000 \text{ mg} : 1 \text{ mL}$$

4. Multiply the 2 inside numbers. Multiply the 2 outside numbers.

$$1000X = 750$$

5. Solve for X:

$$X = \frac{750}{1000} = 0.75 \text{ mL}$$

IV Drip Rate

$$\frac{\text{Total number of milliliters to be infused}}{\text{Total number of minutes infusion}} \times \text{Drop factor} = \text{Rate (Drops per minute)}$$

Techniques of Administration
Angles of Injection

M

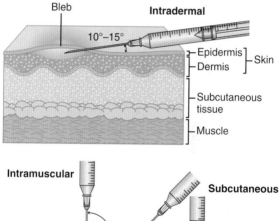

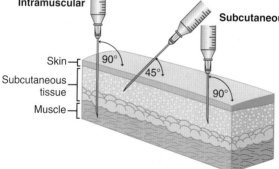

Injection Sites
Subcutaneous

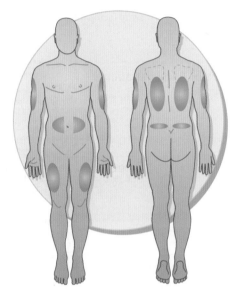

Intramuscular: Ventrogluteal Muscle

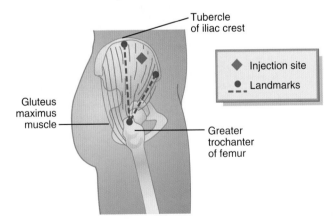

Intramuscular: Dorsogluteal Muscle

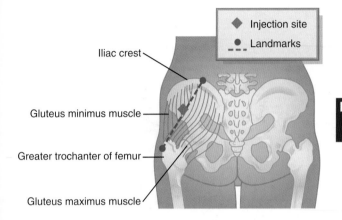

Intramuscular: Deltoid Muscle

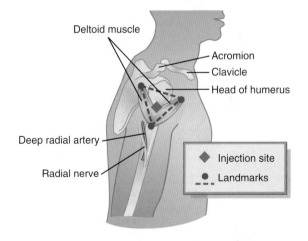

Intramuscular: Vastus Lateralis Muscle

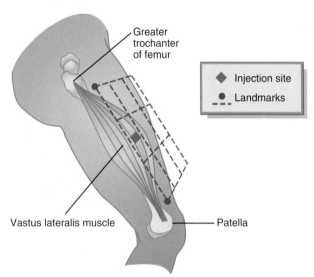

Greater trochanter of femur

◆ Injection site
●--- Landmarks

Vastus lateralis muscle

Patella

Z-Track Technique

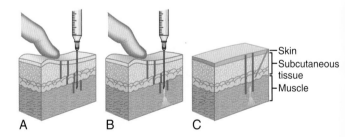

Skin
Subcutaneous tissue
Muscle

A   B   C

IV Site Complications

	Infiltration	Phlebitis
Assessment		
Color	Pale	Red
Temperature	Cool to cold	Warm to hot
Swelling	Rounded	Cordlike vein path
Pain	Yes, usually	Yes
Flow	Slowed or stopped	No change or may be slowed
Nursing Actions		
	Tourniquet proximally (flow continues—infiltration)	Discontinue IV infusion; usually call IV team
	Lower bag (blood in tubing—no infiltration)	Note irritating solution (diazepam [Valium], cephalothin sodium, potassium chloride [KCl] running too fast)
	Discontinue IV infusion	Warm compresses; elevate and immobilize part
	Call IV team	
	Get order for warm compresses and elevate part	

M

TEMPERATURE EQUIVALENTS

°C	°F	°C	°F	°C	°F
34.0	93.2	37.2	99.0	40.2	104.4
34.2	93.6	37.4	99.3	40.4	104.7
34.4	93.9	37.6	99.7	40.6	105.2
34.6	94.3	37.8	100.0	40.8	105.4
34.8	94.6	38.0	100.4	41.0	105.9
35.0	95.0	38.2	100.8	41.2	106.1
35.2	95.4	38.4	101.1	41.4	106.5
35.4	95.7	38.6	101.5	41.6	106.8
35.6	96.1	38.8	101.8	41.8	107.2
35.8	96.4	39.0	102.2	42.0	107.6
36.0	96.8	39.2	102.6	42.2	108.0
36.2	97.2	39.4	102.9	42.4	108.3
36.4	97.5	39.6	103.3	42.6	108.7
36.6	97.9	39.8	103.6	42.8	109.0
36.8	98.2	40.0	104.0	43.0	109.4
37.0	98.6	—	—	—	—

°C, Celsius (centigrade) degrees; *°F,* Fahrenheit degrees.

Conversion Factors

To convert from °C to °F:

$$\left(°C \times {}^9/_5\right) + 32 = °F$$

To convert from °F to °C:

$$\left(°F - 32\right) \times {}^5/_9 = °C$$

TNM CLASSIFICATION SYSTEM

Primary Tumor (T)

T_0	No evidence of primary tumor
T_{is}	Carcinoma in situ
T_{1-4}	Ascending degrees of increase in tumor size and involvement
T_x	Tumor cannot be measured or found

Regional Lymph Nodes (N)

N_0	No evidence of disease in lymph nodes
N_{1-4}	Ascending degrees of nodal involvement
N_x	Regional lymph nodes unable to be assessed clinically

Distant Metastases (M)

M_0	No evidence of distant metastases
M_{1-4}	Ascending degrees of metastatic involvement, including distant nodes
M_x	Cannot be determined

ENGLISH/SPANISH COMMON MEDICAL TERMS

Hints for Pronunciation of Spanish Words

- *h* is silent.
- *j* is pronounced as *h*.
- *ll* is pronounced as a *y* sound.
- *r* is pronounced with a trilled sound, and *rr* is trilled even more.
- *v* is pronounced with a *b* sound.
- A *y* by itself is pronounced with a long *e* sound.
- Accent marks over the vowel indicate the syllable that is to be stressed.

T

Common Words/Phrases for Clinical Situations

Introductory

I am _____.	Soy _____.
What is your name?	¿Cómo se llama usted?
I would like to examine you now.	Quisiera examinarlo(a) ahora.

General

How do you feel?	¿Cómo se siente?
Good	Bien
Bad	Mal
Do you feel better today?	¿Se siente mejor hoy?
Where do you work?	¿Dónde trabaja? (¿Cuál es su profesión o trabajo?) (¿Qué hace usted?)
Are you allergic to anything?	¿Es usted alérgico(a) a algo?
Medications, foods, insect bites?	¿Medicinas, alimentos, picaduras de insectos?
Do you take any medications?	¿Toma usted algunas medicinas?
Do you have any drug allergies?	¿Es usted alérgico(a) a algún médicamento?
Do you have a history of:	¿Ha sufrido antes:
Heart disease?	Del corazón?
Diabetes?	De diabetes?
Epilepsy?	De epilepsia?
Bronchitis?	De bronquitis?
Emphysema?	De enfisema?
Asthma?	De asma?

Pain

Have you any pain?	¿Tiene dolor?
Where is the pain?	¿Dónde le duele?
Do you have any pain here?	¿Le duele aquí?
How severe is the pain?	¿Qué tan fuerte es el dolor?
Mild, moderate, sharp, or severe?	¿Ligero, moderado, agudo, severo?
What were you doing when the pain started?	¿Qué estaba haciendo cuando le comenzó el dolor?
Have you ever had this pain before?	¿Ha tenido este dolor antes?

Common Words/Phrases for Clinical Situations—cont'd

Do you have a pain in your side?	¿Tiene usted dolor en el costado?
Is it worse now?	¿Es peor ahora?
Does it still pain you?	¿Le duele todavía?
Did you feel much pain at the time?	¿Sintió mucho dolor entonces?
Show me where.	Muéstreme dónde.
Does it hurt when I press here?	¿Le duele cuando aprieto aquí?

Head

Head	La cabeza
Face	La cara
Eye	El ojo

Ears/Nose/Throat

Ears	Los oídos
Eardrum	El tímpano
Laryngitis	La laringitis
Lip	El labio
Mouth	La boca
Nose	La naríz
Tongue	La lengua

Cardiovascular

Heart	El corazón
Heart attack	El ataque del corazón
Heart disease	La enfermedad del corazón
Heart murmur	El soplo del corazón
High blood pressure	Presión alta

Respiratory

Chest	El pecho
Lungs	Los pulmones

Gastrointestinal

Abdomen	El abdomen
Intestines/bowels	Los intestinos
Liver	El hígado
Nausea	Náusea

T

Continued

Common Words/Phrases for Clinical Situations—cont'd

Gastric ulcer	La úlcera gástrica
Stomach	El estómago, la panza, la barriga
Stomachache	El dolor de estómago

Genitourinary

Genitals	Los genitales
Kidney	El riñón
Penis	El pene, el miembro
Urine	La orina

Musculoskeletal

Ankle	El tobillo
Arm	El brazo
Back	La espalda
Bones	Los huesos
Elbow	El codo
Finger	El dedo
Foot	El pie
Fracture	La fractura
Hand	La mano
Hip	La cadera
Knee	La rodilla
Leg	La pierna
Muscles	Los músculos
Rib	La costilla
Shoulder	El hombro
Thigh	El muslo

Neurologic

Brain	El cerebro
Dizziness	El vértigo, el mareo
Epilepsy	La epilepsia
Fainting spell	El desmayo
Unconsciousness	Pérdida del conocimiento (inconsciente, sin sentido)

Reproductive

Uterus	El útero, la matríz
Vagina	La vagina

U

Continued

URINALYSIS

Test	Normal	Abnormal Finding	Possible Etiology and Significance
Color	Amber yellow	Dark, smoky color	Hematuria
		Yellow-brown to olive green	Excessive bilirubin
		Orange-red or orange-brown	Normal side effect of phenazopyridine
		Cloudiness of freshly voided urine	Urinary tract infection (UTI)
		Colorless urine	Excessive fluid intake, kidney disease, or diabetes insipidus
Odor	Aromatic	Ammonia-like odor	Urine allowed to stand
		Unpleasant odor	UTI
Protein	Random protein (dipstick): 0–trace 0–8 mg/dL	Persistent proteinuria	Acute and chronic kidney disease, heart failure
	24-hr protein (quantitative): 50–80 mg/day		Heart failure, inflammatory process of urinary tract, nephritis, nephrosis, strenuous exercise
Glucose	None	Glycosuria	Diabetes mellitus, pituitary disorders

URINALYSIS—cont'd

Test	Normal	Abnormal Finding	Possible Etiology and Significance
Ketones	None	Present	Diabetes mellitus, starvation, dehydration
Bilirubin	None	Present	Liver disorders
Specific gravity	1.005–1.030	Low	Diabetes insipidus
	Maximum concentrating ability of kidney in morning urine (1.025–1.030)	High	Dehydration, albuminuria, glycosuria
		Fixed at about 1.010	Renal inability to concentrate urine; end-stage kidney disease
Osmolality	50–1200 mOsm/kg (50–1200 mmol/kg)	<50 mOsm/kg (<50 mmol/kg)	Aldosteronism, diabetes insipidus, hypokalemia, pyelonephritis.
		>1200 mOsm/kg (>1200 mmol/kg)	Heart failure, liver disease, shock, SIADH.
pH	4.6–8.0	4.6–8.0	UTI, urine allowed to stand at room temperature.
			Respiratory or metabolic acidosis

hpf, High-power field; *SIADH,* syndrome of inappropriate antidiuretic hormone secretion.

INDEX

Note: Page numbers followed by *f* indicate figures and *t* indicate tables.